Immunological Approaches To Cancer Therapeutics

Immunological Approaches To Cancer Therapeutics

Edited by

ENRICO MIHICH

Roswell Park Memorial Institute
Buffalo, New York

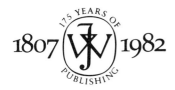

1807 1982
175 YEARS OF PUBLISHING

A Wiley-Interscience Publication

JOHN WILEY & SONS

New York · Chichester · Brisbane · Toronto · Singapore

Library of Congress Cataloging in Publication Data:

Main entry under title:

Immunological approaches to cancer therapeutics.

"A Wiley-Interscience publication."
Includes index.
1. Immunotherapy. 2. Cancer—Treatment.
3. Cancer—Immunological aspects. I. Mihich,
Enrico.

RC271.I45I46	616.99'4061	81-19801
ISBN 0-471-06049-6		AACR2

Printed in the United States of America

10 9 8 7 6 5 4 3 2 1

Preface

Considerable progress has been made since 1950 in the management of various types of human neoplasias with chemotherapeutic agents alone or in combination, or with other modalities of treatment. Patients with certain tumors can be brought into complete remission by chemotherapy or radiotherapy and are free of detectable disease five years or longer after diagnosis. In other cases, adjunctive treatments after surgical excision of primary tumors significantly increase the percentage of long term survivors. The list of tumors which in some cases can be successfully treated include acute leukemias, lymphomas—particularly Hodgkin's disease—certain types of choriocarcinoma, testicular tumor, Wilm's tumor, certain tumors of the skin, osteosarcoma of the limb, and certain clinical types of breast tumors, ovarian carcinoma, oat cell carcinoma of the lung, and thyroid tumors.

Despite the obvious advances achieved, major limitations must still be overcome before effective treatment of many neoplastic diseases can be achieved. Chemotherapy, for example, suffers from such limitations as insufficient selectivity for the target tumors and toxicity to normal tissues. Therefore, in most cases a relatively minor degree of tumor resistance to a drug cannot be overcome without unacceptable toxicity. Many approaches are being pursued in efforts to develop more effective anticancer treatments; these include the development of new drugs and new modalities of treatments based on increased knowledge of the biochemical and biological basis of selectivity of antitumor action as well as the development of new types of treatment that may modify the interactions between host and tumor.

Based on the assumption that tumor-associated antigens would elicit relatively specific host responses, many attempts have been made recently to develop immunotherapies to utilize this potential. It was postulated that these treatments would have minimal toxicity, because they were to exploit physiological host reactions, and could be used without additional toxicity in cooperation with less selective cytoreductive modalities. Largely because of the empiricism which pervaded the design of the early immunotherapy trials, the initial optimism, which was reinforced by what later appeared to have been premature reports, was followed by substantial skepticism about the potential value of this approach. However, solid evidence has indeed been obtained in experimental systems and, to a limited extent, in humans indicating that alteration of tumor–host relationships may be therapeutically exploitable. It is therefore appropriate to review the knowledge gained in this area so that the potentialities and limitations of this approach can be carefully assessed. The

v

74756

purpose of this book is to provide a critical review of the experience gained to date in the pursuit of immunological approaches in cancer therapeutics and to propose areas in which opportunities for further development can be reasonably expected to be realized in the future.

With the acquisition of more knowledge concerning the mechanisms of immune functions and their regulation, it now seems possible to develop new approaches in immunotherapy and to better utilize the new agents that recently have become available. It has become increasingly apparent that many of the immunomodulating, immunostimulating, and immunorestorative agents may cause different effects depending on the status of immune systems at the time they are exposed to these agents. It is reasonable to postulate, therefore, that the success of a certain immunotherapeutic regimen may depend partly on the development and appropriate utilization of methodologies to assess the status of antitumor host defense systems in individual patients. Through this assessment it should be possible to acquire further knowledge of the regulation of the immune response in humans. This would provide additional opportunities for the development of improved treatments.

The existence of tumor-specific or tumor-associated antigens is a central prerequisite for achieving antitumor selectivity through the exploitation of specific immune defense mechanisms against tumor. Knowledge in this area is expanding. However, the existence of tumor antigens does not necessarily imply that an effective antitumor response can be elicited; indeed untoward immune responses and/or tumor escape mechanisms need to be understood if effective immunotherapy is to be designed. Active immunotherapy with tumor cells or a tumor antigen preparation has been a major goal of immunotherapy which to date has escaped full realization in the face of the difficulties surrounding the identification of tumor-specific antigens. Immunotherapy with modified tumor cells, which stimulate a host response, has been achieved in numerous animal systems and is being verified in humans.

Modification of immune responses to tumor may be obtained through augmentation or restoration of the effector mechanisms of host defenses, or through immunomodulation leading to the establishment of a favorable balance between therapeutically desirable and undesirable components of host reactions. Such modifications may be achieved through the use of microbial products, chemical compounds, thymic hormones and interferons, or nutritional control. The possibility of transferring immunological responsiveness through the administration of such products as immune RNA or Transfer Factor might deserve future study toward possible applications in cancer therapeutics.

The use of hybridomas as "factories" of monoclonal antibodies has a potential in therapeutics which is just beginning to be studied. In fact, based on the assumption that tumor has distinctive antigens, monoclonal antibodies directed against them may provide, upon passive transfer, the means of attacking the tumor directly, or may serve as a vector for selective delivery of cytotoxic agents to the tumor. The transfer of cells represents an area where major progress has been made both in terms of reconstitution of immune potential through the therapeutic transfer of bone marrow cells to heavily irradiated and immunosuppressed patients and in terms of adoptive transfer of immune lymphocytes. The latter approach has been facilitated recently by the isolation of specific factors allowing the growth in culture of sensitized cells which can then be used in adoptive transfer trials.

Although the clinical value of most of the immunotherapeutic regimens tested to date has not yet been unequivocally proven or has been found to be at best relatively limited, it is reasonable to expect that treatments capable of increasing the efficacy of host responses to tumor will be developed and will ultimately provide essential tools in the definitive management of certain forms of cancer. To this end, it is essential to acquire further basic knowledge of the host defense systems and the mechanisms by which they may be perturbed, particularly in humans. It also seems important to continue to develop new agents aimed at the exploitation of immune systems in cancer therapeutics. I hope that the information discussed in this book will be a source of stimulation and a basis for rational planning toward the further development of novel cancer immunotherapies.

ENRICO MIHICH

Buffalo, New York
March 1982

Contents

Immunological Approaches To Cancer Therapeutics

Serologic Analysis of Human Solid Tumor Antigens

JOHN M. BROWN
STEVEN A. ROSENBERG
Surgery Branch, National Cancer Institute
National Institutes of Health
Bethesda, Maryland

1. INTRODUCTION

A central issue in studies of human tumor immunology deals with whether human cancer cells express antigens not present in normal adult tissues of the host. The identification and characterization of these putative tumor antigens may be of use in the development of new diagnostic and therapeutic strategies and could significantly add to our understanding of malignant transformation and the host response to it.

The existence of tumor-associated antigens has been clearly established in many experimental animal systems. Animal experimentation has utilized primarily *in vivo* manipulations such as immunization and tumor cell challenge. The use of inbred animal strains and transplantable tumors induced by carcinogenic agents and viruses has provided valuable reproducibility of both host and tumor. A variety of antigen types have been described in experimental tumors (Table 1). With the use of *in vivo* transplantation techniques, tumors induced with chemical carcinogens have generally been found to express unique antigens, although antigens common to a variety of tumors have also been detected (1). Serologic (antibody) techniques have also been utilized to detect tumor antigens in carcinogen-induced tumors, and both unique and cross-reacting antigens have been described (2). In contrast to carcinogen-induced tumors, tumors induced by the same virus have been shown most often to express common or virus-associated group-specific antigens (3,4). Antigens normally expressed only during fetal development have been detected in many animal tumors, including those induced with chemical carcinogens as well as with viruses (5,6).

Human tumors have also been extensively analyzed over the last decade for the presence of tumor-associated antigens. In studies in humans, of course, it has been impossible to employ the kinds of *in vivo* transplantation test with viable cells that have formed the basis for the identification of tumor-associated antigens in animal systems. Although some studies have involved *in vivo* skin

TABLE 1.   Types of Antigens that May Be Present on Experimental Tumors

Tumor associated
  Unique
  Common
  Viral (etiologic)
  Fetal

Tissue specific

Allospecific

Species specific

Artifactual (method of antigen preparation, culture conditions, contaminating virus, etc.)

testing with nonviable tumor cells or antigen preparations, most have relied on *in vitro* tests of lymphocyte or antibody reactivity to tumor cells or antigen preparations. A major problem with human testing has been the difficulty in obtaining sufficient and reproducible quantities of tissue. This has led to the extensive use of cultured tumor cells as a source of antigen. As is discussed more thoroughly in a subsequent section, the use of cultured cells has been accompanied by a host of problems that have impeded progress in this field.

Despite these difficulties, many serologic studies have claimed the demonstration of tumor-associated antigens in human tumors. An important aspect of the serologic study of tumor antigens is the simultaneous testing of both tumor tissues and normal adult tissues to define the tumor specificity of the involved antigens. Much of the early work in this field did not sufficiently address questions of tissue specificity. In many instances when putative tumor-associated antigens were more thoroughly studied and more sensitive assays developed, the antigens were detected, sometimes in lower quantities, in normal adult tissues as well. Many other serologic analyses, however, have provided seemingly strong evidence for the existence of tumor-associated antigens in human malignancy. In this chapter we present an overview of serologic studies of human solid tumors, with particular emphasis on melanoma and sarcoma.

2. METHODS OF ANALYSIS

2.1. Sources of Antigens and Antibodies

Whole tissues, tissue-cultured cells, tissue homogenates, and various soluble antigen preparations have been used as sources of human tumor antigens. Although cultured cells provide a convenient and reproducible source of antigen, several problems are associated with their use (Table 2). Irie et al. (7,8)

TABLE 2.   Problems with Use of Tissue-Cultured Tumor Cells in Serologic Studies of Human Tumor Antigens

Identification of cells as malignant (overgrowth of normal cells)

Change of cells with passage (overgrowth of tumor subpopulations)

Expression of neoantigens not expressed *in vivo*

Loss of *in vivo* antigens on establishment in tissue culture

Altered antigenicity with variations in

　　Culture conditions (medium, serum source, CO_2 concentration, temperature)

　　Growth stage (cell cycle, state of confluency, time from last medium change)

　　Use of proteolytic enzymes in cell preparation

Binding of medium components to cells (heterologous serum antigens)

Contamination of cultures with antigenic organisms (PPLO, viruses, etc.)

described the ability of cultured cells to incorporate foreign antigens present in heterologous sera used in culture media, and such antigens are a potential source of confusion in serologic analyses. The expression of antigens can be highly variable, depending on cell cycle and culture conditions (9–13). An even greater problem is the difficulty in establishing the malignant nature of the cultured cells. Although various approaches have been taken, including growth of cells in immunosuppressed animals, karyotype analysis, ultrastructural studies, marker analysis, and growth characteristics in culture, no single criterion appears sufficient to characterize a cultured cell as malignant (13). Normal cells may overgrow in cultures derived from tumor tissue, and this finding may be a source of confusion in many studies.

Antibodies to human tumors have been obtained both from human sources and after immunization of animals with various tumor preparations. Although sera from cancer patients have been a major source of human antibodies, elution of antibodies from tumor specimens has also been achieved (14). Antibodies from human as opposed to xenogeneic sources are of particular interest because they may reflect a response by the host to immunologically relevant tumor antigens. However, there are drawbacks to the study of human tumor antigens with the use of sera from cancer patients. Human sera have generally been found to yield low concentrations of antibodies, and highly sensitive tests are required for their detection. Such tests have often been confused by the finding that normal human sera possess antibodies directed against certain antigens present on the cell surface (15). Xenogeneic antisera, on the other hand, can usually be obtained with much higher titers. However, such preparations react with a variety of nonrelevant antigens, and extensive absorption with normal tissues must be performed. A recent approach to overcome this problem has involved the use of somatic cell hybrids to produce high-titered monoclonal antibodies reacting with a single antigenic specificity (16). Although such work is still in early stages, this technique has great potential for obtaining large quantities of highly specific antibodies against tumor-associated antigens.

2.2. Methods of Assay

Various methods have been used to detect antibody binding to tumor antigens (Table 3), and a compendium of this methodology has recently been compiled (17). The most extensively used assay has utilized immunofluorescence to measure antibody binding to the surface of viable cells and to the cytoplasm and nucleus of fixed cells. Several other highly sensitive assays that also measure antibody binding to cell membranes involve the use of indicator red blood cells, as in the immune adherence and mixed hemadsorption tests. Assays involving the ability of bound antibody to induce cell lysis include complement-dependent cytotoxicity and antibody-dependent, lymphocyte-mediated cytotoxicity. Complement fixation and immunoprecipitation assays have been used in many studies to detect reactivity to solubilized antigens. Recently,

TABLE 3.   Assays Used in Serologic Analysis of Human Solid Tumor Antigens

Assays measuring antibody binding to cells
   Immunofluorescence (direct and indirect)
   Immune adherence
   Mixed hemadsorption
   Isotopic antiglobulin
   Protein A (radiolabeled and erythrocyte tagged)
Assays measuring antibody function
   Complement-dependent cytotoxicity
   Antibody-dependent cell-mediated cytotoxicity
Assays utilizing soluble antigen
   Complement fixation
   Immunoprecipitation (immunodiffusion, immunoelectrophoresis, radioimmunoassay)

radioimmunoassays have been employed in many different systems to measure antibody binding to both cells and solubilized antigens. These assays can be highly sensitive and are also readily quantifiable, an advantage over more subjective tests such as those involving immunofluorescence or indicator cells that must be assessed by microscopic examination.

Depending on the assay and the reagents employed, a test will be sensitive only for certain classes of immunoglobulin. For example, an indirect immunofluorescence assay may be designed to detect IgG antibodies, whereas a complement fixation assay will be sensitive to those immunoglobulin classes able to fix complement, primarily IgM and IgG. Because important reactivities might be missed with single assays, the use of a battery of serologic tests has been recommended (18).

Absorption analyses, utilizing both whole tissues and solubilized antigens, have been a common feature in most serologic studies. Such analyses allow for the detection of tissue antigens that cross-react with those present in the test preparation and thus are vital to determining antigen specificity. Absorptions are also useful with tissues that are not suitable for direct tests. In addition, absorption analyses may detect antigens that were not detected in direct tests (19). Absorption analyses have drawbacks, however. Tissue preparations may nonspecifically absorb immunoglobulins or release substances that interfere with the assay. Furthermore, the preparation of tissues for absorption may alter their antigenicity. These problems continue to plague most serologic studies.

3.   ONCOFETAL ANTIGENS

Some tumors appear to express antigens or synthesize proteins normally expressed only by fetal and not by adult tissue. Many of these oncofetal antigens have been described, including serum proteins, cell surface antigens, intracellular enzymes, and ectopic hormones [recently reviewed by Sell (5) and Uriel (6)]. However, most of these fetal antigens are not strictly tumor-associated, and with the use of sensitive assays, they have also been detected in small amounts in nonmalignant adult cells. The two best-studied oncofetal antigens are alphafetoprotein (AFP) and carcinoembryonic antigen (CEA). These antigens have been analyzed with the use of xenogeneic antisera raised against tumor or fetal preparations. Alphafetoprotein is a serum protein associated with normal fetal and neonatal development and with the growth of hepatocellular tumors (5,6). However, it is also produced during liver regeneration, and low-serum AFP levels have been found in the normal adult. Carcinoembryonic antigen is a fetal colon cell-surface glycoprotein that is produced by tumors of ectodermal origin—intestinal, pulmonary, pancreatic, gastric, and mammary adenocarcinoma (5,6). Elevated serum CEA levels are also associated with smoking and with inflammatory diseases of bowel, lung, and pancreas. Low-serum CEA is present in normal adults.

Several oncofetal antigens have been described that appear to be specific for fetal and tumor tissue, although more extensive analyses or more sensitive tests may identify such antigens on normal adult tissues. Avis and Lewis (20), using an approach similar to that used to detect CEA, raised rabbit antisera to perchloric acid extracts of human fetuses. The sera, which were absorbed with normal tissue components, reacted by membrane and cytoplasmic immunofluorescence with fetal tissues and with certain human tumors. No reactivity was observed with several normal adult tissues.

This concept of a common oncofetal antigen was further supported by the work of Irie et al. (21). Using an immune adherence assay, those investigators found that sera from several melanoma patients reacted with a melanoma cell line in tissue culture. An extensive absorption analysis indicated that a common antigen was present on the surface of a variety of histologic types of biopsied and cultured tumors and on human fetal brain. A number of biopsied normal tissues were negative for the antigen. However, when muscle and skin were placed in tissue culture, they became positive for the antigen, indicating that normal adult tissues may reexpress fetal antigens under conditions of tissue culture. This common oncofetal antigen (OFA) appeared to be immunogenic because melanoma patients receiving therapy with allogeneic melanoma cells bearing OFA displayed increased titers of anti-OFA (22). However, anti-OFA reactivity has also been found in normal individuals (23).

A similar fetal-associated antigen has been described by Rosenberg and co-workers with the use of a complement-dependent cytotoxicity assay. Most human sera were found to possess antibodies reactive with common antigens expressed on cultured sarcomas, cultured normal skin fibroblasts, and first-trimester human fetal tissue (24–26). Normal adult tissues prior to culture did not express fetal antigens. Similar antibody levels were found in sarcoma patients when compared to normal individuals (24,27), and this finding raises several possibilities: (1) the fetal antigen may cross-react with a common environmental antigen; (2) the antifetal reactivity may be the result of an immune surveillance mechanism against malignant transformation in normal individuals; or (3) the reactivity may be an autoantibody directed against an undetected normal tissue antigen.

Salinas et al. (28,29) have presented evidence for the existence of a common interspecies OFA. With the use of radiolabeled antiglobulin and membrane immunofluorescence assays, human sera were found to react with both human and mouse fetal liver cells. Sera from patients with various types of cancer showed a markedly higher incidence of reactivity (71–92%) than did normal sera (11–31%). However, because an extensive absorption analysis was not performed, the tissue specificity of the xenogeneic antigen was not well established.

Blood group antigens are determined by carbohydrate chains present on the cell surface. The loss or gain of these chains is a common occurrence in fetal erythrocytes. Several studies have demonstrated, in isolated cases, the appearance of illegitimate blood group antigens, that is, normal blood group antigens that are nevertheless different from those present on normal tissues of the host (30). T antigen, the precursor of blood group MN antigens, is an antigen not found on normal adult erythrocytes. Springer et al. (31) demonstrated the presence of T antigen on all breast cancers studied, whereas benign mammary glands taken from the same individuals did not express T antigen. Anti-T antibodies were found in all human sera tested.

Numerous other studies have identified OFAs. Many of these are discussed in the following sections dealing with specific tumor types.

4. MELANOMA ANTIGENS

The antigenicity of malignant melanoma has been more extensively studied than that of any other human solid tumor. This may be due in part to the clinical impression that immunologic factors play a role in the natural history of the disease. Little evidence exists to support this impression, however. The immunology of melanoma has recently been reviewed (32,33).

4.1. Tests with Human Sera

Membrane Antigens.   Many workers have utilized human sera as a source of antibody to study melanoma cells for the presence of cell-surface tumor-associated antigens (Table 4). Several classes of antigen have been detected: unique antigens reactive only with autologous sera, common antigens cross-reactive with some or all other melanomas tested, and OFAs. Lewis and coworkers (34,35), using cytotoxicity and membrane immunofluorescence tests, detected reactivity in patient sera directed solely against autologous melanoma cells. The antibodies could be absorbed only with autologous tumor, and not with autologous normal cells or allogeneic tumor. Immunofluorescence and

TABLE 4.   Detection of Cell Surface Melanoma Antigens with Use of Melanoma Patient Sera

Assay	Antigen-Positive Tissues	Antigen-Negative Tissues	Comments	Ref.
Immunofluorescence	Fresh autologous and allogeneic melanoma		Fifty-seven percent of melanoma patients and 13% of normal sera reactive	40
Cytotoxicity, immunofluorescence	Fresh and cultured autologous melanoma	Allogeneic melanoma, autologous skin	One-third of patients sera gave autologous reactions	34, 35
Cytotoxicity, immunofluorescence	Cultured autologous melanoma	Most cultured allogeneic melanoma, autologous skin, epidermal and colonic tumors	Normal sera unreactive; several melanoma sera reacted weakly with allogeneic melanoma	36
Cytotoxicity	Cultured allogeneic melanoma and breast carcinoma		Thirty percent of melanoma patients and 7% of control sera reactive to melanoma	42
Immune adherence	Cultured autologous and allogeneic melanoma	Allogeneic skin fibroblasts, lymphocytes, cultured breast carcinoma line	Eighteen percent of melanoma patients and no normal or other tumor sera reactive with allogeneic melanoma	10
Complement fixation	Fresh autologous and allogeneic melanomas	Fresh sarcoma, carcinoma, normal muscle, kidney, lung	Test antibodies were eluted from fresh melanomas	14
Cytotoxicity	Cultured autologous melanoma	Most cultured allogeneic melanoma	Fifty percent of patient sera gave autologous reactions; 14% of positive sera reacted with allogeneic melanoma	37
Immune adherence	Fresh and cultured melanoma and other tumors, cultured normal skin, muscle	Fresh normal skin, muscle, other tissues, fresh and cultured lymphocytes	Termed *oncofetal antigen* (OFA)	21

TABLE 4.   (Continued)

Assay	Antigen-Positive Tissues	Antigen-Negative Tissues	Comments	Ref.
Mixed hemadsorption, immune adherence, anti-C3 mixed hemadsorption, protein A	Three classes of antigen detected I Unique antigen on autologous cultured melanoma only II Common antigen on autologous and allogeneic cultured melanoma only III Normal antigen on various fresh and cultured normal and malignant cells of human and animal origin		Studies utilized melanoma patient sera reactive with autologous tumor	18, 19, 49, 50
Cytotoxicity	Cultured allogeneic melanoma		Thirty-four percent of melanoma patients and 21% of normal sera reactive	41
Immunofluorescence, mixed hemadsorption	Autologous and allogeneic cultured melanoma	Autologous and allogeneic fibroblasts, cultured nonmelanoma tumors, human and monkey kidney, fresh fetal	Melanoma patient reactivity seen only after immunization with autologous or allogeneic melanoma cells	52, 53
Immune adherence	Cultured allogeneic melanoma, brain tumor, adult fibroblasts, fresh human fetal	Red blood cells, pooled platelets	Melanoma sera were preabsorbed with red cells and platelets	55
Radioimmune precipitation	Two membrane antigens solubilized from a fresh melanoma 80,000 MW[a] allogeneic 124,000 MW autologous		Four normal sera unreactive with solubilized antigens	38, 39

TABLE 4.   (Continued)

Assay	Antigen-Positive Tissues	Antigen-Negative Tissues	Comments	Ref.
Immunofluorescence, immune adherence	Autologous and allogeneic cultured melanoma	Autologous and allogeneic fibroblasts and lymphoblasts	Melanoma sera were preabsorbed with virus-transformed fibroblasts or lymphoblasts	54
Immunofluorescence	Two antigens detected OFA—autologous and allogeneic fresh and cultured melanoma, other cultured tumors and fibroblasts, fetal brain	Fresh autologous and allogeneic skin and kidney		45
	After fetal brain absorption—autologous and allogeneic fresh and cultured melanoma	Sarcoma, breast carcinoma, fibroblasts, fetal brain		
Immune adherence, complement fixation	Two antigens detected OFA—autologous and allogeneic fresh and cultured melanoma sarcoma, carcinoma, fibroblasts	Fresh liver, lung, lymphoblastoid cell line	Test antibodies isolated by serum-affinity chromatography on melanoma membranes	46
	After absorption with sarcoma—autologous and allogeneic melanoma	Sarcoma, fibroblasts		
Complement fixation, immune adherence, protein A radioassay	Two antigens isolated from melanoma culture medium OFA-cultured allogeneic melanoma and fibroblasts, fetal brain	Allogeneic lymphoblastoid cell line	Fifty-six percent of melanoma patient sera and 12 to 23% of normal and other tumor sera reacted with TAA	47, 48

TABLE 4.   (Continued)

Assay	Antigen-Positive Tissues	Antigen-Negative Tissues	Comments	Ref.
	Tumor-associated antigen (TAA)—cultured allogeneic melanoma, breast carcinoma, teratoma, ovarian carcinoma	Cultured sarcoma, renal cell carcinoma, lung carcinoma, fetal fibroblasts		
Mixed hemadsorption protein A	Autologous cultured melanoma	Allogeneic cultured melanoma autologous fibroblasts	Class I typing serum used to identify papain-solubilized antigen	51
Immune adherence	Cultured autologous and allogeneic melanoma, fetal and adult fibroblasts	Sera lost all reactivity after absorption with fetal fibroblasts or fetal calf serum	Fourteen percent of Stage II melanoma patients and 3% of normal sera reactive	43
Cytotoxicity	Cultured autologous and allogeneic melanoma, fetal and adult fibroblasts	Sera lost all reactivity after absorption with fetal fibroblasts	Higher level of reactivity in Stage II melanoma patients than normal sera	44

aMolecular weight.

cytotoxicity studies by Nairn et al. (36) and Bodurtha et al. (37) have also demonstrated primarily autologous tumor reactivity in the sera of melanoma patients. In more recent studies by Lewis and associates, melanoma membrane antigens were isolated on affinity columns of autologous serum IgG (38,39). Two antigens were isolated—a unique antigen of 124,000 molecular weight precipitable only by autologous serum, and a common antigen of 80,000 molecular weight precipitable by allogeneic melanoma sera, but not normal sera. However, the characterization of this reactivity was incomplete in that few sera were tested and control normal tissues were not similarly analyzed.

In contrast to the results reported by Lewis et al. (34,35), Morton et al. (40) —using a similar membrane immunofluorescence assay—detected serum reactivity against allogeneic melanoma cells. A higher incidence of melanoma reactivity was observed in melanoma patients (57%) than in normal donors (13%). Higher levels of reactivity in melanoma patients than in normals to allogeneic melanoma were also found by Ferrone and Pellegrino (41), Canevari et al. (42), Cornain et al.(10), Sener et al. (43), and Brown et al.(44). Gupta and Morton (14) eluted antibodies from the surface of fresh melanoma cells and found that they reacted by complement fixation with a number of melanoma tissues, but not with other normal or malignant tissues. Melanoma reactivity could not be eluted from either normal or malignant nonmelanoma tissues.

As mentioned previously, Irie et al. (21) demonstrated by membrane immunofluorescence an OFA present on certain tumors, normal cells in culture, and human fetal brain, but not on fresh normal adult tissues. In a subsequent study several melanoma sera were absorbed with fetal brain to remove reactivity to OFA (45). The absorbed sera possessed residual reactivity to a common melanoma antigen. Gupta et al. (46) isolated patient serum immunoglobulins on affinity columns prepared from biopsied melanoma membranes and also demonstrated reactivities against OFA and a common melanoma antigen. In a further analysis of these reactivities Gupta et al. (47) utilized melanoma sera to identify antigens shed by melanoma cells into the culture medium. Extraction of the medium with chloroform:methanol (C:M) led to the identification of OFA activity in the C:M-insoluble fraction and a common melanoma antigen in the C:M-soluble fraction. Absorption analysis indicated that although the C:M-soluble antigen was present on a majority of melanomas, it was also present on several other nonmelanoma tumors but not on normal tissues (48), suggesting the presence of a more broadly distributed common tumor antigen.

Old and co-workers have analyzed membrane antigens on cultured autologous melanoma cells (18,19,49,50) by using a battery of serologic tests, including immune adherence, mixed hemadsorption, C3-mixed hemadsorption, and protein A hemadsorption (see also Chapter 12). Multiple assays were used to increase the likelihood of detecting significant reactions, whereas autologous testing eliminated possible interference due to alloantibodies. For detection of cross-reactive antigens, absorption tests were performed. The authors categorized three classes of antigens: Class I, unique tumor antigens restricted to autologous cultured tumor; Class II, shared tumor antigens present on allogeneic cultured tumor cells; and Class III, common antigens present on both normal and malignant cultured cells of human and animal origin. The studies identified 22 sera reactive with autologous cultured melanoma. Three sera recognized Class I antigens, two sera recognized Class II antigens (restricted to allogeneic melanoma cells, but not present on other tumor types), whereas 17 recognized Class III antigens. The Class II typing sera detected a common antigen present on some, but not all, melanoma cells tested. In several cases the same serum detected different antigen classes, depending on the assay employed. These studies lend support to the presence of at least two tumor-associated antigens—a unique antigen and a common melanoma antigen. One problem with these studies is that most of the tissues used for analysis were cultured and were thus a potential source of culture artifacts (see Table 3). Carey et al. (51) used a Class I melanoma typing serum to isolate and characterize a unique antigen solubilized from autologous melanoma by papain treatment. The antigen is a glycoprotein of molecular weight 20,000–50,000, is not associated with β_2-microglobulin or HLA antigens and cannot be solubilized from other melanoma or nonmelanoma cells.

Krementz and co-workers (52,53) analyzed reactivity in melanoma patient sera by using membrane immunofluorescence and mixed hemadsorption assays and could observe no reactivity against cultured melanoma cells prior to immunization with autologous or allogeneic melanoma cells. However, after start of immunotherapy, the patients' sera developed antibodies against a common tumor antigen present on a majority of the melanomas tested, but not on other tumor types, normal cells, or fetal cells. Common melanoma antigens have also been described by Cornain et al. (10) and Saxton et al. (54). Seibert et al. (55), using an immune adherence assay, were unable to detect any unique or common melanoma-specific antigens. However, common tumor-associated fetal antigens were readily identified on the cultured melanoma target cells.

Intracellular Antigens.   A number of workers have also detected the presence of intracellular melanoma antigens using antibodies in patient sera (Table 5). Although both unique and common antigens have been detected on the

TABLE 5.   Detection of Intracellular Melanoma Antigens with Use of Melanoma Patient Sera

Assay	Antigen-Positive Tissues	Antigen-Negative Tissues	Comments	Ref.
Immunofluorescence on acetone-fixed imprints	Fresh autologous and allogeneic melanoma	Fresh breast cancer, colon cancer, spleen, animal tissue	Sixty-one percent of melanoma sera and 20% of normal sera were reactive; both cytoplasmic and nuclear staining observed	40
Immunofluorescence on acetone-fixed cells	Cultured allogeneic melanoma	Cultured allogeneic skin, leukemia, lymphoma, breast carcinoma	Sixty-one percent of melanoma sera 0 to 11% of normal and other tumor sera were reactive	56
Immunofluorescence on fixed cells	Cultured fixed allogeneic melanoma	Cultured live melanoma, fixed or live benign nevus, HeLa, human and guinea pig kidney	One hundred percent of melanoma sera and 0% of normal or other tumor sera were reactive	57
Immunofluorescence on fixed cells	Fresh and cultured autologous and allogeneic melanoma	Lymphoid cells, bronchial carcinoma		34

TABLE 5.   (Continued)

Assay	Antigen-Positive Tissues	Antigen-Negative Tissues	Comments	Ref.
Immunofluores-cence on fixed cells	Fresh and cultured autologous and allogeneic mela-noma	Fresh benign nevus, cerebral cortex	Sixty-six percent of melanoma sera and 22% of normal sera were reactive; cytoplasmic and nuclear antigens detected	58
Immunofluores-cence, immuno-diffusion	Melanoma patient antibodies separ-ated into those reacting with cell surface and with cytoplasm			60
Immunofluores-cence on fixed cells	Fresh autologous and allogeneic melanoma	Normal tissues, tumor lines KB, HeLa, HEp-2	Nucleolar staining	62
Immunofluores-cence on fixed cells, complement fixation	Fresh and cultured autologous and allogeneic mela-oma			59
Immunofluores-cence on fixed imprints	Fresh allogeneic melanoma, squa-mous cell carcino-ma, neuroblastoma, sarcoma, lung carcinoma	Lymphocytes	Higher levels of reactivity in mela-noma sera than in normals	61

cell membrane, intracellular melanoma antigens are invariably of the common type. Morton et al. (40) examined immunofluorescent reactivity of patient sera against acetone-fixed melanoma and found a higher incidence of antibodies in melanoma patients (61%) than in normal donors (20%). Both nuclear and cytoplasmic staining were detected. Cross-reactive antibodies were found in four of six sera tested, and absorption analysis indicated a common tumor antigen in three of five melanomas tested, but not in other tumors or normal cells. The results with cytoplasmic staining were supported by Oettgen et al. (56), Muna et al. (57), Romsdahl and Cox (58), and Bourgoin and Bourgoin (59). Lewis and co-workers also detected reactivity to a common cytoplasmic antigen in melanoma sera (34) and were able to separate the antibodies against autologous membrane antigens from those against common cytoplasmic antigens by cell homogenate affinity techniques (60). Wood and Barth (61) detected multiple common tumor-specific, rather than melanoma-specific, cytoplasmic antigens. Common nuclear antigens have also been described by Romsdahl and Cox (58) and McBride et al. (62).

4.2. Tests with Xenogeneic Sera

Unlike studies with human sera that have detected both unique and common tumor antigens, studies with xenogeneic sera have detected primarily common melanoma antigens (Table 6). Goodwin et al. (63) immunized rabbits with fresh melanoma tissue and tested sera for cytoplasmic immunofluorescence after extensive absorption with normal tissues. The resultant antisera detected a common melanoma antigen not present in other tumors or normal tissues, including a benign pigmented mole. Carrel and Theilkaes (64), using rabbit antibodies, found a common melanoma antigen in the urine of melanoma patients, but not in the urine of other cancer patients, except those with neuroblastoma and ganglioneuroma. The positive patients had tumors derived from the embryonic neural crest, thus suggesting that these tumors may share a common fetal antigen.

Several studies have provided additional evidence that melanoma cells express common fetal antigens. Viza and Phillips (65) raised rabbit antisera to papain-solubilized melanoma membranes. After absorption with normal tissue antigens, the antisera reacted with several pools of melanoma extracts and with first-trimester fetal extracts, but not with extracts from other tumors or with normal tissue antigens. Fritze et al. (66) produced guinea pig antisera to cultured melanoma and demonstrated cytotoxic specificity for common antigens on melanoma and fetal skin. Bystryn and Smalley (67), using a rabbit antimelanoma serum, also detected a common fetal antigen on melanoma cells.

In a series of studies involving rabbit antisera, Ferrone and co-workers identified both common melanoma and common tumor antigens. Antisera were raised against spent melanoma culture media and against 3 M KCl extracts of melanomas (68). After absorption with human red blood cells and lymphoblastoid cell lines, the sera retained reactivity only to melanoma. The melanoma antigens were separable from HLA antigens, and in a subsequent study (69) the antigens were shown not to be genetically linked to HLA A and B antigens. Although DR (Ia-like) lymphocyte-associated antigens have been detected on melanoma (70,71), preabsorption of the antisera with DR-positive lymphoblastoid lines eliminated this as a possible source of confusion (72). Immunoprecipitation of spent culture media indicated the presence of two non-cross-reacting antigens (72). One antigen, with a molecular weight of 170,000, was produced only by melanoma cells, whereas the other antigen, molecular weight 94,000, was produced by a number of tumor types, including melanoma.

A number of studies have utilized nonhuman primates as a source of antisera. This approach has the advantage that serum proteins and blood group and histocompatibility antigens are similar, thus increasing the possibility of raising a specific response to tumor antigens (73). Seigler and associates (74) reported that several monkey antisera to human melanoma, after absorption

TABLE 6.   Detection of Melanoma Antigens with Use of Xenogeneic Sera

Xenogeneic Species, Immunogen	Tissues Used for Preabsorption	Assay	Antigen Positive Tissues	Antigen Negative Tissues	Ref.
Rabbit, fresh melanoma	Whole skin, kidney powder, extracts of skin and lymph node	Immunofluorescence in fixed cells	Fresh and cultured autologous and allogeneic melanoma	Benign moles, carcinomas, sarcoma, normal tissues	63
Rabbit, fresh melanoma and patient urine	Plasma, normal urine, skin extracts, red blood cells	Double diffusion	Urine from patients with melanoma, neuroblastoma, and and ganglioneuroma	Urine from normals and nonmelanoma tumor patients	64
Rabbit, fetal extracts	Human serum, extracts of pooled adult tissue	Immunofluorescence	Fetal cells, and melanoma, other tumors (colon, breast, and kidney neuroblastoma, etc.)	Adult normal tissues including lymphocytes, skin, and gut	20
Monkey, cultured melanoma	Erythrocytes, leukocytes, HeLa	Cytotoxicity, mixed hemadsorption	Cultured and fresh autologous and allogeneic melanoma	Allogeneic cultured fibroblasts, four nonmelanoma tumor lines, normal allogeneic lymphocytes	74
Rabbit, solubilized melanoma membranes	Human serum, spleen extracts	Double diffusion, immunoelectrophoresis	Fresh autologous and allogeneic melanoma, fetal tissue, melanoma patient sera	Lung tumor, leukemia, normal and nonmelanoma tumor sera	65
Chimpanzee, fresh melanoma	Autologous lymphocytes	Cytotoxicity	Cultured allogeneic melanoma, fetal fibroblasts	Autologous and allogeneic lymphocytes, allogeneic adult fibroblasts, eight nonmelanoma tumor lines	73, 75
Guinea pig, cultured melanoma	Pooled lymphoid cells	Cytotoxicity	Cultured autologous and allogeneic melanoma, fresh fetal skin	Cultured autologous and allogenic fibroblasts, carcinomas, fresh fetal viscera	66

TABLE 6.   (Continued)

Xenogeneic Species, Immunogen	Tissues Used for Preabsorption	Assay	Antigen Positive Tissues	Antigen Negative Tissues	Ref.
Rabbit, fresh melanoma	Placenta	Radioimmune precipitation	Cultured allogeneic melanoma, fetal cells	Fresh allogeneic lymphocytes, liver and spleen cells, cultured HeLa, colon adenocarcinoma	67
Rabbit, cultured melanoma extracts and spent culture medium	Red cells and lymphoblastoid cell lines	Radiolabeled protein A	Cultured melanomas	Cultured lymphoblastoid lines	68
Monkey, cultured melanoma	Erythrocytes and platelets	Immune adherence	Cultured autologous and allogeneic melanoma, fetal fibroblasts, adult fibroblasts, two nonmelanoma tumor lines, fresh fetal cells	Fetal calf serum, mycoplasma, BCG	76
Mouse monoclonal hybridomas, cultured melanoma		Isotopic antiglobulin, mixed hemadsorption	Cultured autologous and allogeneic melanoma, fresh allogeneic melanoma, cultured astrocytoma	Cultured colorectal tumor lines, allogeneic fibroblasts, fresh allogeneic skin, hepatocytes, red blood cells, giant hairy nevus	78–80
Monkey, cultured melanoma	Erythrocytes, platelets, kidney, oral carcinoma cell line	Mixed hemadsorption	Cultured autologous and allogeneic melanoma, adult fibroblasts, retinoblastoma, fresh fetal tissue	Five nonmelanoma tumor lines, fetal lung fibroblasts, some adult fibroblasts, fresh adult skin, spleen, BCG	77
Mouse monoclonal hybridomas, cultured melanoma		Radiolabeled protein A	Primarily autologous melanoma	Allogeneic cultured melanoma, autologous and allogeneic fibroblasts, cultured nonmelanoma tumors, normal lymphoid cells	81

TABLE 6.   (Continued)

Xenogeneic Species, Immunogen	Tissues Used for Preabsorption	Assay	Antigen Positive Tissues	Antigen Negative Tissues	Ref.
Rabbit, cultured melanoma, soluble extracts, spent culture medium	Lymphoblastoid cell lines	Protein A, immunoprecipitation	Two melanoma antigens solubilized 170,000 MW melanoma specific 94,000 MW broad tumor specificity		72

with normal cells and nonmelanoma tumors, reacted with all cultured and fresh melanomas tested, but not with any other tumor or normal tissues. This finding of a common melanoma antigen was studied further (73). A chimpanzee was hyperimmunized to a fresh human melanoma and the resultant serum absorbed with the tumor donor's lymphocytes. The antiserum was reactive with 14 of 14 melanoma lines and 8 of 8 fetal fibroblast lines, but not with any other tumor or normal adult cells. Further absorption with fetal fibroblasts removed reactivity to all fetal cells but left reactivity to 2 of 2 melanoma lines. The results were interpreted to indicate the presence of both a common oncofetal antigen and a common melanoma antigen. Both the melanoma and fetal antigens were solubilized by pronase digestion of cultured and fresh melanoma and were partially separated from each other and from HLA antigens (75). In contrast to these results, Brüggen et al. (76), using monkey antisera, detected reactivities directed primarily against fetal antigens. Cross-reactivity and absorption studies indicated the presence of multiple tumor-associated antigens on different melanomas, and no antigen was uniformly expressed on all melanomas. Similar evidence for multiple partially cross reactive antigens, both melanoma-specific and fetal-associated, was provided by Liao et al. (77).

A recent approach to the study of melanoma antigens has involved the use of monoclonal antibodies produced by hybridomas. Koprowski and associates were able to generate four hybridomas, obtained by the fusion of sensitized mouse splenocytes with mouse myeloma cells, which produced antibodies with apparent specificity for melanoma cells (78,79). When clones of these hybridomas were examined in further detail, the secreted antibodies reacted strongly with most melanoma cell lines tested and with two astrocytoma lines, but not with colorectal tumor lines or with normal fibroblasts (79). The monoclonal antibodies were also found to bind to fresh melanoma cells, but not to freshly prepared normal autologous skin fibroblasts, hepatocytes, red blood cells, or melanocytes from a giant hairy nevus (80). Subsequent studies indicated that two of three of the hybridoma clones tested did not exhibit the desired tumor specificity and were reacting with Ia-like antigens expressed on melanoma cells and normal lymphoid cells (79).

Using techniques similar to those of Koprowski and associates, Yeh et al. (81) produced three mouse monoclonal antibodies that reacted with the donor melanoma cells, but not with autologous normal skin fibroblasts. The antibodies reacted strongly only with the donor melanoma cells; weak reactivity was observed with 2 of 11 allogeneic melanomas, but no reactivity was observed with a number of other tumor types or normal cells, including lymphoid cells bearing Ia-like antigens. The results, unlike those of Koprowski and co-workers, demonstrate the generation of antibodies against antigens with a much more restricted range of expression on different melanomas. Because the melanoma cells used in this study were cultured, one cannot exclude the possibility that antigens were lost or altered during the course of growth in tissue culture.

5. SARCOMA ANTIGENS

Studies of sarcomas have been limited primarily to the use of human sera as antibody source and to the use of tissue cultured tumor as antigen source. The latter has been due, in part, to the difficulty of obtaining suitable cell preparations for analysis from fresh sarcoma tissues and to the ease of growing sarcomas in tissue culture. Unlike melanoma, the studies have demonstrated the presence of common sarcoma and fetal antigens but not individually specific antigens.

5.1. Membrane Antigens

A number of studies have examined sarcoma cell-surface antigens (Table 7). Wood and Morton (82), using a complement-dependent cytotoxicity assay on cultured osteosarcoma cells, found a high incidence of reactivity in sera of patients with a variety of sarcomas (70%) and in sera of their family members (58%) and low reactivity in sera of normal donors (8%). The sarcoma sera reacted both with autologous and allogeneic sarcomas and showed lower but significant levels of reactivity with a normal fibroblast line. Positive absorption was obtained with two different sarcoma lines, but not with several nonsarcoma tumor lines and normal cells. The results were confirmed in another study by Wood and Morton (83), who also demonstrated an increase in sarcoma reactivity after a patient received immunotherapy with autologous sarcoma cells. The studies indicated the presence of a common sarcoma antigen, and the high incidence of reactivity in the sera of family members suggested that a common viral agent might be involved. Bloom (9), in a similar study, also detected cytotoxic reactivity to a common antigen shared by most sarcoma cell lines tested but not present on nonsarcoma cells. However, a similar

TABLE 7. Detection of Cell Surface Sarcoma Antigens with Use of Sarcoma Patient Sera

Assay	Antigen-Positive Tissues	Antigen-Negative Tissues	Comments	Ref.
Cytotoxicity	Cultured autologous and allogeneic osteosarcoma, liposarcoma, some reactions with cultured fibroblasts	Some cultured fibroblasts, tumor lines KB, HeLa, Chang liver cells	Seventy percent of sarcoma patients and 8% of normals reactive to sarcoma	82, 83
Cytotoxicity	Cultured autologous and allogeneic sarcomas, non-sarcoma tumor lines	Normal fibroblast line	Ninety-seven percent of sarcoma patients and 85% of normals reactive to sarcoma	9
Immunofluorescence	Cultured allogeneic neurogenic sarcoma	Cultured allogeneic lymphoma, melanoma, adenocarcinoma	Seventy-three percent of sarcoma sera and 6% of normal sera reactive	85
Immunofluorescence	Cultured allogeneic neurogenic sarcoma	Cultured allogeneic lymphoma, colon carcinoma, melanoma, skin fibroblasts, fresh erythrocytes, nerve tissue	Nineteen of 21 sarcoma sera remained reactive after absorption with nonsarcoma tumors and fibroblasts	86
Immunofluorescence, immunodiffusion	Cultured allogeneic osteosarcoma	Cultured allogeneic liposarcoma, fetal lung	Only osteosarcoma sera reactive; sera from breast adenocarcinoma, liposarcoma, and normals unreactive	87
Cytotoxicity	Cultured autologous and allogeneic osteosarcomas and skin fibroblasts	Fetal calf serum	Ninety percent of sarcoma sera lysed tumor and skin; 66% of normal sera reactive	24
Cytotoxicity	Cultured allogeneic skin fibroblasts, fresh fetal tissue	Fresh adult allogeneic lymphocytes, decidua, skin, muscle, fetal calf serum	Normal adult cells in tissue culture express fetal antigens	25
Cytotoxicity	Four of 11 cultured autologous and allogeneic osteosarcomas	Eleven of 11 cultured autologous and allogeneic skin fibroblasts, 7 of 11 cultured	Sera were preabsorbed with fetal tissue; 90% of osteosarcoma sera and 0% of	13, 26, 84

TABLE 7.   (Continued)

Assay	Antigen-Positive Tissues	Antigen-Negative Tissues	Comments	Ref.
		osteosarcomas, fresh and cultured fetal cells	normal sera were reactive after pre-absorption	
Cytotoxicity	Cultured alloge-neic skin fibro-blasts		Similar levels of reactivity in osteo-sarcoma, soft tissue sarcoma, and and normal sera	27

incidence and levels of reactivity were found in sera of sarcoma patients, their families, nonsarcoma patients, and normal donors.

An extensive analysis of complement-dependent serum cytotoxicity has also been performed by Rosenberg and associates. Unlike the previous studies, it was found that sera from osteosarcoma patients were equally reactive against cultured osteosarcoma cells and normal skin fibroblasts, both autologous and allogeneic (24). In addition, a majority of normal sera also possessed similar levels of cytotoxicity to these cells (24,27). When these natural antibodies in normal sera against skin fibroblasts were examined further, it was found that they could be removed by absorption with first-trimester human fetal tissue, but not by a variety of fresh normal adult tissues, including maternal decidua, skin, muscle, and lymphocytes (25). It thus appeared that normal adult cells in tissue culture were expressing a fetal antigen not present on fresh adult tissue. The expression of the antigen was not related to the use of fetal bovine serum in the culture medium (24,25).

The ability to remove the natural antibodies by absorption with fetal tissue was then used as a tool to analyze normal and osteosarcoma sera for the presence of tumor-specific reactivity. Absorption with fetal cells, but not with adult normal tissues, resulted in the removal of all reactivity from a normal serum when tested against allogeneic osteosarcoma as well as normal skin fibroblasts (26). However, when serum from a tumor-bearing osteosarcoma patient was exhaustively absorbed with fetal cells, significant reactivity against the patient's osteosarcoma cells remained although all reactivity against autologous normal cells was removed (26). Sera from 11 osteosarcoma patients and nine normal donors were analyzed by this technique (84). Following absorption with human fetal tissue cultured lines, sera from all 11 patients lost reactivity to autologous and allogeneic normal skin fibroblasts. However, sera from four patients retained reactivity against both their autologous tumor and an allogeneic osteosarcoma, sera from five patients retained reactivity to the allogeneic tumor but not their autologous tumor, and sera from two patients lost all reactivity to tumor. Sera from all nine normal donors lost reactivity to both normal and osteosarcoma cells after fetal absorption. The results indicate that most osteosarcoma patients possess antibodies to a common tumor antigen expressed on some, but not all, osteosarcoma cells in tissue culture. To further define the antigen specificity, direct tests and absorption analyses must be performed on other normal and nonosteosarcoma tumor tissues, both fresh and cultured.

Even among those cultured osteosarcoma cells that did express a common tumor-associated antigen, antigen expression was found to be variable (13). Two distinct cell lines cultured from separate fragments of the same tumor were analyzed, and sarcoma antigen was consistently detected on cells derived from one primary culture, but not from the other. This finding, along with the previously described observation that tumor lines derived from 7 of 11 osteosarcoma patients did not express a common sarcoma antigen, suggests several possible explanations: (1) the antigen-negative cultures were not derived from malignant cells; (2) the cultured lines were malignant, but there was a heterogeneity of cells *in vivo,* and the malignant cells that grew in these cultures were not capable of expressing the antigen; or (3) the cultured lines were malignant but the culture conditions were such that antigen expression was limited.

Drewinko et al. (85,86) analyzed the antigen expression on a cultured neurogenic sarcoma line by using membrane immunofluorescence. Sera from patients with a variety of sarcomas showed a high incidence of reactivity (64%) with these cells, whereas sera from nonsarcoma tumor patients and normal donors were significantly lower (14 and 4%, respectively) (85,86). Absorption analyses indicated that most of the sarcoma sera retained reactivity after absorption with a number of nonsarcoma tumor and normal cells, whereas nonsarcoma sera lost reactivity (86). Although the results suggest the presence of a common sarcoma antigen on the neurogenic sarcoma line, direct tests or absorption analyses were not performed with other sarcoma cells, and the conclusion must be considered tentative. Antigen expression on the neurogenic sarcoma line was found to be cell-cycle-dependent, with maximum levels expressed during mid-G_1 phase and lowest levels in S and G_2 phases (11,12).

Membrane immunofluorescence was also utilized by Blakemore and associates to analyze antigens on a cultured osteosarcoma line. Osteosarcoma patient sera, but not sera from several other nonsarcoma patients and normals, were found to react with the tumor line (87). Antigens were solubilized from osteosarcoma plasma membranes and found to react by immunoprecipitation only with the sarcoma sera. Antigens similarly solubilized from liposarcoma or fetal lung cultures were unreactive. Although a limited number of sera and cells were tested, the results implicate a common osteosarcoma antigen. This was examined further with xenogeneic sera (88). Soluble plasma membrane osteosarcoma antigens were used to raise antisera in rabbits. The antisera absorbed with normal tissues reacted only with osteosarcoma cells, and not with other sarcomas, nonsarcoma tumors, fetal cells, or normal adult cells, giving further support to the existence of a common osteosarcoma antigen.

5.2 Intracellular Antigens

Table 8 summarizes the results of studies analyzing sarcoma intracellular antigens. Morton and associates examined fixed preparations of osteosarcomas by using direct and indirect immunofluorescence assays. When tumor imprints were examined, osteosarcoma patient sera were found to react with both autologous and allogeneic osteosarcomas, producing a diffuse cytoplasmic and weak nuclear staining (89). The sera did not react with three nonsarcoma tumors. A high incidence of antibodies was found in osteosarcoma patients (100%), their family members (85 to 100%) and close associates (89 to 91%), and a low incidence in normal donors (25 to 29%), once again suggesting a viral etiology in sarcoma. Blocking studies in direct tests indicated that a common antigen was involved. The epidemiologic results were confirmed in a subsequent study (90). However, it was found that the osteosarcoma sera also reacted with soft tissue sarcomas and with two of four melanomas tested, implicating a more broadly specific antigen than first believed. Complement-fixation studies were also employed by using homogenates of tissue cultured cells as antigen source (91). When sera were tested against antigens of a liposarcoma line, a higher incidence and higher levels of reactivity were found in sarcoma patients and their families than in nonsarcoma cancer patients and normal donors. The sarcoma sera also reacted with most osteosarcoma and fibrosarcoma lines tested, but not with cultured skin, muscle, other normal tissues, or nonsarcoma tumors. The results indicate the presence of a common sarcoma antigen in the cells tested. Byers et al. (92), using an immunofluorescence assay with fixed fresh and cultured cells, detected a common antigen in osteogenic sarcomas and giant cell tumors of bone.

Hirshaut and co-workers have performed an extensive analysis of intracellular antigens in sarcoma cells (93). When sarcoma patient sera were tested against fixed cultured sarcoma lines by indirect immunofluorescence assay, a punctate cytoplasmic fluorescence was observed. On further analysis it was found that the incidence of reactive antibodies was 94% in sarcoma patients, 31 to 90% in nonsarcoma cancer patients, and 58% in normal donors (94). The antigen, apparently present in lysosomes and termed S_1 by the authors, was also detected in cultured breast and colon carcinomas and melanomas, but not in any fresh tumor specimens. Similar results were obtained by Moore et al. (95). However, they could not detect the antigen in nonsarcoma tissues including normal adult, carcinoma, and embryonic. More recent studies indicate that the S_1 antigen is heterogeneous and also heterophilic, as it is found by absorption analysis in bovine and guinea pig tissues (96). Additionally, it was found that preparations of fresh colon and lung cancers and several adult normal tissues were also able to absorb S_1 reactivity (96). This makes it unlikely that S_1 is a true tumor-associated antigen.

A second antigen type was also detected by Hirshaut and associates using immunofluorescence and designated S_2 (97). Cultured sarcomas were found to

TABLE 8.   Detection of Intracellular Sarcoma Antigens with Use of Sarcoma Patient Sera

Assay	Antigen-Positive Tissues	Antigen-Negative Tissues	Comments	Ref.
Immunofluorescence on fixed imprints	Fresh autologous and allogeneic osteosarcoma	Melanoma, breast and colon carcinomas	Diffuse cytoplasmic fluorescence. 100% of osteosarcoma sera, and 29% of normal sera reactive	89
Immunofluorescence on fixed cells	Fresh autologous and allogeneic osteosarcoma, soft-tissue sarcomas, two of four melanomas	Breast and colon carcinomas	Eighty percent of osteochondrosarcoma sera and 26% of normal sera reactive	90
Complement fixation	Cultured allogeneic liposarcoma, osteosarcoma, fibrosarcoma	Cultured allogeneic carcinomas, embryonic cell lines, adult liver, muscle, skin	Ninety-five percent of sarcoma sera and 25% of normal sera reactive	91
Immunofluorescence on fixed cells	Cultured autologous and allogeneic sarcomas, breast and colon carcinomas, melanomas, preparations of fresh colon and lung cancer, adult brain, colon, and lung, bovine tissue, guinea pig kidney, sheep erythrocytes	Fresh sarcomas, human erythrocytes	Punctate, cytoplasmic fluorescence, termed S_1 antigen; 96% of sarcoma sera and 58% of normal sera reactive	93, 94, 96
Immunofluorescence on fixed cells	Fresh and cultured autologous and allogeneic sarcomas, giant cell tumors	Cultured allogeneic Ewing's sarcoma, nonsarcoma tumor and normal cell lines, sheep erythrocytes, guinea pig kidney	Diffuse fluorescence; 50% of sarcoma sera and 0% of normal sera reactive	98
Immunofluorescence on fixed cells	Cultured allogeneic sarcomas	Fresh tumor tissues, cultured breast, lung, and colon carcinomas	Punctate fluorescence; 38% of sarcoma sera reactive	95
Immunofluorescence on fixed cells	Cultured allogeneic osteosarcomas, benign	Cultured allogeneic soft tissue sarcomas, carci-	Diffuse fluorescence, termed S_2 antigen; 72% of	96, 97

TABLE 8.   (Continued)

Assay	Antigen-Positive Tissues	Antigen-Negative Tissues	Comments	Ref.
	giant cell tumors, fetal lines, adult skin lines	nomas of pancreas, ovary, and lung, human and sheep erythrocytes	sarcoma sera and 11% of normal sera reactive	
Immunofluorescence on fixed cells	Fresh and cultured autologous and allogeneic osteosarcoma, giant cell tumor of bone	Fresh and cultured autologous and allogeneic skin, muscle, soft-tissue sarcomas, other tumors	Positive reactions only with sera from osteosarcoma and giant cell tumor patients	92
Complement fixation	Cultured autologous and allogeneic sarcomas, fresh adult brain and muscle preparations, guinea pig kidney	Fresh allogeneic sarcomas, cultured melanomas, breast carcinomas, adult skin, bovine tissue, human and sheep erythrocytes	Termed S_3 antigen; 84% of sarcoma sera and 7% of normal sera reactive	96, 99, 100

yield a diffuse cytoplasmic fluorescence when reacted with patient sera. The antigen was found only in early passages of cultured cells and was most easily detected in giant cell tumors of bone. A high incidence of reactivity to S_2 was found in sarcoma patients (72%) and their families (30%) and in carcinoma patients (20 to 53%), and a low incidence was observed in patients with lymphoproliferative malignancies (7 to 13%) and in normal donors (11%). On further analysis, S_2 was found to be present in most sarcoma and benign giant cell tumor lines, in cultured fetal tissue and cultured normal adult skin, but not in three cultured carcinomas tested. Although the results suggest that S_2 may be an oncofetal antigen also expressed by normal adult cells in culture, fresh adult tissues were not tested. Therefore, one cannot rule out the possibility that S_2 is a normal tissue antigen. The frequency of the antibody in sarcoma patients and their families and the morphology of the antigen suggest a close resemblance with those sarcoma antigens described by Morton et al. (89,90) and Priori et al. (98). Although the epidemiologic studies might support the theory of a common viral etiology, Mukherji and Hirshaut (97) also found an increased antibody incidence against S_2 in carcinoma patients. The authors felt it unlikely that a single viral agent would be the cause of such a wide variety of tumors.

Hirshaut and co-workers described a third antigen, designated S_3, with a complement-fixation assay (99,100). With the use of sarcoma patient sera, S_3 was detected only in homogenates of cultured sarcomas, and not in carcinomas, melanomas, or normal skin, either fresh or cultured. A high incidence of reactivity was found in the sera of sarcoma patients (84%), their families (40%), and carcinoma patients (30 to 60%), and a low incidence in normal donors (7%). Strong evidence that the antigen is tumor-associated comes from the finding that antibody titers consistently rose in sarcoma patients after surgical removal of their tumors. However, recent absorption analyses indicate that several normal adult tissue preparations, including brain and muscle, possess a cross-reactive antigen (96).

6. OTHER TUMOR ANTIGENS

Several studies have demonstrated that sera from patients with brain tumors have a higher incidence of reactivity to tumor cells than do sera from normal donors. Thus Kornblith and associates (101–103), using a complement-dependent cytotoxicity assay with a glioblastoma cell line, showed that 82% of astrocytoma patients reacted, versus 9% of normal donors. Sheikh et al. (104) demonstrated increased incidence in glioma patients of antibodies reacting with cytoplasmic glioma antigens. Old and co-workers (18,105), in an analysis similar to their melanoma studies, detected both unique and common tumor antigens on the membrane of cultured astrocytoma cells. Similar results have recently been reported by Coakham and Kornblith (106) with glioma cells. Xenogeneic antisera have also been used to define brain tumor antigens. Rabbit antisera have detected common glioma antigens (107,108) and common astrocytoma antigens (109,110). Hybridoma techniques have recently been used by Kennett and Gilbert (111) to produce mouse monoclonal antibodies against neuroblastomas. One antibody clone specifically reacted with neuroblastomas, a retinoblastoma, a glioblastoma, and with fetal brain cells, but not with other tumors or normal cells. The reactive cells all share a common neuroectodermal origin, indicating that the antibody may be detecting a fetal antigen expressed on tumors with a common embryonic origin. In a preliminary study Miyake and Kitamura (112), using a rabbit antiglioma serum, also described a fetal brain antigen expressed strongly on gliomas and neurinomas, tumors derived from tissues of common neuroectodermal origin.

Serologic analysis of lung tumors has been limited primarily to the use of xenogeneic antisera. When the sera have been sufficiently well characterized, most studies have been unable to detect lung tumor-associated antigens not present on normal adult tissues. Bell et al. (113), using a rabbit antiserum against oat cell carcinoma, detected two distinct lung tumor antigens not present on normal adult lung. However, one of the antigens was found to cross-react with antigens present on certain endodermally derived normal epithelial cells of the digestive system, and the other antigen was present on neural crest-derived Schwann cells (114,115). Like Ia antigens on melanoma (70,71), this is another example of a tumor cell expressing normal differentiation antigens not present on the cell of origin. When the antisera were absorbed with normal colon and nerve tissues to remove reactivity to the normal tissue antigens, a common tumor antigen was detected on all oat cell carcinomas tested, but not on other tumors or normal tissues (116). McIntire and associates generated rabbit antisera against saline extracts of lung adenocarcinomas. The sera were absorbed with normal tissues and used in the isolation of a common soluble lung tumor antigen from two different adenocarcinomas (117,118). Using immunodiffusion techniques, the antigen was found to be present only in lung tumor extracts, and not in normal tissues or sera. However, when a more sensitive radioimmunoassay was developed, a cross-reactive antigen was detected in the sera of normal donors (119). The normal serum protein was subsequently identified as α_1-antichymotrypsin (120). The lung tumor antigen and the normal serum protein are physically distinct but possess common antigenic determinants. Despite the cross-reactivity, the radioimmunoassay was able to detect higher antigen levels in sera of patients bearing lung cancer than in normal sera (119,120). Veltri et al. (121), in an early study, characterized three lung tumor antigens by using rabbit antisera. All three antigens were found to cross-react with normal serum proteins α-1-globulin, ferritin, and lactoferrin. In a more recent study, two additional antigens have been described (122). One membrane antigen was detected on 70% of all lung tumors, and not on other tumors or normal tissues. The other membrane antigen was present on 80% of lung tumors and also on two of three colon carcinomas tested. Neither antigen cross-reacted with CEA or normal serum proteins.

Serologic studies of a variety of other tumors have been performed and are mentioned only briefly in this review. Bhattacharya and Barlow (123,124) raised antisera in rabbits against extracts of ovarian cystadenocarcinomas. After absorption of the sera with normal tissues, two cytoplasmic tumor antigens were detected. One antigen, termed OCAA, was present only in extracts of ovarian cystadenocarcinomas, and not in extracts of other normal or malignant tissues. The other antigen was found to be common to a variety of tumor types. A radioimmunoassay was developed for OCAA, and serum levels of the antigen showed a good correlation with tumor burden in a majority of cases studies (125,126). However, with the more sensitive assay, cross-reacting antigens were detected in sera of patients with colon, breast, and cervical carcinomas. In a similar type of analysis, Imamura et al. (127) detected a number of antigens in ovarian cystadenocarcinomas. One of them, termed OvC-6, was apparently unique for the immunizing tumor. Another antigen, termed OvC-2, was present in 8 of 93 ovarian epithelial cancers, one dysgerminoma, placenta, amniotic fluid, and fetal intestine, but not in any other tumors or normal tissues, indicating that it may be an OFA (128).

Leung et al. (129,130) recently described a breast tumor antigen, MTGP, detected with rabbit antisera and present on the membrane surface and in the cytoplasm of breast carcinoma cells, but not in other tumor or normal tissues. Antigens cross-reacting with mouse mammary tumor virus have been detected in human breast carcinoma cells by several groups (131,132).

Old and co-workers, using an assay system similar to their melanoma studies, detected both unique and common renal carcinoma antigens with autologous human sera (18,133). In several other recent studies, using xenogeneic sera, common renal tumor antigens have also been detected (134–136).

Monoclonal antibodies produced by hybridomas have been used to detect common colorectal carcinoma antigens not expressed on other tumors or normal cells and not related to CEA (79,137).

7. COMMENTS

Serologic analyses have indicated the presence of a variety of human tumor-associated antigens. Although the conclusions of the various studies should be considered tentative, some generalizations may be attempted (Table 9). Tumor-associated antigens on the cell surface can be categorized as unique antigens, common tumor histologic or organ type-specific antigens, antigens common to a variety of tumor histologies, and fetal antigens, both common and restricted to cells of similar embryonic tissue origin. Although unique antigens have been reported to exist on melanoma, astrocytoma, and renal carcinoma, common and fetal antigens have been detected on most tumors studied. Intracellular antigens have been characterized as both common and fetal, although unique antigens have not been detected. Human sera have revealed unique, common, and fetal antigens, whereas xenogeneic sera have in general revealed only common and fetal antigens. In addition, most studies that have revealed common histologic type-specific or common fetal antigens have been unable to reveal their presence in all relevant tumors or have revealed multiple patterns of common antigen expression (76,77).

How convincing are the studies in support of the existence of tumor-associated antigens? Although much circumstantial evidence has been provided by a variety of groups, little exists in the way of confirmatory findings in any single disease studied. The strongest studies to date are those in which a large variety of tissues have been examined, both normal and malignant, for antigen specificity. Studies that have shown higher reactivity in cancer patient sera than in normal sera, when tested against tumor cells, should be considered inconclusive without further tissue specificity experiments. In addition, studies

TABLE 9. Classification of Antigens that May Be Present on Human Solid Tumors

Unique

Common

   Histologic or organ type-specific

   Broadly expressed

Fetal

   Tissue specific

   Broadly expressed

Viral?

that have relied solely on the use of tissue-cultured cells as source of antigen run the risk of being obscured by culture artifacts and are less convincing than those studies that have also examined fresh tissue. Many of the epidemiologic studies with sarcoma have implicated a common viral etiology by virtue of increased antibody levels in both cancer patients and their families and associates. Although this is an interesting possibility that might explain the presence of common sarcoma antigens analogous to virus-associated sarcoma antigens in animal models (3,4), further support for this hypothesis has not been forthcoming.

The two major problems that have confronted the serologic analysis of human tumor antigens are (1) the lack of a suitable reproducible source of tumor tissue for use in assays and (2) the low titer of antibodies to putative tumor antigens found in human sera. The use of tissue-cultured human tumor introduces substantial difficulties and artifacts into serologic studies. Little progress has been made, however, in developing techniques for making viable single-cell suspensions of fresh tumor. The introduction of techniques utilizing hybridoma-synthesized antibodies can provide the serologist with high-titered specific antisera to human tumor-associated antigens, although this still remains a hope rather than a reality.

If past history is a guide, it is to be expected that many of the antigens described in this review will be found not to be uniquely tumor associated on further analysis. As more tissues are studied, and as more sensitive assays are developed, antigens may be detected in normal tissues as well. This might be especially true for OFAs as evidenced by the studies with AFP, CEA, and other oncofetal markers (5,6). Indeed, fetal antigens may always be present in low amounts in normal adult tissues and in many nonmalignant disease states.

Many problems remain with the use of serologically defined tumor antigens in the immunotherapy of cancer. Studies with xenogeneic sera may reveal antigens that are not immunogenic in humans and thus of no use in active immunotherapy. Tumor-associated antigens and their corresponding antibodies might play a role in the way in which tumors evade the host's immune system (138), and therapy directed at these antigens may result in tumor enhancement. Although studies have revealed both cell-surface and intracellular antigens, the relevance to immunotherapy of intracellular antigens that are not exposed to the immune system in live tumor cells remains to be established. Finally, because many of the antigens described have been found to be restricted in expression, as exemplified by unique antigens and by common antigens present on some, but not all, tumors of the same histologic type, it may be necessary to develop separate immunotherapeutic reagents for each individual tumor to be treated.

REFERENCES

1. R. W. Baldwin, Immunological aspects of chemical carcinogenesis. *Adv. Cancer Res.,* **18,** 1 (1973).

2. G. A. Parker and S. A. Rosenberg, Serologic identification of multiple tumor-associated antigens on murine sarcomas. *J. Natl. Cancer Inst.,* **58,** 1303 (1977).

3. D. P. Bolognesi, Structural components of RNA tumor viruses. *Adv. Virus Res.,* **19,** 315 (1974).

4. R. Kurth, E. M. Fenyo, E. Klein, and M. Essex, Cell-surface antigens induced by RNA tumour viruses. *Nature,* **279,** 197 (1979).

5. S. Sell, The biologic and diagnostic significance of oncodevelopmental gene products. In H. Waters, Ed., *The Handbook of Cancer Immunology,* Vol. 3, Garland STPM Press, New York, 1978, p. 1.

6. J. Uriel, Retrodifferentiation and the fetal patterns of gene expression in cancer. *Adv. Cancer Res.,* **29,** 127 (1979).

7. R. F. Irie, K. Irie, and D. L. Morton, Natural antibody in human serum to a neoantigen in human cultured cells grown in fetal bovine serum. *J. Natl. Cancer Inst.,* **52,** 1051 (1974).

8. R. F. Irie, K. Irie, and D. L. Morton, Characteristics of heterologous membrane antigen on cultured human cells. *J. Natl. Cancer Inst.,* **53,** 1545 (1974).

9. E. T. Bloom, Further definition by cytotoxicity tests of cell surface antigens of human sarcomas in culture. *Cancer Res.,* **32,** 960 (1972).

10. S. Cornain, J. E. DeVries, J. Collard, C. Vennegoor, I. van Wingerden, and P. Rumke. Antibodies and antigen expression in human melanoma detected by the immune adherence test. *Internatl. J. Cancer,* **16,** 981 (1975).

11. K. H. Burk, B. Drewinko, B. Lichtiger, and J. M. Trujillo, Cell cycle dependency of human sarcoma-associated tumor antigen expression. *Cancer Res.,* **36,** 1278 (1976).

12. K. H. Burk and B. Drewinko, Cell cycle dependency of tumor antigens. *Cancer Res.,* **36,** 3535 (1976).

13. S. A. Rosenberg, J. M. Brown, W. P. Thorpe, C. Hyatt, P. Shoffner, and S. Tondreau, Serologic studies of the antigens on human osteogenic sarcoma. In S. A. Rosenberg, Ed., *Serologic Analysis of Human Cancer Antigens,* Academic, New York, 1980, p. 93.

14. R. K. Gupta and D. L. Morton, Suggestive evidence for in vivo binding of specific antitumor antibodies of human melanomas. *Cancer Res.,* **35,** 58 (1975).

15. J. M. Brown, M. S. Catapano, and S. A. Rosenberg, Natural antibodies in human sera which react with tissue cultured cells. In S. A. Rosenberg, Ed., *Serologic Analysis of Human Cancer Antigens,* Academic, New York, 1980, p. 463.

16. G. Kohler and C. Milstein, Continuous cultures of fused cells secreting antibody of predefined specificity. *Nature,* **256,** 495 (1975).

17. S. A. Rosenberg, Ed., *Serologic Analysis of Human Cancer Antigens,* Academic, New York, 1980, pp. 583–710.

18. H. Shiku, T. Takahashi, T. Carey, L. Resnick, M. Pfreundschuh, R. Ueda, H. F. Oettgen, and L. J. Old, Definition of cell surface antigens of human malignant melanoma, astrocytoma and renal cancer by typing with autologous serum. In S. A. Rosenberg, Ed., *Serologic Analysis of Human Cancer Antigens,* Academic, New York, 1980, p. 305.

19. H. Shiku, T. Takahashi, L. A. Resnick, H. F. Oettgen, and L. J. Old, Cell surface antigens of human malignant melanoma. III. Recognition of autoantibodies with unusual characteristics. *J. Exp. Med.,* **145,** 784 (1977).

20. P. Avis and M. G. Lewis, Tumor-associated fetal antigens in human tumors. *J. Natl. Cancer Inst.,* **51,** 1063 (1973).

21. R. F. Irie, K. Irie, and D. L. Morton, A membrane antigen common to human cancer and fetal brain tissues. *Cancer Res., 36,* 3510 (1976).

22. R. F. Irie, A. E. Giuliano, and D. L. Morton, Oncofetal antigen: A tumor-associated fetal antigen immunogenic in man. *J. Natl. Cancer Inst., 63,* 367 (1979).

23. M. J. Lucas, R. F. Irie, and D. L. Morton, A case/control study of antibody to oncofetal antigen. *Proc. Am. Assoc. Cancer Res., 19,* 134 (1978).

24. S. A. Rosenberg, Lysis of human normal and sarcoma cells in tissue culture by normal human serum: Implications for experiments in human tumor immunology. *J. Natl. Cancer Inst., 58,* 1233 (1977).

25. W. P. Thorpe, G. A. Parker, and S. A. Rosenberg, Expression of fetal antigens by normal human skin cells grown in tissue culture. *J. Immunol., 119,* 818 (1977).

26. W. P. Thorpe and S. A. Rosenberg, Serologic analysis of human tumor antigens. I. Anti-sarcoma antibodies in the sera of patients with osteogenic sarcomas. *J. Natl. Cancer Inst., 62,* 1143 (1979).

27. M. S. Catapano, J. M. Brown, and S. A. Rosenberg, Levels of cytotoxic reactivity to cultured normal skin fibroblasts in sera from normal and sarcoma-bearing patients. *Cancer Res., 40,* 979 (1980).

28. F. A. Salinas, K. M. Sheikh, and S. B. Chandor, Serological reactivity in cancer patients to human and mouse fetal liver cells. *Cancer Res., 38,* 401 (1978).

29. F. A. Salinas, K. H. Wee, and H. K. B. Silver, Detection and characterization of antibodies to xenogeneic oncofetal antigen (XOFA) in human neoplasia. In S. A. Rosenberg, Ed., *Serologic Analysis of Human Cancer Antigens,* Academic, New York, 1980, p. 539.

30. P. Levine, Illegitimate blood group antigens P_1, A, and MN (T) in malignancy—A possible therapeutic approach with anti-Tj^a, anti-A, and anti-T. *Ann. N. Y. Acad. Sci., 277,* 428 (1976).

31. G. F. Springer, P. R. Desai, and E. F. Scanlon, Blood group MN precursors as human breast carcinoma-associated antigens and "naturally" occurring human cytotoxins against them. *Cancer, 37,* 169 (1976).

32. S. Ferrone and M. A. Pellegrino, Antigens and antibodies in malignant melanoma. In H. Waters, Ed., *The Handbook of Cancer Immunology,* Vol. 3, Garland STPM Press, New York, 1978, pp. 291.

33. G. M. Stuhlmiller and H. F. Seigler, Immunology and immunotherapy of melanoma. In H. Waters, Ed., *The Handbook of Cancer Immunology,* Vol. 5, Garland STPM Press, New York, 1978, p. 315.

34. M. G. Lewis, R. L. Ikonopisov, R. C. Nairn, T. M. Phillips, G. H. Fairley, D. C. Bodenham, and P. Alexander. Tumour-specific antibodies in human malignant melanoma and their relationship to the extent of the disease. *Brt. Med. J., 3,* 547 (1969).

35. M. G. Lewis and T. M. Phillips, The specificity of surface membrane immunofluorescence in human malignant melanoma. *Internatl. J. Cancer, 10,* 105 (1972).

36. R. C. Nairn, A. P. P. Nind, E. P. G. Guli, and D. J. Davies. Anti-tumour immunoreactivity in patients with malignant melanoma. *Med. J. Aust., 1,* 397 (1972).

37. A. J. Bodurtha, D. O. Chee, J. F. Laucius, M. J. Mastrangelo, and R. T. Prehn, Clinical and immunological significance of human melanoma cytotoxic antibody. *Cancer Res., 35,* 189 (1975).

38. E. Preddie, D. Hartmann, and M. G. Lewis, Human melanoma tumor specific antigens: (1) An allogeneic antigen from patient "PY" melanoma tumor cell plasma membranes. *Cancer Biochem. Biophys., 2,* 161 (1978).

39. E. Preddie, D. Hartmann, S. Persad, M. Khosravi, and M. Lewis, Isolation of an autologous tumor-specific antigen from tumor cell plasma membranes of a human melanoma patient. *Cancer Biochem. Biophys., 2,* 199 (1978).

40. D. L. Morton, R. A. Malmgren, E. C. Holmes, and A. S. Ketcham, Demonstration of antibodies against human malignant melanoma by immunofluorescence. *Surgery,* **64**, 233 (1968).

41. S. Ferrone and M. A. Pellegrino, Cytotoxic antibodies to cultured melanoma cells in the sera of melanoma patients. *J. Natl. Cancer Inst.,* **58**, 1201 (1977).

42. S. Canevari, G. Fossati, G. D. Poria, and G. P. Balzarim, Humoral cytotoxicity in melanoma patients and its correlation with the extent and course of the disease. *Internatl. J. Cancer,* **16**, 722 (1975).

43. S. F. Sener, J. M. Brown, C. L. Hyatt, W. D. Terry, and S. A. Rosenberg, Serologic analysis of human tumor antigens. III. Reactivity of patients with melanoma and osteogenic sarcoma to cultured tumor cells and fibroblasts using the immune adherence assay. *Cancer Immunol. Immunother.,* **11**, 243 (1981).

44. J. M. Brown, P. C. Shoffner, S. P. Tondreau, E. J. Matthews, W. D. Terry, and S. A. Rosenberg, Cytotoxic reactivity in the sera of melanoma patients to paired autologous and allogeneic cultured tumor and skin fibroblasts. *Cancer Res.,* (in press).

45. K. Irie, R. F. Irie, and D. L. Morton, Humoral immune response to melanoma-associated membrane antigen and fetal brain antigen demonstrated by indirect membrane immunofluorescence. *Cancer Immunol. Immunother.,* **6**, 33 (1979).

46. R. K. Gupta, H. K. B. Silver, R. A. Reisfeld, and D. L. Morton, Isolation and immunochemical characterization of antibodies from the sera of cancer patients which are reactive against human melanoma cell membranes by affinity chromatography. *Cancer Res.,* **39**, 1683 (1979).

47. R. K. Gupta, R. F. Irie, D. O. Chee, D. H. Kern, and D. L. Morton, Demonstration of two distinct antigens in spent tissue culture medium of a human malignant melanoma cell line. *J. Natl. Cancer Inst.,* **63**, 347 (1979).

48. R. K. Gupta, Antigenic complexity in human malignant melanoma tumors detected by allogeneic antibody. In S. A. Rosenberg, Ed., *Serologic Analysis of Human Cancer Antigens,* Academic, New York, 1980, p. 339.

49. T. E. Carey, T. Takahashi, L. A. Resnick, H. F. Oettgen, and L. J. Old, Cell surface antigens of human malignant melanoma: Mixed hemadsorption assays for humoral immunity to cultured autologous melanoma cells. *Proc. Natl. Acad. Sci.,* **73**, 3278 (1976).

50. H. Shiku, T. Takahashi, H. F. Oettgen, and L. J. Old, Cell surface antigens of human malignant melanoma. II. Serological typing with immune adherence assays and definition of two new surface antigens. *J. Exp. Med.,* **144**, 873 (1976).

51. T. E. Carey, K. O. Lloyd, T. Takahashi, L. R. Travassos, and L. J. Old, AU cell-surface antigen of human malignant melanoma: Solubilization and partial characterization. *Proc. Natl. Acad. Sci.,* **76**, 2898 (1979),

52. S. P. L. Leong, C. M. Sutherland, and E. T. Krementz, Immunofluorescent detection of common melanoma membrane antigens by sera of melanoma patients immunized against autologous or allogeneic cultured melanoma cells. *Cancer Res.,* **37**, 4035 (1977).

53. S. K. Liao, S. P. L. Leong, C. M. Sutherland, P. B. Dent, P. C. Kwong, and E. T. Krementz, Common human melanoma membrane antigens detected by mixed hemadsorption microassay with serum from a patient undergoing immunotherapy with autologous tumor cells. *Cancer Res.,* **38**, 4395 (1978).

54. R. E. Saxton, R. F. Irie, S. Ferrone, M. A. Pellegrino, and D. L. Morton, Establishment of paired tumor cells and autologous virus-transformed cell lines to define humoral immune responses in melanoma and sarcoma patients. *Internatl. J. Cancer,* **21**, 299 (1978).

55. E. Seibert, C. Sorg, R. Happle, and E. Macher, Membrane associated antigens of human malignant melanoma. III. Specificity of human sera reacting with cultured melanoma cells. *Internatl. J. Cancer,* **19**, 172 (1977).

56. H. F. Oettgen, T. Aoki, L. J. Old, E. A. Boyse, E. DeHarven, and G. M. Mills, Suspension culture of a pigment-producing cell line derived from a human malignant melanoma. *J. Natl. Cancer Inst.,* **41**, 827 (1968).

57. N. M. Muna, S. Marcus, and C. Smart, Detection by immunofluorescence of antibodies specific for human malignant melanoma cells. *Cancer,* **23**, 88 (1969).

58. M. M. Romsdahl and I. S. Cox, Human malignant melanoma antibodies demonstrated by immunofluorescence. *Arch. Surg.,* **100**, 491 (1970).

59. J. J. Bourgoin and A. Bourgoin, Cytoplasmic antigens in human malignant melanoma cells. *Pigment Cell,* **1**, 366 (1973).

60. M. G. Lewis and T. M. Phillips, Separation of two distinct tumor-associated antibodies in the serum of melanoma patients. *J. Natl. Cancer Inst.,* **49**, 915 (1972).

61. G. W. Wood and R. F. Barth, Immunofluorescent studies of the serologic reactivity of patients with malignant melanoma against tumor-associated cytoplasmic antigens. *J. Natl. Cancer Inst.,* **53**, 309 (1974).

62. C. M. McBride, J. M. Bowen, and L. L. Dmochowski, Antinucleolar antibodies in the sera of patients with malignant melanoma. *Surg. Forum,* **23**, 92 (1972).

63. D. P. Goodwin, M. O. Hornung, S. P. L. Leong, and E. T. Krementz, Immune responses induced by human malignant melanoma in the rabbit. *Surgery,* **72**, 737 (1972).

64. S. Carrel and L. Theilkaes, Evidence for a tumour-associated antigen in human malignant melanoma. *Nature,* **242**, 609 (1973).

65. D. Viza and J. Phillips, Identification of an antigen associated with malignant melanoma. *Internatl. J. Cancer,* **16**, 312 (1975).

66. D. Fritze, D. H. Kern, C. R. Drogemuller, and Y. H. Pilch, Production of antisera with specificity for malignant melanoma and human fetal skin. *Cancer Res.,* **36**, 458 (1976).

67. J. C. Bystryn and J. R. Smalley, Identification and solubilization of iodinated cell surface human melanoma associated antigens. *Internatl. J. Cancer,* **20**, 165 (1977).

68. R. P. McCabe, S. Ferrone, M. A. Pellegrino, D. H. Kern, E. C. Holmes, and R. A. Reisfeld, Purification and immunologic evaluation of human melanoma-associated antigens. *J. Natl. Cancer Inst.,* **60**, 773 (1978).

69. R. A. Curry, V. Quaranta, M. A. Pellegrino, and S. Ferrone, Serologically detectable human melanoma-associated antigens are not genetically linked to HLA-A and B antigens. *J. Immunol.,* **122**, 2630 (1979).

70. R. J. Winchester, C. Y. Wang, A. Gibofsky, H. G. Kunkel, K. O. Lloyd, and L. J. Old, Expression of Ia-like antigens on cultured human malignant melanoma cell lines. *Proc. Natl. Acad. Sci.,* **75**, 6235 (1978).

71. B. S. Wilson, F. Indiveri, M. A. Pellegrino, and S. Ferrone, DR (Ia-Like) antigens on human melanoma cells. Serological detection and immunochemical characterization. *J. Exp. Med.,* **149**, 658 (1979).

72. S. Ferrone, K. Imai, R. P. McCabe, G. A. Molinaro, D. R. Galloway, and R. A. Reisfeld, Production, characterization and use of xenoantisera to human melanoma associated antigens. In S. A. Rosenberg, Ed., *Serologic Analysis of Human Cancer Antigens,* Academic, New York, 1980, p. 445.

73. G. M. Stuhlmiller and H. F. Seigler, Characterization of a chimpanzee anti-human melanoma antiserum. *Cancer Res.,* **35**, 2132 (1975).

74. R. S. Metzgar, P. M. Bergoc, M. A. Moreno, and H. F. Seigler, Melanoma-specific antibodies produced in monkeys by immunization with human melanoma cell lines. *J. Natl. Cancer Inst.,* **50**, 1065 (1973).

75. G. M. Stuhlmiller, R. W. Green, and H. F. Seigler. Solubilization and partial isolation of human melanoma tumor-associated antigens. *J. Natl. Cancer Inst.,* **61**, 61 (1978).

76. J. Brüggen, C. Sorg, and E. Macher. Membrane associated antigens of human malignant melanoma. V: Serological typing of cell lines using antisera from nonhuman primates. *Cancer Immunol. Immunother.,* **5**, 53 (1978).

77. S. K. Liao, P. C. Kwong, J. C. Thompson, and P. B. Dent, Spectrum of melanoma antigens on cultured human malignant melanoma cells as detected by monkey antibodies. *Cancer Res.,* **39**, 183 (1979).

78. H. Koprowski, Z. Steplewski, D. Herlyn, and M. Herlyn. Study of antibodies against human melanoma produced by somatic cell hybrids. *Proc. Natl. Acad. Sci.,* **75**, 3405 (1978).

79. H. Koprowski, Monoclonal Antibodies in the Study of Melanoma and Colorectal Carcinoma. In S. A. Rosenberg, Ed., *Serologic Analysis of Human Cancer Antigens,* Academic, New York, 1980, p. 423.

80. Z. Steplewski, M. Herlyn, D. Herlyn, W. H. Clark, and H. Koprowski, Reactivity of monoclonal anti-melanoma antibodies with melanoma cells freshly isolated from primary and metastatic melanoma. *Eur. J. Immunol.,* **9**, 94 (1979).

81. M. Y. Yeh, I. Hellstrom, J. P. Brown, G. A. Warner, J. A. Hansen, and K. E. Hellstrom, Cell surface antigens of human melanoma identified by monoclonal antibody. *Proc. Natl. Acad. Sci.,* **76**, 2927 (1979).

82. W. C. Wood and D. L. Morton, Microcytotoxicity test: Detection in sarcoma patients of antibody cytotoxic to human sarcoma cells. *Science,* **170**, 1318 (1970).

83. W. C. Wood and D. L. Morton, Host immune response to a common cell-surface antigen in human sarcomas. Detection by cytotoxicity tests. *New Engl. J. Med.,* **284**, 569 (1971).

84. S. A. Rosenberg, S. C. Tondreau, P. C. Shoffner, C. Hyatt, J. M. Brown, W. Thorpe, and W. Sindelar, Serologic analysis of human tumor antigens. II. Reactivity of sera from eleven osteogenic sarcoma patients against autologous and allogeneic tumor cells. *Surgery,* **86**, 258 (1979).

85. B. Drewinko, C. T. Montgomery, and J. M. Trujillo, Demonstration of common sarcoma-associated antigen(s) in an established human neurogenic sarcoma cell line. *Cancer Res.,* **33**, 601 (1973).

86. B. Lichtiger, J. M. Trujillo, K. H. Burk, and B. Drewinko, Identification and subcellular localization of a sarcoma-associated antigen(s) in a human cell line. *Cancer,* **37**, 1788 (1976).

87. I. Singh, K. Y. Tsang, and W. S. Blakemore, Isolation and partial purification of plasma membrane-associated antigens from human osteosarcoma (TE-85) cells in tissue culture. *Cancer Res.,* **36**, 4130 (1976).

88. I. Singh, K. Y. Tsang, and W. S. Blakemore, Serologic analysis of tumor-associated surface antigens on human osteosarcoma cells. In S. A. Rosenberg, Ed., *Serologic Analysis of Human Cancer Antigens,* Academic, New York, 1980, p. 161.

89. D. L. Morton and R. A. Malmgren, Human osteosarcomas: Immunologic evidence suggesting an associated infectious agent. *Science,* **163**, 1279 (1968).

90. D. L. Morton, R. A. Malmgren, W. T. Hall, and G. Schidlovsky, Immunologic and virus studies with human sarcomas. *Surgery,* **66**, 152 (1969).

91. F. R. Eilber and D. L. Morton, Sarcoma-specific antigens: Detection by complement fixation with serum from sarcoma patients. *J. Natl. Cancer Inst.,* **44**, 651 (1970).

92. V. S. Byers, A. S. Levin, J. O. Johnston, and A. J. Hackett, Quantitative immunofluorescence studies of the tumor antigen-bearing cell in giant cell tumor of bone and osteogenic sarcoma. *Cancer Res.,* **35**, 2520 (1975).

93. G. Giraldo, E. Beth, Y. Hirshaut, T. Aoki, L. J. Old, E. A. Boyse, and H. C. Chopra, Human sarcomas in culture. Foci of altered cells and a common antigen; Induction of foci and antigen in human fibroblast cultures by filtrates. *J. Exp. Med.,* **133**, 454 (1971).

94. Y. Hirshaut, D. T. Pel, R. C. Marcove, B. Mukherji, A. R. Spielvogel, and E. Essner, Seroepidemiology of human sarcoma antigen (S_1). *New Engl. J. Med.,* **291**, 1103 (1974).

95. M. Moore, P. J. Witherow, C. H. G. Price, and S. A. Clough, Detection by immunofluores-cence of intracytoplasmic antigens in cell lines derived from human sarcomas. *Internatl. J. Cancer,* **12**, 428 (1973).

96. Y. Hirshaut, J. K. Sethi, and C. Feit, Human sarcoma antigens provoking patient immune responses. In S. A. Rosenberg, Ed., *Serologic Analysis of Human Cancer Antigens,* Aca-demic, New York, 1980, p. 123.

97. B. Mukherji and Y. Hirshaut, Evidence for fetal antigen in human sarcoma. *Science,* **181**, 440 (1973).

98. E. S. Priori, J. R. Wilbur, and L. Dmochowski, Immunofluorescence tests on sera of patients with osteogenic sarcoma. *J. Natl. Cancer Inst.,* **46**, 1299 (1971).

99. J. Sethi and Y. Hirshaut, Complement-fixing antigen of human sarcomas. *J. Natl. Cancer Inst.,* **57**, 489 (1976).

100. J. K. Sethi and Y. Hirshaut, Variation in expression of S_3 antigen in human sarcoma cell lines: Influence of passages and medium on generation of S_3. *Eur. J. Cancer,* **14**, 1229 (1978).

101. P. L. Kornblith, F. C. Dohan, Jr., W. C. Wood, and B. O. Whitman, Human astrocytoma: Serum-mediated immunologic response. *Cancer,* **33**, 1512 (1974).

102. W. C. Wood, P. L. Kornblith, E. A. Quindlen, and L. A. Pollock, Detection of humoral immune response to human brain tumors. *Cancer,* **43**, 86 (1979).

103. P. L. Kornblith, L. A. Pollock, H. B. Coakham, E. A. Quindlen, and W. C. Wood, Cyto-toxic antibody responses in astrocytoma patients. An improved allogeneic assay. *J. Neuro-surg.,* **51**, 47 (1979).

104. M. A. Khalid, L. J. Michael, K. Apuzzo, R. Kochsiek, and M. H. Weiss, Malignant glial neoplasms: Definition of a humoral host response to tumor-associated antigen(s). *Yale J. Biol. Med.,* **50**, 397 (1977).

105. M. Pfreundschuh, H. Shiku, T. Takahashi, R. Ueda, J. Ransohoff, H. F. Oettgen, and L. J. Old, Serological analysis of cell surface antigens of malignant human brain tumors. *Proc. Natl. Acad. Sci.,* **75**, 5122 (1978).

106. H. Coakman and P. L. Kornblith, Serologic analysis of solid tumor antigens: Immune adherence studies on human gliomas. In S. A. Rosenberg, Ed., *Serologic Analysis of Human Cancer Antigens,* Academic, New York, 1980, p. 65.

107. T. Wahlstrom, E. Linder, E. Saksela, and B. Westermark, Tumor-specific membrane antigens in established cell lines from gliomas. *Cancer,* **34**, 274 (1974).

108. C. J. Wikstrand and D. D. Bigner, Surface antigens of human glioma cells shared with normal adult and fetal brain. *Cancer Res.,* **39**, 3235 (1979).

109. H. Coakham, Surface antigen(s) common to human astrocytoma cells. *Nature,* **250**, 328 (1974).

110. H. B. Coakham and M. S. Lakshmi, Tumour-associated surface antigen(s) in human astrocytomas. *Oncology,* **31**, 233 (1975).

111. R. H. Kennett and F. Gilbert, Hybrid myelomas producing antibodies against a human neuroblastoma antigen present on fetal brain. *Science,* **203**, 1120 (1979).

112. E. Miyake and K. Kitamura, An attempt to detect cell surface antigens in cultured human brain tumors by mixed hemadsorption test. *Acta Neuropathol.,* **37**, 27 (1977).

113. C. E. Bell, Jr., S. Seetharam, and R. C. McDaniel, Endodermally-derived and neural crest-derived differentiation antigens expressed by a human lung tumor. *J. Immunol.,* **116**, 1236 (1976).

114. C. E. Bell, Jr. and S. Seetharam, Identification of the Schwann cell as a peripheral nervous system cell possessing a differentiation antigen expressed by a human lung tumor. *J. Im-munol.,* **118**, 826 (1977).

115. C. E. Bell, Jr. and S. Seetharam, Expression of endodermally derived and neural crest-derived differentiation antigens by human lung and colon tumors. *Cancer,* **44**, 13 (1979).

116. C. E. Bell, Jr. and S. Seetharam, A plasma membrane antigen highly-associated with oat-cell carcinoma of the lung and undetectable in normal adult tissue. *Internatl. J. Cancer,* **18**, 605 (1976).

117. J. A. Braatz, K. R. McIntire, G. L. Princler, K. H. Kortright, and R. B. Herberman, Purification and characterization of a human lung tumor-associated antigen. *J. Natl. Cancer Inst.,* **61**, 1035 (1978).

118. S. A. Gaffar, J. A. Braatz, K. H. Kortright, G. L. Princler, and K. R. McIntire, Further studies on a human lung tumor-associated antigen. Comparison of antigens from different tumors. *J. Biol. Chem.,* **254**, 2097 (1979).

119. K. R. McIntire, J. A. Braatz, S. A. Gaffar, G. L. Princler, and K. H. Kortright, Development of a radioimmunoassay for a lung tumor associated antigen. In F. G. Lehmann, Ed., *Carcino-Embryonic Proteins,* Vol. 2, Elsevier, New York, 1979, p. 533.

120. J. A. Braatz, S. A. Gaffar, G. L. Princler, and K. R. McIntire, Description of a human lung tumor associated antigen. In S. A. Rosenberg, Ed., *Serologic Analysis of Human Cancer Antigens,* Academic, New York, 1980, p. 181.

121. R. W. Veltri, H. F. Mengoli, P. E. Maxim, S. Westfall, J. M. Gopo, C. W. Huang, and P. M. Sprinkle, Isolation and identification of human lung tumor-associated antigens. *Cancer Res.,* **37**, 1313 (1977).

122. R. W. Veltri, P. E. Maxim, and J. M. Boehlecke, Tumor associated membrane antigens (TAMA) isolated from human squamous cell carcinoma of the lung. In S. A. Rosenberg, Ed., *Serologic Analysis of Cancer Tumor Antigens,* Academic, New York, 1980, p. 211.

123. M. Bhattacharya and J. J. Barlow, Immunologic studies of human serous cystadenocarcinoma of ovary. *Cancer,* **31**, 588 (1973).

124. M. Bhattacharya and J. J. Barlow, Tumor-associated antigen for cystadenocarcinomas of the ovary. *Natl. Cancer Inst. Monogr.,* **42**, 25 (1975).

125. M. Bhattacharya and J. J. Barlow, Ovarian tumor antigens. *Cancer,* **42**, 1616 (1978).

126. M. Bhattacharya and J. J. Barlow, Tumor-specific antigens associated with human ovarian cystadeno-carinoma. In H. Waters, Ed., *The Handbook of Cancer Immunology,* Vol. 4, Garland STPM Press, New York, 1978, p. 277.

127. N. Imamura, T. Takahashi, K. O. Lloyd, J. L. Lewis, Jr., and L. J. Old, Analysis of human ovarian tumor antigens using heterologous antisera: Detection of new antigenic systems. *Internatl. J. Cancer,* **21**, 570 (1978).

128. K. O. Lloyd, Human ovarian tumor antigens. In S. A. Rosenberg, Ed., *Serologic Analysis of Human Cancer Antigens,* Academic, New York, 1980, p. 515.

129. J. P. Leung, E. F. Plow, R. M. Nakamura, and T. S. Edgington, A glycoprotein set specifically associated with the surface and cytosol of human breast carcinoma cells. *J. Immunol.,* **121**, 1287 (1978).

130. J. P. Leung, G. M. Bordin, R. M. Nakamura, D. H. DeHeer, and T. S. Edgington, Frequency of association of mammary tumor glycoprotein antigen and other markers with human breast tumors. *Cancer Res.,* **39**, 2057 (1979).

131. N. S. Yang, C. M. McGrath, and P. Furmanski, Presence of a mouse mammary tumor virus-related antigen in human breast carcinoma cells and its absence from normal mammary epithelial cells. *J. Natl. Cancer Inst.,* **61**, 1205 (1978).

132. R. M. Tejada, I. Keydar, M. Ramanarayanan, T. Ohno, C. Fenoglio, and S. Spiegelman, Detection in human breast carcinomas of an antigen immunologically related to a group-specific antigen of mouse mammary tumor virus. *Proc. Natl. Acad. Sci.,* **75**, 1529 (1978).

133. R. Ueda, H. Shiku, M. Pfreundschuh, T. Takahashi, L. T. C. Li, W. F. Whitmore, H. F. Oettgen, and L. J. Old, Cell surface antigens of human renal cancer defined by autologous typing. *J. Exp. Med.,* **150**, 564 (1979).

134. M. Waghe and S. Kumar, Demonstration of a Wilms' tumour associated antigen using xenogeneic antiserum. *Eur. J. Cancer,* **13**, 993 (1977).

135. T. Ghose, P. Belitsky, J. Tal, and D. T. Janlgan, Production and characterization of xeno-geneic antisera to a human renal cell carcinoma-associated antigen. *J. Natl. Cancer Inst.,* **63**, 301 (1979).

136. S. Okada, K. Itaya, and Y. Kurata, Identification of a tumor-specific antigen in the in-soluble fraction of human nephroblastoma. *Eur. J. Cancer,* **15**, 1085 (1979).

137. M. Herlyn, Z. Steplewski, D. Herlyn, and H. Koprowski, Colorectal carcinoma-specific antigen: Detection by means of monoclonal antibodies. *Proc. Natl. Acad. Sci.,* **76**, 1438 (1979).

138. K. E. Hellström, I. Hellström, and J. T. Nepom, Specific blocking factors—are they im-portant? *Biochim. Biophys. Acta,* **473**, 121 (1977).

2

Tumor Immunity and Escape Mechanisms in Humans

HOWARD OZER
Department of Medical Oncology
Roswell Park Memorial Institute
Buffalo, New York

1. INTRODUCTION

As discussed in several chapters throughout this book, an enormous effort has already been invested in the search for tumor-specific antigens, initially in animal and subsequently in human systems. The future commitment to this search in terms of funding and the numbers of investigators involved is, in addition, rapidly increasing. The logarithmic growth of this field reflects the confidence of the scientific community not only that such antigenic specificities associated with most human tumors do exist, but also that tumor immunity can be enhanced or manipulated in ways that will ultimately provide therapeutic benefits. The existence of tumor associated antigens per se does not mean, however, that these antigens will invariably elicit an effective antitumor immune response. Although an immunosurveillance mechanism directed against such antigens may indeed be responsible for the elimination of transformed tumor cells in most normal individuals, the basis for immunosurveillance remains essentially hypothetical. The observation that immunosuppressed patients develop certain tumors at an increased incidence and rate has been cited as confirmation of the theory of immunosurveillance (1). Nonetheless, it is also apparent that tumors grow successfully in individuals without detectable abnormalities of their immune system and in some in whom tumor-specific immunity can be demonstrated. The mechanisms by which tumors may "escape" or evade immune destruction remain imperfectly understood, although the tumor-host relationship clearly bears directly on the fundamentals of immunoregulation of syngeneic determinants or "self" in both cell-mediated and humoral responses.

The concept that immunosurveillance protects against tumor cell transformation that occurs constantly and at high frequency was first suggested by Ehrlich in 1909 (2). With the demonstration that chemically induced tumors were strongly antigenic in the autologous host (3–6), it became obvious that certain tumors carried tumor-specific, or at least tumor-associated, antigens. It was Thomas (7), however, who first suggested that the ability to reject skin allografts was in fact a reflection of an immunosurveillance mechanism directed against neoplastic cells, one that had actually evolved in vertebrate systems to deal with incipient tumor cell transformation. The theory and eponym of "immunosurveillance" was subsequently put forth by Burnet (8), and an impressive array of evidence was marshaled in its support (7–9). It is, therefore, not surprising that immunosurveillance was unquestionably accepted by most oncologists as the primary line of defense against tumorigenesis in humans. During the last decade, however, emerging evidence on the biological mechanisms of immunoregulation and the recognition that tumor cell populations retain both heterogeneity and the ability to interact with the host's immunological response to their proliferation have undermined the immunosurveillance theory to such an extent that it is currently being reinterpreted and heavily criticized (10–13).

Nevertheless, as is discussed in Chapter 1, it is clear that both tumor-specific and tumor-associated antigens can be demonstrated for many human tumors and probably will be identified for virtually all tumors that are adequately studied. Some of these antigens are highly immunogenic in autochthonous hosts, and others could potentially be modified to elicit cellular and/or humoral immunity *in vivo*. Even in the unlikely event that specific immunity could not be induced for some tumor antigens, the advent of monoclonal antibody technology (see Chapter 9) and particularly the recent development of human hybridomas offers immuno-oncologists the potential for inducing immunity *in vitro* and passively transferring antibody or even cytotoxic T-cell hybrids specific for an individual tumor. The purpose of this chapter is to examine the means by which human tumors have been shown to interact with their host's immunoregulatory responses and may thereby escape destruction.

2. AVOIDANCE OF IMMUNE REJECTION BY "SNEAKING THROUGH"

The simplest way to avoid punishment is to avoid capture. This is the basic premise behind the concept of "sneaking through" as originally proposed by Old and his colleagues (14). This postulate argues that tumors that are weakly immunogenic (such as naturally occurring human cancers) cannot be recognized as "foreign" (i.e., alien to the host system) until the tumor load is too great for the host immune system to mount an effective response. In actuality, the dose response curve for chemically induced murine sarcomas transplanted into syngeneic recipients is biphasic: a very low or a very high cell inoculum will produce growth, whereas intermediate doses do not result in tumor engraftment (14). This phenomenon has been ascribed to a "failure" of the immune system to recognize very small numbers of tumor cells in a manner analogous to low-zone tolerance induction, whereas very large tumor cell inocula may saturate the immunologic response through a mechanism similar to the induction of high-zone tolerance. Although this theory is attractive and frequently quoted as a viable mechanism of tumor escape from surveillance, it contains a number of inherent difficulties. The primary difficulty is that "sneaking through" can be demonstrated with only a few experimental tumors, the best examples of which are chemically induced sarcomas and lymphomas, although it has been demonstrated with some solid tumors as well. (19).

The argument that incipient weakly antigenic tumors can avoid immune destruction by simply escaping detection in their early stages of growth has been cited in support of the theory of immunosurveillance, since immunosuppressed patients have an increased incidence of tumorigenesis. It is argued, for example, that the very high incidence of neoplasia in renal transplant patients is a result of the immunosuppressive therapy that reduces their normal immunosurveillance mechanisms (16,17). However, if this were the case, one would expect an increase in the incidence of a wide variety of tumors. In fact, the majority of the tumors have been of epithelial origin, whereas the remainder have been reticulum cell sarcomas and other lymphomas. It is now clear that at least a proportion of these tumors can be ascribed to the direct carcinogenic effects of azathioprine, cyclophosphamide, x-irradiation, and perhaps steroids as well (18) and that more secondary malignancies are likely to occur as renal and other transplant recipients enjoy increasingly longer survival. But what of the similar association of leukemias and lymphomas in patients with immunodeficiency diseases (19–22) who are not routinely exposed to known carcinogenic therapy? Again, the representation of reticulum cell sarcomas in these patients is abnormally high (19), as it is in congenitally athymic nude mice (20). Since those tumors are of B-cell origin (21), Schwartz (22) has argued that the lymphomas and leukemias associated with immunodeficiency might result not from weakened immunosurveillance permitting transformed tumor cells to escape detection, but rather from an immunoregulatory abnormality in an already pathologically disturbed immunologic circuit. Thus the phenomenon of "sneaking through" would represent not a failure of immunologic recognition, but rather an interaction between tumor cells and immunologically competent lymphocytes that results in a shutdown of the cytotoxic response. This interpretation was originally provided by Prehn and Lappé (23–25), who suggested that low doses of tumor cells stimulated a weak immunologic response that promotes tumor growth. Naor (15) has pointed to the possible involvement of suppression in potentiating nascent tumor growth by suggesting that small tumor inocula or weak tumor antigens might preferentially activate suppressor cells that restrict the antitumor immune response and thereby enhance tumor progression.

Therefore, the process by which tumor cells initially escape immunologic control mechanisms is more complicated than a failure of the host immune system to recognize weak tumor antigens. It is now clear from a large body of experimental evidence that the most critical of these factors concern the host's immunoregulatory circuit. Successful evasion by neoplastic cells of immunologic destruction is almost certainly not the result of passively "sneaking through" but rather results from abberations in immune regulatory mechanisms as they attempt to define and eliminate nascent tumor development.

3. EVIDENCE OF HUMAN TUMOR IMMUNITY

If the host's immunologic system is fully capable of recognizing autochthonous tumor growth as foreign, why, then, is the tumor allowed to grow successfully rather than being rejected? This paradox has become the focal point for research in human tumor immunology since the demonstration in the 1960s that autologous tumor cells could be rejected when inoculated subcutaneously in small doses but would form nodules when injected in higher dosages (26–29). In Winn-type neutralization assays, autologous leukocytes inhibited nodule formation in about 50% of patients, whereas normal control leukocytes were unable to do so (27,29). Although specificity and clinical correlation could not be established because of inadequate controls, these results may represent an equivalent finding in human systems to that of "concomitant immunity" to animal tumors. In the latter situation animals with a large primary tumor mass are protected from artificial metastases introduced by the intravenous route (30,31). Concomitant immunity has been convincingly demonstrated to be mediated by sensitized T cells rather than by antibody (32–34) and thus can be abrogated by treatment with antilymphocyte globulin (35). In addition, the persistence of concomitant immunity is evidently critically dependent on the presence of a large primary tumor mass (36,34) since it rapidly declines following removal of the primary lesion.

Delayed skin reactions to intradermally inoculated antigens prepared from autologous tumors have more recently been employed to demonstrate immunity *in vivo*. Delayed skin reactions to extracts of a variety of human tumors have been described. In early experiments with crude extracts, positive reactions were observed in a minority of patients with certain tumors, although neither specificity nor correlation with clinical status could be established (37–39). Subsequent studies have demonstrated characteristic histologic findings in reactions to autologous extracts (40), and a clinical correlation between positive reactions and remission duration has been described in patients with Burkitt's lymphoma receiving autologous tumor extracts (41,42).

The major problem with skin testing to autologous tumors is to design adequate controls that exclude nonspecific reactivity to contaminants, bacterial products, or excess foreign protein. As pointed out in a review on lymphocyte-mediated cytotoxicity by the Hellströms (46), the only appropriate controls that can be performed are in those few patients with two different types of tumor in whom extracts of each neoplasm can be administered to the same individual. Moreover, clinical correlations such as those published in Burkitt's lymphoma (41) and malignant melanoma (43,44) are much needed. Finally, correlation between observed skin reactions *in vivo* with determinations of specific reactivity *in vitro,* preferably in the T-cell-mediated ^{51}Cr-release-type assay, must be established to confirm the validity of skin testing in any tumor system.

Although an enormous body of evidence has now been accumulated in a variety of *in vitro* assays attempting to demonstrate tumor-specific recognition and cytolysis or inhibition, the *in vitro,* like the *in vivo,* data are fraught with problems of specificity, appropriate controls, and correlation with clinical status (see references 45–47 for detailed reviews). In most of these studies allogeneic lymphocytes from patients with the same histologic tumor type gave positive reactions, whereas controls consisting of cell lines from different tumors or freshly harvested tumor cells did not. Unfortunately, many of the target cells or cell lines examined were incompletely characterized, and specificity of the reactions was thus uncertain. In addition, a number of investigators have reported positive *in vitro* reactivity by lymphocytes isolated from patients with different tumors as well as some normal individuals. This "nonspecific reactivity" by control lymphocytes has been estimated at approximately 15% of normal individuals examined (46), although Takasugi et al. (48) have found that up to 90% of normal donors' lymphocytes may react with either short-term or established tumor cell lines.

The majority of these *in vitro* recognition assays have employed mixed lymphocyte-tumor cell cultures in which responder lymphocytes are obtained from patients in chemotherapy-induced remissions, and the autologous tumor cells or cell lines are irradiated and used as stimulators. Because these mixed tumor and lymphocyte cultures measure only the afferent or recognition arm of the immune response, they do not directly address the issue of whether the host is capable of subsequently responding to autochthonous tumor cells with an effector arm in the form of cytotoxic T lymphocytes (CTL). Since cellular T-cell-mediated immunity may be critical in effective tumor rejection, the steps between immune recognition and the generation of specific CTL are those that must be subverted by a successfully growing tumor. The best *in vitro* assay of specific T-cell-mediated immunity is the ^{51}Cr-release assay. When this assay has been examined in human tumor systems, however, there has not been convincing evidence that specific circulating cytotoxic cells do indeed exist. Cytotoxicity has been demonstrated in only a fraction of patients studied, and in those experiments describing positive results, the degree of cytotoxicity has usually been 10% or less. In addition, no correlations between a positive test and a favorable prognosis have been demonstrated. Zarling et al. have recently provided the best evidence to date that specific CTL can be induced to human leukemia cells (49). Utilizing the fact that a mixed lymphocyte culture (MLC) can enhance the generation of cytotoxic lymphocytes to third-party antigens, they performed "three-way" MLCs by coculturing remission lymphocytes, mitomycin-C-treated allogeneic lymphocytes, and autologous leukemic blast cells from the patients with acute myelogenous leukemia. Cultured lymphocytes were found to be cytotoxic for the autologous leukemic cells. Cytotoxic T lymphocytes were not generated when the allogeneic lymphocytes were omitted or when allogeneic leukemia cells were employed in a standard two-way MLC. Thus this report demonstrates not only that tumor-associated antigens exist, but also that both the recognition arm and the effector CTL arm of the immune response can be generated to them *in vitro*. In a recent modification of this experiment in a murine system, Zarling and her colleagues have demonstrated the generation in three-way MLCs of both CTL and another cytotoxic cell type capable of lysing syngeneic tumor cells (50). This latter cytotoxic cell type is particularly intriguing since it is evidently a non-T natural killer (NK) cell and thus a likely candidate to share the function of causing tumor cytolysis with specific cytotoxic T cells and macrophages.

The evidence for macrophage participation *in vivo* in human tumor immunity remains more substantial than for K or NK cells, however. Several investigators have reported systems in which macrophages are the predominant cytolytic cells *in vitro* and perhaps also *in vivo* (51–53). Both specific cytolysis by armed macrophages and a nonspecific cytotoxic effect of activated macrophages have been described (54). Tumor cell neutralization by immune lymphoid cells has been found to occur less effectively in mice treated with the macrophage toxin silica (54). The evidence for lymphoreticular cell infiltration into tumors *in vivo* and its correlation with more favorable prognosis have been discussed by Underwood (55). In addition, neoplastic cells may have a greater sensitivity than do their normal counterparts to the nonspecific cytotoxic effect of activated macrophages (56). As pointed out in a review by North et al. on mechanisms of macrophage-mediated immunity to tumor cells (13), the *in vivo* interactions of macrophages with other cell types are likely to be complex. Recruitment and arming of Fc receptors with specific antibody may impart specific cytotoxic capability, whereas release of lymphokines may attract and activate macrophages directly within tumors.

In addition to macrophages and T and B cells, "null" lymphoid cells can have cytotoxic effects against tumor cells regardless of whether the targets are coated with specific antibody. The concept of natural cell-mediated cytotoxicity in humans has derived from observations that the peripheral lymphocytes of normal healthy donors as well as those of cancer patients mediate direct cytolysis against a variety of neoplastic and normal cell lines (see reference 57 for review). Until recently, NK activity was thought to be mediated by lymphocytes devoid of detectable cell surface markers (null cells) and thus distinct from activated monocytes or from cells capable of mediating antibody-dependent cellular cytotoxicity (ADCC). More recent studies have demonstrated that human NK cells bear Fc receptors, lack Ia-like determinants in common with K cells (58–60), and cannot be separated from K lymphocytes. It has been suggested that K-NK cytotoxic activities are mediated by the same cell through different mechanisms, thus stressing their potential importance for *in vivo* tumor defense (60). At present the cellular origin of K-NK effector cells remains uncertain, although both T cell (58,61) and monocyte (62) surface markers have been suggested, implicating what may be either a third lymphocyte type or a more primitive differentiation step in the mononuclear cell pathway. The demonstration that K and NK cells are particularly cytotoxic against transformed tumor cells has to a certain extent revived the surveillance concept, particularly in view of the fact that NK cells do not require recognition of determinants coded for by histocompatibility genes and are thus appropriate defenders against sygeneic or authocthonous tumors. Since athymic mice or patients with DiGeorge syndrome are fully competent with respect to NK and K cells, as well as macrophage activity, an explanation is provided for the their relatively unimpaired tumor resistance. It should be emphasized, however, that there are a multitude of tumor defense mechanisms in the intact host, each apparently capable of retarding or preventing tumorigenesis. This redundancy may be critical to successful defense against neoplastic growth. Nevertheless, as described later, the nascent tumor may itself have a variety of redundant systems at its disposal to counteract immune recognition and destruction. Since the relative importance of a particular escape mechanism may vary with different tumors, patients, or clinical stages, it becomes necessary to define the operant escape mechanism(s) to design effective immunotherapy.

4. EVASION OF SPECIFIC TUMOR IMMUNITY

4.1. Masking of Cell-Surface Antigens

The cytotoxic effect of sensitized lymphocytes and macrophages on tumor cells appears to involve two steps: (1) a specific adhesion process and (2) cytolysis of the target cells. One of the simplest concepts of tumor escape from specifically immune lymphocytes was based on the evidence that certain molecules, such as sialomucin, which are frequently bound to the surfaces of tumor cells, are able to mask tumor antigens from complete exposure *in vivo* and also to prevent adhesion of sensitized lymphocytes (63,64). The cell surface sialic acid content varies during the cell cycle (65) with the highest levels in mitotic and transformed blast cells (66). Tumor cells reportedly have an increased negative net surface charge and lower mutual adhesiveness than normal cells (67), although they exhibit an increase in nonspecific stickiness with a tendency to adhere to foreign substances (68). It is conceivable that a partial explanation for the phenomenon of concomitant immunity and the successful escape of metastatic disease from its control might be related to the ability of established bulky tumors to successfully mask their surface antigens whereas metastatic cells might be more likely to expose tumor-specific surface antigens. The enzyme neuraminidase extracted from *Vibrio cholerae* removes sialic acid residues from cell membranes, a procedure that results in increased exposure of other surface determinants and thereby facilitates immunologic recognition. This provided the rationale for the treatment of autochthonous tumor cells with neuraminidase *in vitro* to increase immunogenicity and their subsequent reinfusion to achieve specific immunization (63,69,70) (see also Chapter 14).

Mathe et al. (71) first reported the encouraging results of active specific immunotherapy using allogeneic leukemia cells plus BCG in children with acute lymphoblastic leukemia (71). Since then a number of studies utilizing nonspecific immunotherapy with BCG, MER, or *C. parvum,* active specific immunotherapy with autologous or allogenic tumor cells plus or minus BCG, or passive specific immunotherapy with "immune" RNA or transfer factor in a variety of neoplastic disease in humans have been reported. Holland and Bekesi (72) have also reported early encouraging results using active specific immunotherapy with neuraminidase-treated myeloid leukemic cells in patients with acute myeloblastic leukemia, and additional positive results have been reported in bronchogenic carcinoma (73). Success with the use of any of these maneuvers has, however, not been reproducible, and they have yet to become acceptable adjuncts to chemotherapy.

4.2. Shedding of Tumor Antigens

The failure to elicit an immune response to a tumor in an immunologically competent host may result from the induction of tolerance to tumor-specific antigens through either a high- (large tumors) or low-zone (metastases or nascent tumors) mechanism. Acquisition of tolerance renders normally antigen-reactive T and B cells insensitive to the appropriate activation signals by either altering the cells' reactivity to antigen, saturating antigen receptors on the cell surface with antigen of low immunogenicity and thus preventing stimulation of the cell by highly immunogenic antigen, or the elimination of specifically reactive clones through direct antigen contact (74). Polymeric, highly immunogenic antigens in high doses may induce tolerance in effector T and B cells, possibly by direct attachment to the cell surface. Soluble, oligovalent, and poorly immunogenic antigens may suppress afferent immune recognition by clonal deletion or activation of specific suppressor T lymphocytes. Antigen-antibody complexes are apparently capable of inducing tolerance in both T and B effector function.

The presence of circulating soluble tumor antigens has been demonstrated in the sera of tumor-bearing animals (76–78) as well as humans (79,80), and the subject has been reviewed by Alexander (81). The mechanism by which shed soluble tumor antigens may interfere with the antitumor response has been investigated in methylcholanthrene-induced fibrosarcomas of the rat by Currie and Alexander (82). Culture supernatants of a highly metastatic, non-immunogenic fibrosarcoma strain were shown to neutralize specific cytotoxicity by draining lymph node cells, whereas a highly immunogenic, poorly metastatic strain had no neutralizing activity in culture supernatants, thus indicating an absence of spontaneously shed tumor antigens. The biological role of shed tumor antigens proposed by Currie and Alexander was to assist metastatic spread of the tumor by saturation of the effector limb of T-cell-mediated immunity in the tumor microenvironment (82). Because such antigens may be shed into the circulation in large quantities from large progressive primary tumors, Baldwin et al. (83) have suggested that antigen-antibody complexes within a large tumor would paralyze the localized effector response by swamping cytotoxic lymphocytes with specific tumor antigen. Similar results have been demonstrated *in vitro* with sensitized lymphocytes from patients with colon carcinoma. Cytotoxicity by these lymphocytes was specifically inhibited following incubation with tumor membrane preparations, thus suggesting that cell-mediated immunity was similarly inhibited *in vivo* by circulating antigen (84).

An explanation for tumor escape based on the trapping of localized immunocompetent cells within tumor draining lymph nodes has been discussed by Hawrylko (85). Rapid antigen release by poorly immunogenic tumors may occur during their early stages of growth, resulting in the development of large numbers of specifically reactive cells within draining nodes, a small proportion of which may circulate in the peripheral blood. The continued localized exposure to high doses of tumor antigens, however, results in saturation of specifically reactive cell receptors, tolerance of the localized immune response, and homing of circulating immunocompetent cells to the medulla of the draining node (86). Such "lymph node paralysis" could then persist while distant nodes and circulating cells responded normally to other antigens. Following excision of the primary tumor, the percentage of specific immunoblasts in the thoracic duct lymph can increase within one day (86). As pointed out by Hawrylko (85), the difficulty with this proposition is the demonstration, particularly in human systems, that large numbers of specific cytotoxic lymphocytes *can* be demonstrated in the peripheral circulation of patients with advanced tumors (46). As discussed earlier, however, controversy remains regarding the correlation of circulating cytotoxic cells with clinical stage or metastatic spread (87–90).

The potential inhibitory role of circulating tumor antigen on effector function of cytotoxic lymphocytes has been suggested by Currie and collaborators for patients with malignant melanoma (91–93). Only 15% of melanoma patients in their series had circulating lymphocytes with demonstrable cytotoxicity, and the presence of these lymphocytes was correlated with minimal tumor burden (93). The proportion of reactive cell populations was shown to be increased, however, simply by repeated washing (92). In a series of 14 patients only three had lymphocytes cytotoxic for their autologous tumor cells prior to washing, whereas all 14 cell populations were cytotoxic following extensive washing (91). Cells from patients that required extensive washing to demonstrate cytotoxic activity were readily inhibited by the addition of autologous serum; those that expressed cytotoxicity without washing were not inhibited in the presence of autologous serum (92). The inhibitory activity of the autologous sera on lymphocyte cytotoxicity was also shown to correlate with the patients' clinical stage.

4.3. Blocking Factors in Tumor Enhancement

Despite the many descriptions of antigen shedding in animal and human tumor systems, it is far more likely that the role that shed antigens play in enhancing tumor growth is due to interaction with host-produced specific immunoglobulin to form antigen-antibody complexes. Factors produced in the serum of tumor-bearing hosts that can passively block cytotoxic activity by autologous immunocompetent cells have been known for many years. Kaliss (94) initially interpreted enhancement as a physiologic adaption of the tumor induced by its interaction with antiserum that rendered it more resistant to the host immune response. The mechanism of blocking activity has been extensively studied and is the subject of a number of excellent reviews (46,47,75,85,95,96). The original concept that antibody could abrogate the cytotoxic effects of lymphocytes by binding to tumor cell surfaces was based on studies that showed that blocking activity could be absorbed by incubation with suspensions of target cells, separated with 7S globulin fractions by chromatography, and could be inhibited by antibody to IgG (97). The observation that blocking activity in serum decayed within 72 hours of surgical tumor removal, however, suggested that blocking could not be due purely to specific immunoglobulin (98). It is now known that blocking activity is not demonstrable with sera from animals bearing regressing tumors, and these sera may even counteract the protective influence of blocking sera (99,100). The rapid decay and neutralization of blocking activity by sera from animals, called "unblocking factors," suggested that the effect was due to antigen-antibody complexes. The most likely interpretation, therefore, is that blocking activity is caused by soluble tumor antigens (101) and/or antigen-antibody complexes shed into the circulation (46,83,102,

103) and that "unblocking" regressor sera represent a shift on the binding curve from antigen to antibody excess as a consequence of tumor decline (64).

A variety of mechanisms have been proposed whereby specific antibody or antigen-antibody complexes may inhibit the host immune response resulting in tumor enhancement. Kaliss has categorized these theories into central and peripheral inhibition to describe the probable step in lymphoid cell differentiation at which the feedback inhibition might occur (104). Peripheral inhibition could result from an efferent blockade in which the host develops both cellular and humoral immunity to autochthonous tumor antigens, but immunocompetent cells and cytolytic antibodies are ineffective because antigenic tumor sites are saturated with noncytolytic antibody (75,105,106). Alternatively, peripheral inhibition might result from afferent enhancement in which antibodies bound to tumor cells decrease immunogenicity, presumably by antigen sequestration. A classical example of afferent enhancement was described by Snell et al. (107), who showed that lymph nodes draining the site of a grafted tumor were less reactive to the tumor if the mice were injected with immune serum prepared against the tumor prior to tumor transplantation. In central enhancement it is presumed that antibody or antigen-antibody complexes act directly on the differentiation or proliferation of immunocompetent cells (108–110). Most investigators agree that an antibody must combine with a specific tumor antigen before inhibition of differentiation or cytolysis can occur (102).

Because blocking and enhancement phenomena are difficult to examine *in vivo* in human systems, the *in vitro* effects on a wide variety of cellular assays have received the most attention (46,47). Most of the studies have been performed with the colony inhibition or ^{51}Cr-release assays in which the autologous tumor targets are pretreated with sera and cocultured with lymphocytes. Blocking activity has been described in the sera of patients with several types of tumors (111–116). Antibodies that block in vitro assays for cell-mediated immunity have also been found to be associated with and can be eluted from resected tumors (102). In the study by Sjögren et al. (102), these resected tumors were shown to contain both low- and high-molecular-weight fractions that individually failed to block cytotoxicity by patients' lymphocytes but were effective when recombined in a 1:1 ratio. In assays in which each fraction was added separately to tumor cells, treatment with the low-molecular-weight fraction followed by the high-molecular-weight one failed to inhibit cytotoxicity. If the sequence was reversed, blocking occurred. Therefore, the high- and low-molecular-weight fractions were interpreted as containing specific antibody and tumor antigen, respectively. These data may be analogous to the demonstration that eluates of Burkitt lymphoma cells at a low pH have been shown to contain IgG with specificity for the surface antigens of Burkitt cells (117).

A similar correlation with *in vivo* activity was suggested by the results obtained by Vánky et al. (118) using the lymphocyte blast transformation assay. A blocking effect with sera from patients with sarcomas was demonstrated for autologous tumor cells. The specificity of the inhibitory effect was demonstrated by testing the effects of a large number of allogeneic sera, in addition to autologous sera taken at different time points in the clinical course (119). Thirty-seven of 46 autologous sera and 25 of 40 allogeneic sera from patients with similar tumors had inhibitory effects. In contrast, only 3 of 17 sera from allogeneic patients with unrelated tumors and 7 of 45 sera from normal individuals had inhibitory effects. In several instances, a correlation was noted between the blocking activity and the clinical course. Fresh tumor biopsies taken directly from the patients did not stimulate lymphocyte transformation, whereas stimulation was seen after incubation of the biopsy cells at pH 3.1 so as to elute blocking factors; addition of the eluates blocked lymphocyte transformation (119,120). These findings suggested that blocking factors demonstrated *in vitro* were bound to specific tumors *in vivo*.

The studies by the Hellströms and their collaborators also represent an attempt to directly relate observations in *in vitro* assays to *in vivo* tumor growth in humans (46,121,122). Lymphocytes from patients with surgically excised, localized melanoma were shown to have a strong cytotoxic effect on autochthonous and allogeneic melanoma cells, whereas their sera had no blocking activity. In contrast, sera from patients with widespread metastatic disease were usually found to have blocking activity, and the degree of lymphocyte-mediated cytotoxicity was less than that of the first group. In those patients who subsequently relapsed with metastatic disease, serum blocking activity was frequently found several months prior to clinical evidence of metastases and was eventually noted in all relapsed patients. Patients were also described in whom blocking activity was found to decline in conjunction with surgical removal of small metastatic masses and who then remained in remission; a return of blocking activity was subsequently associated with relapse. One patient whose melanoma underwent spontaneous remission was devoid of serum blocking activity, but his serum was able to potentiate cytotoxicity by the lymphocytes of other patients with melanomas (121,122).

Although these experiments tend to support the contention that blocking and unblocking factors play a significant *in vivo* role in human tumor enhancement, they do not provide direct proof that tumor-specific antigens complexed to antibody mediate such enhancement *in vivo,* or even that this mechanism represents a viable means of tumor escape from immune destruction. Sera obtained at a particular time may contain a variety of antibodies and other serum components, and it is possible that *in vitro* and *in vivo* effects are due to entirely different factors. Moreover, even when clinical and experimental observations have been correlated, the results have not been uniformly positive, indicating either that other mechanisms of enhancement are involved as well as blocking or that the *in vitro* observations are simply artifact related to the presence of circulating antibodies to tumor antigens.

Furthermore, as pointed out by North et al. (13), it is possible that the action of blocking factors may not be expressed systemically, but limited to the site of the primary tumor itself. Otherwise, it would be difficult to explain why the presence of these factors in serum does not inhibit the expression in tumor bearers of high levels of concomitant immunity. For this reason it is difficult to reconcile the evidence for the expression of concomitant immunity with the blocking effects of infusions of relatively small amounts of blocking serum (123). It is not unlikely that the effects of blocking factors observed *in vitro,* rather than being the result of directly inhibiting lymphocyte attachment and cytolysis at the binding site, are due to lymphokines or other factors that have indirect effects on cytotoxicity or blast transformation.

4.4. Antigenic Modulation

Although a direct blockade of cytotoxic lymphocytes resulting from masking of tumor antigen binding sites by noncytolytic antibody *in vivo* remains to be established, another possible mechanism of antibody-mediated escape may involve the complete or partial loss of tumor antigens or the suppression of their expression *in vivo* as a result of antigenic modulation. Antigenic modulation, shedding as antigen-antibody complexes, and internalization of antigenic structures may account for some or even most of the *in vitro* cytotoxicity data previously interpreted as supporting an efferent blocking mechanism in preventing cytotoxicity. The subject of antigenic modulation has been extensively reviewed recently by Stackpole and Jacobson (124), and an attempt is made here only to highlight the major findings supporting a role for modulation in tumor enhancement and in human systems.

In 1963 Old and his colleagues described a cell-surface antigen that was present only on certain mouse leukemias and on thymocytes from some, but not all, mouse strains (125,126). The antigen, designated thymus leukemia (TL) because of this restricted occurrence, was produced in the mouse strain C57Bl/6, a TL−strain, by immunization with mouse leukemia cells. The resulting antiserum was cytotoxic in the presence of guinea pig complement for passaged leukemic cells, but not for C57Bl/6 thymocytes, spleen, lymph node, or bone marrow cells. Two other mouse strains, A and C58, as well as F_1 hybrids of these strains were shown to possess TL antigen exclusively on their thymocytes, whereas spleen, lymph node, bone marrow, and other tissues were negative for TL antigen in these strains (126). The genetic locus for TL determinants was shown to be located on the mouse chromosome 17 and is closely linked with H-2, the murine major histocompatibility locus (127–130). Because of the genetic association and strong immunogenicity of H-2 antigens, TL antisera raised by immunization of TL − mice with TL + thymocytes could be distinguished only when host and donor histocompatibilities were chosen so as to avoid production of antibodies to H-2 as well (126).

When it was initially discovered that TL + leukemias often arise in TL − animals, it was felt that hyperimmunization of these mice with TL + leukemias was an ideal way to immunize against subsequent leukemia transplants. However, when Boyse et al. (131) inoculated the immunized mice with tumor transplants, the leukemic cells grew progressively and killed their hosts despite the continued presence of high levels of cytotoxic TL antibody in their serum. When tumor cells transplanted to immunized mice were removed, they were found to be completely insensitive to the cytotoxic effects of TL antiserum and complement; that is, the TL+ leukemia cells had become TL−. The leukemic cells remained TL− while they were passaged in immunized mice, but the original TL+ phenotype was restored by a single transplant in normal unimmunized mice. The disappearance of TL antigenicity was not accompanied by any decrease in H-2 antigens, indicating that modulation of TL was both specific and reversible (126). Modulation of TL determinants on leukemic cells and thymocytes was also found to be induced in the intact host by passive administration of antiserum, (132) indicating that both leukemic cells and normal lymphcytes will modulate their surface antigens in response to passive immunotherapy with specific antiserum.

Subsequent studies revealed that TL antigenic modulation is completely reversible regardless of whether the cells are treated *in vitro* or *in vivo* (133,134) and that modulation will occur in the absence of complement or with the use of univalent Fab fragments of TL antibody (135). Modulation of TL determinants is a temperature- and energy-dependent process, and pretreating TL+ leukemic cells with actinomycin D or iodoacetamide will prevent modulation, suggesting that it is an active metabolic process requiring protein synthesis (131,134). Taken together, these data proved to be a major milestone in our understanding of the nature of tumor antigens and in the way leukemic cells (and possibly solid tumors) might avoid immune destruction by modulating recognizable surface determinants. The following points need to be emphasized: (1) modulation of TL antigen is clearly not due to the emergence of a resistant subpopulation of leukemic cells (136) since virtually 100% of the inoculated cells are positive and the growth kinetics during and after modulation *in vivo* reflect proliferation by the large majority of inoculated cells; and (2) the *in vitro* data demonstrate that modulation is an adaptive phenotypic change of the leukemic cell membrane rather than a passive blocking or masking of TL antigens (137). As summarized by Stackpole and Jacobsen (124), modulation of TL antigens is now known to be the result of capping, membrane redistribution, and some endocytosis of antigen-antibody complexes (138–140). The inability to detect TL determinants by standard antibody and complement-mediated lysis appears to be the result of antibody-induced lateral displacement of antigen within the fluid cell membrane into "microaggregates" that are resistant to subsequent cytolysis by antibody and complement (124). When more sensitive cytotoxicity, immunofluorescence, or radioimmunoassay techniques are utilized, retention of most of the original quantity of TL surface antigens in a redistributed pattern on the leukemic cell surface can be demonstrated (124,141,142). Thus TL antigenic modulation (as well as modulation of MHC-encoded determinants) is a completely distinct process from immunoglobulin capping on B lymphocytes in which antigen-antibody complexes cap and *completely* disappear from B cell surfaces, resulting in irreversible differentiation of the reactive cells. The loss of immunoglobulin determinants after ligand binding on normal or malignant B cells appears to result in endocytosis and shedding of all detectable immune complexes (143–148).

Although demonstrations of antigenic modulation of other than immunoglobulin determinants on human cells or malignant cell lines have been limited largely to specific viral antigens (149–151), there are several reports of antibody-induced antigenic suppression that are likely to prove to be due to a modulation-type mechanism. Smith et al. (152) have reported that incubation of cell lines derived from Burkitt's lymphoma cells with sera obtained from patients resulted in a marked decrease in detectable tumor-specific cell-surface antigenicity. If the cells were washed, they recovered the ability to specifically bind antibody within two to three cell divisions (12 to 24 hours). This reversible decrease in antigenicity did not occur at 0°C and was blocked at 37°C by antimetabolites (153). Interestingly, another potential example of antigenic modulation in humans may involve myasthenia gravis. The pathophysiology of myasthenia gravis involves depletion of functional acetylcholine receptors at neuromuscular junctions and is thought to involve receptor-specific autoantibody (154,155). *In vitro,* IgG from myasthenic immune serum produces a depletion of acetylcholine receptors with characteristics similar to *in vitro* TL modulation (154).

Although true modulation of human leukemic antigens has yet to be convincingly demonstrated, a potential human equivalent of the murine TL determinant has been described by Levy et al. (156). The antigen is present in high concentration on 100% of both T cell and common acute lymphatic leukemia (ALL) cells as well as on a subpopulation of normal cortical thymocytes, but only in low quantities on spleen, bone marrow, or lymph node cells. This tissue distribution is thus reminiscent of that of murine TL. It is unlike murine TL, however, in that it separates in a higher-molecular-weight region on sodium dodecyl sulfate (SDS)-polyacrylamide gel electrophoresis and is not associated with $\beta 2$ microglobulin in the cell surface as is murine TL (156). Finally, Schlossman and his colleagues have prepared a cytotoxic monoclonal antibody specific for the putative tumor antigen of common non-T acute leukemia (157). When this antibody was passively infused in milligram quantities in a patient with common ALL, the leukemic cell population became antigen negative within 18 hours, and antigenic expression reappeared following completion of the therapy (S. F. Schlossman, personal communication). If true antigenic modulation of common ALL determinants by specific monoclonal antibody can be confirmed *in vitro* and *in vivo,* this escape mechanism might have significant and potentally grave implications for the therapeutic application of monoclonal antibodies to the lymphoblastic malignancies.

It is apparent that antigenic modulation involves antigen shedding, endocytosis, and redistribution within the cell membrane without a complete loss of determinants from the cell surface. Nonetheless, in the classical TL system the end result of modulation is an insensitivity of the leukemic population to cytolysis in the immune host. Whether this is a general phenomenon in human leukemias, lymphomas, or solid tumors and whether it represents a viable immunologic escape option to the growing or metastasizing tumor population requires further investigation.

4.5.   Miscellaneous Mechanisms of Immune Escape

When Kaliss (94) initially interpreted the mechanism of tumor enhancement, he suggested that it was due to a physiological adaption of tumor cells that was induced by a "preenhancement" exposure to antibody before the host immune response was sufficiently strong enough to effect rejection. Although we now suspect that persistent tumor growth occurs as a direct result of tumor cell or antigenic interactions with immunoregulatory components of the host, there are several reports suggesting that tumor cells may undergo physiological or biochemical evolution in the face of immunologic attack. Gorer (158,159) has suggested that specific antibody may result in direct stimulation of mitotic activity in allogeneic tumor systems. Although there have been other reports of tumor growth stimulation by antibody (160), this effect seems to be the result of cytolytic injury accompanied by uncoupling of oxidative phosphorylation followed by a rebound of increased tumor cell division (161). Biochemical mutational changes in the tumor cell population have also been suggested (161,162), although they also may be a result of initial cell insult and have not been related to a tumor-specific immune response. The best evidence of directly enhanced tumor growth in response to antibody has been presented by Shearer and his colleagues (163–167). They demonstrated that, at low doses, either antibody or antibody plus complement will increase nucleoside incorporation and DNA synthesis by murine L cells both *in vitro* and *in vivo*. Increased doses of antibody would then result in cytotoxicity. Tumors themselves may also release factors that act locally in the microenvironment to promote their own growth. Production of lysozomal enzymes that may alter the complement-fixing capacity of specific antibodies has been demonstrated (168). Noncytotoxic antibodies thus produced might then remain able to complex antigen, resulting in efferent blockade. Finally, solid tumors have been shown to produce a ribonucleoprotein of approximately 100,000 molecular weight known as the *tumor angiogenesis factor* (TAF) (169). This mediator is capable of stimulating capillary endothelial cell mitosis, resulting in neovascularization of the growing tumor fraction. Whether it is produced as a result of immunoregulatory mechanisms remains uncertain. As discussed previously, however, there can be no doubt that other immunoregulatory host-tumor cell interactions have profound influences on the growth and metastatic potential of neoplasms.

4.6.   Interaction Between Neoplastic Cells and the Host's Immunoregulatory Apparatus

In contrast to the original concept of the vertebrate immune system as having its primary function in the simple recognition and destruction of bacterial or viral pathogens by production of specific antibody, it is now clear that most of the biological energy of the immune system is invested in self-regulation. These immunoregulatory functions have been found to be quite complex and are not unlike regulation within the endocrine system for the production of its own hormonal products. Thus the products of an effector arm of the immunologic network such as cytotoxic antibody or cytolytic T cells can regulate the entire immune system by feedback inhibition or augmentation of the induction phase of the specific immune response. The ultimate expression of specific immunity, whether to a simple hapten or a transformed and proliferating tumor cell population, is thus the end product of this interplay between positive and negative regulatory interactions. A number of such regulatory signals within the immunological network have been described. Antibody itself may exert feedback control for its own production by binding specific circulating antigen and eliminating its immunogenic stimulus (170). Antigen-antibody complexes may directly block the receptor sites on afferent immunocompetent cells (171) or may induce tolerance of the specific response after binding to afferent or efferent receptors (172). Feedback signals may also be delivered by effector T cells and may stimulate either suppression or activation of the specific cellular response (173). Phagocytic macrophages can exert a dual role both as effector cells and regulatory cells by delivering either activating or suppressor signals to the immunoregulatory network (174). Moreover, each of these feedback signals is itself rigorously controlled in that it may act in a nonspecific fashion (175), may regulate a particular immunoglobulin isotype (176), may exhibit genetic restrictions (177), or may regulate only the idiotype-specific response while having no effect on other antigenic responses (178). It is apparent, then, that the mechanisms by which tumors avoid immune destruction are far more complicated than merely "sneaking through" and must be closely linked to the host's immunoregulatory apparatus with potential interactions involving tumors, specific antibody, recognition and effector lymphocytes, macrophages, and inflammatory factors. Among the most successful escape mechanisms that tumors are known to exhibit is the ability to interact with the regulatory network so as to induce unresponsiveness, both specific and general, and, in turn, to be at least partially regulated by the immune system themselves.

The fact that some cancer patients demonstrate a generalized decrease in cell-mediated immunity has been known for some time. The evidence consists primarily of a depressed ability of tumor bearers to mount delayed skin reactions to recall antigens or of their lymphocytes to respond to mitogens or antigens *in vitro*. In patients with carcinomas, impaired reactivity to recall antigens has been seen primarily in individuals with advanced disseminated disease (179). Such patients may also show impaired reactivity to contact sensitization *de novo* with such agents as dinitrochlorobenzene (DNCB). For patients with malignancies of their cellular immune system, such as leukemias and lymphomas, it has been argued that they demonstrate impaired *in vitro* and *in vivo* cell-mediated immunity even prior to metastatic dissemination or advanced tumor burden (180–182) and that decreased reactivity correlates with prognosis in acute leukemia (182). The importance of immune responsiveness to *de novo* skin sensitization with DNCB in demonstrating a subsequently favorable prognosis for carcinoma patients has been clearly demonstrated (183–185), although again this may be related to tumor burden rather than to a primary immunologic deficit. The best evidence for an early defect in immune responsiveness has been found in Hodgkin's disease (186). Several reports have indicated that circulating, nonspecific suppressor cells may be partially responsible for the *in vivo* hyporesponsiveness associated with this lymphoma (187–189), and it has also been suggested that this suppressor cell activity may be restricted by gene products of the MHC (188,189). There is additional evidence that the sera of tumor bearers may contain soluble factors that nonspecifically inhibit lymphocyte responses both *in vivo* and *in vitro,* and these factors may be of either host or tumor origin (190–192). Prostaglandins, which act pharmacologically as suppressor factors, have been shown to be produced by both tumor cells (193) and host mononuclear suppressor cells in patients with Hodgkin's disease (194).

It should be emphasized, however, that each of these experimental systems lacks specificity. Therefore, it is somewhat difficult to interpret enhanced tumor growth in patients who have excessive nonspecific suppressor activity but, at the same time, may demonstrate specific cytotoxic T cells for the autochthonous tumor *in vitro.* Indeed, Johnson et al. (195–197) have shown that failure to elicit delayed responses to DNCB in cancer patients is more likely the result of an inability to mount inflammatory responses in general, rather than the result of suppressor-cell-mediated immunity. Evidence from a number of investigations in humans has shown that macrophages from tumor bearers may be defective in their ability to respond to chemotactic stimuli *in vitro* (198–200) and *in vivo* (201), although these findings may in fact also be related to tumor-produced suppressive factors (202). Direct support for the role of circulating tumor antigen in suppressing "specific" monocyte function in advanced tumors has been presented by Grosser and Thompson and their colleagues (203–205). They demonstrated that patient monocytes in early disease stages were specifically reactive with their own tumor through cytophilic IgG arming of the monocyte Fc receptors. Nonreactive monocytes from patients with metastatic disease failed to bind cytophilic antibody since the monocytes were coated with antigen and were thus unable to react. Sera from these unreactive advanced cancer patients were specifically inhibitory for monocytes of reactive patients, indicating saturation of cytophilic IgG receptors with soluble tumor antigens. It is thus evident that tumor-induced immunosuppression can be mediated through several mechanisms and may induce immunoregulatory deficits at the afferent or efferent level and probably in each cytotoxic cell population capable of tumor destruction.

The concept that tumors might escape immune destruction as a direct result of the immunoregulatory function of the host's suppressor T cells in response to the tumor presence is a relatively new one (206). Nonetheless, the literature on suppressor T cells and non-T cells is expanding at an enormous rate and the subject in relation to tumor immunity has recently been extensively reviewed (207,208). Evidence for the fine specificity of T-cell responses or for genetic restrictions remain largely confined to animal systems. As mentioned earlier, Hillinger and Herzig (189) have described T cells that nonspecifically inhibited autologous MLC responses to allogeneic cells in the blood of two patients with Hodgkin's disease. Fujimoto et al. have demonstrated that the peripheral blood of patients with osteogenic sarcoma may simultaneously contain both cytotoxic and suppressor T cells (209). Twelve of 28 patients studied demonstrated cytotoxicity by null lymphoid cells *in vitro* for osteogenic sarcoma cells. When lymphocytes from those patients who failed to demonstrate cytotoxicity were fractionated on bovine serum albumin gradients, however, a tumor-specific cytotoxic subpopulation could be isolated in 11 of 13 patients, and a cytotoxic suppressor subset was identified in a different density fraction in 4 of 10 patients. The suppressor subset could inhibit autologous tumor-specific cytolysis, formed E rosettes, and was nylon-adherent (a characteristic of murine suppressor T cells). The presence of suppressor cells in each of the four patients was associated with pulmonary metastases, whereas only one of six patients without suppressor T cells was reported to have metastatic disease. These data appear to resemble those in murine methylcholanthrene-induced sarcomas in which tumor growth has been shown to be promoted by suppressor T cells (209,210).

Impairment of the host's immunoregulatory apparatus is not, however, limited to suppression of cell-mediated immune function or inhibition of inflammatory responses, but, in certain malignancies, can result in profound inhibition of humoral immunity or even of nonlymphoid hematopoiesis. Excessive host suppressor cell activity is thought to be the basis for depression of polyclonal B-cell function and the anemias of spindle-cell thymoma and of multiple myeloma (211–213), whereas the malignant cell population of some T-cell acute leukemias and a subset of patients with the Sézary syndrome may retain their own immunoregulatory function following blast transformation (214–217). Certain patients with thymoma have an associated syndrome consisting of hypogammaglobulinemia, B-cell, and, occasionally, red-cell aplasia (211,218). Waldmann, et al. (211) have shown that the majority of these patients have circulating suppressor T cells that can block the maturation of polyclonal B cells stimulated *in vitro* with pokeweed mitogen. Whether the *in vivo* hypogammaglobulinemia and pancytopenias of spindle-cell thymoma are the direct consequence of these peripheral T suppressor cells or represent an immunoregulatory response in patients with a primary hematopoietic stem cell defect remains unknown.

Multiple myeloma is clinically defined as a malignant plasma cell proliferation resulting in bone marrow replacement, paraprotein production, osteolytic bone lesions, decreased polyclonal immunoglobulin synthesis, and a concomitant increase in susceptibility to certain bacterial pathogens (219–221). The immunodeficiency of myeloma is distinct from that of other malignancies in that both myeloma patients and mice bearing plasmacytomas exhibit impaired primary responses to antigenic challenge whereas secondary responses as well as delayed hypersensitivity are less severely affected (219, 221–225). A variety of hypotheses have been proposed to explain the impaired host polyclonal immunoglobulin synthesis, including alteration of antigen-binding cells by infective RNA subunits from the malignant plasma cells (226), the influence of mitotic inhibitors or chalones that block polyclonal B-cell differentiation (227), and the presence of circulating immunosuppressive factors such as those produced by murine plasmacytoma cells (228). In contrast to studies attributing the depressed humoral responses to an immunosuppressive product of the expanding population of tumor cells, Broder et al. (229) originally suggested the potential abnormality of host immunoregulatory cells. They demonstrated suppressor activity by unfractionated myeloma peripheral leukocytes that was mediated primarily by phagocytic mononuclear cells and not by T lymphocytes. Similar adherent cell suppressor mechanisms have been demonstrated in the murine plasmacytoma model (223,230), and, in addition, an augmenting role for tumor cell factors on macrophage-mediated suppression has been suggested. Knapp and Baumgartner (231), however, demonstrated that adherent cell suppressor activity is present in healthy individuals as well as myeloma patients, suggesting that monocyte-mediated suppression of B-cell differentiation is neither a disease-specific phenomenon nor an explanation of decreased *in vivo* or *in vitro* polyclonal immunoglobulin synthesis in myeloma. Paglieroni and MacKenzie, in contrast, have shown that a significant amount of suppressor activity in myeloma patients is present in a nonadherent null lymphoid subset bearing Fc receptors that does not appear to be thymus derived as defined by the presence of receptors for sheep erythrocytes (232,233). Furthermore, the suppression of differentiation of immunoglobulin-synthesizing cells in multiple myeloma appears distinct from the depressed immunoglobulin secretion seen *in vivo* and *in vitro* with leukemic B-cell populations from patients with chronic lymphocytic leukemia (CLL). In those patients neither B-cell proliferation nor subsequent immunoglobulin secretion occurs, even in the absence of suppressor cells, unless the patients are in remission (234), indicating instead an intrinsic functional deficit of the circulating leukemic B-cell population of all but a minor subset (235) of CLL patients.

The malignant cell populations of some patients with lymphoproliferative malignancies have also been shown to retain immunoregulatory properties leading to profound aberration of the host's immunologic defense mechanisms and thus potentially promoting their own growth. An example of neoplasia of suppressor T cells has been described by Broder et al. (214) in a child with acute lymphoblastic leukemia and hypogammaglobulinemia. Following systemic chemotherapy, this patient's immunoglobulin levels returned to normal in association with clinical remission and declined again during leukemic relapse. The leukemic blast population could suppress normal T-cell-induced B-cell differentiation in the presence of pokeweed mitogen, but only when added to the culture together with normal unirradiated T cells. The suppressor leukemic cells were themselves sensitive to x-irradiation. Broder et al. (214)

have suggested that these data indicate the requirement for T-T interaction in the generation of human suppressor effector cells. Regulatory activity by leukemic cells has also been described by Uchiyama et al. (215), who reported that three of six Japanese patients with adult T-cell leukemia had neoplastic cells with suppressorlike properties. Immunoregulatory neoplastic cellular function is not restricted to suppression of B-cell differentiation, however. The leukemic populations of some, but not all, patients with the Sézary syndrome appear to retain inducerlike function for B-cell differentiation (216,217). In addition, factors produced by some solid tumors may play a role in regulation of host hematopoietic differentiation. Suda et al. (236) recently described a patient with a poorly differentiated squamous cell carcinoma and associated granulocytosis that resolved during chemotherapy. The patient's serum, as well as an extract of his tumor cells, was found to contain a potent colony-stimulating factor capable of promoting macrophage-granulocyte colony growth *in vitro*. The fact that this regulatory factor was produced by the tumor cells *in vivo* has been indicated by the demonstration that the factor is continually produced by the tumor cells following transplantation into nude mice. Moreover, the nude mice bearing this tumor demonstrated overwhelming neutrophilic granulocytosis that could be eliminated by surgical extirpation of the tumor (236). These results strongly suggest that the tumor secreted a colony-stimulating factor with biological activity similar to that produced by PHA-stimulated leukocytes *in vitro* and resulted in granulocytosis in the patient. Although it remains uncertain whether the retention of any of these regulatory functions by neoplastic cells serves to promote their escape from immune destruction, it is apparent that patients with, for example, suppressor T-cell leukemias might fall into a poor prognostic category as a result of an inability to mount immune responses to either the tumor itself or bacterial or viral pathogens (208).

Just as neoplasms may induce host-cell immunoregulatory abnormalities or may retain regulatory properties after transformation, certain lymphoproliferative malignancies have themselves been shown to have both their growth characteristics and their differentiation under host immunoregulatory control. This has been elegantly demonstrated in the murine myeloma model by Lynch and his colleagues (237), who have shown that myeloma cells differentiate during *in vivo* growth and that their growth and differentiation are under strict control by host regulatory T cells in a manner paralleling that of normal B-cell differentiation. Recent evidence in human myeloma also points in this direction: both surface-idiotype-bearing B cells and early B-cell precursors containing cytoplasmic idiotypic immunoglobulin only have been identified in patients with multiple myeloma, indicating several differentiation steps within the malignant cell population of a single individual (238). Evidence for both heterogeneity and differentiation of the malignant cell population *in vivo* and in vitro had also been described for CLL by Fu and his colleagues (239,240). They have shown that CLL cells from some patients can differentiate *in vivo* to plasma cells (239) and that the rate of differentiation can be accelerated *in vitro* by inducer T cells (240). Similar regulation has been demonstrated for other lymphoproliferative malignancies (241,242) as well as for myeloid leukemia cells (243). The fact that the tumor-bearing host can influence the growth and differentiation of lymphoproliferative malignancies is perhaps not surprising in view of the elaborate immunoregulatory apparatus that orchestrates the expansion, contraction, and differentiation of normal B-cell clones (173). Nonetheless, it is clear that the original concept of a tumor population as the monoclonal expansion of monotonously identical cells "frozen" in a single differentiated state is no longer valid. Rather, it is becoming clear that neoplastic cell populations are continuously differentiating *in vivo* and, at least in the lymphoproliferative malignancies, are also capable of both sending and receiving regulatory signals between themselves and nonmalignant immunocompetent cells. This ability to communicate with the host's immune defense network may prevent their identification as "nonself" and lead to an effective escape from immune destruction.

5. CONCLUSION

It is apparent that tumor cell transformation, growth, and proliferation succeed not because the nascent tumor population is secretive or because all neoplasms possess only one overwhelmingly effective escape mechanism. Instead, there is increasing evidence that each transformed cell is interrogated, recognized, and responded to by the host immune system. Those that grow successfully do so because they are themselves able to respond to this immunologic probing, not just at one point on their growth curves, but throughout the entire course. Collectively, and perhaps individually, tumor cell populations have an array of defense mechanisms. Each defense mechanism may operate in the tumor microenvironment, systemically, or both, and some may function simultaneously. Tumor cell antigens shed into the circulation appear to play a critical role in immune escape, probably in the form of antigen-antibody complexes. Although the role of antigen-antibody complexes in blocking effector function of immunocompetent cells has been emphasized in the past, complexes as well as other tumor-produced factors may also act on the afferent arm of the immunoregulatory network to increase suppression of effector function or to block differentiation of cytolytic effectors. Other humoral factors act nonspecifically to impair inflammatory responses, chemotaxis, the complement cascade or to augment angiogenesis within solid tumors. They may be produced by tumor cell populations or by regulatory cells in the presence of immune complexes. Finally, the tumor cell population itself is more protean than had been previously believed. It can differentiate, modulate its surface antigenicity in response to antibody binding, and, in certain cases, regulate host immunologic function and hematopoietic differentiation. The successful application of immunotherapy to neoplastic disease is critically dependent on these immunoregulatory interactions between tumor and host.

As our understanding of the biology of tumor-host interactions improves, our options and opportunities for intervention in the human immunoregulatory apparatus will also improve. Pharmacologic or immunologic manipulation of specific regulatory deficits will provide the future strategies necessary to counter tumor escape mechanisms and to individually tailor therapy for malignant disease.

REFERENCES

1. O. Stutman, Immunodepression and malignancy. I. *Adv. Cancer Res.,* **22**, 261–422 (1975).

2. P. Ehrlich, Über den jetzigen Stand der Karzinom-forschung. In F. Himmelweit, Ed., *The Collected Papers of Paul Ehrlich,* Vol. II, *Immunology and Cancer Research,* Pergamon, New York, 1957, pp. 550–562.

3. L. Gross, Intradermal immunization of C3H mice against a sarcoma that orginated in an animal of the same line. *Cancer Res.,* **3**, 326–333 (1943).

4. R. W. Baldwin, Immunity to methylcholanthrene-induced tumours in inbred rats following atrophy and regression of the implanted tumours. *Brt. J. Cancer,* **9**, 652–657 (1955).

5. R. T. Prehn and J. M. Main, Immunity to methylcholanthrene-induced sarcomas. *J. Natl. Cancer Inst.,* **18**, 769–778 (1957).

6. G. Klein, H. O. Sjögren, E. Klein, and K. E. Hellström, Demonstration of resistance against methylcholanthrene-induced sarcomas in the primary authochthonous host. *Cancer Res.,* **20**, 1561–1572 (1960).

7. L. Thomas, Reactions to homologous tissue antigens in relation to hypersensitivity. In H. S. Lawrence, Ed., *Cellular and Humoral Aspects of the Hypersensitive States,* Hoeber, New York, 1959, pp. 529–532.

8. F. Burnet, The Concept of immunological surveillance. *Progr. Exp. Tumor Res.,* **13**, 1–27 (1970).

9. R. A. Good and T. Finstad, Essential relationship between the lymphoid system, immunity, and malignancy. *Natl. Cancer Inst. Monogr.,* **31**, 41–58 (1969).

10. R. T. Prehn, Immunlogical surveillance: Pro and Con. *Clin. Immunobiol.,* **2**, 191–203 (1974).

11. G. Möller and E. Möller, Considerations of some current concepts of cancer research. *J. Natl. Cancer Inst.,* **55**, 755–759 (1975).

12. R. S. Schwartz, Another look at immunologic surveillance. *New Engl. J. Med.,* **293**, 181–184 (1975).

13. R. J. North, G. L. Spitalny, and D. P. Kirstein, Antitumor defense mechanisms and their subversion. In H. Waters, Ed., *The Handbook of Cancer Immunology,* Garland STPM Press, New York, 1978, pp. 187–224.

14. L. J. Old, E. A. Boyse, D. A. Clarke, and E. Carswell, Antigenic properties of chemically induced tumors. *Ann. N. Y. Acad. Sci.,* **101**, 80–106 (1961).

15. D. Naor, Suppressor Cells: Permitters and promoters of malignancy? *Adv. Cancer Res.,* **29**, 45–125 (1979).

16. I. Penn and T. E. Starzl, Malignant tumors arising *de novo* in immunosuppressed organ transplant recipients. *Transplantation,* **14**, 407–417.

17. R. Hoover and J. F. Fraumeni, Risk of cancer in renal-transplant recipients. *Lancet,* **2**, 55–57 (1973).

18. S. M. Sieber, The action of antitumor agents: a double-edge sword? *Medi. Pediatr. Oncol.,* **3**, 123–131 (1977).

19. C. J. M. Melief and R. S. Schwartz, In F. F. Becker, Ed., *Immunocompetence and Malignancy: A Comprehensive Treatise,* Vol. 1, Plenum, New York, 1975, pp. 121–160.

20. H. C. Outzen, R. P. Custer, G. J. Eaton, and R. T. Prehn, Spontaneous and induced tumor incidence in germ-free "nude" mice. *J. Reticuloendothel. Soc.,* **17**, 1–9 (1975).

21. R. J. Lukes and R. D. Collins, Immunologic characterization of human malignant lymphomas. *Cancer,* **34**, 1488–1503 (1974).

22. R. S. Schwartz, Another look at immunological surveillance. *New Engl. J. Med.,* **293**, 181–184 (1975).

23. R. T. Prehn, Perspectives on oncogenesis; Does immunity stimulate or inhibit neoplasia? *J. Reticuloendothel. Soc.,* **10**, 1–16 (1971).

24. R. T. Prehn and M. A. Lappé, An immunostimulation theory of tumor development. *Transplant. Rev.,* **7**, 26–54 (1971).

25. R. T. Prehn, Tumor progression and homeostasis. *Adv. Cancer Res.,* **23**, 203–233 (1976).

26. C. M. Southam and A. Brunschwig, Quantitative studies of autotransplantation of human cancer. *Cancer,* **14**, 971–978 (1961).

27. A. Brunschwig, C. M. Southam, and A. G. Levin, Host resistance to cancer. Clinical experiments by homotransplants, autotransplants, and admixture of autologous leucocytes. *Ann. Surg.,* **162**, 416 (1965).

28. J. T. Grace, D. Perese, R. S. Metzgar, T. Sasabe, and B. Holdrige, Tumor autograft response in patients with glioblastoma multiforme. *J. Neurosurg.,* **28**, 759 (1961).

29. C. M. Southam, The immunologic states of patients with nonlymphomatous cancer. *Cancer Res.,* **28**, 1433–1440 (1968).

30. L. Milas, M. Hunter, K. Mason, and H. R. Withers, Immunological resistance to pulmonary metastases in C3Hf/BU mice bearing syngeneic fibrosarcoma of different sizes. *Cancer Res.,* **34**, 61–71 (1974).

31. J. M. Yuhas, H. G. Pazimino, and E. Wagner, Development of concomitant immunity in mice bearing the weakly immunogenic line one lung carcinoma. *Cancer Res.,* **35**, 237–241 (1971).

32. R. K. Gershon, R. L. Carter, and J. Kondo, On concomitant immunity in tumor-bearing hamsters. *Nature,* **213**, 674–676 (1967).

33. R. Kearney, A. Basten, and D. S. Nelson, Cellular basis for the immune response to methylcholanthrene-induced tumors in mice. Heterogeneity of effector cells. *Internatl. J. Cancer,* **15**, 438–450 (1975).

34. R. J. North and D. P. Kirstein, T-Cell-mediated concomitant immunity to syngeneic tumors. I. Activated macrophages as expressors of nonspecific immunity to unrelated tumors and bacterial parasites. *J. Exp. Med.,* **145**, 275 (1977).

35. S. E. James and A. J. Salsbury, Facilitation of metastasis by antithymocyte globulin. *Cancer Res.,* **34**, 367–370 (1973).

36. G. Crile and S. D. Deodhar, Role of preoperative irradiation in prolonged concomitant immunity and preventing metastasis in mice. *Cancer,* **27**, 629–634 (1971).

37. L. E. Hughes and B. Lytton, Antigenic properties of human tumours: Delayed cutaneous hypersensitivity reactions. *Brt. Med. J.,* **I**, 209 (1964).

38. T. H. M. Stewart, The presence of delayed hypersensitivity reactions in patients towards cellular extracts of their malignant tumors. 1. The role of tissue antigen, non specific reactions of nuclear material, and bacterial antigen as a cause for this phenomenon. *Cancer,* **23**, 1368 (1969).

39. T. M. Stewart and M. Orizaga, The presence of delayed hypersensitivity reactions in patients toward cellular extracts of their malignant tumors. *Cancer,* **28**, 1472 (1972).

40. M. E. Oren and R. B. Herberman, Delayed cutaneous hypersensitivity reactions to membrane extracts of human tumor cells. *Clin. Exp. Immunol.,* **9**, 45 (1971).

41. L. Fass, R. B. Herberman, and J. Ziegler, Delayed cutaneous hypersensitivity reactions to autologous extracts of Burkitt-lymphoma cells. *New Engl. J. Med.,* **282**, 776 (1970).

42. A. Z. Bluming, J. L. Ziegler, L. Fass, and R. B. Herberman, Delayed cutaneous sensitivity reactions to autologous Burkitt lymphoma protein extract. *Clin. Exp. Immunol.,* **9**, 713 (1971).

43. L. Fass, R. B. Herberman, J. L. Ziegler, and J. W. M. Kiryabwire, Cutaneous hypersensitivity reactions to autologous extracts of malignant melanoma cells. *Lancet,* **I**, 116 (1970).

44. A. Z. Bluming, C. L. Vogel, J. L. Ziegler, and I. W. Kiryabwire, Delayed cutaneous sensitivity reactions to extracts of autologous malignant melanoma: A second look. *J. Natl. Cancer Inst.,* **48**, 17 (1972).

45. R. B. Herberman, M. E. Nunn, D. H. Lavrin, and R. Asofsky, Effect of antibody to theta antigen on cell-mediated immunity induced in syngeneic mice by murine sarcoma virus. *J. Natl. Cancer Inst.,* **51**, 1509 (1973).

46. K. E. Hellström and I. Hellström, Lymphocyte-mediated cytotoxicity and blocking serum activity to tumor antigens. *Adv. Immunol.,* **18**, 209–277 (1974).

47. R. B. Herberman, Cell-mediated immunity to tumor cells. *Adv. Cancer Res.,* **19**, 207–263 (1974).

48. M. Takasugi, M. R. Mickey, and P. I. Terasaki, Reactivity of lymphocytes from normal persons on cultured tumor cells. *Cancer Res.,* **33**, 2898 (1973).

49. J. M. Zarling, P. C. Raich, M. McKeough, and F. H. Bach, Generation of cytotoxic lymphocytes *in vitro* against autologous human leukaemia cells. *Nature,* **262**, 691–693 (1976).

50. F. H. Bach, P. A. Paciucci, S. Macphail, P. M. Sondel, B. J. Alter, and J. M. Zarling, Antitumor cytoxic T cells and non-T-cells generated by allosensitization *in vitro. Transpl. Proc.,* **XII**, 2–7 (1980).

51. M. S. Tosi and R. S. Weiser, Mechanisms of immunity of sarcoma I allografts in the C57B1-Ks mouse. I. Passive transfer studies with immune peritoneal macrophages in x-irradiated hosts. *J. Natl. Cancer Inst.,* **40**, 37 (1968).

52. R. Evans and P. Alexander, Cooperation of immune lymphoid cells with macrophages in tumour immunity. *Nature (Lond.),* **228**, 620 (1970).

53. R. Evans and P. Alexander, Mechanism of immunologically-specific killing of tumour cells by macrophages. *Nature (Lond.),* **236**, 168 (1972).

54. J. M. Zarling and S. S. Tevethia, Transplantation immunity to simian virus 40-transformed cells in tumor-bearing mice. II. Evidence for macrophage participation at the effector level of tumor cell rejection. *J. Natl. Cancer Inst.,* **50**, 149 (1973).

55. J. C. E. Underwood, Lymphoreticular infiltration in humor tumors: Prognostic and biological implications: A review. *Br. J. Cancer,* **30**, 538–547 (1974).

56. J. B. Hibbs, Jr., L. H. Lambert, and J. S. Remington, Possible role of macrophage-mediated nonspecific cytotoxicity in tumour resistance. *Nature New Biol..,* **235**, 48–50 (1972).

57. R. B. Herberman and H. T. Holden, Natural cell-mediated immunity. *Adv. Cancer Res.,* **27**, 309 (1978).

58. W. H. West, C. B. Cannon, H. D. Kay, G. D. Bonnard, and R. B. Herberman, Natural cytotoxic reactivity of human lymphocytes against myeloid cell lines: Characterization of effector cells. *J. Immunol.,* **118**, 355–361 (1977).

59. H. D. Kay, G. D. Bonnard, W. H. West, and R. B. Herberman, A functional comparison of human Fc-receptor-bearing lymphocytes active in natural cytotoxicity and antibody-dependent cellular cytotoxicity. *J. Immunol.,* **118**, 2058–2066 (1977).

60. H. Ozer, A. J. Strelkauskas, R. T. Callery, and S. F. Schlossman, The functional dissection of human peripheral null cells with respect to antibody-dependent cellular cytoxicity and natural killing. *Eur. J. Immunol.,* **9**, 112–118 (1979).

61. E. P. Rieber, J. G. Saal, M. Hadam, H. Rodt Rietmüller, and M. P. Dierich, Effector cells of natural cytotoxicity against human melanoma cells. In G. Rietmuller, P. Wernet, G. Cudkowicz, Eds., *Natural and Induced Cell-Mediated Cytotoxicity,* Academic, New York, 1979, pp. 43–55.

62. E. L. Reinherz, L. Moretta, M. Roper, J. M. Breard, M. C. Mingari, M. D. Cooper, and S. F. Schlossman, Human T lymphocyte subpopulations defined by Fc receptors and mono-clonal antibodies. *J. Exp. Med.,* **151**, 969–974 (1980).

63. B. Sanford, An alteration in tumor histocompatability induced by neuraminidase. *Transplantation,* **5**, 1273 (1967).

64. E. Watkins, Y. Ogata, L. Anderson, and M. Waters, Activation of host lymphocytes cultured with cancer cells treated with neuraminidase. *Nature,* **231**, 83 (1971).

65. C. A. Buck, M. C. Glick, and L. Warren, Glycopeptides from the surface of control and virus-transformed cells. *Science,* **172**, 169 (1971).

66. T. O. Fox, J. R. Sheppard, and M. M. Burger, Cyclic membrane changes in animal cells: Transformed cells permanently display a surface architecture detected in normal cells only during mitosis. *Proc. Natl. Acad. Sci. (USA),* **68**, 244 (1971).

67. D. R. Coman, Mechanism responsible for the origin and distribution of blood-borne tumor metastases. A review. *Cancer Res.,* **13**, 397 (1953).

68. D. R. Coman, Adhesiveness and stickiness. Two independent properties of cell surfaces. *Cancer Res.,* **21**, 1436 (1961).

69. G. A. Currie and K. D. Bagshawe, The role of sialic acid in antigenic expression: further studies of the Landschütz ascites tumor. *Brt. J. Cancer,* **22**, 843–853 (1968).

70. G. A. Currie and K. D. Bagshawe, Tumour specific immunogenicity of methylcholanthrene-induced sarcoma cells after incubation in neuraminidase. *Brt. J. Cancer,* **23**, 141–149 (1969).

71. G. Mathé, J. L. Amiel, and L. Schwarzenberg, Active immunotherapy for acute lympho-blastic leukemia. *Lancet,* **1**, 697–699 (1969).

72. J. F. Holland and J. G. Bekesi, Immunotherapy of human leukemia with neuraminidase-modified cells. *Med. Clin. North Amr.,* **60**, 539–549 (1976).

73. H. Takita, T. Han, and P. Marabella, Immunotheraphy in bronchogenic carcinoma: Effects on cellular immunity. *Surg. Forum,* **25**, 235–236 (1974).

74. G. J. V. Nossal, Principles of immunological tolerance and immunocyte receptor blockade. *Adv. Immunol.,* **20**, 93–130 (1974).

75. K. E. Hellström and I. Hellström, The role of cell-mediated immunity in control and growth of tumors. *Clin. Immunobiol.,* **2**, 233–265 (1974).

76. D. M. P. Thomson, V. Sellens, S. Eccles, and P. Alexander, Radioimmunoassay of tumour specific transplantation antigen of a chemically induced rat sarcoma: Circulating soluble tumour antigen in tumour bearers. *Brt. J. Cancer,* **28**, 377–388 (1973).

77. A. Wolf, K. A. Steele, and P. Alexander, Estimation in sera by radioimmunoassay of a specific membrane antigen associated with a murine lymphoma. *Brt. J. Cancer,* **33**, 144–153 (1976).

78. R. W. Baldwin, J. G. Bowen, and M. R. Price, Detection of circulating hepatoma D23 antigen and immune complexes in tumour bearer serum. *Brt. J. Cancer,* **28**, 16–24 (1973).

79. D. M. P. Thomson, J. Krupey, S. O. Freedman, and P. Gold, The radioimmunoassay of circulating carcinoembryonic antigen of the human digestive system. *Proc. Natl. Acad. Sci. (USA),* **54**, 161–167 (1969).

80. J. S. Tatarinov, Presence of embryonal α-globulin in the serum of patients with primary hepatocellular carcinoma. *Vopr. Med. Khim,* **10**, 90–91 (1964).

81. P. Alexander, Escape from immune destruction by the host through shedding of surface antigens: Is this a characteristic shared by malignant and embryonic cells? *Cancer Res.,* **34**, 2077–2082 (1974).

82. G. A. Currie and P. Alexander, Spontaneous shedding of TSTA by viable sarcoma cells: Its possible role in facilitating metastatic spread. *Brt. J. Cancer,* **29,** 72–75 (1974).

83. R. W. Baldwin, M. R. Price, and R. A. Robins, Inhibition of hepatoma-immune lymph-node cells cytotoxicity by tumour-bearer serum, and solubilized hepatoma antigen. *Internatl. J. Cancer,* **11,** 527–535 (1973).

84. R. W. Baldwin, M. J. Embleton, and M. R. Price, Inhibition of lymphocyte cytotoxicity for human colon carcinoma by treatment with solubilized hepatoma antigen. *Internatl. J. Cancer,* **12,** 84–92 (1973).

85. E. Hawrylko, Mechanisms by which tumors escape immune destruction. In H. Waters, Ed., *The Handbook of Cancer Immunology,* Vol. 2, Garland STPM Press, New York, 1978, pp. 1–53.

86. P. Alexander and J. G. Hall, The role of immunoblasts in host resistance and immuno-theraphy of primary sarcomata. *Adv. Cancer Res.,* **13,** 1–37 (1970).

87. M. A. Bean, H. Pees, J. E. Fogh, H. Gradstald, and H. F. Oettgen, Cytotoxicity of lympho-cytes from patients with cancer of the urinary bladder: Detection by a ³H-proline micro-cytotoxicity test. *Internatl. J. Cancer,* **14,** 186–197 (1974).

88. C. O'Toole, P. Perlmann, B. Unsgaard, G. Moberger, and F. Edsmyr, Cellular immunity to human urinary bladder carcinoma. I. Correlation to clinical stage and radiotherapy. *Internatl. J. Cancer,* **10,** 77–91 (1972).

89. R. W. Baldwin, M. J. Embleton, J. S. P. Jones, and M. J. S. Langman, Cell-mediated and humoral immune reactions to human tumors. *Internatl. J. Cancer,* **12,** 73–83 (1973).

90. G. H. Heppner, L. Stolbach, M. Bryne, F. J. Cummings, E. McDonough, and P. Calabresi, Cell-mediated and serum blocking reactivity to tumor antigens in patients with malignant melanoma. *Internatl. J. Cancer,* **11,** 245–260 (1973).

91. G. Currie, The role of circulating antigen as an inhibition of tumour immunity in man. *Brt. J. Cancer,* **28, Suppl. I,** 153–161 (1973).

92. G. A. Currie and C. Baham, Serum-mediated inhibition of the immunological reactions of the patient to his own tumour: A possible role for circulating antigen. *Brt. J. Cancer,* **26,** 427–438 (1972).

93. G. A. Currie, F. Lejeune, and G. H. Fairley, Immunization with irradiated tumour cells and specific lymphocyte cytotoxicity in malignant melanoma. *Brt. Med. J.,* **II,** 305–310 (1971).

94. N. Kaliss, Immunlogical enhancement of tumor homografts in mice: A review. *Cancer Res.,* **18,** 992 (1958).

95. V. V. Likhite, Review of tumor enhancement. In H. Waters, Ed., *The Handbook of Cancer Immunology,* Vol. 4, Garland STPM Press, New York, pp. 235–276.

96. R. B. Faanes, Antibody, lymphocyte and tumor cell interactions. In ibid., Vol. 5, pp. 1–28.

97. I. Hellström and K. E. Hellström, Studies in cellular immunity and its serum-mediated inhibition in Moloney virus-induced mouse sarcomas. *Internatl. J. Cancer,* **4,** 587–600 (1969).

98. R. W. Baldwin, M. J. Embleton, and R. A. Robins, Cellular and humoral immunity to rat hepatoma-specific antigens correlated with tumour status. *Internatl. J. Cancer,* **11,** 1–10 (1973).

99. L. Hellström, K. E. Hellström, H. O. Sjögren, and G. A. Warner, Serum factors in tumor-free patients cancelling the blocking of cell-mediated tumor immunity. *Internatl. J. Cancer,* **8,** 185–191 (1971).

100. H. O. Sjögen, I. Hellström, S. C. Bansal, and K. E. Hellström, Suggestive evidence that the "blocking antibodies" of tumor-bearing individuals may be antigen-antibody com-plexes. *Proc. Natl. Acad. Sci. (USA),* **68,** 1372–1375 (1971).

101. R. J. Brawn, *In vitro* desensitization of sensitized murine lymphocytes by a serum factor (soluble antigen?). *Proc. Natl. Acad. Sci. (USA),* **68,** 1634 (1971).

102. H. O. Sjögen, I. Hellström, S. C. Bansal, G. A. Warner, and K. E. Hellström, Elution of "blocking factors" from human tumors, capable of abrogating tumor-cell destruction by specifically immune lymphocytes. *Internatl. J. Cancer,* **9,** 274–283 (1972).

103. R. W. Baldwin, M. R. Price, and R. A. Robins, Blocking of lymphocyte-mediated cytotoxicity for rat hepatoma cells by tumour-specific antigen-antibody complexes. *Nat. New Biol.,* **238,** 185–187 (1972).

104. N. Kaliss, Immunological enhancement. *Internatl. Rev. Exp. Pathol.,* **8,** 242–273 (1969).

105. G. Möller, Studies on the mechanism of immunological enhancement of tumor homografts. II. Effect of isoantibodies on various tumor cells. *J. Natl. Cancer Inst.,* **30,** 1177 (1963).

106. B. H. Berne, Immunological homograft enhancement. Interactions of antiserum and skin and tumor homografts. *Proc. Soc. Exp. Biol. Med.,* **118,** 228 (1965).

107. G. D. Snell, H. J. Winn, J. H. Stimpfling, and S. J. Parker, Depression by antibody of the immune response to homografts and its role in immunological enhancement. *J. Exp. Med.,* **112,** 293–314 (1960).

108. M. Takasugi and W. H. Hildemann, Regulation of immunity toward allogeneic tumors in mice. I. Effect of antiserum fractions on tumor growth. *J. Natl. Cancer Inst.,* **43,** 843 (1969).

109. D. B. Amos, I. Cohn, and W. T. Klein, Mechanisms of immunological enhancement. *Cancer Res.,* **32,** 825 (1970).

110. M. S. Mitchell, Central inhibition of cellular immunity to leukemia L1210 by isoantibody. *Cancer Res.,* **32,** 825 (1972).

111. I. Hellström, K. E. Hellström, H. O. Sjögren, and G. A. Warner, Serum factors in tumor-free patients cancelling the blocking of cell-mediated tumor immunity. *Internatl. J. Cancer,* **8,** 185 (1971).

112. J. Bubenik, P. Perlmann, K. Helmstein, and G. Moberger, Cellular and humoral immune response to human urinary bladder carcinomas. *Internatl. J. Cancer,* **5,** 310 (1970).

113. J. E. de Vries, P. Rumke, and J. L. Berukeim, Cytotoxic lymphocytes in melanoma patients. *Internatl. J. Cancer,* **9,** 567 (1972).

114. M. Byrne, G. Heppner, L. Stolbach, F. Cummings, E. McDonough, and P. Calabresi, Tumor immunity in melanoma patients as assessed by colony inhibition and microcytotoxicity methods: A preliminary report. *Natl. Cancer Inst. Monogr.,* **37,** 3 (1973).

115. J. G. Sinkovics, W. J. Reeves, and J. R. Caviness, Cell-and antibody-meidated immune reactions of patients to cultured cells of breast carcinoma. *Cancer,* **30,** 1428 (1971).

116. N. L. Levy, Use of an *in vitro* microcytotoxicity test to assess human tumor-specific cell-mediated immunity and its serum-mediated abrogation. *Natl. Cancer Inst. Monogr.,* **37,** 85 (1973).

117. G. Klein, Immunological aspects of Burkitt's lymphoma. *Adv. Immunol.,* **14,** 187 (1971).

118. F. Vánky, J. Stjernswärd, G. Klein, and V. Nilsonne, Serum-mediated inhibition of lymphocyte stimulation by autochthonous human tumors. *J. Natl. Cancer Inst.,* **47,** 95 (1971).

119. J. Stjernswärd and F. Vánky, Stimulation of lymphocytes by autochthonous cancer. *Natl. Cancer Inst. Monogr.,* **35,** 237 (1972).

120. F. Vánky, J. Stjernswärd, G. Klein, L. Steiner, and L. Lindberg, Tumor-associated specificity of serum-mediated inhibition of lymphocyte stimulation by autochthonous human tumors. *J. Natl. Cancer Inst.,* **51,** 25 (1973).

121. I. Hellström, H. O. Sjögren, G. A. Warner, and K. E. Hellström, Blocking of cell-mediated tumor immunity by sera from patients with growing neoplasms. *Internatl. J. Cancer,* **7,** 226 (1971).

122. I. Hellström, G. A. Warner, K. E. Hellström, and H. O. Sjögren, Sequential studies on cell-mediated tumor immunity and blocking serum activity in ten patients with malignant melanoma. *Internatl. J. Cancer,* **11,** 280 (1973).

123. S. C. Bansal, R. Hargreaves, and H. O. Sjögren, Facilitation of polyoma tumor growth in rats by blocking sera and tumor eluate. *Internatl. J. Cancer,* **9**, 97-108 (1972).

124. C. W. Stackpole and J. B. Jacobson, Antigenic modulation. In H. Waters, Ed., *The Handbook of Cancer Immunology,* Vol. 2, Garland STPM Press, 1978, pp. 55-160.

125. L. J. Old, E. A. Boyse, and E. Stockert, Antigenic properties of experimental leukemias. I. Serological studies *in vitro* with spontaneous and radiation-induced leukemias. *J. Natl. Cancer Inst.,* **31**, 977-986 (1963).

126. E. A. Boyse, L. J. Old, and E. Stockert, The TL (thymus leukemia) antigen: A review. In P. Grabar and P. A. Miescher, Eds., *Immunopathology, 4th International Symposium, Monte Carlo,* Schwabe, Basel, 1965, pp. 23-40.

127. E. A. Boyse, L. J. Old, and E. Stockert, An approach to the mapping of antigens on the cell surface. *Proc. Natl. Acad. Sci. (USA),* **60**, 886-893 (1968).

128. E. A. Boyse, W. Stockert, and L. J. Old, Isoantigens of the H-2 and TLa loci of the mouse: Interactions affecting their representation on thymocytes. *J. Exp. Med.,* **128**, 85-95 (1968).

129. E. A. Boyse, L. J. Old, and E. Stockert, The relation of linkage group IX to leukemogenesis in the mouse. In P. Emmelot and P. Bentuelsen, Eds., *RNA Viruses and Host Genome on Oncogenesis,* North-Holland, New York, 1972, pp. 171-185.

130. J. Klein, *Biology of the Mouse Histocompatibility-2 Complex,* Springer Verlag, New York, 1975.

131. E. A. Boyse, L. J. Old, and E. Stockert, The TL (thymus leukemia) antigen: A review. In P. Graber and P. A. Miescher, Eds., *Immunopathology: IVth International Symposium,* Grune and Stratton, New York, pp. 23-46.

132. E. A. Boyse, E. Stockert, and L. J. Old, Modification of the antigenic structure of the cell membrane by thymus-leukemia (TL) antibody. *Proc. Natl. Acad. Sci. (USA),* **58**, 954-957 (1967).

133. J. B. Jacobson, S. Galuska, and C. W. Stackpole, *In vivo* modulation of TL antigens on mouse leukemia cells and thymocytes: Modulating antibody remains on the cell surface. *J. Natl. Cancer Inst.,* **61**, 819 (1978).

134. E. A. Boyse, L. J. Old, and E. Stockert, Antigenic modulation. In H. Peeters, Ed., *Protides of the Biological Fluids, Proc. 17th Colloquium, Bruges,* Pergamon, New York, 1969, pp. 225-227.

135. M. E. Lamm, E. A. Boyse, L. J. Old, B. Lisowska-Bernstein, and E. Stockert, Modulation of TL (thymus-leukemia) antigens by Fab-fragments of TL antibody. *J. Immunol.,* **101**, 99-103 (1968).

136. E. A. Boyse, L. J. Old, and S. Luell, Antigenic properties of experimental leukemias. II. Immunological studies *in vivo* with C57BL/6 radiation-induced leukemias. *J. Natl. Cancer Inst.,* **31**, 987-995 (1963).

137. E. A. Boyse, E. Stockert, and L. J. Old, Properties of four antigens specified by the Tla locus. Similarities and differences. In N. R. Rose and F. Milgrom, Eds., *International Convocation Immunology,* Buffalo, N. Y., Karger-Basel, New York, 1968, pp. 353-357.

138. F. Doljanski and M. Kapeller, Cell surface shedding-the phenomenon and its possible significance. *J. Theor. Biol.,* **62**, 253-270 (1976).

139. C. W. Stackpole, J. B. Jacobson, and M. P. Lardis, Antigenic modulation *in vitro.* I. Fate of thymus-leukemia (TL) antigen-antibody complexes following modulation of TL antigenicity from the surfaces of mouse leukemia cells and thymocytes. *J. Exp. Med.,* **140**, 939-953 (1974).

140. A. Yu, and E. P. Cohen, Studies on the effect of specific antisera on the metabolism of cellular antigens. II. The synthesis and degradation of TL antigens of mouse cells in the presence of TL antiserum. *J. Immunol.,* **112**, 1296-1307 (1974).

141. N. L. Esmon and J. R. Little, An indirect radioimmunoassay for thymus-leukemia (TL) antigens. *J. Immunol.,* **117**, 911-918 (1976).

142. N. L. Esmon and J. R. Little, Different mechanisms for the modulation of TL antigens on murine lymphoid cells. *J. Immunol.,* **117**, 919–926 (1976).

143. T. Takahashi, Possible examples of antigenic modulation affecting H-2 antigens and cell surface immunoglobulins. *Transplant. Proc.,* **3**, 1217–1220 (1971).

144. T. Takahashi, L. J. Old, K. R. McIntire, and E. A. Boyse, Immunoglobulin and other surface antigens of cells of the immune system. *J. Exp. Med.,* **134**, 815–832 (1971).

145. S. de Petris and M. C. Raff, Distribution of immunoglobulin on the surface of mouse lymphoid cells as determined by immunoferritin electron microscopy. Antibody-induced, temperature-dependent redistribution and its implications for membrane structure. *Eur. J. Immunol.* **2**, 523–535 (1972).

146. C. W. Stackpole, L. T. DeMilio, J. B. Jacobson, U. Hammerling, and M. P. Lardis, A comparison of ligand-induced redistribution of surface immunoglobulins, alloantigens, and concanavalin A receptors on mouse lymphoid cells. *J. Cell. Physiol.,* **82**, 441–448 (1974).

147. R. E. Cone, J. J. Marchalonis, and R. T. Rolley, Lymphocyte membrane dynamics. Metabolic release of cell surface proteins. *J. Exp. Med.,* **134**, 1373–1384 (1971)

148. J. D. Wilson, G. J. V. Nossal, and H. Lewis, Metabolic characteristics of lymphocyte surface immunoglobulin. *Eur. J. Immunol.,* **2**, 225–232 (1972).

149. B. S. Joseph and M. B. A. Oldstone, Immunologic injury in measles virus infection. II. Suppression of immune injury through antigenic modulation. *J. Exp. Med.* **142**, 864–876 (1975).

150. L. J. Old, E. Stockert, E. A. Boyse, and J. H. Kim, Antigenic modulation. Loss of TL antigen from cells exposed to TL antibody. Study of the phenomenon *in vitro. J. Exp. Med.,* **127**, 523–529 (1968).

151. M. B. A. Oldstone, Role of antibody in regulating virus persistence: Modulation of viral antigens expressed on the cell's plasma membrane and analysis of cell lysis. *National Institute of Child and Human Development Conference on Development of Host Defenses,* Elkridge, Md., May 1976.

152. R. T. Smith, G. Klein, E. Klein, and P. Clifford, Studies of the membrane phenomenon in cultured and biopsy cell lines from the Burkitt lymphoma. In J. Dausset, J. Hamburger, and G. Mathé, Eds. *Advances in Transplantation,* Williams and Wilkins, Baltimore, 1968, pp. 483–493.

153. R. T. Smith, Comment. In M. Landy and W. Braun, Eds., *Immunological Tolerance,* Academic, New York, 1969, pp. 50–52.

154. I. Kao and D. B. Drachman, Myasthenic immunoglobulin accelerates acetylcholine receptor degradation. *Science,* **196**, 527–529 (1977).

155. K. V. Toyka, D. E. Drachmam, A. Pestronk, J. A. Winkelstein, K. H. Fischbeck, Jr., and I. Kao, Myasthenia gravis. Study of humoral immune mechanisms by passive transfer to mice. *New Engl. J. Med.,* **296**, 125–131 (1977).

156. R. Levy, J. Dilley, R. I. Fox and R. Warnke, A human thymus-leukemia antigen defined by hybridoma monoclonal antibodies. *Proc. Natl. Acad. Sci. (USA),* **76**, 6552–6556 (1979).

157. J. M. Pesando, J. Ritz, H. Lazarus, S. B. Costello, S. Sallan, and S. F. Schlossman, Leukemia-associated antigens in ALL. *Blood,* **54**, 1240–1248 (1979).

158. P. A. Gorer, Some reactions of H-2 antibodies *in vitro* and *in vivo. Ann. N.Y. Acad. Sci.,* **73**, 707–721 (1958).

159. P. A. Gorer, Interactions between sessile and humoral antibodies. In G. E. W. Wolstenholme and M. O'Connor, Eds., *Ciba Foundation Symposium on Cellular Aspects of Immunity* Little, Brown, Boston, 1960, pp. 330–346.

160. D. B. Amos and J. D. Wakefield. Growth of mouse ascites tumor cells in diffusion chambers. II. Lysis and growth inhibition by diffusible antibody. *J. Natl. Cancer. Inst.,* **22**, 1077 (1959).

161. D. B. Amos, W. H. Prioleau, and P. Hutchin, Biochemical changes during growth of C3H ascites tumor BP8 in C57B1 mice. *J. Surg. Res.*, **8**, 122–127 (1968).

162. P. Hutchin, D. B. Amos, and W. H. Prioleau, Interactions of humoral antibodies and immune lymphocytes. *Transplantation* **5**, 68 (1967).

163. M. P. Fink, C. W. Parker, and W. T. Shearer, Antibody stimulation of tumour growth in T-cell depleted mice. *Nature*, **255**, 404–405 (1975).

164. W. R. Shearer, J. P. Atkinson, M. M. Frank, and C. W. Parker, Humoral immunostimulation. IV. Role of complement. *J. Exp. Med.,* **141**, 736–752 (1975).

165. W. T. Shearer, G. W, Philpott, and C. W. Parker, Stimulation of cells by antibody. *Science*, **182**, 1357–1359 (1973).

166. W. T. Shearer, G. W. Philpott, and C. W. Parker, Humoral immunostimulation. I. Increased (^{125}I) iododeoxyuridine, and (^{3}H) thymidine into TNP-cells treated with anti-TNP antibody. *J. Exp. Med.*, **139**, 367–379 (1974).

167. W. T. Shearer, G. W. Philpott, and C. W. Parker, Humoral immunostimulation. II. Increased nucleoside incorporation, DNA synthesis, and cell growth in L cells treated with anti-L cell antibody. *Cell. Immunol.*, **17**, 447–462 (1975).

168. M. J. Dauphinee, N. Talal, and I. P. Witz, Generation of noncomplement fixing, blocking factors by lysozomal extract treatment of cytotoxic antitumor antibodies. *J. Immunol.,* **113**, 948 (1974).

169. J. Folkman, Tumour angiogenesis. *Adv. Cancer Res.*, **19**, 331–358 (1974).

170. J. W. Uhr and G. Möller, Regulatory effect of antibody on the immune response. *Adv. Immunol.*, **8**, 81–127 (1968).

171. R. Gorczynski, S. Kontiainen, N. A. Mitchison, and R. E. Tigelaar, In G. M. Edelmam, Ed., *Cellular Selection and Regulation in the Immune Response,* Raven, New York, 1974, pp. 143–154.

172. E. Diener and M. Feldmann, Relationship between antigen and antibody-induced suppression of immunity. *Transplant. Rev.*, **8**, 76–103 (1972).

173. R. K. Gershon, T cell control of antibody production. *Contemp. Top. Immunobiol.*, **3**, 1 (1974).

174. B. H. Waksman and Y. Namba, On soluble mediators of immunologic regulation. *Cell. Immunol.*, **21**, 161–176 (1976).

175. T. A. Waldmann and S. Broder, Suppressor cells in the regulation of the immune response. *Prog. Clin. Immunol.*, **3**, 155–199 (1977).

176. T. Tada, Regulation of reaginic antibody formation in animals. *Prog. Allergy*, **19**, 122–194 (1975).

177. B. Benacerraf and M. Dorf, The nature and function of specific H-linked immune response genes and immune suppression genes. In D. H. Katz and B. Benacerraf, Eds., *The Role of Products of the Histocompatibility Gene Complex in Immune Response,* Academic, New York, 1976, pp. 225–248.

178. K. Rajewsky and K. Eichmann, Antigen receptors of T helper cells. *Contemp. Top. Immunobiol.*, **7**, 69–112 (1977).

179. J. Harris and D. Copeland, Impaired immunoresponsiveness in tumor patients. *Ann. N. Y. Acad. Sci.*, **230**, 56–85 (1974).

180. D. Lamb, F. Pilney, W. D. Kelly, and R. A. Good, A comparative study of the incidence of anergy in patients with carcinoma, leukemia, Hodgkin's disease and other lymphomas. *Immunology*, **89**, 555 (1962).

181. G. W. Santos, G. M. Mullins, W. B. Bias, T. N. Anderson, K. D. Grasiano, D. L. Klein, and P. J. Burkem, Immunologic studies in acute leukemia. *Natl. Cancer Inst. Monogr.*, **37**, 69 (1973).

182. E. M. Hersh, J. P. Whitecar, K. B. McCredie, G. P. Bodey, and E. J. Freireich, Chemotherapy, immunocompetence, immunosuppression and prognosis in acute leukemia. *New Engl. J. Med.*, **285**, 1211 (1971).

183. F. R. Eilber and D. L. Morton, Impaired reactivity and recurrence following cancer surgery. *Cancer*, **25**, 362–367 (1970).

184. C. M. Pinsky, H. F. Oettgen, A. El Domeiri, L. J. Old, E. J. Beattie, and J. H. Burchenal, Delayed hypersensitivity reactions in patients with cancer. *Proc. Am. Assoc. Cancer Res.*, **12**, 100 (1971).

185. S. A. Wells, J. S. Burdicki, C. Christiansen, A. S. Ketcham, and P. C. Adkins, Demonstration of tumor-associated delayed cutaneous hypersensitivity reactions in patients with lung cancer and in patients with carcinoma of the cervix. *Natl. Cancer Inst. Monogr.*, **2**, 113 (1973).

186. H. S. Kaplan, Role of immunologic disturbance in human oncogenesis: some facts and fancies. *Br. J. Cancer*, **25**, 620 (1971).

187. J. J. Twomey, A. H. Laughter, S. Farrow, et al., Hodgkin's disease: An immunodepleting and immunosuppressive disorder. *J. Clin. Invest.*, **56**, 467–475 (1975).

188. E. G. Engleman, R. Hoppe, H. Kaplan, J. Comminskey, and H. O. McDevitt, Suppressor cells of the mixed lymphocyte reaction in healthy subjects and patients with Hodgkin's disease and sarcoidosis. *Clin Res.*, **26**, 513A (1978).

189. S. M. Hillinger, and G. P. Herzig, Impaired cell-mediated immunity in Hodgkin's disease mediated by suppressor lymphocytes and monocytes. *J. Clin. Invest.*, **61**, 1620–1627 (1978).

190. W. H. Brooks, M. G. Netshy, D. E. Normansell, and D. A. Horwitz, Depressed cell-mediated immunity in patients with primary intracranial tumors: Characterization on a humoral immunosuppressive factor. *J. Exp. Med.*, **136**, 1631–1647 (1972).

191. A. H. Glasgow, R. B. Nimberg, J. O. Menzoiam, I. Saporoschetz, S. R. Cooperband, K. Schmid, and J. A. Mannick, Association of anergy with immunosuppressive peptide faction in the serum of patients with cancer. *New Engl. J. Med.*, **291**, 1263–1267 (1974).

192. R. B. Nimberg, A. H. Glasgow, J. O. Menzoian, M. B. Constantain, S. R. Cooperband, J. A. Mannick, and K. Schid, Isolation of immunosuppressive peptide faction from the serum of cancer patients. *Cancer Res.*, **35**, 1489–1494 (1975).

193 O. J. Plescia, A. H. Smith and K. Grinwich, Subversion of immune system by tumor cells and role of prostaglandins. *Proc. Natl. Acad. Sci. (USA)*, **72**, 1848–1851 (1975).

194. J. S. Goodwin, R. P. Messner, A. D. Bankhurst, G. L. Peake, J. H. Saiki, and R. C. Williams, Prostaglandin-producing suppressor cells in Hodgkin's disease. *New Engl. J. Med.*, **297**, 963–968 (1977).

195. M. W. Johnson, H. I. Maibach, and S. E. Salmon, Impaired delayed sensitivity or faulty inflammatory response. *New Engl. J. Med.*, **284**, 1255–1257 (1971).

196. M. W. Johnson, H. I. Mailbach, and S. E. Salmon, Dinitrochlorobenzene: Inflammatory response and delayed cutaneous hypersensitivity. *New Engl. J. Med.*, **286**, 1162–1165 (1972).

197. M. W. Johnson, H. I. Mailbach, and S. E. Salmon, Quantitiative impairment of primary inflammatory response in patients with cancer. *J. Natl. Cancer Inst.*, **51**, 1075–1076 (1973).

198. D. A. Boetcher and E. J. Leonard, Abnormal monocyte chemotactic response in cancer patients. *J. Natl. Cancer Inst.*, **52**, 1091–1099 (1974).

199. M. S. Hausman, A. Brosman, R. Synderman, M. R. Mickey, and J. Fahey, Defective monocyte function in patients with genitourinary carcinoma. *J. Natl. Cancer Inst.*, **55**, 1047–1054 (1975).

200. R. H. Rubin, A. B. Cosimi, and E. Goetzl, Defective human mononuclear leukocyte chemotaxis as an index of host resistance to malignant melanoma. *Clin. Immunol. Immunopathol.*, **6**, 376–388 (1976).

201. Q. S. Dizon and C. M. Southam, Abnormal cellular response to skin abrasions in cancer patients. *Cancer*, **14**, 1288–1292 (1963).

202. T. Ruutu, P. Ruutu, P. Vuopio, K. Franssila, and E. Lindem, An inhibitor of chemotaxis and phagocytosis in reticulum cell sarcoma. *Scand. J. Haematol.*, **15**, 27–34 (1975).

203. N. Grosser, J. H. Marti, J. W. Proctor, and D. M. P. Thomson, Tube leukocyte adherence inhibition assay for the detection of anti-tumor immunity. I. Monocyte is the reactive cell. *Internatl. J. Cancer*, **18**, 39–47 (1976).

204. N. Grosser and D. M. P. Thomson, Tube leukocyte (monocyte) adherence inhibition assay for the detection of antitumor immunity. III. "Blockade" of monocyte reactivity by excess free antigen and immune complexes in advanced cancer patients. *Internatl. J. Cancer*, **18**, 58–66 (1976).

205. J. H. Marti, N. Grosser, and D. M. P. Thomson, Tube leukocyte adherence inhibition assay for the detection of anti-tumor immunity. II. Monocyte reacts with tumor antigen via cytophilic anti-tumor antibody. *Internatl. J. Cancer*, **18**, 48–57 (1976).

206. J. M. Kirkwood and R. K. Gershon, A role for suppressor T cells in immunological enhancement of tumor growth. *Prog. Exp. Tumor Res.*, **19**, 157–179 (1974).

207. D. Naor, Suppressor cells: Permitters and promoters of malignancy? *Adv. Cancer Res.*, **29**, 45–125 (1979).

208. S. Broder and T. A. Waldmann, The suppressor-cell network in cancer. *New Engl. J. Med.*, **299**, 1281–1341 (1978).

209. S. Fujimoto, M. Greene, and A. H. Sehon, Regulation of the immune response to tumor antigens. I. Immunosuppressor cells in tumor-bearing hosts. *J. Immunol.*, **116**, 791 (1976).

210. S. Fujimoto, M. Greene, and A. H. Sehon, Regulation of the immune response to tumor antigens. II. The nature of immunosuppressor cells in tumor-bearing hosts. *J. Immunol.*, **116**, 800 (1976).

211. T. A. Waldmann, S. Broder and M. Durm, Suppressor T cells in the pathogenesis of hypogammaglobulinemia associated with thymoma. *Trans. Assoc. Am. Physicians,* **88**, 120–134 (1975).

212. T. A. Waldmann and W. Strober, Metabolism of immunoglobulins. *Progr. Allergy,* **13**, 1–110 (1969).

213. S. Broder, R. Humphrey, M. Durm, M. Blackman, B. Meade, C. Goldman, W. Strober, and T. A. Waldmann, Impaired synthesis of polyclonal (non-paraprotein) immunoglobulins by circulating lymphocytes from patients with multiple myeloma: Role of suppressor cells. *New Engl. J. Med.*, **293**, 887–892 (1975).

214. S. Broder, D. Poplack, J. Whang-Peng, M. Durm, C. Goldman, L. Muul, and T. A. Waldmann, Characterization of a suppressor-cell leukemia: Evidence for the requirement of an interaction of two T cells in the development of human suppressor effector cells. *New Engl. J. Med.*, **298**, 66–72 (1978).

215. T. Uchiyama, K. Sagawa, K. Takatsuki, et al., Effect of adult T-cell leukemia cells on pokeweed mitogen-induced normal B-cell differentiation. *Clin. Immunol. Immunopathol.*, **10**, 24–34 (1978).

216. S. Broder, E. L. Edelson, M. A. Lutzner, D. L. Nelson, R. P. MacDermott, M. E. Durm, C. K. Goldman, B. D. Meade, and T. A. Waldmann, The Sézary syndrome: A malignant proliferation of helper T cells. *J. Clin. Invest.*, **58**, 1297–1306 (1976).

217. S. Broder, E. Lawrence, M. Durm, C. Goldman, L. Muul, and T. A. Waldmann, Further characterization of neoplastic helper T cells from patients with the Sézary syndrome. In D. O. Lucas, Ed., *Regulatory Mechanisms in Lymphocyte Activation*, Academic, New York, 1977, pp. 689–691.

218. F. S. Jeunet and R. A. Good, Thymoma immunologic deficiencies, and hematological abnormalities. *Birth Defects*, **4**, 192–206 (1968).

219. J. L. Fahey, R. Scoggins, J. P. Uts, and C. F. Szwed, Infection, antibody response and gamma globulin components in multiple myeloma and macroglobulinemia. *Am. J. Med.*, **39**, 698–707 (1963).

220. L. Cone and J. J. Uhr, Immunological deficiency disorders associated with chronic lymphocytic leukemia and multiple myeloma. *J. Clin. Invest.*, **43**, 2241–2248 (1961).

221. S. E. Salmon, Paraneoplastic syndromes associated with monoclonal lymphocyte and plasma cell proliferation. *Ann. N. Y. Acad. Sci.*, **230**, 228–239 (1974).

222. S. Zolla, D. Naor, and P. Tanapatchaiyapong, Cellular basis of immunodepression in mice bearing plasmacytomas. *J. Immunol.*, **112**, 2068–2076 (1974).

223. J. Kolb, S. Arria, and S. Zolla-Pazner, Suppression of the humoral immune response by plasmacytomas: Mediation by adherent mononuclear cells. *J. Immunol.*, **118**, 702–709 (1977).

224. S. Zolla, The effect of plasmacytomas on the immune response of mice. *J. Immunol.*, **108**, 1039–1048 (1972).

225. R. S. Krakauer, W. Strober, and T. A. Waldmann, Hypogammaglobulinemia in experimental myeloma: The role of suppressor mononuclear phagocytes. *J. Immunol.*, **118**, 1385–1390 (1977).

226. N. V. Boopalam, V. Yakulis, N. Costea and P. Heller, Surface immunoglobulins in circulating lymphocytes in mouse plasmacytoma. II. The influence of plasmacytoma RNA on surface immunoglobulins of lymphocytes. *Blood*, **39**, 465–471. (1972).

227. S. E. Salmon, Immunoglobulin synthesis and tumor kinetics of multiple myeloma. *Semin. Hematol.*, **10**, 135–147 (1973).

228. P. Tanapatchaiyapong and S. Zolla, Humoral immunosuppressive substance in mice bearing plasmacytomas. *Science*, **186** 748–750 (1974).

229. S. Broder, R. Humphrey, M. Durm, M. Blackman, B. Meade, C. Goldman, W. Strober, and T. A. Waldmann, Impaired synthesis of polyclonal (non-paraprotein) immunoglobulins by circulating lymphocytes from patients with multiple myeloma: Role of suppressor cells. *New Engl. J. Med.*, **293**, 887–892 (1975).

230. J. Kennard and S. Zolla-Pazner, Origin and function of suppressor macrophages in myeloma. *J. Immunol.*, **124**, 268–273 (1980).

231. W. Knapp and G. Buamgartner, Monocyte-mediated suppression of human B lymphocyte differentiation *in vitro*. *J. Immunol.*, **121**, 1177–1183 (1978).

232. T. Paglieroni and M. R. MacKenzie, Studies on the pathogenesis of the immune defect in multiple myeloma. *J. Clin. Invest.*, **59**, 1120–1133 (1977).

233. T. Paglieroni and M. R. MacKenzie, Multiple myeloma: An immunologic profile. III. Cytotoxic and suppressive effects of the EA rosette-forming cell. *J. Immunol.*, **124**, 2563 (1980).

234. T. Han and B. Dadey, *In vitro* functional studies of mononuclear cells in patients with CLL, Evidence for functionally normal T lymphocytes and monocytes and abnormal B lymphocytes. *Cancer*, **43**, 109–117 (1979).

235. S. M. Fu, N. Chiorazzi, and H. G. Kunkel, Differentiation capacity and other properties of the leukemic cells of chronic lymphocytic leukemia. *Immunol. Rev.*, **48**, 22 (1979).

236. T. Suda, Y. Miura, H. Mizoguchi, K. Kubota, and F. Takaku, A case of lung cancer associated with granulocytosis and production of colony-stimulating activity by the tumor. *Br. J. Cancer*, **41**, 980 (1980).

237. R. G. Lynch, J. W. Rohrer, B. Odermatt, H. M. Gebel, J. R. Autry, and R. G. Hoover, Immunoregulation of murine myeloma cell growth and differentiation: A monoclonal model of B cell differentiation. *Immunol. Rev.*, **48**, 45 (1979).

238. H. Kubagawa, L. B. Vogler, J. D. Capra, M. E. Conrad, A. R. Lawton, and M. D. Cooper, Studies on the clonal origin of multiple myeloma. *J. Exp. Med.*, **150**, 792 (1979).

239. S. M. Fu, R. J. Winchester, T. Feizi, P. D. Walzer, and H. J. Kunkel, Idiotype specificity of surface immunoglobulin and the maturation of leukemic bone-marrow derived lymphocytes. *Proc. Natl. Acad. Sci. (USA)*, **71** 4487 (1974).

240. S. M. Fu, N. Chiorazzi, H. J. Kunkel, J. P. Halper, and S. R. Harris, Induction of *in vitro* differentiation and immunoglobulin synthesis of human B leukemic lymphocytes. *J. Exp. Med.*, **148**, 1570 (1978).

241. S. Sugai, D. W. Palmer, N. Talal, and I. P. Witz, Protective and cellular immune responses to idiotypic determinants on cells from a spontaneous lymphoma of NZB/NZW$_{F1}$ mice. *J. Exp. Med.*, **140**, 1547 (1974).

242. G. Haughton, L. L. Lanier, G. F. Babcock, and M. A. Lynes, Antigen-induced murine B cell lymphomas. II. Exploitation of surface idiotype as tumor specific antigen. *J. Immunol.*, **121**, 2358 (1978).

243. J. Lotem and L. Sachs, *In vivo* induction of normal differentiation in myeloid leukemia cells. *Proc. Natl. Acad. Sci. (USA)*, **75**, 3781 (1978).

3

Immunotherapy with
Microbial Products

MICHAEL J. MASTRANGELO
DAVID BERD
Department of Medicine
Fox Chase Cancer Center
Philadelphia, Pennsylvania

This work was supported by USPHS Grants CA-13456, CA-06927, and RR-05539 from the National Institutes of Health and by an appropriation from the Commonwealth of Pennsylvania.

1. INTRODUCTION

Regression of neoplastic disease had been reported in patients with acute bacterial infections. Thus in 1893 W. B. Coley initiated treatment of human cancers with the toxic products of bacterial metabolism. The results of therapy with Coley's toxins were reviewed by Nauts (1). Tumor regressions were reported for a large percentage of patients with histologically confirmed malignant disease. Therapy appeared most effective when toxin was administered directly into tumors. Despite these encouraging early results, this area of therapeutic research remained dormant until 1965, when Villasor (2) reported on the use of bacillus Calmette-Guerin (BCG) in combination with chemotherapy in patients with advanced cancer. Since that time there has been a dramatic proliferation of clinical trials with microbial products. The majority of these trials have employed BCG and *Corynebacterium parvum* (or their fractions), and thus these materials serve as the focus for this review. Other microbial adjuvants, such as *Nocardia rubra* cell-wall skeletons, have not been studied sufficiently to allow conclusions regarding their clinical utility and thus are not considered.

Bacillus Calmette-Guerin is an attenuated strain of *Mycobacterium bovis* that Calmette and Guerin developed from a virulent culture in 1908 by the addition of bile to the medium. Although all cultures of BCG have originated from this strain, various vaccines are not identical as a result of differences in preparation, cultural methods, and genetic drift.

The efficacy of BCG for treating neoplasia is probably related to the ability of the microbe to nonspecifically stimulate the immune system. Bacillus Calmette-Guerin enhances resistance to intracellular parasites, antibody production, and cellular immunity. These areas have been extensively reviewed by Laucius et al. (3) and Mitchell and Murahata (4). Among the earliest demonstrations of the antitumor effects of BCG were the animal studies of Zbar and associates (5). Working with an inbred strain of guinea pigs and a transplantable hepatocarcinoma, these investigators demonstrated that intralesional BCG can induce regression of established dermal tumor transplants and microscopic regional nodal metastasis as well as stimulate tumor-specific cell-mediated immunity. They found that tumor regression requires an intact immune system and direct contact between BCG and tumor cells. Although BCG modulates a wide variety of immune functions, the antitumor effect is felt to be due mainly to macrophage activation.

Bacillus Calmette-Guerin toxicity has been defined and is directly related to the dose, the amount of debris in the preparation employed, and the route of administration. The systemic reaction consists of fever, chills, anorexia, nausea, vomiting (rarely), and myalgias that occur within 4 to 6 hours after injection and subside within 36 to 48 hours. With intralesional injection, BCG bacteremia was observed (6). Scarification causes the fewest systemic side effects.

Prevost (7) was the first to observe that organs of animals and humans naturally infected with anaerobic coryneforms or injected with killed suspensions of these organisms displayed "histioreticulosis with large multinuclear macrophages showing intense hyperergia." Although many strains of anaerobic coryneforms produced this effect, Prevost chose one of these for more intensive study, strain 936 B, which he identified as *Corynebacterium parvum.* Subsequent studies have raised considerable doubt about the existence of *C. parvum* as a taxonomic entity. The designation *C. parvum* indicates only a preparation (usually killed) of one of a number of anaerobic coryneforms with biologic activity. Almost all the work to be discussed in this review involved suspensions of killed organisms supplied by either the Burroughs-Wellcome Company or the Merieux Institute.

The immunologic effects of *C. parvum* are diverse (antibody production, delayed hypersensitivity, antitumor immunity), involve modification of several cell types (macrophages, T lymphocytes, B lymphocytes), and may be positive (stimulatory) or negative (inhibitory). Berd (8) has extensively reviewed the effects of *C. parvum* on various aspects of immunity.

Clinical interest in *C. parvum* emanates from its ability to inhibit the growth of malignant animal tumors. Woodruff and Boak (9) first described the use of *C. parvum* in the therapy of transplanted syngeneic murine tumors. They observed that intravenous administration 2 days before or 8 to 12 days after tumor inoculation significantly delayed the appearance of a palpable tumor and prolonged survival. A host of investigators have achieved similar results. *Corynebacterium parvum* is most effective when given before, simultaneous with or shortly after tumor transplantation. This antitumor effect is thought to be mediated through macrophage activation.

The side effects of *C. parvum* are related to route of administration. Acute toxicities are most common following intravenous administration and include fever, chills, headache, and alterations in cardiorespiratory status (10). These symptoms may be followed by feelings of malaise or influenzalike symptoms for several days. Subcutaneous administration is further complicated by local hypersensitivity reactions that may be severe and develop into sterile abscesses.

There is a large clinical experience with both BCG and *C. parvum.* Unfortunately, these studies were conducted without adequate preliminary data to identify the best route, dose, or schedule of administration. Further, many of these trials were poorly designed and/or inadequately controlled. Despite these shortcomings, a number of evaluable trials have been published and some successes noted. This brief review focuses on lung and bladder cancers, melanoma, and the hematologic malignancies, as these are the tumors in which BCG and *C. parvum* have been most systematically evaluated.

2. LUNG CANCER

2.1. Adjuvant Studies

McKneally et al. (11) were the first to evaluate the therapeutic efficacy of intrapleural BCG (Tice strain, 10^7 viable units) in patients with operable, non-oat cell, Stage I (primary <3.0 cm diameter ± hilar node metastases or primary > 3 cm without hilar node metastases) lung cancer. The results of this and similar trials are presented in Table 1. Although a clear improvement in survival was demonstrated for BCG treated patients, recurrences were not significantly reduced, and it has not yet been determined if intrapleural BCG improves the surgical cure rate. Although randomized in design, this trial has been the subject of criticism because the control group did not perform as well as similarly treated patients elsewhere. However, it must be assumed that treated patients would have done as poorly as controls if left untreated.

A number of other investigators are currently evaluating intrapleural BCG in similar patient populations (Table 1). Wright et al. (12) have not been able to demonstrate a decrease in recurrence rate, but disease-free intervals may be improved in the BCG-treated group. Lowe et al. (13) noted fewer deaths in Glaxo BCG-treated patients than in controls. Attempts to draw definitive conclusions from these two trials are compromised by the small patient populations and the brevity of follow-up. The Lung Cancer Study Group has in progress a large randomized trial of intrapleural BCG. This study should provide an accurate assessment of the clinical utility of this therapeutic modality.

Stjernsward (14) reported the results of the Ludwig Lung Cancer Study Group by comparing intrapleural *C. parvum* (204 patients) with placebo (196 patients) in operable, Stages I and II, non-small-cell, bronchogenic carcinoma. No differences were noted between placebo- and *C. parvum*-treated groups in relapse rates (55/196 vs. 71/204) or deaths (44/196 vs. 51/204). Fever and chest pain were common complications in the treated patients. A fever greater than 38°C was associated with a decreased disease-free interval.

TABLE 1.   Adjuvant Intrapleural BCG in Operable Stage I Non-Oat Cell Carcinoma of the Lung

	McKneally et al. (11)		
Treatment	Tice BCG	Control	
Patients (no.)	30	36	
Recurrences: 1 year	2/30	10/36	$p = .78$
2 years	6/28	9/26	$p = .69$
3 years	1/22	2/17	$p = .46$
Median survival (months)	52	24	$p = .006$
	Wright et al. (12)		
Treatment	Tice BCG	Control	
Patients (no.)	48	33	
Recurrences	13	12	
	Lowe et al. (13)		
Treatment	Glaxo BCG	Control	
Patients (no.)	22	23	
Deaths	2	7	

A multicenter Canadian trial evaluated oral BCG as an adjuvant to treatment of resectable carcinoma of the bronchus (Stage I, II, or III) (15). One hundred and fifty-five patients received oral BCG (Connaught; 120 mg/dose; weekly × 4, every 2 weeks up to 3 months and then every 3 months up to 18 months) while 153 patients were randomized to an untreated control group. No differences were noted between the two groups in disease-free interval and survival rates. This study differed from the intrapleural BCG trials discussed previously in that it included some patients with operable oat cell carcinoma. Further, outcome by stage of disease was not reported.

Several studies have employed the cutaneous route in evaluating BCG as an adjuvant to surgery in lung cancer (Table 2). Pouillart and co-workers (16) randomized 55 patients with operable Stages I and II squamous cell carcinoma of the bronchus to receive BCG or serve as untreated controls. Actuarial disease free survival curves show no difference with a median follow-up of 40 months. However, subset analysis shows an improved survival for BCG treated Stage I patients. Edwards and colleagues (17) alternately allocated 500 patients with lung cancer to receive BCG or serve as untreated controls. Patients were eligible for study regardless of histologic type of tumor or stage of disease as long as all macroscopic tumor tissue could be removed at surgery. No differences were noted in survival at 2 years. Roscoe et al. (18) randomly allocated 92 patients with lung cancer deemed suitable for resection to BCG (multipuncture or intradermal) or placebo treatment. All histologic types were included. Overall survival was not prolonged. However, data were not analyzed by stage of disease or histologic type. After lobectomy or pneumonectomy, 45 patients with Stage I and 6 with Stage II non-small-cell carcinoma of the lung were randomized by Perlin et al. (19) to receive intradermal BCG (± allogeneic tumor cells) or serve as untreated controls. Stage I patients treated with BCG displayed a trend toward fewer relapses. Further, the median disease-free survival of this group was 1500 + days, compared with 700 days in the untreated control (p = .051).

Jansen et al. (20) evaluated the therapeutic efficacy of systemic and intrapleural BCG in patients with locally advanced but operable primary squamous cell bronchial carcinoma. Thirty-four patients received BCG (RIV strain) by scarification (weekly × 6 then twice every 3 months at weekly intervals for 30 months). Of these, 14 patients were randomly chosen to receive a single intrapleural injection of BCG (35 × 10^6 viable units). Although only 6 of 14 patients receiving the combined treatment relapsed compared with 13 of 20 patients receiving only BCG by scarification, there was no difference in survival curves. Subset analysis by disease stage was not presented.

Another approach to the postsurgical adjuvant immunotherapy of lung cancer is the administration of an allogeneic tumor antigen extract in combination with complete Freund's adjuvant. Following lung resection, Takita and co-workers (21) randomized 80 Stage I and II patients to control, Freund's adjuvant + pooled allogeneic tumor antigen or Freund's adjuvant alone. Actuarial survival analysis estimates a 3-year survival of 34% for control patients, 89% for patients treated with Freund's adjuvant alone, and 94% for those

TABLE 2. Systemic BCG as a Post Surgical Adjuvant in Operable Lung Cancer

	Pouillart et al. (16)		
Treatment	Pasteur BCG[a]	Control	
Stages I and II			
Patients (no.)	28	27	
Relapses	15	19	
Median survival (months)	28	24	
Stage I only			
Patients (no.)	12	13	
Median survival (months)	48+	36	$p < .05$

	Edwards (17)	
Treatment	Glaxo BCG[b]	Control
Patients (no.)	250	250
Alive at 2 years	119 (48%)	114 (46%)

	Roscoe et al. (18)		
Treatment	Glaxo BCG[b]		Control
	Multipuncture	Intradermal	
Patients (no.)	29	26	37
Median survival (months)	33+	24	24

	Perlin et al. (19)	
Treatment	Pasteur BCG ± TC[d]	Control
Stages I and II		
Patients (no.)	30	21
Relapses	7	9
Stage I only		
Patients (no.)	24	17
Relapses	5	8

[a] 75 mg per scarification; weekly × 52, then every 2 weeks.

[b] 5 × 10^6 organisms subdermally 10 days postoperative.

[c] Multipuncture (50 to 250 × 10^6 viable units) and intradermal (0.4 to 0.9 × 10^6 viable units) vaccinations at 1, 2, 5, 9, 13, and 26 weeks after operation and every 26 weeks thereafter.

[d] 3–5 × 10^8 organisms intradermally (Heaf gun) twice monthly for 24 months; allogeneic (fresh-frozen) tumor cells (TC) (5 × 10^7) intradermally and subcutaneously proximal to a BCG injection site.

patients who received tumor antigen in addition to Freund's adjuvant. Both treatment arms differed significantly ($p < .05$) from the control. These results confirm those of an earlier trial by Stewart et al. (22) that was not fully randomized.

Taken as a whole, the data suggest that BCG, especially through the intrapleural route, may prolong disease-free interval and survival when used as a postsurgical adjuvant for Stage I lung cancer. However, this improvement is clinically modest, and there is as yet no evidence to indicate that this treatment significantly improves the surgical curve rate. The studies of Perlin et al. (19) and Takita et al. (21) indicate that the addition of allogeneic tumor antigen does not improve the result. Therapeutic outcome may be improved by newer routes of administration, particularly injection of the primary tumor. Holmes et al. (23) and Matthay et al. (24) have proved the feasibility of this approach. Therapy trials are currently in progress.

2.2. Macroscopic Residual Disease Trials

Immunotherapy has been combined with chemotherapy for the treatment of inoperable lung cancer (Table 3). Israel and Edelstein (25) randomized lung

TABLE 3.   Chemoimmunotherapy in Advanced Lung Cancer

	Israel and Edelstein (25)		
Treatment	Chemo[a]	Chemo ∣ C. parvum	
Squamous cell			
Patients (no.)	75	68	
Median survival (months)	4	9	$p < .001$
Oat cell			
Patients (no.)	20	21	
Median survival (months)	5	7	$p < .02$
	Dimitrov et al. (26)		
Treatment	Chemo[b]	Chemo + C. parvum	
Patients (no.)	29	37	
Responses	6	5	
Median survival (months)	7.8	10.7	$p = .06$
	Bjornsson et al. (27)		
Treatment	Chemo[c]	Chemo + C. parvum	
Patients (no.)	17	27	
Responses	5	3	
Median survival (weeks)	20	28	$p = .05$
	McCracken et al. (28)		
Treatment	Chemo[d]	Chemo + BCG	
Patients (no.)	130	144	
Response rate	46%	50%	
Median duration response (weeks)	20	23	
Median survival (weeks)	28	29	

[a] Cyclophosphamide + 5-fluorouracil + methotrexate + vincristine + rufocromycin.

[b] Adriamycin.

[c] Cyclophosphamide + adriamycin + platinum + vincristine.

[d] See text.

cancer patients to treatment with chemotherapy alone or supplemented with *C. parvum* [4 mg subcutaneously (sc) weekly]. For both squamous cell and oat cell carcinoma of the lung, *C. parvum*-treated patients survived longer than those treated with chemotherapy alone. Similarly, Dimitrov et al. (26) randomized 66 patients to chemotherapy alone or in combination with weekly subcutaneous *C. parvum*. The data suggest an improved survival for *C. parvum*-treated patients.

Bjornsson et al. (27) randomized 44 patients to chemotherapy alone or in combination with *C. parvum* [intravenously (iv) starting at a dose of 0.25 mg and escalating to 3.0 mg subsequently]. Response rates were not altered; however, *C. parvum*-treated patients survived significantly longer.

The studies just cited suggest that the addition of *C. parvum* to chemotherapy in Stage III lung cancer can modestly improve survival. The use of BCG in combination with chemotherapy has been even less effective. A Southwest Oncology Group (28) protocol for extensive small cell carcinoma added BCG (Pasteur, 5×10^8 per scarification on day 8 and 15 of each cycle) to chemotherapy with either cyclophosphamide, adriamycin, or vincristine or cyclophosphamide, methotrexate, vincristine, or 5-fluorouracil. Local radiotherapy and prophylactic brain radiation were also administered. The results are shown in Table 3. No improvements were noted in response rate or duration or in survival.

3. MELANOMA

3.1. Local Immunotherapy

In 1970 Morton (29) demonstrated that the injection of live BCG organisms directly into cutaneous melanoma deposits could induce tumor regression in immunocompetent patients. Following his example intralesional BCG therapy for metastatic malignant melanoma was adopted by a large number of investigators. The pooled data of 14 investigators (Table 4) reveal that in approximately 66% of patients treated by intralesional BCG, there was regression of injected nodules, and in 21% of patients there was also regression of uninjected nodules (the latter were mainly in close proximity to injected lesions). Twenty-seven percent of patients experienced complete remission of all clinically evident disease, and this group was composed almost exclusively of immunocompetent individuals with small tumor burdens limited to the dermis. Many investigators have demonstrated that this modality can cause regression of injected and uninjected lesions. These observations are the most clearly demonstrable and readily reproducible evidence for an antitumor effect of immunotherapy.

Immunostimulants other than BCG have been employed intralesionally in the treatment of dermal lesions of recurrent malignant melanoma. The results are summarized in Table 5. The agents, in these small series of patients, have some efficacy and response rates appear similar to those obtained with intra-

TABLE 4. Immunotherapy of Melanoma with Intralesional BCG

| | Regression of Nodules[a] | | Complete | |
Source BCG	Injected	Uninjected	Responders	Reference
Glaxo, Tice	25/90[b]	6/36	11/36	30
?	1/4	1/4	1/4	31
Tice	7/9	2/9	2/9	32
Glaxo	0/1	0/1	0/1	33
Tice, Glaxo	15/25	2/25	2/25	34
Tice, Glaxo	12/15	11/14[c]	7/15	35
Tice	3/7	1/7	?	36
?	2/8?	?	?	37
Tice	1/2	0/2	?	38
Connaught	2/3	1/3	?	39
Tice	4/6	2/6?	3/6	40
Pasteur	7/11?	0/11	?	41
Glaxo	1/2	0/2	0/2	42
Glaxo, Tice	5/5	?	?	43
	85/127 (66%)	26/120 (21%)	26/98 (27%)	

[a] Number of patients showing regression of nodules/total number of patients treated.
[b] Regression on a per patient basis available on only 29 patients.
[c] One patient had only a single nodule.

lesional BCG. It is likely that PPD, MER, CWS + P3, and *C. parvum* have mechanisms of action similar to that of BCG. An obvious advantage over BCG is that these are nonviable materials.

3.2. Systematic Immunotherapy

Adjuvant Studies.   Several historically controlled trials have suggested that postoperative adjuvant BCG was effective in prolonging remission duration and/or survival. These conclusions have been questioned because of the difficulty in demonstrating the comparability of current treatment and historical control groups. Further, it is not possible to compensate for changes in conventional treatment over time. Results of randomized trials are presented in Table 6. Pinsky et al. (49) have conducted a randomized prospective comparison of BCG (Tice; 4 to 6 × 10^7 viable units; Tine technique; weekly × 52, every other week × 26, monthly × 12) versus no treatment following surgery in Stage II melanoma. No benefit was detected. It must be pointed out that the patient population was sufficiently small that a clinical benefit may have been overlooked. Further, the dose of BCG was substantially less than that for which benefit was claimed in earlier historically controlled trials.

Morton (50) performed a randomized prospective trial in Stage II melanoma patients following surgery comparing no treatment with BCG (Tice, 1 to 2 × 10^8 by Tine weekly × 12, then biweekly). Bacillus Calmette-Guerin did not prolong remission duration but favorably influenced survival following re

TABLE 5. Local Immunotherapy of Melanoma with Miscellaneous Microbial Adjuvants

Microbial Adjuvant	Regression of Nodules[a]		Complete Responders	Reference
	Injected	Uninjected		
PPD	1/1	1/1	?	44
MER	12/18	?	6/18	45
C. parvum	6/14[c]	0/14	3/14	46
C. parvum	31/86[d]	?	?	43
CWS + P3[b]	11/23[c]	0/23	?	47
CWS + P3	6/15	4/15	?	48

[a] Number of patients showing regression of nodules per total number patients treated.

[b] CWS + P3: Mycobacterium cell wall skeleton + trehalose dimycolate.

[c] Several patients had tumors other than melanoma.

[d] Number of nodules showing regression in a total of 5 patients.

currence. This has been attributed to an alteration of recurrence patterns towards less ominous sites in BCG-treated patients. Quirt et al. (51) evaluated DTIC + BCG versus an untreated control and found no benefit in Stage I patients. However, as in the study of Morton, treated Stage II patients had improved survival after relapse and experienced fewer systemic relapses than did the control group. Wood et al. (52) evaluated DTIC, BCG, and DTIC + BCG in Stages I and II melanoma patients. Survival of patients treated with DTIC + BCG was superior to that of patients treated with either agent alone. An untreated control was not included. These data suggest a therapeutic advantage for DTIC + BCG. The International Group for the Clinical Study of Melanoma is conducting a four-arm study in Stages I and II melanoma: no treatment versus BCG (lyophylized Pasteur, 75 mg percutaneously) versus DTIC versus DTIC + BCG. All three treatment arms are performing better than the untreated control. This trial has 696 patients entered and should clearly define the role of these adjuvant therapies in the treatment of melanoma.

A new approach is preoperative intralesional adjuvant immunotherapy. Rosenberg et al. (54) randomized 26 high risk Stage I patients to conventional surgical therapy (wide excision plus regional node dissection) with or without preoperative intralesional BCG. With a median follow-up of 3.3 years, significantly fewer recurrences were noted in the BCG-treated patients. These preliminary results, combined with the results of intralesional BCG in dermal melanoma metastases, make this a promising approach to adjuvant therapy.

Macrometastatic Residual Disease Trials

Immunotherapy Alone. Laucius et al. (55) treated 18 patients with surgically incurable metastatic malignant melanoma with a mixture of irradiated (15,000 rads) autologous tumor cells (1 to 2 × 10^8) and BCG (Glaxo, 2 to 4.5

TABLE 6.   BCG Immunostimulation in the Maintenance of Remission in Stages I and II Melanoma Patients

	Pinsky et al. (49)		
Treatment	BCG	Control	
Stage II			
Patients (no.)	24	23	
Median duration remission (weeks)	69	76	
Median survival (weeks)	125	125	
	Morton (50)		
Treatment	BCG	Control	
Stage II			
Patients (no.)	45	46	
Recurrences	26 (57%)	27 (59%)	
Median duration remission (months)	14.4	10.1	
Median survival (months)	23.7	13.8	$p < .01$
	Quirt et al. (51)		
Treatment	DTIC + BCG	Control	
Stage I			
Patients (no.)	29	28	
Relapse rate	33%	43%	
Survival	73%	50%	
Stage II			
Patients (no.)	18	19	
Relapse rate	65%	68%	
Survival	60%	37%	$p = .1$
	Wood et al. (52)		
Treatment	DTIC	BCG	DTIC + BCG
Stages I and II			
Patients (no.)	20	65	56
Recurrences	9 (45%)	17 (26%)	7 (13%)
Deaths	6 (30%)	11 (17%)	3 (5%)
	Rosenberg et al. (54)		
Treatment	BCG	Control	
Stage I			
Patients (no.)	13	13	
Recurrences	5 (38%)	10 (77%)	$p < .05$
Deaths	3 (23%)	6 (46%)	

$\times$ 10^6 organisms), which was injected intradermally every 2 weeks ($\times$ 5). Four of 18 (22%) evaluable patients achieved objective remissions. It was concluded that this treatment regimen does not have general clinical application because the remissions were infrequent, of short duration (median 3 months) and occurred only in patients with minimal, nonvisceral tumor burdens. Nonetheless, biological activity was demonstrated.

Nineteen patients with Stage III melanoma were treated with IV BCG by Orefice et al. (56). A single dose of lyophilized Pasteur BCG ranging from 2×10^7 to 3×10^8 viable units was given in 500 ml of saline infused over 5 to 6 hours. Three of 16 evaluable patients showed objective regression of more than 50% of the original volume lasting 2 to 5 months. The objective remissions were induced at the higher (2×10^8) BCG doses, although toxicity was severe. Only skin, subcutaneous, and lung metastases responded. Israel et al. (57) also observed partial remissions in two of four patients with advanced melanoma treated with IV *C. parvum* (4 mg/day, 5 days/week).

Falk et al. (58) noted objective tumor regression in two of seven patients with disseminated melanoma, treated repeatedly with oral BCG. Of interest is the fact that one of these two responders had bone metastases.

Overall the results achieved with systemic immunotherapy alone are modest. The most encouraging antitumor effects were achieved with IV BCG or *C. parvum.* The fact that any response to biological response modification was seen is impressive.

Chemoimmunotherapy.   The results of relevant chemoimmunotherapy trials in melanoma patients with disseminated diseases are summarized in Table 7. Gutterman and co-workers (59) evaluated the efficacy of dimethyl triazeno imidazole carboxamide (DTIC) plus Pasteur BCG by scarification in 89 patients, using as controls a retrospective group of 111 patients treated with DTIC alone. Patients receiving DTIC-BCG exhibited a response rate significantly greater than patients treated with DTIC alone ($p = .05$). Survival was also greater in the chemoimmunotherapy group ($p = .001$). Patients with lymph node metastases and no evidence of visceral disease were particularly benefited by the DTIC-BCG regimen, demonstrating a remission rate of 55% compared with 18% for controls ($p = .025$). An augmented response in metastatic nodules regional to BCG scarification sites was also noted. The authors speculated that drainage of BCG into regional lymphatics and local tissue potentiated chemotherapy at those sites.

Randomized, prospective studies have yielded conflicting results regarding the efficacy of chemoimmunotherapy regimens compared with chemotherapy alone in melanoma patients. Costanzi et al. (60) evaluated the contribution of BCG to a triple drug regimen (BHD) of 1,3-bis(2-chloroethyl)-1-nitrosourea (BCNU), hydroxyurea, and DTIC. Addition of BCG to the BHD regimen did not result in an enhanced overall response rate. However, BCG patients over age 60 and patients with predominantly pulmonary or lymph node metastases had significantly higher response rates. Analysis by age, sex, and site of disease

TABLE 7.   Chemoimmunotherapy in Disseminated Melanoma[a]

	Gutterman et al. (59)		
Treatment	DTIC-BCG	DTIC	
Patients (no.)	89	111	
Response rate	27%	14.4%	$p = .05$
Median duration remission (months)	6	5	
Median survival (months)	7	5	$p = .001$
Remission rate (1 year)	20%	0	

	Costanzi et al. (60)		
Treatment	DTIC-BCG	BHD-BCG	BHD
Patients (no.)	119	150	82
Response rate	19%	29%	35% NS

	Presant et al. (61)		
Treatment	DTIC-C-CP	DTIC-C	
Patients (no.)	27	29	
Response rate	29%	18%	NS
Median duration remission (weeks)	13	15.6	NS
Median survival (months)	5.7	6.1	NS

	Mastrangelo et al. (62)		
Treatment	M-V-BCG-TC	M-V	
Patients (no.)	31	31	
Response rate	19%	23%	NS
Median duration remission (months)	8	6	NS
Median survival (months)	8.0	6.5	NS

[a] Abbreviations: C, cyclophosphamide; CP, *Corynebacterium parvum;* BHD, BCNU + hydroxyurea + DTIC; M, MeCCNU; V, vincristine; TC, allogeneic tumor cells; NS, $p > .05$.

indicated that patients with pulmonary metastases had significantly longer remission ($p = .04$) and survival ($p = .05$) on BCG. Further, BCG seemed to yield longer survival in patients over 60 years of age ($p = .01$). These observations need confirmation in trials specifically designed to evaluate these points, particularly since only the above-described subsets of patients were shown to benefit from immunotherapy.

Presant and co-workers (61) evaluated *C. parvum* added to a drug regimen of DTIC and cyclophosphamide and observed no difference in response or survival between treatment groups. Mastrangelo and co-workers (62), in a regimen that included BCG and allogeneic tumor cells, failed to demonstrate a greater efficacy of the chemoimmunotherapy regimen.

The addition of currently available immunotherapies to chemotherapy regimens may yield a small biologic effect that is significant in some subgroups and that is of sufficient magnitude to be of continued clinical research interest particularly when more active cytotoxic agents are available.

4. BLADDER CANCER

Morales and co-workers (63) were the first to employ BCG in the prophylaxis and treatment of superficial bladder cancer. Patients who, after resection or fulguration, had at least two recurrences in the preceeding 12 months were eligible for study. Within 10 days after cystoscopy and documentation of recurrence, BCG (Institut Armand Frappier) treatment was started. Bacillus Calmett-Guerin (120 mg in 50 ml of saline) was instilled into the bladder through a catheter and retained for at least 2 hours. At the same time 5 mg of BCG was administered intradermally (Heaf gun). This treatment was repeated weekly for 6 consecutive weeks. Follow-up was by cystoscopy every 3 months. As can be seen from Table 8, there was a sharp decrease in episodes of tumor recurrence following BCG treatment, and 14 of 16 patients remained disease free. Lamm et al. (64) and Camacho et al. (65) used the same strain, dose, route, and schedule of BCG to treat patients with recurrent superficial bladder can-

TABLE 8.   Intravesical BCG in the Treatment of Recurrent Superficial Bladder Cancer

	Morales et al. (63)		
Treatment	Pre-BCG	Post-BCG	
Patients (no.)	16	16	
Median follow up (months)	11	11	
Disease free (no.)	0	14	
Episodes recurrence	47	2	
	Lamm et al. (64)		
Treatment	BCG	Control	
Patients (no.)	23	24	
Disease free (no.)	18	13	
Episodes recurrence	8	19	
Mean time to recurrence (months)	19.4	12	$p = .039$
	Camacho et al. (65)		
Treatment	BCG	Control	
Patients (no.)	22	22	
Tumors per month			
Prestudy	3.60	2.97	
Poststudy	0.75	2.37	
	$p = .001$	$p = .59$	

cer. Experimental design differed in that a randomized conventionally treated control group was included. This permitted comparison of pre- and poststudy episodes of recurrence in individual patients, as was done by Morales, and also afforded an opportunity to compare poststudy recurrence rates in BCG and conventionally treated patients. The results of these two studies, detailed in Table 8, indicate that BCG increases the mean time to recurrence and decreases the number of recurrences and are thus confirmatory of the observations by Morales and co-workers (63). Thus it appears that BCG is of benefit when combined with conventional therapy in the management of recurrent superficial bladder cancer. A more precise estimate of the magnitude of this benefit must await the treatment of a greater number of patients and more prolonged follow-up.

5. HEMATOLOGIC MALIGNANCIES

5.1. Acute Myelogenous Leukemia

Until recently, it was unusual to obtain complete remissions in acute myelogenous leukemia (AML) and difficult to maintain them. With the development of chemotherapy regimens capable of inducing a significant percentage of complete remissions, studies were undertaken to evaluate methods of maintaining these remissions. The results of these trials are summarized in Tables 9 and 10. Crowther et al. (66) investigated four maintenance therapies in 45 patients with AML in whom complete remissions were induced with daunorubicin and cytosine arabinoside. In the first trial maintenance immunotherapy (three, autologous leukemia cells; two, BCG and allogeneic cells; four, BCG alone) was compared to chemotherapy with mercaptopurine and methotrexate (13 patients). Patients who received immunotherapy had remission durations similar to those achieved by patients who received chemotherapy. This trial failed to demonstrate a therapeutic advantage for either remission maintenance regimen or their equivalence. The two longest remissions in the immunotherapy group were patients who received BCG plus irradiated allogeneic tumor cells. This finding prompted the design of trials 2 and 3, in which maintenance chemotherapy (daunorubicin and cytosine arabinoside alternately with thioguanine and cytosine arabinoside, 10 patients) was compared with the same chemotherapy plus BCG (10^6 Glaxo BCG by Heaf gun) and irradiated allogeneic leukemia cells (10^9) weekly (13 patients). The median remission duration for the patients who received only chemotherapy was 30 weeks, whereas patients who received chemoimmunotherapy had a median remission duration in excess of 40 weeks.

These studies were continued and additional trials were designed (4A and 4B) that involved slightly modified ways of administering the induction chemotherapy. Powles et al. (67) reported results 2.5 years after entry of the last patient (Table 9). Remission durations were similar, but overall survival was

TABLE 9.   BCG plus Allogeneic Tumor Cells in Remission Maintenance in Acute Myelogenous Leukemia

	Crowther et al. (66)	
Treatment	BCG and/or TC	MP + MTX
Patients (no.)	9	13
Median duration remission (months)	45	63

	Powles et al. (67)		
Treatment	BCG + TC + DCT	DCT	
Patients (no.)	28	22	
Median duration remission (months)	10	6.4	NS
Median survival (months)	17	9	$p = .03$
Survival after ½ first relapse (months)	5.5	2.5	

	Galton and Peto (68)		
Treatment	BCG + TC + DCT	DCT	
Patients (no.)	47	24	
Median duration remission (months)	8.5	7.0	NS
Median survival (months)	16	13	NS
Survival after first relapse (months)	5.5	3.5	NS

	Reizenstein (69)		
Treatment	BCG + TC + RCT	RCT	
Patients (no.)	(Total of 111)		
Median duration remission (months)	10	6	$p < .05$
Median survival (months)	23	13.6	$p < .001$

	Harris et al. (70)		
Treatment	BCG + TC	Unmaintained	
Patients (no.)	21	20	
Median duration remission (months)	8.8	4.9	$p = .05$
Median survival (months)	22.5	11.5	$p = .032$

[a] Abbreviations: TC, allogeneic tumor cells; MP, mercaptopurine; MTX, methotrexate; DCT, daunomycin + cytosine arabinoside + thioguanine; RCT, rubidomycin + thioguanine + cytosine arabinoside; NS, $p > .05$.

TABLE 10.   BCG in the Maintenance of Remission in Acute Myelogenous Leukemia[a]

	Vogler et al. (72)			
Treatment	BCG[b]	CD	CA + BCG	
Patients (no.)	17	21	22	
Median duration remission (months)	17	10	9	NS
Median survival (months)	18	19	NR	NS

	Omura et al. (73)			
Treatment	BCG[c]	BA	NT	
Patients (no.)	30	35	32	
Median duration remission (months)	6	7	6	NS
Median surival (months)	22	16	16	NS

	Vogler et al. (74)		
Treatment	MTX + BCG[d]	MTX	
Patients (no.)	25	33	
Median duration remission (months)	6.3	3.3	$p < .05$
Median survival (months)	23.3	19.5	NS

	Hewlett et al. (75)		
Treatment	OAP + BCG[e]	OAP	
Patients (no.)	20	25	
Median duration remission (months)	13.5	13.8	NS
Median survival (months)	18.7	30+	NS

	Fiere et al. (76)		
	CMVC +		
Treatment	BCG[f]	CMVC	
Patients (no.)	20	24	
Median duration remission (months)	10	8.6	NS
Median survival (months)	21+	13	NS

	Whittaker and Slatter (77)		
Treatment	CD + BCG[g]	CD	
Patients (no.)	18	17	
Median duration remission (months)	7	5	NS
Median survival (months)	15	11	$p < .02$

[a] Abbreviations: NR, not reached; NT, no treatment; CD, cytosine arabinoside + daunorubicin; BA, BCNU + cytosine arabinoside; MTX, methotrexate; OAP, vincristine + cytosine arabinoside + prednisone; CMVC, cyclophosphamide + methylglyoxal-bis(guanylhydrazone) + vincristine + cytosine arabinoside; NS, $p > .05$.

[b] Tice strain by Heaf gun twice weekly $\times$ 4 weeks, then once every 4 weeks for 1 year.

[c] Tice strain by Tine in all four extremities, twice weekly $\times$ 4, then monthly $\times$ 11.

[d] Tice strain by Tine twice weekly $\times$ 4 weeks.

[e] Pasteur by scarification on day 7, 14, and 21 of each chemotherapy cycle for 1 year, then on days 7 and 21.

[f] Pasteur by Heaf gun at weekly intervals between cycles of chemotherapy.

[g] Glaxo, intravenously, monthly.

significantly improved for patients receiving chemoimmunotherapy. This improvement in overall survival was due to a prolongation of survival after first relapse in the chemoimmunotherapy-treated patients.

In 1973 the British Medical Research council initiated a randomized trial using the same therapies as in the St. Bartholomew's-Royal Marsden trials reported by Powles et al. (67). Seventy-one patients were entered. The results are detailed in Table 9 (68). There is a trend toward improved remission duration and survival in patients receiving chemoimmunotherapy, but these differences are not statistically significant. Similarly, survival after first relapse seems to be prolonged in this group. Two hundred days after relapse, 9 of 34 patients were alive in the chemoimmunotherapy group, compared with 3 of 21 patients maintained with chemotherapy alone.

The Leukemia Group of Central Sweden initiated a randomized trial comparing remission maintenance with chemotherapy alone (cytosine arabinoside plus rubidomycin or thioguanine) or in combination with BCG (Glaxo, 10^6 viable units) plus allogeneic myeloblasts (10^9, nonirradiated, viable). Using a large number of patients, this group (69) was able to demonstrate clear improvements in remission duration and survival for patients who were maintained on chemoimmunotherapy.

These trials suggest that maintenance chemoimmunotherapy modestly prolongs remission duration and survival when compared with maintenance chemotherapy. Only Crowther et al. (66) compared immunotherapy alone with chemotherapy. Despite its randomized design, the small number of patients in the immunotherapy arm and the use of three different immunotherapies hamper interpretation of the results. Harris et al. (70) compared immunotherapy alone with no maintenance therapy. Remission was induced in 41 adults with the use of daunorubicin and cytosine arabinoside. Following consolidation with cyclophosphamide and 6-thioguanine, patients were randomized to maintenance with BCG plus allogeneic leukemic cells or to no maintenance. The results are presented in Table 9. Bacillus Calmette-Guerin + tumor cells were clearly superior to no maintenance. Comparison of immunotherapy alone with the best available maintenance chemotherapy has not been accomplished. Further, since all studies except Crowther et al. (66) involved the use of both BCG and allogeneic cells, it is not possible to determine the contribution of the individual components. However, preliminary results suggest that the addition of neuraminidase-treated allogeneic myeloblasts to maintenance chemotherapy improves remission duration (median 22 months, 30 patients) when compared to chemotherapy alone (median 6 months, 17 patients) in a randomized trial (71).

Studies employing BCG in the maintenance of remission in acute myelogenous leukemia are detailed in Table 10. Vogler et al. (72) and Omura et al. (73) compared percutaneous BCG with chemotherapy alone and found the treatments to be equally effective. Omura et al. (73) included an untreated control group that performed as well as the treated groups, thus suggesting that neither treatment regimen added significantly to the therapeutic efficacy of intensive induction and consolidation chemotherapy. Other investigators (74–76) have combined percutaneous BCG with chemotherapy. Only Vogler et al. (74) were able to demonstrate a therapeutic effect. This study differed from the other two in that BCG treatment was limited to a 4-week period before the initiation of maintenance chemotherapy. Whittaker and Slater (77) have reported on the use of intravenous BCG in combination with chemotherapy. Patients treated with BCG experienced a statistically significant increase in survival of 4 months. None of the chemoimmunotherapy trials included an unmaintained control. It must be concluded from these studies that a therapeutic benefit from percutaneous BCG, if present, is modest. The clinical utility of intravenous BCG requires additional study.

5.2. Acute Lymphatic Leukemia

Although chemotherapy has long been successful in inducing remissions in patients with acute lymphatic leukemia (ALL), until the mid-1960s the duration of first remission and survival were poor, especially in adults. Many investigators initiated trials with BCG in an effort to improve remission duration and survival. The results of these studies are summarized in Table 11. Mathe et al. (78) evaluated active immunotherapy in 30 patients (24 of whom were less than 15 years of age) with ALL. Complete remissions were induced with either prednisone alone or in combination with vincristine and rubidomycin. To further reduce tumor burden, remission induction was followed by sequential complementary chemotherapy. At the end of this phase, all chemotherapy and steroid therapy were terminated. Ten of these patients were then randomly allocated to a control group to which no additional therapy was administered. The remaining 20 patients were randomly allocated to one of the active immunotherapy remission maintenance programs: BCG (Pasteur, 150 mg of fresh pellicle grown) by scarification every fourth day for 1 month and then weekly thereafter (eight patients), allogeneic leukemic lymphoblasts (4×10^7 cells pretreated with formalin or irradiated *in vitro*) subcutaneously weekly (five patients), or both (seven patients). By day 130 all 10 control patients relapsed, whereas only 9 of 20 patients who received some form of immunotherapy relapsed ($p<.02$). Seven of 20 patients in the immunotherapy group have remained in remission for periods of 7 to 10 years (79).

Although no single type of immunotherapy proved superior to the other two, all subsequent trials have included BCG plus allogeneic leukemia cells. In an attempt to further improve results, chemotherapy was intensified, and central nervous system disease was treated prophylactically with intrathecal methotrexate and whole brain irradiation. Different immunostimulants have been added to the standard regimen of BCG plus allogeneic lymphoblasts. Mathe et al. (80) reported the results of the first 100 patients treated with BCG + allogeneic lymphoblasts. The overall 5-year survival is about 50%, and half of these 50 patients are still in first complete unmaintained remission 5 to 10 years after the initiation of immunotherapy. Further, 94% of patients who

TABLE 11.   Immunotherapy in the Maintenance of Remission in Patients with Acute Lymphatic Leukemia[a]

	Mathe et al. (78)		
Treatment	TC and/or BCG	NT	
Patients (no.)	20	10	
Median duration remission (weeks)	36	10.4	$p < .02$

	Mathe et al. (79)		
Treatment	TC + BCG		
Patients (no.)	168		
Median survival (weeks)	138.6		

	BMRC (81)		
Treatment	MTX	BCG or NT	
Patients (no.)	52	52 18	
Median duration remission (weeks)	52	27 17	$p = .01$

	CCSGA (82)		
Treatment (early)	MPV	BCG or NT	
Patients evaluable (no.)	247	28 28	
Relapses	18%	79% 74%	$p < 10^{-6}$
Treatment (late)	MPV	BCG or NT	
Patients evaluable (no.)	48	44 49	
Relapses (6 months)	14%	55% 46%	$p = .006$

	Eckert et al. (83)		
Treatment	MP + CTX + BCG	MP + CTX	
Patients (no.)	8	12	
Relapses (3 years)	3/8	6/12	

	Poplack et al. (84)		
	BCG + TC + Chemo	Chemo [b]	
Treatment			
Patients (no.)	21	35	
Median duration remission (months)	40	38	NS

	Leventhal et al. (85)		
Treatment	MTX + TC	BCG + TC	
Patients (no.)	7	9	
Median duration remission (weeks)	21.6	13.0	NS

TABLE 11.   (Continued)

	Sacks et al. (86)		
Treatment	COAP + RAJI	COAP	
Patients (no.)	8	8	
Median duration remission (weeks)	20.7	24.3	NS

	EORTC (87)		
Treatment	BCG + TC	MP + MTX	
Patients (no.)	28	29	
Median duration remission (weeks)	100	130+	NS
Survival (120 weeks)	88%	81%	NS

[a] Abbreviations: BRMC, British Medical Research Council; CCSGA, Children's Cancer Study Group A; TC, allogeneic tumor cells; NT, no treatment; MTX, methotrexate; MPV, methotrexate + prednisone + vincristine; MP, 6-mercaptopurine; CTX, cyclophosphamide; COAP, cyclophosphamide + cytosine arabinoside + vincristine + prednisone; NS, $p > 0.05$.

[b] See text.

relapsed obtained a second remission. Mathe has emphasized that the morbidity of active immunotherapy has been minimal.

Additional trials were conducted in an attempt to assess the efficacy of BCG alone in the maintenance of remission in patients with ALL (Table 11). The British Medical Research Council (BMRC) (81) studied 122 previously untreated patients (80% less than 10 years of age) with ALL in whom complete remissions were induced with prednisone, vincristine, mercaptopurine, L-asparaginase, and high-dose methotrexate followed by folinic acid. These patients were randomized to three remission maintenance regimens: BCG (Glaxo, freeze dried), one ampule administered by Heaf gun weekly (52 patients); methotrexate twice weekly (52 patients); or no treatment (18 patients). Median remission lengths are presented in Table 11. These data indicate that BCG, when used in this fashion, was no more effective in maintaining remission than was no treatment. On the other hand, methotrexate maintenance appeared superior to both no treatment and BCG.

Between 1970 and 1973 Children's Cancer Study Group A (CCSGA) (82) conducted a randomized controlled trial to evaluate the merits of BCG or chemotherapy at maintaining a drug-induced remission at both "early" and "late" periods during remission. A total of 372 of 502 previously untreated children (less than 16 years old) achieved complete remission after chemotherapy with prednisone, vincristine, and methotrexate. These children were then randomized to one of three primary maintenance arms: no therapy; BCG (Tice strain), 75 mg biweekly for 4 weeks, then weekly until relapse with the multiple puncture technique; or chemotherapy with methotrexate, prednisone, and vincristine. At 7 months 26% of the patients who received no treatment remained in remission, as compared with 21% of patients who received BCG. Patients who received chemotherapy did significantly better, with 82% in remission at 7 months. The median duration of remission was similar (about 4 months) for the BCG and the no-treatment groups.

If BCG or any immunotherapy is more effective when leukemia cells are fewer, one would anticipate a better result when immunotherapy is applied to patients who have remained in chemotherapeutically induced remission for 8 months as opposed to patients who have just completed remission induction and consolidation. To test this point, CCSGA rerandomized patients who maintained their initial remission through 8 months of chemotherapy. Forty-nine patients received no additional maintenance therapy, 44 received BCG, and 48 continued on chemotherapy. At 6 months 45% of the BCG-treated patients and 54% of the untreated patients remained in remission, as compared to 86% of drug-treated patients ($p = .006$).

The studies conducted by the BMRC and the CCSGA failed to confirm the results of Mathe et al. (78). However, the treatment protocols differed from that of the French group in several respects. Although the initial report by Mathe et al. (78) indicated that BCG alone was as effective as BCG plus leukemia cells (3/8 vs. 4/7) in producing long-term remission, all subsequent studies by the French group involved the use of allogeneic tumor cells in addition to BCG. The trials conducted by the other investigators did not employ leukemia cells. Differences in the chemotherapeutic induction regimens are also apparent. For example, in the CCSGA trial the induction regimen was less intense than in the French studies, and, in addition, prophylactic treatment to the central nervous system was not given. The CCSGA and BMRC studies involved the use of lyophilized strains of BCG administered by the multiple puncture technique, whereas Mathe et al. (78) used fresh Pasteur BCG given by scarification; the relative merit of various strains and preparations of BCG and different modes of administration is still questionable, however. A proper test of Mathe's hypothesis that BCG and allogeneic leukemia cells are effective in maintaining remission in ALL patients must await a randomized prospective trial in previously untreated patients that compares optimum chemotherapy, immunotherapy with BCG plus allogeneic cells, and both.

Eckert et al. (83) combined BCG with chemotherapy. Twenty children (median age 5.5 years) with ALL were maintained in complete remission for 1 year with 6-mercaptopurine and cyclophosphamide. At the end of this period 8 patients were assigned to receive intermittent BCG (Pasteur) in addition to the chemotherapy, and the remaining 12 children continued on maintenance chemotherapy alone. At 36 months 5 of 8 chemoimmunotherapy patients and 6 of 12 chemotherapy patients remained in complete remission. In this small study the addition of BCG to chemotherapy did not improve remission duration.

Several groups have included tumor cells plus BCG in their maintenance immunotherapy regimens. Patients with ALL who were less than 20 years of age were induced into complete remission by Poplack et al. (84) with the use of POMP (prednisone, vincristine, methotrexate, 6-mercaptopurine). Once remission was obtained, patients were consolidated with cytosine arabinoside and 6-thioguanine, cranial irradiation, and intrathecal chemotherapy. Maintenance therapy consisted of two parts, A and B. For all patients, part A of maintenance was chemotherapy (vincristine, prednisone, 6-mercaptopurine, methotrexate). Part B was a randomization to (1) methotrexate twice weekly, (2) methotrexate daily × 5 days with 10-day rest intervals, or (3) allogeneic leukemia cells collected from a single donor (4×10^7 intradermal) plus BCG (fresh Pasteur, 1×10^9 over injection site with Heaf gun) weekly × 4. Maintenance parts A and B were alternated for five cycles lasting 34 months. The results of this study indicate that neither the relapse rate nor the duration of remission were statistically different (Table 11). At 48 months of follow-up 42% of the patients were in complete remission and the remission duration curves had plateaued. Although this study was similar to those of Mathe in that it used Pasteur BCG and allogeneic tumor cells, the immunotherapy was intermittent and combined with chemotherapy.

Leventhal et al. (85) used allogeneic tumor cells in two modes of maintenance therapy in a group of 16 previously treated ALL patients (median age 10 years) who achieved a second complete remission. Patients were randomly allocated to maintenance therapy with either BCG (0.5 to 1.0 ml of fresh Pasteur by scarification) plus allogeneic leukemic cells (4×10^7 injected intradermal at a site between BCG vaccination and regional lymph nodes) weekly × 4 and every 4 weeks thereafter or methotrexate (days 1 to 5) plus allogeneic tumor cells (4×10^7) (days 13, 15, 17, and 19 of each 30-day cycle). Remission duration was 21.6 weeks in the methotrexate plus tumor cell group compared with 13.6 weeks in the immunotherapy-alone group. The difference was not statistically significant.

A second study was conducted in patients with at least one relapse. This was based on an apparent antigenic cross-reactivity between ALL cells and the Raji cell line developed from Burkitt's lymphoma. All patients received maintenance chemotherapy with cyclophosphamide, cytosine arabinoside, vincristine, and prednisone. Half were randomized to also receive immunotherapy with 1×10^8 Raji cells (intradermal and subcutaneous) on days 15, 17, and 19 of each 36-day cycle. The results as reported by Sacks (86) show no benefit from immunization.

The European Organization for Research and Treatment of Cancer (EORTC) Hemopathies Working Party (87) initiated a trial in 1971 to compare the best available maintenance chemotherapy (6-mercaptopurine plus methotrexate) with maintenance immunotherapy similar to that of Mathe and his co-workers (78). Two milliliters of fresh Pasteur BCG was administered by scarification twice weekly for 6 months and weekly thereafter. In addition, patients received 4×10^7 allogeneic nonirradiated leukemic blasts every week for 3 months and then once monthly. Eleven of 28 patients on immunotherapy have relapsed, compared with 4 of 29 patients on chemotherapy. However, four of the patients on chemotherapy died in complete remission, and three expired from infections. Further, patients who have relapsed on immunotherapy have had second long-term remissions induced with chemotherapy. Thus, in terms of survival, there is little difference: 26 of 28 on immunotherapy as opposed to 25 of 29 on chemotherapy.

It seems clear that, as studied, BCG either alone or in combination with chemotherapy does not improve remission duration or survival in ALL. The therapeutic efficacy of tumor cells (with or without chemotherapy) has not been adequately evaluated. Mathe's contention that tumor cells plus BCG prolong survival in ALL has been validated in part by the EORTC trial, which has demonstrated the equivalence of this regimen with maintenance chemotherapy. The question that remains is whether these maintenance regimens alone or in combination add to the survival benefits achieved with modern induction and consolidation chemotherapy.

5.3. Lymphomas

Hoerni et al. (88) induced complete remissions in patients with non-Hodgkin's lymphoma of an aggressive histology (e.g., immunoblastic) or advanced (Stage III or IV) using cyclophosphamide and prednisone (with or without adriamycin or VM-26). Radiotherapy was also employed. Following induction of complete remission patients were randomized to serve as unmaintained controls or to receive BCG (Pasteur by scarification weekly for 3 years). Response data are shown in Table 12. There were significantly fewer relapses in BCG maintained Stage I patients. Further, the death rate overall was significantly lower in the BCG-maintained patients.

TABLE 12. BCG in the Treatment of Lymphomas[a]

	Hoerni et al. (88)		
Treatment	BCG	NT	
Patients (no.)	20	23	
Relapses: Stage I	0/9	5/9	
II	2/5	4/6	
III and IV	1/6	4/8	
Overall	3	13	$p < .025$
Deaths	1	8	

	Jones et al. (89)		
Treatment	CHOP + BCG	CHOP + Bl	COP + Bl
Patients (no.)	65	66	75
Complete responders	75%	67%	71%
Median duration remission (weeks)	104	130	104	NS
Survival (130 weeks)	95%	70%	35%	NS

[a]Abbreviations: NS, $p > .05$; CHOP, cyclophosphamide, adriamycin, vincristine, prednisone; COP, cyclophosphamide, vincristine, prednisone; Bl, Bleomycin.

Although this was a randomized trial, these encouraging data must be evaluated with a consideration of other problems in study design: clinical staging was not optimal, chemotherapy regimens varied, and sex distribution was not equal between groups.

Previously untreated (with chemotherapy) patients with Stages III and IV non-Hodgkin's nodular lymphoma were randomly assigned to one of three induction regimens: CHOP + BCG, CHOP + Bleomycin, or COP + Bleomycin. Highly viable Pasteur BCG was reconstituted from lyophilized vaccine $(6 \pm 4 \times 10^8$ viable units) just prior to use and administered by scarification on days 8 and 15 of each 21-day treatment cycle. The response data as reported by Jones et al. (89), detailed in Table 12, reveal that BCG did not improve response rates or increase remission duration. There is a trend toward improved survival when CHOP + BCG is compared with CHOP + bleomycin ($p = .08$). The results, although not yet significant at the $p<.05$ level, are encouraging.

6. SUMMARY

The regression of injected and uninjected dermal melanoma metastases is the most clearly demonstrable and readily reproducible evidence for an antitumor effect of immunotherapy.

The role of microbial products as postsurgical adjuvants is slowly being resolved. It appears that a slight therapeutic effect is discernable. Intrapleural BCG appears to increase survival in Stage I non-oat cell carcinoma of the lung with minimal cost and negligible morbidity.

A seemingly bewildered array of trials have been conducted to evaluate BCG (with or without allogeneic tumor cells) as maintenance therapy in the treatment of leukemias. Despite this, firm conclusions remain elusive.

An overall assessment of the chemoimmunotherapy data in patients with disseminated disease suggests a modest biological effect as evidenced by improved survival.

On the basis of the guinea pig hepatoma model and encouraging results in dermal melanoma metastases, intralesional BCG has been extended to treatment of the primary tumor. Studies in cutaneous melanoma and superficial bladder cancer suggest that this is a promising new direction for research with microbial adjuvants.

REFERENCES

1. H. C. Nauts, The apparently beneficial effects of bacterial infections on host resistance to cancer: End results in 435 cases. *N. Y. Cancer Res. Inst. Monogr.*, **8**, 1 (1969).
2. R. P. Villasor, The clinical use of BCG vaccine in stimulating host resistance to cancer. *J. Philippine Med. Assoc.*, **41**, 619 (1965).
3. J. F. Laucius, A. J. Bodurtha, M. J. Mastrangelo, and R. H. Creech, Bacillus Calmette-Guerin in the treatment of neoplastic disease. *J. Reticuloendothel. Soc.*, **16**, 347 (1974).

4. M. S. Mitchell and R. I. Murahata, Modulation of immunity by Bacillus Calmette-Guerin. *Pharmacol. Ther.*, **4**, 329 (1979).

5. B. Zbar, I. D. Bernstein, and H. J. Rapp, Suppression of tumor growth at the site of injection and living Bacillus Calmette-Guerin. *J. Natl. Cancer Inst.*, **46**, 831 (1971).

6. C. Pinsky, Y. Hirshaut, and H. Oettgen, Treatment of malignant melanoma by intratumoral injection of BCG. *Proc. Am. Assoc. Cancer Res.*, **13**, 21 (1972).

7. A. R. Prevot, Bacteriological Aspects of anaerobic corynebacteria in relation to RES stimulation. In B. Halpern, Ed., *Corynebacterium parvum. Applications in Experimental and Clinical Oncology*, Plenum, New York, 1975, pp. 3–10.

8. D. Berd, Effects of *Corynebacterium parvum* on immunity. *Pharmac. Ther. A.*, **2**, 373 (1978).

9. M. F. A. Woodruff and J. C. Boak, Inhibitory effect of injection of *Corynebacterium parvum* on the growth of tumor transplants in isogeneic hosts. *Br. J. Cancer*, **20**, 345 (1966).

10. H. F. Oettgen, C. M. Pinsky, and L. Delmonte, Treatment of cancer with immuno-modulators *Corynebacterium parvum* and levamisole. *Med. Clin. North Am.*, **60**, 511 (1976).

11. McKneally, C. Maver, L. Lininger, H. W. Kausel, M. B. McIlduff, T. M. Older, E. D. Foster, and R. D. Alley, Four year follow-up on the Albany experience with intrapleural BCG in lung cancer, *J. Thor. Cardiovasc. Surg.*, **81**, 485 (1981).

12. P. W. Wright, L. D. Hill, A. V. Peterson, R. P. Anderson, S. P. Hammer, L. P. Johnson, E. H. Morgan, and R. D. Pinkham, Adjuvant immunotherapy with intrapleural BCG and levamisole in patients with resected, non-small cell lung cancer. In *Proceedings of the Second International Conference on the Immunotherapy of Cancer*, Bethesda, Md., 4/28–30/80.

13. J. Lowe, P. B. Iles, D. R. Shore, M. J. S. Langman, and R. W. Baldwin, Intrapleural BCG in operable lung cancer. In *Proceedings of the Second International Conference on the Immunotherapy of Cancer*, Bethesda, Md., 4/28–30/80.

14. J. Stjernsward, Adjuvant immunotherapy in operable lung cancer. In *Proceedings of the Second International Conference on the Immunotherapy of Cancer*, Bethesda, Md., 4/28–30/80.

15. A. B. Miller, H. E. Taylor, M. A. Baker, D. J. Dodds, R. Falk, A. Frappier, D. P. Hill, A. Jindani, S. Landi, A. S. MacDonald, J. W. Thomas, and C. Wall. Oral administration of BCG as an adjuvant to surgical treatment of carcinoma of the bronchus. *Can. Med. Assoc. J.*, **121**, 45 (1979).

16. P. Pouillart, T. Palangie, M. Jouve, and E. Garcia-Giralt, Systemic BCG in squamous cell lung cancer. In S. E. Jones and S. E. Salmon, Eds., *Adjuvant Therapy of Cancer II*, Grune and Stratton, New York, 1979, pp. 553–560.

17. F. R. Edwards, Use of BCG as an immunostimulant after resection of carcinoma of the lung: A two year assessment of a trial of 500 patients. *Thorax*, **34**, 801 (1979).

18. P. Roscoe, S. Pearce, S. Ludgate, and N. W. Horne, A controlled trial of BCG immunotherapy in bronchogenic carcinoma treated by surgical resection. *Cancer Immunol. Immunother.*, **3**, 115 (1977).

19. E. Perlin, R. K. Oldham, J. L. Weese, W. Heim, J. Reid, M. Mills, C. Miller, J. Blom, D. Green, S. Bellinger, G. B. Cannon, I. Law, R. Connor, and R. B. Herberman, Carcinoma of the lung: Immunotherapy with intradermal BCG and allogeneic tumor cells. *Internatl. J. Rad. Oncol. Biol. Phys.*, **6**, 1033 (1980).

20. H. M. Jansen, T. H. The, and N. G. M. Orie, Adjuvant immunotherapy with BCG in squamous cell bronchial carcinoma. *Thorax*, **35**, 781 (1980).

21. H. Takita, A. C. Hollinshead, F. Edgerton, J. N. Bhagava, R. M. Moskowitz, R. H. Adler, M. Ramundo, T. Han, R. G. Vincent, D. Conway, and L. Takita, Adjuvant active immunotherapy of squamous cell lung carcinoma. In *Proceedings of the Second International Conference on the Immunotherapy of Cancer*, Bethesda, Md., 4/28–30/80.

22. T. H. M. Stewart, A. C. Hollinshead, J. E. Harris, S. Raman, R. Belanger, A. Crepeau, A. F. Crook, W. E. Hirte, D. Hooper, D. Klaassen, E. F. Rapp, and H. J. Sachs, Specific active immunochemotherapy in lung cancer: A survival study. *Can. J. Surg.*, **20**, 370 (1977).

23. E. C. Holmes, K. P. Ramming, M. E. Bein, and W. F. Coulson, Intralesional BCG immunotherapy of pulmonary tumors. *J. Thor. Cardiovasc. Surg.*, **77**, 362 (1979).

24. R. A. Matthay, D. A. Mahler, M. S. Mitchell, D. H. Carter, J. Loke, H. Y. Renolds, and A. E. Baue, Intratumoral BCG immunotherapy prior to surgery for lung cancer. In *Proceedings of the Second International Conference on the Immunotherapy of Cancer*, Bethesda, Md., 4/28–30/80.

25. L. Israel and R. L. Edelstein, Non-specific immunostimulation with *Corynebacterium parvum* in human cancer. In *Immunological Aspects of Neoplasia*, Williams and Wilkins, Baltimore, 1975, pp. 489–493.

26. N. V. Dimitrov, J. Conroy, L. G. Suhrland, T. Singh, and H. Teitlebaum, Combination therapy with *Corynebacterium parvum* and doxorubicin hydrochloride in patients with lung cancer. In W. D. Terry and D. Windhorst, Eds., *Immunotherapy of Cancer: Current Status of Trials in Man*, Raven, New York, 1978, pp. 181–190.

27. S. Bjornsson, H. Takita, N. Kuberka, H. Preisler, H. Catane, D. Higby, and E. Henderson. Combination chemotherapy plus methanol extracted residue of Bacillus Calmette-Guerin or *Corynebacterium parvum* in stage III lung cancer. *Cancer Treat. Rep.*, **62**, 505 (1978).

28. J. D. McCracken, L. Heilbrum, J. White, R. Reed, M. Samson, J. H. Saiexs, R. Stephens, W. J. Stuckey, J. Bickers, and R. Livingston, Combination chemotherapy, radiotherapy, and BCG immunotherapy in extensive (metastatic) small cell carcinoma of the lung. A Southwest Oncology Group study. *Cancer,* **46**, 2335 (1980).

29. D. L. Morton, F. R. Eilber, W. L. Joseph, W. C. Wood, E. Trahan, and A. S. Ketcham. Immunological factors in human sarcomas and melanomas. *Ann. Surg.*, **172**, 740 (1970).

30. D. L. Morton, F. R. Eilber, R. A. Malmgren, and W. C. Wood, Immunological factors which influence response to immunotherapy in malignant melanoma. *Surgery*, **68**, 158 (1970).

31. E. T. Krementz, M. S. Samuels, and J. H. Wallace, Clinical experience in the immunotherapy of cancer. *Surg. Gynecol. Obstet.*, **133**, 209 (1971).

32. L. Nathanson, Regression of intradermal melanoma after intralesional injection of Mycobacterium bovis strain BCG. *Cancer Chemother. Rep.*, **56**, 659 (1972).

33. N. L. Levy, M. S. Mahaley, Jr., and E. D. Day, Serum-mediated blocking of cell-mediated antitumor immunity in a melanoma patient: Association with BCG immunotherapy and clinical deterioration. *Internatl. J. Cancer*, **10**, 44 (1972).

34. C. M. Pinsky, Y. Hirshaut, and H. F. Oettgen, Treatment of malignant melanoma by intratumoral injection of BCG, *Natl. Cancer Inst. Monogr.*, **39**, 225 (1973).

35. M. J. Mastrangelo, H. L. Sulit, L. M. Prehn, R. S. Bornstein, J. W. Yarbro, and R. T. Prehn, Intralesional BCG in the treatment of metastatic malignant melanoma. *Cancer*, **37**, 684 (1976).

36. G. V. Smith, P. A. Morse, Jr., G. D. Deraps, S. Raju, and J. D. Hardy, Immunotherapy of patients with cancer. *Surgery*, **74**, 59 (1973).

37. J. R. Minton, Mumps virus and BCG vaccine in metastatic melanoma. *Arch. Surg.*, **106**, 503 (1973).

38. M. A. Baker and R. N. Taub, BCG in malignant melanoma. *Lancet*, **1**, 1117 (1973).

39. E. Klein, O. A. Holterman, B. Papermaster, H. Milgrom, D. Rosner, L. Klein, M. J. Walker, and B. Zbar, Immunologic approaches to various types of cancer with the use of BCG and purified protein derivatives. *Natl. Cancer Inst. Monogr.*, **39**, 229 (1973).

40. R. Lieberman, J. Wybran, and W. Epstein, The immunologic and histopathologic changes in BCG-mediated tumor regression in patients with malignant melanoma. *Cancer*, **35**, 756 (1975).

41. L. Israel, A. Depierre, and R. Edelstein, Effect of intranodular BCG in 22 melanoma patients. In *Proceedings IV International Symposium on the Locoregional Treatment of Tumors*, Turin, Italy, UICC, 9/19-21/73.

42. R. M. Grant, R. Mackie, A. J. Cochran, E. L. Murray, D. Hoyle, and C. Ross, Results of administering BCG to patients with melanoma. *Lancet*, **2**, 1096 (1974).

43. M. H. Cohen, E. Felix, J. Jessup, and S. Rosenberg, Treatment of metastatic melanoma by intralesional injection of BCG, organic chemicals and *C. parvum*. In R. G. Crispen, Ed., *Neoplasm Immunity Mechanism*, Franklin Institute Press, Philadelphia, 1975, pp. 121-134.

44. G. Tisman, S. J. G. Wu, and G. E. Safire, Intralesional PPD in malignant melanoma. *Lancet*, **1**, 161 (1975).

45. S. E. Krown, E. Y. Hilal, C. M. Pinsky, Y. Hirshaut, H. S. Wanebo, J. A. Hansen, A. G. Huvos, and H. F. Oettgen, Intralesional injection of the methanol extraction residue of Bacillus Calmette-Guerin (MER) into cutaneous metastases of malignant melanoma. *Cancer*, **42**, 2648 (1978).

46. W. F. Cunningham-Rundles, Y. Hirshaut, C. M. Pinsky, and H. F. Oettgen, Phase I trial of intralesional *C. parvum*. *Clin. Res.*, **26**, 337A (1978).

47. S. P. Richman, J. U. Gutterman, E. M. Hersh, and E. E. Ribi, Phase I-II study of intratumor immunotherapy with BCG cell wall skeleton plus P3. *Cancer Immunol. Immunother.*, **5**, 41 (1978).

48. G. J. Vosika, J. R. Schmidtke, A. Goldman, E. Ribi, R. Parker, and G. R. Gray, Intralesional immunotherapy of malignant melanoma with *Myobacterium smegmatis* cell wall skeleton combined with trehalose dimycolate (P3). *Cancer*, **44**, 495 (1979).

49. C. M. Pinsky, Y. Hirshaut, H. J. Wanebo, E. Y. Hilal, J. G. Fortner, V. Mike, D. Schottenfeld, and H. F. Oettgen, Surgical adjuvant immunotherapy with BCG in patients with malignant melanoma: Results of a prospective randomized trial. In W. D. Terry and D. Windhorst, Eds., *Immunotherapy of Cancer: Current Status of Trials in Man,* Raven, New York, 1978, pp. 27-33.

50. D. L. Morton, Adjuvant immunotherapy of malignant melanoma: Results of a randomized trial. In *Proceedings of the Second International Conference on the Immunotherapy of Cancer,* Bethesda, Md., 4/28-30/80.

51. I. Quirt, P. Kersey, M. Baker, A. Bodurtha, M. King. S. Norvell, D. Osoba, P. Dent, and P. McCulloch, A comparison of adjuvant chemoimmunotherapy with observation alone in patients with poor prognosis primary melanoma and completely resected recurrent melanoma. In *Proceedings of the Second International Conference on Immunotherapy of Cancer,* Bethesda, Md., 4/28-30/80.

52. W. C. Wood, A. B. Cosimi, R. W. Carey, and S. D. Kaufman, Adjuvant chemoimmunotherapy in stage I and II melanoma. In *Proceedings of the Second International Conference on the Immunotherapy of Cancer,* Bethesda, Md., 4/28-30/80.

53. G. Beretta, Randomized study of prolonged chemotherapy, immunotherapy and chemoimmunotherapy as an adjuvant to surgery for Stage I and II malignant melanoma. In *Proceedings of the Second International Conference on the Immunotherapy of Cancer,* Bethesda, Md., 4/28-30/80.

54. S. A. Rosenberg, H. Rapp, W. Terry, B. Zbar, J. Costa, C. Seipp, and R. Simon, Intralesional BCG therapy of patients with primary stage I melanoma. In *Proceedings of the Second International Conference on the Immunotherapy of Cancer,* Bethesda, Md., 4/28-30/80.

55. J. F. Laucius, A. J. Bodurtha, M. J. Mastrangelo, and R. E. Bellet, A phase II study of autologous irradiated tumor cells plus BCG in patients with metastatic melanoma. *Cancer*, **40**, 2091 (1977).

56. S. Orefice, N. Cascinelli, M. Vaglini, and U. Veronesi, Intravenous administration of BCG in advanced melanoma patients. *Tumori*, **64**, 437 (1978).

57. L. Israel, R. Edelstein, A. Depierre, and N. Dimitrov, Daily intravenous infusions of *Corynebacterium parvum* in twenty patients with disseminated cancer. *J. Natl. Cancer Inst.*, **55**, 29 (1975).

58. R. E. Falk, P. Mann, and B. Largen, Cell-mediated immunity to human tumors. *Arch. Surg.*, **107**, 261 (1973).

59. J. U. Gutterman, G. Mavligit, J. A. Gottlieb, M. A. Burgess, C. E. McBride, L. Einhorn, E. J. Freireich, and E. M. Hersh, Chemoimmunotherapy of disseminated malignant melanoma with dimethyl triazeno imidazole carboxamide and Bacillus Calmette-Guerin. *New Engl. J. Med.*, **291**, 529 (1974).

60. J. J. Costanzi, M. Al-Sarraf, and D. O. Dixon, Chemoimmunotherapy of disseminated melanoma. *Proc. Am. Assoc. Clin. Oncol.*, **20**, 362 (1979).

61. C. A. Presant, A. A. Bartolucci, R. V. Smalley, and W. R. Vogler, Cyclophosphamide plus 5-(3,3-dimethyl-1-triazeno) imidazole-4-carboxamide (DTIC) with or without *Corynebacterium parvum* in metastatic malignant melanoma. *Cancer,* **44**, 899 (1979).

62. M. J. Mastrangelo, R. E. Bellet, and D. Berd, A phase II comparison of methyl-CCNU + vincristine with or without BCG + allogeneic tumor cells in malignant melanoma. *Cancer Immunol. Immunother.*, **6**, 231 (1979).

63. A. Morales, D. Eidinger, and A. W. Bruce, Adjuvant BCG immunotherapy in recurrent superficial bladder cancer. In W. D. Terry and D. Windhorst, Eds., *Immunotherapy of Cancer: Current Status of Trials in Man*, Raven, New York, 1978, pp. 225–230.

64. D. Lamm, D. E. Thor, S. C. Harris, V. D. Stogdill, and H. M. Radwin, Intravesical and percutaneous BCG immunotherapy of recurrent superficial bladder cancer. In *Proceedings of the Second International Conference on the Immunotherapy of Cancer*, Bethesda, Md., 4/28–30/80.

65. F. Camacho, C. Pinsky, D. Kerr, W. Whitmore, and H. Oettgen, Treatment of superficial bladder cancer with intravesical BCG. In *Proceedings of the Second International Conference on the Immunotherapy of Cancer*, Bethesda, Md., 4/28–30/80.

66. D. Crowther, R. L. Powles, C. J. T. Bateman, M. E. J. Beard, C. J. Gauci, P. F. M. Wrigley, J. S. Molpas, G. Hamilton-Fairley, and R. B. Scott, Management of adult acute myelogenous leukemia. *Br. Med. J.*, **1**, 131 (1973).

67. R. L. Powles, J. Russell, T. A. Lister, T. Oliver, J. M. A. Whitehouse, J. Malzar, B. Chapuis, D. Crowther, and P. Alexander, Immunotherapy for acute myelogenous leukemia: Analysis of a controlled clinical study 2½ years after entry of the last patient. In W. D. Terry and D. Windhorst, Eds., *Immunotherapy of Cancer: Present Status of Trials in Man*, Raven, New York, 1978, pp. 315–327.

68. D. A. G. Galton and R. Peto, Immunotherapy of acute myeloid leukemia. *Br. J. Cancer,* **37**, 1 (1978).

69. P. Reizenstein, BCG plus leukemic cell therapy of patients with acute myeloid leukemia. In *Proceedings of the Second International Conference on the Immunotherapy of Cancer*, Bethesda, Md., 4/28–30/80.

70. R. Harris, S. R. Zuhrie, A. P. Read, C. B. Freeman, J. E. McIver, C. C. Geary, I. W. Delamore, and J. A. Tooth, A randomized trial of immunotherapy alone versus no maintenance treatment in adult acute myelogenous leukemia. In *Proceedings of the Second International Conference on the Immunotherapy of Cancer*, Bethesda, Md., 4/28–30/80.

71. J. F. Holland, J. G. Bekesi, J. Cuttner, and O. Glidewell, Chemoimmunotherapy of acute myelocytic leukemia with neuraminidase treated allogeneic myeloblasts. In *Proceedings of the Second International Conference on the Immunotherapy of Cancer*, Bethesda, Md., 4/28–30/80.

72. W. R. Vogler, E. F. Winton, D. S. Gordon, R. Jarrell, and L. Lefante, A phase III trial comparing BCG, cytosine arabinoside and daunorubicin for maintenance therapy in acute myeloblastic leukemia. In *Proceedings of the Second International Conference on the Immunotherapy of Cancer*, Bethesda, Md., 4/28–30/80.

73. G. A. Omura, W. R. Vogler, and J. Lefante, BCG immunotherapy of acute myelogenous leukemia. In *Proceedings of the Second International Conference on the Immunotherapy of Cancer,* Bethesda, Md., 4/28-30/80.

74. W. R. Vogler, A. A. Bartolucci, G. A. Omura, D. Miller, R. V. Smalley, W. H. Knospe, and A. S. Goldsmith, A randomized clinical trial of BCG in myeloblastic leukemia. In W. D. Terry and D. Windhorst, Eds., *Immunotherapy of Cancer: Present Status of Trials in Man,* Raven, New York, 1978, pp. 365-373.

75. J. S. Hewlett, S. Balcerzak, J. U. Gutterman, E. J. Freireich, E. A. Gehan, and A. Kennedy, Remission maintenance in adult acute leukemia with and without BCG. A Southwest Oncology Group study. In W. D. Terry and D. Windhorst, Eds., *Immunotherapy of Cancer: Present Status of Trials in Man,* Raven, New York, 1978, pp. 323-391.

76. D. Fiere, M. Doillon, C. Martin, T. VuVan, and L. Revol, Chemoimmunotherapy versus chemotherapy in acute myeloid leukemia. Preliminary results. *Biomedicine, 25,* 318 (1976).

77. J. A. Whittaker and A. J. Slater, Immunotherapy of acute myelogenous leukemia using intravenous BCG. In W. D. Terry and D. Windhorst, Eds., *Immunotherapy of Cancer: Present Status of Trials in Man,* Raven, New York, 1978, pp. 393-404.

78. G. Mathe, J. L. Amiel, L. Schwarzenberg, M. Schneider, A. Cattan, J. R. Schlumberger, M. Hayat, and F. DeVassal, Active immunotherapy for acute lymphoblastic leukemia. *Lancet, 1,* 697 (1969).

79. G. Mathe, L. Schwarzenberg, J. L. Amiel, P. Pouillart, M. Hayat, F. DeVassal, C. Rosenfeld, and E. Jasmin, New experimental and clinical data on leukemia immunotherapy. *Proc. Roy. Soc. Med., 68,* 211 (1975).

80. G. Mathe, F. DeVassal, M. Delgado, P. Pouillart, D. Belpomme, R. Joseph, L. Schwarzenberg, J. L. Amiel, M. Schneider, A. Cattan, M. Musset, J. L. Misset, and C. Jasmin, Current results of the first 100 cytologically typed acute lymphoid leukemia submitted to BCG active immunotherapy. *Cancer Immunol. Immunother., 1,* 77 (1976).

81. Medical Research Council, Treatment of acute lymphoblastic leukemia, Comparison of immunotherapy (BCG), intermittent methotrexate and no therapy after a five month intensive cytotoxic regimen (Concord Trial). Preliminary report to the Medical Research Council by the Leukemia Committee and the Working Party on Leukemia in Childhood. *Br. Med. J., 4,* 189 (1971).

82. R. M. Heyn, P. Joo, M. Karon, M. Nesbit, N. Shore, N. Breslow, J. Weiner, P. H. Reed, H. Sather, and D. Hammond, BCG in the treatment of acute lymphocytic leukemia. In W. D. Terry and D. Windhorst, Eds., *Immunotherapy of Cancer: Present Status of Trials in Man,* Raven, New York, 1978, pp. 503-512.

83. H. Eckert, D. G. Jose, F. C. Wilson, R. N. Matthews, and H. Lay, Intermittent chemotherapy and immunotherapy with BCG in remission maintenance of children with acute lymphocytic leukemia: Effects upon immunological function. *Internatl. J. Cancer, 16,* 103 (1975).

84. D. G. Poplack, B. G. Leventhal, R. Simon, T. Pomeroy, R. G. Graw, and E. S. Henderson, Treatment of acute lymphatic leukemia with chemotherapy alone or chemotherapy plus immunotherapy. In W. D. Terry and D. Windhorst, Eds., *Immunotherapy of Cancer: Current Status of Trials in Man,* Raven, New York, 1978, pp. 497-501.

85. B. G. Leventhal, A. LePourhiet, R. H. Halterman, E. S. Henderson, and R. B. Herberman, Immunotherapy in previously treated acute lymphatic leukemia. *Natl. Cancer Inst. Monogr., 39,* 177 (1973).

86. K. L. Sacks, C. Olweny, D. L. Mann, R. Simon, G. E. Johnson, D. G. Poplack, and B. G. Leventhal, A clinical trial of chemotherapy and RAJI immunotherapy in advanced acute lymphatic leukemia. *Cancer Res., 35,* 3715 (1975).

87. J. M. Andrien, M. P. Beumer-Jockmans, J. Bury, J. L. David, G. Delalieux, M. J. Delbeke, R. Denolin, P. DePoree, D. Fiere, G. Flowerdew, S. L. George, H. Hainaut, J. Hughes, Y.

Kenis, R. Masure, R. Maurus, J. Michel, J. Otten, M. E. Peetermans, M. Reginster-Bous, P. A. Stryckmans, R. Sylvester, M. Van Glabbeke, W. Van Hove, L. Verbist, A. Wenner-holm, and H. Williaert, Immunotherapy versus chemotherapy as maintenance treatment of acute lymphoblastic leukemia. In W. D. Terry and D. Windhorst, Eds., *Immunotherapy of Cancer: Current Status of Trials in Man,* Raven, New York, 1978, pp. 471–481.

88. B. Hoerni, M. Durand, P. Richaud, A. DeMascarel, G. Hoerni-Simon, J. Chauvergne, and C. Lagardi, Successful immunotherapy by BCG of non-Hodgkin's malignant lymphoma. *Br. J. Haematol.*, **42**, 507 (1979).

89. S. E. Jones, S. E. Salmon, and R. Risher, Adjuvant Immunotherapy with BCG in non-Hodgkin's lymphoma: A Southwest Oncology Group controlled clinical trial. In S. E. Jones and S. E. Salmon, Eds., *Adjuvant Therapy of Cancer II,* Grune and Stratton, New York, 1979, pp. 163–171.

Immunomodulation by Synthetic Muramyl Peptides and Trehalose Diesters

E. LEDERER
L. CHEDID
Laboratoire de Biochimie, CNRS, Gif sur Yvette
and Institut de Biochimie
Université de Paris-Sud, Centre d'Orsay
Laboratoire d'Immunothérapie Expérimentale
Institut Pasteur Paris

1. INTRODUCTION

The immune system is responsive to an unlimited number of endogenous and exogenous stimulations. Several exogenous products have been found to influence the immune response without the host having been directly or phylogenetically exposed to them previously. Such is the case of various immunosuppressors such as cyclophosphamide and certain adjuvants such as aluminum hydroxide. Another class of exogenous products that interact continuously with the host is represented by various parasitic agents; among these bacteria, viruses, and to a lesser degree fungi have been extensively investigated. Microorganisms or microbial products have been studied intensively and repeatedly shown to enhance the natural resistance of the host to various tumors. Since immunotherapy with microbial products or other synthetic agents are reviewed in separate chapters, we have chosen to focus our attention on synthetic immunostimulants structurally derived from bacterial cell walls. We limit ourselves to a review of *muramyl peptides* and *trehalose diesters.*

Bacillus Calmette-Guerin (BCG) has been widely used in the laboratory and in clinics as an adjuvant for the stimulation of host immunity, in particular in cancer therapy. However, since viable BCG (1,2) even killed mycobacteria (3) can lead to untoward effects, research for active nonviable mycobacterial components has been actively pursued. A methanol extraction residue (MER) of BCG has been widely studied by Weiss et al. (4) and is presently in limited clinical use; it is, however, also not completely free of side effects (5).

The first well-defined immunoactive mycobacterial constituent that was identified is "cord factor" isolated in 1950 as "toxic lipid" by Bloch (6). It was shown to be a 6,6′-dimycolate of trehalose (7), and analogous trehalose diesters were found in related microorganisms, such as Nocardiae (8,9) and Corynebacteria (10). However, interesting immunoadjuvant properties of "cord factor" were discovered only much later by Bekierkunst (11).

The further identification of active components of mycobacterial cells was greatly facilitated by the finding that carefully purified mycobacterial cell walls had full adjuvant activity in Freund's incomplete adjuvant (12). Bacillus Calmette-Guerin cell walls can also replace whole living BCG for complete tumor regression in guinea pigs by intralesional injection in emulsion with paraffin oil (13).

A detailed study of the chemical structure of mycobacterial cell walls (14) and their hydrolysis products then led to the isolation of the first water-soluble adjuvant (WSA) (15,16) and finally to the preparation of smaller peptidoglycan fragments in which a *N*-acylated muramic acid moiety was linked to typical cell wall peptides containing an L-alanyl-D-glutamyl moiety (17). It was shown in 1974 that synthetic *N*-acetyl-muramyl-L-alanyl-D-isoglutamine* (MDP, for muramyl dipeptide) (**1**) was the minimal structure capable of replacing whole killed mycobacteria in complete Freund's adjuvant (18,19). The chemistry of these structures has been reviewed by several investigators (20–26). Here we restrict ourselves to a short description of the basic facts about structure-activity relationships of these compounds and their mechanism of action at the cellular level and dwell in more detail on their application to experimental tumor models.

MDP

1

2. MURAMYL DIPEPTIDES

2.1. Structure-Activity Relationships of MDP and Derivatives

Since the first synthesis of MDP several hundred analogues and derivatives have been synthesized; the extraordinary flexibility of the molecule has allowed the tailoring of compounds having various types of biological activity. The chemistry of these agents has been discussed in detail in recent reviews (24–26).

---

*Muramic acid, a typical constituent of bacterial cell walls, is the 3-*O*-D-lactyl ether of D-glucosamine. In most bacterial cell walls it is *N*-acetylated, and in mycobacteria and Nocardiae it is *N*-glycolylated (14).

The *carbohydrate* moiety can be simplified, giving nor-MDP (in which the methyl group of the lactyl side chain of muramic acid is replaced by a hydrogen atom (27). Although less active in some tests, this molecule is also less toxic (21). Some disaccharide dipeptides containing the MDP moiety seem more active than MDP (28,29) but are difficult to prepare. Larger peptidoglycan fragments, such as tetra- to hexasaccharides of di- to pentapeptides, have greater activity for inducing arthritogenicity (30) and for inhibiting plasminogen activator secretion from macrophages (31).

The *peptide moiety* is essential for the immunologic activities of MDP; L-Ala can be replaced by other L-amino acids (e.g., the L-seryl and L-valyl derivatives are more active than MDP) (21,32), but the replacement of L-Ala by D-Ala gives an inactive or even an immunosuppressive molecule (33,34). The replacement of the D-glutamic acid residue by either D-Asp or L-Glu gives again inactive compounds (35). The α and γ substituents of the D-Glu residue of MDP can be varied in different ways (21,23).

Until the discovery of the first WSA proved the contrary (15,16), it was postulated that a mycobacterial adjuvant must be liposoluble. Indeed, earlier studies had established that adjuvant active chloroform-soluble wax D fractions of mycobacteria contain a peptidoglycan moiety linked to an arabinogalactan esterified by mycolic acids (36). Therefore, lipophilic derivatives of MDP have been studied extensively in view of potentiating the glycopeptide's activity.

Japanese authors (37–41) have described many 6-*O*-acylesters of MDP; they showed that 6-*O*-mycolyl-MDP, 6-*O*-nocardomycolyl-MDP, and 6-*O*-corynomycolyl-MDP have interesting antitumor properties and are less pyrogenic than MDP (see paragraphs that follow). Later, lipophilic MDP derivatives bearing a mycolyl group at the end of the peptide chain, such as MurNAc-L-Ala-D-isoGln-L-Ala-glycerol-mycolate (42), were shown to stimulate strongly adjuvant activity and nonspecific antibacterial resistance (43). Surprisingly the corresponding "desmuramyl" compound, that is, L-Ala-D-isoGln-L-Ala-glycerol-mycolate, is as active as the MurNAc derivative in stimulating antibacterial resistance but entirely inactive for increasing humoral antibodies (43) (Figure 1). This shows the important role played by the MurNAc moiety in the latter activity, for this series at least.

Indeed, an active peptidoglycan derivative has been obtained by *N*-laurylation of an inactive diaminopimelic acid containing tetrapeptide of a Streptomyces strain (44). A synthetic lauryl-tetrapeptide analogue (N^2-[*N*-(*N*-lauryl-L-alanyl)- γ -D-glutamyl]-N^6-glycyl-DD-LL-diamino-2,6-pimelamic acid) is adjuvant active and protects mice against *Listeria monocytogenes.* The lipophilic nonapeptide L-Ala-D-isoGln-L-Lys(Ac)-D-Ala-(Gly)$_5$-OMe has also been reported to produce delayed hypersensitivity when injected in FIA with an antigen (45).

All these compounds contain the sequence L-Ala-D-Glu that thus seems to be specifically recognized by the target cell, most probably the macrophages.

"Small is beautiful": because of its small size, MDP is not antigenic, nor does it react with antipeptidoglycan antibodies (46); it is, however, very rapidly

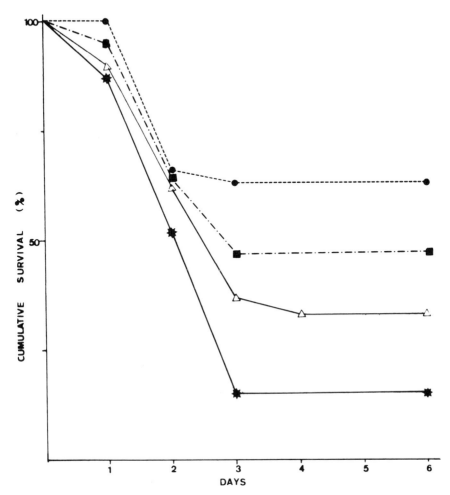

Figure 1. Protective activity of lipophilic MDP derivatives in adult mice infected intramuscularly with 4 • 10⁶ *P. aeruginosa*. Mice were given 300 μg intravenously of each compound 7 days before being infected (43). Symbols: * controls; △ MDP; ▮ *N*-acetyl-muramyl-L-alanyl-D-isoglutaminyl-D-alanyl-glycerolmycolate; ● L-alanyl-D-isoglutaminyl-L-alanyl-glycerol-mycolate.

excreted by the kidney, mainly unchanged. In mice, under appropriate conditions, more than 50% after 30 minutes and more than 90% after 2 hours are recovered in the urine (47). As it is to be expected that larger molecules carrying the MDP unit would have longer lifetimes in the body, various attempts have been made to prepare *oligomers* (26) and *polymers* and to couple MDP to *carriers.*

A *p*-aminophenyl-glycoside of MDP was prepared and cross-linked with glutaraldehyde (48); the resulting polymer of a molecular weight of about 6000 daltons had indeed an increased activity for stimulating antibacterial resistance.

Muramyl dipeptide has been coupled to a synthetic multi(poly) (DL-alanyl)-poly(L-lysine) carrier (referred to as A—L). The resulting conjugate had a hundredfold increased anti-infectious activity but also a very strong pyrogenicity. It was surprising, however, that the conjugate with the inactive MDP-DD isomer was also strongly anti-infectious but nonpyrogenic; it does not sensitize, nor does it induce an immune response to the glycopeptide moiety (49).

2.2. Biological Properties of MDP and Its Derivatives

Adjuvant Activity.   Synthetic MDP and many of its derivatives are capable of increasing the titres of circulating antibodies, even when administered in aqueous solution (50) and by the oral route (51). This capacity was shown with numerous antigens and also with certain bacterial vaccines such as influenza, with either an inactivated virus or a purified subunit (52,53). In certain studies, after the covalent linkage to the MDP-A—L conjugate of a synthetic hapten (54) or of a synthetic viral antigen (55), humoral antibody responses were markedly enhanced, showing that a completely "synthetic vaccine" may be obtained by this procedure.

In early studies the additional presence of a water-in-oil emulsion (FIA) was required to induce specific cellular immunity (delayed hypersensitivity). For instance, immunization of monkeys against malaria has been shown to be possible with MDP and FIA. Protective immunity was produced in Aotus monkeys and in macaques, using MDP or nor-MDP with FIA and merozoites of *Plasmodium falciparum* or *P. knowlesi* as antigens (56,57). Efforts were pursued to find more acceptable vehicles (e.g., liposomes or metabolizable oils) or other derivatives in view of enhancing specific cell-mediated immunity. Thus, Siddiqui et al. (58) went a step further and using liposomes containing a lipophilic 6-O-stearoyl-MDP derivative, obtained full protection of Aotus monkeys, using a *P. falciparum* antigen.

Another fatty acid derivative, MDP-L-Ala-glycerol mycolate, was also shown capable of producing cell-mediated immunity when administered with a protein antigen in liposomes or in squalane and to a lesser degree in an aqueous medium (43,59).

As already mentioned, MDP-DD (N-acetyl-muramyl-D-alanyl-D-isoglutamine) is immunosuppressive (34), but, like other adjuvants, MDP itself can also inhibit immune responses, depending on the timing in relation to the administration of antigen and also on the dosage (60,61). A selective suppression of an IgE response has been obtained with antigen conjugated to lipophilic MDPs since the IgG response was fully maintained. This effect seems to be related to specific IgE suppressor cells (62) and offers an important new therapeutic approach to allergy.

Stimulation of Nonspecific Resistance by MDP.   Muramyl dipeptide and several derivatives increase resistance to bacterial infections in particular by

Klebsiella pneumoniae (63) and are active even in neonate mice, where endotoxin (LPS) is inactive (64). This effect can also be shown after oral administration.

Increased natural resistance to infection was also shown *in vivo* and *in vitro* against parasites. A partial protection of mice against *Trypanosoma cruzi* was obtained by Kierszenbaum and Ferraresi (65) by applying MDP in an Alzet minipump (which releases $1\,\mu l$/hour over several days) or by repeated doses of MDP. The glycopeptide, used either with or without an antigen, was also shown to decrease the degree of infection of rats challenged with *Schistosoma mansoni*; this effect seems due principally to stimulation of nonspecific resistance (66).

Muramyl dipeptide also restores nonspecific immunity in immunosuppressed mice that have a greatly increased susceptibility to various infections (67). Nor-MDP has been shown to counteract the effect of cyclophosphamide and to protect mice with doses of antibiotics smaller than those required for the controls "indicating a potential clinical usefulness of immunostimulation in immunocompromised and infected human patients" (68).

Pharmacological Effects of MDP. Muramyl dipeptide has several untoward effects, such as pyrogenicity (69,70), thrombocytolysis (71), and production of a transitory leukopenia (69). Pyrogenicity of MDP can be obviated by simultaneous administration of indomethacin or by appropriate structural modifications (72). Some adjuvant-active MDPs have also been shown to release serotonin from blood platelets or even to have a direct pharmacologic effect on a strip of guinea pig ileum (73).

The sensitization of BCG-treated mice to endotoxin has been related to cord factor (see Section 3). This increased susceptibility to lipopolysaccharides has also been reported in guinea pigs that received simultaneously MDP (74). (For a review of pharmacological activity of muramyl peptides, see reference 72.)

3. TREHALOSE DIESTERS (CORD FACTOR AND SYNTHETIC ANALOGUES)*

3.1. Adjuvant Activity

The chemistry and biological activities of trehalose esters (cord factor and analogues) have been recently reviewed by Asselineau and Asselineau (75), Brennan and Goren (76), and one of the present authors (77,78). In guinea pigs, contrary to wax D, peptidoglycans, and muramyl peptides, TDM cannot substitute for mycobacteria in FCA; this glycolipid has, however, been shown in certain models to enhance the immune responses. Thus it produces gran-

---

*Nomenclature: the terms "cord factor," P_3, and TDM (for trehalose dimycolate) are synonyms for the mixture of trehalose 6,6'-dimycolates (2) produced by mycobacteria.

ulomas (79) and increases the antibody response to SRBC in mice (80) and is also a good adjuvant in rats (81). The adjuvant activity of synthetic trehalose diesters has also been studied in mice in comparison with the natural TDM (82). A significant prolongation of survival time of mice infected by *Toxoplasma gondii* was obtained by vaccination with protoplasm of disrupted *T. gondii* in an oil-in-water emulsion containing TDM (83).

3.2. Stimulation of Nonspecific Resistance by TDM

Trehalose dimycolate in oil emulsion protects mice against an intraperitoneal (i.p.) challenge with *Salmonella typhi* and *S. typhimurium* (84) and can induce local immunity against an airborne tuberculous infection; this effect has been related to the lung granulomas that TDM produces (85). Aqueous suspensions of TDM are active in mice against *Klebsiella pneumoniae* and *Listeria monocytogenes* infection (86). Moreover, the synthetic lower homologue C_{76} (3) that is less toxic, is as active as TDM in this test (82).

Total carbon number	Structure of $R\text{-}\overset{\displaystyle O}{\overset{\displaystyle \|}{C}}\text{-OH}$	

Mycobacterial mycolic acids, for instance:

2 $\sim C_{180}$
(Cord factor = TDM = P_3)

$$CH_3(CH_2)_{19}CH\text{-}CH(CH_2)_{14}CH\text{-}CH\text{-}(CH_2)_{17}\overset{OH}{\overset{|}{CH}}\text{-}CH\text{-}CO_2H$$

with CH_2, CH_2 bridges and $C_{24}H_{49}$

$C_{84}H_{164}O_3$

3 C_{76}

Synthetic racemic $CH_3(CH_2)_{14}\overset{OH}{\overset{|}{C}}\text{-}CH\text{-}CO_2H$

with H and $C_{14}H_{29}$

$C_{32}H_{64}O_3$

Trehalose dimycolate in aqueous suspension injected 3 to 7 weeks before infection protects mice against the protozoan parasite *Babesia microti* (87). Mice can be partially protected against infection by *Schistosoma mansoni* by injection of aqueous suspensions of TDM, or even by trehalose dipalmitate (in suspension in paraffin oil) (88).

3.3. Pharmacological Activities of TDM

Cord factor (TDM) is toxic for mice when administered in emulsion with 10% paraffin oil; however, $100\,\mu g$ of TDM in emulsion with 1% Bayol F is not toxic (11); TDM is not toxic in rats (89), nor in guinea pigs (15).

Table 1 compares the *in vivo* toxicity of mycobacterial cord factor (TDM) with that of two synthetic C_{76} analogues 3 (isomers of the corynebacterial cord factor). The synthetic analogues are much less toxic but have—in some tests at least—the same immunostimulant activity as TDM (90). They are also much less granulomagenic than TDM (90).

TABLE 1.   Toxicity of Emulsified TDM and Its Synthetic
Analogues (90)

	Number of Deaths/Number Treated	
Material Injected[a]	Exp. 1	Exp. 2
TDM	10/10	10/10
$C_{76}\alpha$	0/10	1/10
$C_{76}\beta$	0/10	1/10
Emulsion	0/10	1/10

[a] Oil (9%)/water emulsions of TDM and its synthetic analogues (0.1 mg/0.2 ml per mouse) or emulsion alone were prepared by grinding and were administered in volumes of 0.2 ml intravenously.

The increase in susceptibility of mice to endotoxin of gram-negative bacteria reported for cord factor by Suter et al. (91) has been confirmed by Parant et al. (86). Under different experimental conditions and with different mouse strains, Yarkoni et al. (92) found no enhancement of endotoxin lethality. This discrepancy has been also ascribed to the use of different proportions of paraffin oil and Tween (93).

4.   ANTITUMOR ACTIVITY OF MDP OR TDM ADMINISTERED SEPARATELY

4.1.   Antitumor Activity of MDP

As previously stated, to enhance cell-mediated immunity, one must use either fatty acid derivatives of MDP or various other components (liposomes, mineral oil, TDM). For instance, MDP itself did not have any antitumor activity *in vivo,* whereas 6-*O*-acyl-esters of MDP were active. In these experiments 100 μ g of the glycopeptides, either in phosphate-buffered saline or attached to oil droplets, was mixed with 1.10^6 fibrosarcoma tumor cells and transplanted intradermally into SWM/MS mice (94). Twenty-three days after inoculation, 6-*O*-mycoloyl-MDP, 6-*O*-nocardomycoloyl-MDP, and 6-*O*-corynomycoloyl -MDP caused suppression of tumor growth in 77 and 37% of the mice, respectively (95). Muramyl dipeptide derivatives containing two mycoloyl groups or linked to an ubiquinonelike moiety are also antitumor active (96) (Table 2).

Having obtained *in vitro* a very large potentiation of the tumoricidal activity of alveolar macrophages by inclusion of MDP in liposomes (see Tables 2 and 3), Fidler et al. (97) have used multiple systemic administration of MDP in such liposomes to study the eradication *in vivo* of established spontaneous pulmonary and lymph node metastases. Of mice thus treated, 74% were free of visible metastases (Table 3).

In another experiment 60% of mice treated with liposome-encapsulated MDP were tumor free 120 days after the last liposome treatment or 110 days after all control mice treated with either free MDP or control liposomes had died of disseminated cancer (Figure 2).

An interesting finding was recently reported concerning MDP-induced cytotoxic antibodies directed against mouse myeloma cells. In these experiments anti-idiotypic antibodies were raised by immunizing mice with MOPC 315 immunoglobulin A administered with Freund's adjuvant or with MDP. Cytotoxicity, however, was not correlated with the amount of anti-idiotypic antibody since it could be found in sera of mice immunized by Freund's adjuvant or by

TABLE 2.   Antitumor Activity of Quinonyl MDP Against the Meth-A System (96)

Compound	Dose (μ g)	Number of Mice Tested	Tumor-Free Mice per Mice Surviving on Day 49
4a	100	10	10/10
4b	100	10	3/10
4c	100	10	6/10
MDP	100	10	0/10
Control	—	10	0/10

4a: Z = L-Val
4b: Z = L-Ser
4c: Z = L-Thr

TABLE 3.   Treatment of Spontaneous B16BL-6 Metastases in C57B1/6 Mice by I.V. Injection of Liposomes containing MDP (97)[a]

| | Pulmonary Metastasis | | | |
Treatment Group	Mice with Metastases/Total	Median	Range	Percentage of Mice without Visible Metastases (%)
PBS, control mice	24/28	49	0 to 107	14
Free MDP (100 μ g)	8/10	55	0 to 94	20
"Empty" liposomes and free MDP (2.5 μ g)	23/26	68	0 to 308	12
Liposome-encapsulated MDP (2.5 μ g)	7/27	0	0 to 7	74

[a] Viable B16BL-6 cells (25,000) were implanted in the footpad of syngeneic C57B1/6 mice. Tumors (10 to 12 mm in diameter) were amputated 4 weeks later. Liposome therapy commenced 3 days following surgery. Each treatment consisted of i.v. injection of 5 μ moles lipid PS/PC MLV liposomes per mouse twice weekly for 4 weeks. Mice were killed 2 weeks after the last treatment and necropsied. Lung metastases were determined microscopically and confirmed histologically. The incidence of metastasis in the group treated with liposome-encapsulated MDP differed significantly from other groups ($p < .001$, χ^2 test). The data represent the combined results of two separate experiments.

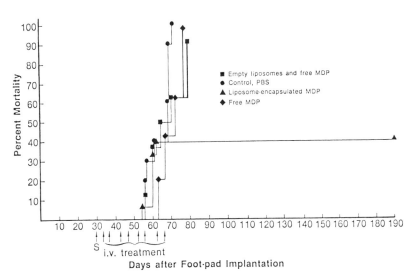

Figure 2.   Survival of mice bearing spontaneous lymph node and pulmonary melanoma metastases following multiple i.v. treatments with PBS (●), 100 μg free MDP per dose (◆), multilaminar vesicle (MLV) 5 μmole total phospholipid per mouse containing PBS and 2.5 μg of free MDP (■), and MLV 5 μmole of total phospholipid per mouse containing 2.5 μg of MDP (▲). The difference in survival between mice treated with liposome-encapsulated MDP and all other treatment groups is significant ($p < .001$, χ^2 test) (15 mice per group) (97).

MDP in the absence of MOPC 315 immunoglobulin A. Studies are being pursued to determine whether there exists a surface antigen that could cross-react with MDP or other mycobacterial components (98).

4.2.   Antitumor Activity of TDM

In mice the intravenous injection of TDM emulsion containing mineral oil and Tween 80 leads to suppression of the development of urethan-induced pulmonary tumors, to a similar degree as viable BCG (99). This effect has also been related to lung granuloma formation. Several investigators have compared the activity of TDM to certain of its synthetic analogues. Thus trehalose-6,6-dipalmitate, sucrose-6,6-dimycolate, methyl-6-mycoloyl- α -D-glucopyranose, methyl-6-mycoloyl- β -D-glucopyranose, and even trehalose monopalmitate injected intravenously in mice inhibited the growth of Ehrlich ascites tumor cells (100). The efficiency of such agents was also shown by use of other syngeneic or chemically induced tumors. In certain experiments metabolizable oils were used. Trehalose dimycolate in Bayol F or in an emulsion of saline and peanut oil was active against L1210 leukemia cells (101). Trehalose dimycolate and the synthetic C_{76} analogue, injected intralesionally into a methylcholanthrene-induced fibrosarcoma inoculated to mice, cause up to 100% regression of the established tumor in presence of 9% paraffin oil (Table 4 and Figure 3).

TABLE 4.   Regression of a Murine Fibrosarcoma by Intralesional Administration of Emulsified TDM or Synthetic Analogues (90)

Experiment Number	Material Injected[a]	Dose (mg)	Number of Tumor-Free Animals/Number of Animals Treated (60 days)	Percentage Regression	p
1	Emulsion	—	1/12	8	—
	TDM	0.15	11/12	92	< .001
	C76 (β)	0.15	10/12	83	< .001
2	No treatment	—	0/12	0	—
	Emulsion	—	0/12	0	
	C76 (a + β)	0.05	12/12	100	< .001
	TDP[c]	0.15	3/12	25	NS[b]
	TDB[d]	0.15	4/12	33	NS
3	No treatment	—	0/12	0	—
	TDM	0.1	11/12	92	< .001
	TDP	0.15	3/10	30	NS
	TDB	0.15	4/10	40	NS

[a] Emulsions (9% oil) were injected into 5- to 6-day-old tumors (3 to 5 mm in diameter).

[b] NS = number of tumor-free animals not significantly different from controls.

[c] TDP = trehalose dipalmitate.

[d] TDB = trehalose dibehenate.

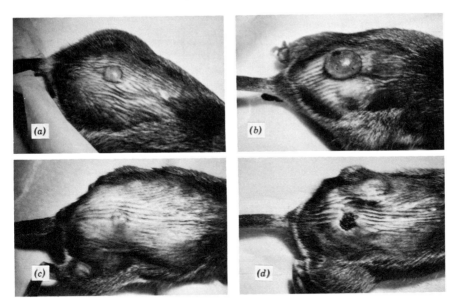

Figure 3. Regression of the methylcholanthrene-induced fibrosarcoma 1023 in male C3H/He N mice after intralesional injection of 100 μg of TDM in 10% Drakeol + 0.2% Tween: (*a*) 7-day-old tumor, no treatment; (*b*) 13-day-old tumor, no treatment; (*c*) 1 day after treatment with TDM of 6-day-old tumor; (*d*) 7 days after treatment with TDM of 6-day-old tumor (90). (Photograph by E. Yarkoni.)

Most of the cured mice are resistant to growth of tumor cells of a challenge inoculum (90). The influence of mineral oil, squalane, and squalene or peanut oil on the antitumor activity of emulsified BCG cell walls or TDM on the regression of the transplanted fibrosarcoma in mice has been studied in detail (102,103). The sulfolipid I studied by Goren et al. (104) emulsified in presence of TDM (equal weights of each) produces regression of the murine fibrosarcoma comparable to TDM alone; the mixtures of sulfolipid I and TDM are less toxic than TDM alone (105).

The growth of an ascitic rat hepatoma is suppressed by i.p. injection of TDM or—to a lesser extent—by some synthetic analogues, when emulsified in peanut oil; paraffin oil gives better results (106) (Figure 4).

Recent results with squalene show that with a small tumor inoculum (10^4 cells), TDM and C_{100}* were equally active, but with a larger challenge (10^5 cells) TDM was definitely more active than synthetic C_{100} (107).

Sukumar et al. (108) have studied the efficacy of BCG cell walls, TDM, and C_{76} for the eradication of pulmonary deposits of intravenously injected syngeneic fibrosarcoma 1023 in C3H mice. The compounds were administered

*The compound C_{100} is a synthetic trehalose 6,6′ diester with two synthetic C_{44} mycolic acids (α - eicosanyl, β hydroxytetracosanoic acids).

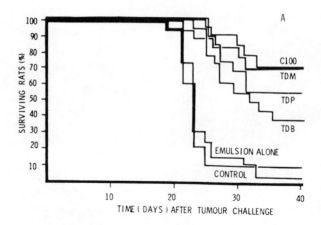

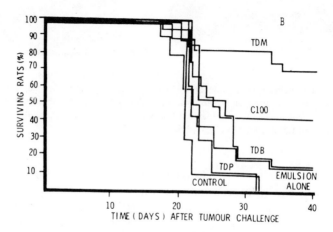

Figure 4. (*a*) Influence of trehalose diesters on growth of ascitic rat hepatoma D23As (10^4 cell challenge). Rats were treated intraperitoneally with 1 mg of material on day of challenge ($p < .005$). All treated groups were compared to emulsion-alone control 18 to 19 rats per group; TDM = trehalose dimycolate; TDB = trehalose dibehenate; TDP = trehalose dipalmitate). (*b*) Influence of trehalose diesters (1 mg) on growth of ascitic rat hepatoma D23As (10^5 cell challenge) ($p < .005$ for TDM-treated rats; other groups not significantly different from emulsion-alone control; 10 to 19 rats per group) (107).

emulsified in 10% Drakeol by three different routes: intraperitoneal, intradermal, or intravenous, 24 hours after intravenous injection of 1023 tumor cells. 100 μg of TDM injected i.p. cured about 50% of treated animals. The other forms of administration were much less effective. Higher doses of C_{76} or BCG cell walls also led to a significant number of cures; however, the routes of optimal activity varied.

Recent unpublished experiments of Yarkoni and Rapp on the guinea pig hepatoma and of Tenu and Petit with mouse peritoneal macrophages have also shown that the synthetic C_{76} is less active than TDM. The synthetic chemist will still have to look for new, easily accessible, fully active trehalose diesters.

In mice the antitumor activity of killed BCG can be increased by addition of TDM (109). Such preparations were active even in the absence of oil (110). Ribi et al. (111,112) had reported that a BCG "cell-wall skeleton" needed addition of P_3 (TDM) or its synthetic analogues (113) to produce regression of the transplanted line 10 hepatocarcinoma in strain 2 guinea pigs.* These experiments have led to *clinical trials* of *M. smegmatis* cell walls + TDM, mainly against malignant melanoma (115-117). An ointment containing killed BCG + TDM has been used with success for treating certain skin cancers (118).

5. ANTITUMOR ACTIVITY OF MDP AND TDM ADMINISTERED TOGETHER

The strong antitumor effect of emulsions of trehalose esters associated with MDP in line 10 dermal tumors of strain 2 guinea pigs has been established independently by McLaughlin et al. (32) and Yarkoni et al. (119). Previous results of Ribi et al. (120,121) had shown that an endotoxin preparation from an O-antigen-deficient (Re) mutant of *Salmonella typhimurium* emulsified with TDM and paraffin oil produced strong regression ($\leqslant 100\%$) after intralesional injection in strain 2 guinea pigs bearing established line 10 dermal tumors. Some synthetic analogues of TDM were shown to be capable of replacing TDM (122). Combination of a purified endotoxin preparation with TDM and a serine analogue of MDP were shown to be even more beneficial (123). More recently McLaughlin et al. (32) have obtained nearly 100% cures, even in the absence of the endotoxic component, by using only an MDP derivative + TDM, in emulsion with 0.75% paraffin oil. It was essential to emulsify both compounds together, since the joint injection of emulsions prepared separately, each containing only one type of compound, gave no cures. "A tertiary complex of muramyl dipeptide, trehalose dimycolate and oil droplets is required" (Table 5).

Parallel experiments of Yarkoni et al. with line 10 hepatocarcinoma in strain 2 guinea pigs have confirmed the antitumor activity of the endotoxin preparation of Ribi et al. (120) combined with TDM or even with the less toxic synthetic C_{76} analogue. More recently Yarkoni et al. (119) have obtained 100% cures using MDP and TDM in 10% paraffin oil. After a detailed study of the optimum percentage and nature of oil, it was shown that a metabolizable oil squalane (2% with 0.2% Tween) gave the best results, and that squalene, or hexadecane, was much less effective. Table 6 shows a dose response study with the use of MDP and TDM emulsified in 2% squalane + 0.2% Tween. The synthetic C_{76} analogue can partially replace TDM (Fig. 5). Again, both MDP

---

*Yarkoni and Rapp (114), however, found killed BCG as well as BCG cell walls fully active in the same guinea pig model (in absence of added TDM).

TABLE 5. Tumor Regression After Treatment[a](32)

Synthetic muramyl dipeptide (150 μ g) Tested with Trehalose Dimycolate (150 μ g)	Observed Tumor Regression
N-Acetylmuramyl-L-alanyl-D-isoglutamine	1/17
N-Acetylmuramyl-D-alanyl-D-isoglutamine	0/9
N-Acetyl-4,6-di-*O*-octanoylmuramyl-L-alanyl-D-isoglutamine	1/9
N-Acetyldesmethylmuramyl-L-alanyl-D-isoglutamine[b]	2/19
N-Acetylmuramyl-L-threonyl-D-isoglutamine	3/9
N-Acetylmuramyl-L-seryl-D-isoglutamine	10/17[c]
N-Acetyldesmethylmuramyl-L-valyl-D-isoglutamine[b]	10/17[c]
N-Glycolyldesmethylmuramyl-L-alanyl-D-isoglutamine	7/9 [c]
N-Acetyl-4,6-di-*O*-octanoylmuramyl-L-valyl-D-isoglutamine	16/18[c]
N-Acetyldesmethylmuramyl-L-α-aminobutyryl-D-isoglutamine	17/18[c]
Trehalose dimycolate alone (control)	0/17
Emulsion of oil, Tween 80, and phosphate-buffered saline (control)	0/14

[a] Values are numbers of guinea pigs cured of dermal and metastatic tumors over numbers of animals treated. Data shown are pooled from two separate experiments. No cures were observed in animals treated with any muramyl dipeptide in the absence of trehalose dimycolate.

[b] These are trivial names for 2-acetamido-2-deoxy-D-gluco-3-*O*-yl-acetyl dipeptides.

[c] Significantly different from the value for trehalose dimycolate-treated controls.

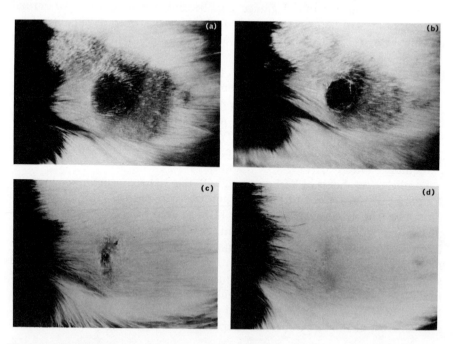

Figure 5. Regression of line 10 hepatocarcinoma in strain 2 guinea pigs after intralesional injection of 1 mg MDP (ser) + 0.5 mg C_{76} emulsified by grinding in 3% Drakeol + 0.2% Tween (Rapp and Yarkoni, unpublished observations). (Photograph by E. Yarkoni.)

TABLE 6. Tumor Regression Induced in Guinea Pigs by Intralesional Injection of Emulsified Mixtures of MDP and TDM: Dose Response (119)

Material Injected[a] (mg)		Number of Cured Animals[b]/Number of Animals Tested (90 days)
MDP	TDM	
0.25	—	0/7
0.25	1	8/8
0.25	0.2	8/8
0.25	0.04	6/8
0.05	0.2	7/8
0.05	0.04	7/8
0.01	1	7/8
0.01	0.2	7/8
0.01	0.2	7/8
0.01	0.04	6/7
	1	0/7

[a] Emulsions were prepared by ultrasonication and contained 2% squalane and 0.2% Tween.

[b] Complete disappearance of the dermal tumor, no clinical evidence of metastatic disease, and rejection of contralateral challenge (10^6 tumor cells) 2 months after the inoculation of the tumor transplant.

and TDM must be emulsified together to cause regression. In all cured animals there was a complete disappearance of the dermal tumor and no evidence of metastases, and all animals rejected a contralateral challenge 2 months after the inoculation of the tumor transplant.

There is still a discrepancy between the experiments of McLaughlin et al. (32) and those of Yarkoni et al. (119) because the former find that, in contrast to certain derivatives, MDP itself is not synergistic (Table 5). This discrepancy could perhaps be due to different experimental conditions, in particular the lower oil content used by McLaughlin et al. (32).

6. POSSIBLE MECHANISMS OF ACTION OF MURAMYL DIPEPTIDES AND TREHALOSE DIESTERS

6.1. *In vitro* Studies with MDP

The primary action of MDP seems to be mediated by the macrophage, leading to the liberation of monokines stimulating B cells and T cells (125–127). Muramyl dipeptide *in vitro* activates macrophages, causing the secretion of prostaglandins, of a collagenase, and of a fibroblast proliferation factor (128). It also inhibits migration of macrophages (129,130). For more details on cellular immunology of MDP, the reader is referred to the reviews of Chedid et al. (20), Dukor et al. (21), and Parant (22).

Resident or thioglycollate-elicited murine macrophages cultivated for 24 hours in the presence of MDP have an increased cytostatic activity against the syngeneic P815 mastocytoma cells (131). Muramyl dipeptide added *in vitro* to strongly cytostatic mouse macrophages obtained 7 days after an i.p. injection of 50 μg of TDM (cord factor) in saline emulsion prevents the decrease of cytostatic activity observed in controls during *in vitro* cultivation (132).

Sone and Fidler (133) have reported an interesting synergistic action of the lymphokine (macrophage activating factor) (MAF) and MDP, measured by the tumoricidal properties of rat alveolar macrophages. These cells are incubated for 15 minutes with a solution of MAF and then treated with subthreshold amounts of MDP (0.001 to 1 μg/ml): they are thus rendered tumoricidal to syngeneic, allogeneic, and xenogeneic tumor cells *in vitro*. The synergism of MAF and MDP could also be demonstrated with both agents encapsulated in liposomes, thus ruling out the primary binding of MAF and/or MDP to the macrophage surface. The possible contamination of MAF or MDP by LPS was ruled out in these experiments by showing that the addition of polymyxin, known to inactivate LPS, did not influence the synergistic activation of the alveolar macrophages. Sone and Fidler (134) have reported recently that alveolar macrophages from lungs of F344 rats are rendered tumoricidal by incubation *in vitro* with MDP alone. These activated macrophages are also cytotoxic against syngeneic, allogeneic, and xenogeneic tumor cells and have no cytotoxic action on cultures of normal cells. Moreover, when encapsulated in multi-lamellar liposomes prepared from phosphatidyl-serine-phosphatidyl-choline (in a 3:7 molar ratio), MDP renders alveolar macrophages tumoricidal at concentrations approximately 4000 times lower than free MDP.

TABLE 7.   Thymocyte Mitogenic Protein[a] Secretion in Supernatants of TDM-Elicited Mouse Peritoneal Macrophages (132)

Macrophage Stimulation		^{3}H-TdR Incorporation in Thymocytes	Relative Effect	Number of Experiments
In vivo	*In vitro*			
None	None	489 $\pm$ 93	1	6
(resident	MDP 10 μg/ml	490 $\pm$ 83	1	6
macrophages)	LPS 50 μg/ml	4868 $\pm$ 632	10	6
Trehalose	None	1767 $\pm$ 245	3.6	12
dimycolate	MDP 10 μg/ml	5769 $\pm$ 749	11.7	12
elicited on	MPP 50 μg/ml	3555 $\pm$ 462	7.3	5
day -7				
(50 μg in	LPS 50 μg/ml	5921 $\pm$ 767	3.4	11
saline i.p.)				

[a] Thymocyte mitogenic protein is assayed at dilution 1/2 on thymocytes of C3H/HeJ mice (8 to 9 weeks) old. Results correspond to the average incorporation of ^{3}H-TdR obtained in the number of experiments indicated.

[b] The relative effect is calculated by determining the ratio of the average value for each assay to the average value for unstimulated resident macrophages.

6.2. *In vitro* Studies with TDM

Most biological effects of natural and synthetic trehalose diesters have been explained by the interaction of these glycolipids with cell membranes and mitochondrial membranes (135,136). Lanéelle and Tocanne (137) have provided evidence for the penetration in liposomes and in mitochondrial membranes of a fluorescent analogue of TDM (137–139). Structural modifications, or simplifications of the trehalose diester model, have led mostly to less active molecules (140). Other types of glycolipids have, however, also been shown to have adjuvant activity, such as N-acyl-D-glucosamines (141) or long-chain 1-thio-β-L-fucopyranosides (142).

The activation of macrophages by TDM has been first shown by Yarkoni et al. (143), who found an increased activity of the lysosomal enzyme acid phosphatase and an increased phagocytosis of *Listeria monocytogenes* by mouse peritoneal macrophages after injections of TDM into the peritoneal cavity. The chemotactic activity of cord factor (TDM) for peritoneal cells as well as for peripheral white blood cells of mice and humans has been reported; at certain concentrations mainly macrophages are attracted (144). The chemotactic activity of P_3 (TDM) for macrophages is plasma dependent, and fibrinogen is considered to be the source of chemotactic activity (145). It was also shown recently that TDM activates the alternative pathway of complement (146).

More recently it was shown that adherent peritoneal cells from mice injected with trehalose dimycolate (50 μg emulsified in water) and collected 7 days afterwards are "activated" as judged by LAF secretion and by their cytostaticity for P815 mastocytoma cells (Table 7); TDM is also active when added *in vitro* to thioglycollate-elicited macrophages in enhancing LAF production and cyto-

TABLE 8. Cytostatic Activity of Resident Macrophages[a] (132)

	In vitro Stimulation with				^{3}H-TdR Incorporation (cpm/Culture)	Growth Inhibition (%)	Number of Experiments
	12 hours (μg/ml)	5% FCS[b]	36 hours (μg/ml)	5% FCS			
P815 alone	–	–	–	–	35,358 ± 3394		14
P815	–	–	–	–	31,695 ± 3042		3
+	–	+	–	+	26,702 ± 3050	0	4
Resident							
macrophages	MDP 10	–	MDP 10	–	17,553 ± 877	34	3
	TDM 10	+	–	+	15,698 ± 941	41	5
	TDM 10	+	MDP 10	+	11,397 ± 3500	57	6
	TDM 10	+	MPP 50	+	14,199 ± 1800	47	3

[a]Sequential stimulation *in vitro* by TDM and MDP as measured by tritiated thymidine incorporation into syngeneic mastocytoma P815 cells.
[b]Fetal calf serum.

staticity; here again MDP acts synergistically, *in vitro* (Table 8). One function of TDM that is important for antitumor activity, might thus be its property of attracting macrophages through production of chemotactic factors from fibrinogen or other plasma constituents.

7. CONCLUSION

Several strategies can be considered for the use of immunoregulating agents in tumor immunology. They can be summarized as follows:

1.   The specific approach: potentiation of immunization by neoantigens.
2.   Enhancement of nonspecific tumor immunity.
3.   Restoration of immunologic imbalance either appearing spontaneously during neoplastic diseases or produced by therapeutic intervention.

Enhancement of specific immunity may become an extremely important approach since neoantigens may progressively become identified and immunogenic preparations may become available because of new technologies (established cell lines, cloning, and production of specific monoclonal antibodies). For the time being enhancement of immune responses is obtained experimentally and clinically assayed mostly by administering irradiated tumor cells or by administering immunostimulants intralesionally. Since it is extremely probable that crude or purified neoantigens will remain weak immunogens, adjuvants should be required.

Enhancement of nonspecific immunity has often been successfully performed in various animal models. Such a record has prompted many therapeutic trials, although it is still very difficult to translate our animal models in clinical terms.

Regarding immunologic imbalance, it is generally recognized that intercurrent infections with fatal outcomes constitute one of the greatest hazards for cancer patients. Therefore, the improvement or even the complete restoration of resistance to infection may possibly represent one of the most realistic goals that can be achieved in a not too distant future.

Because repeated administration of BCG or other organisms can often induce undesirable side effects, synthetic glycopeptides and glycolipids such as those described here should have a potential use in the treatment of human tumors, especially if they can be administered without FIA or other unacceptable vehicles. Since data are emerging showing that certain MDP derivatives and trehalose esters can enhance cell-mediated immune mechanisms, these goals can hopefully be expected.

REFERENCES

1. F. C. Sparks, M. J. Silverstein, J. S. Hunt, C. M. Haskell, Y. H. Pilch, and D. L. Morton, Complications of BCG immunotherapy in patients with cancer. *New Engl. J. Med.,* **289**, 827 (1973).

2. E. M. Hersh, J. U. Gutterman, and G. M. Mavligit, BCG as an adjuvant immunotherapy for neoplasia. *Annu. Rev. Med.,* **28**, 489 (1977).

3. R. Edelman, Vaccine adjuvants, *Rev. Infect. Dis.,* **2**, 370 (1980).

4. D. W. Weiss, Host mechanisms for control of tumor growth that can be modulated by nonspecific immunotherapy. In *Immunotherapy of Human Cancer,* The University of Texas System Cancer M. D. Anderson Hospital and Tumor Institute, 22nd Annual Clinical Conference on Cancer, Raven, New York, 1978, p. 44.

5. R. J. Quesada, I. H. Libshitz, E. M. Hersh, and J. U. Gutterman, Pulmonary abnormalities in patients intravenously receiving the methanol extraction residue of BCG. *Cancer,* **45**, 1340 (1980).

6. H. Bloch, Studies on the virulence of tubercle bacilli. Isolation and biological properties of a constituent of virulent organisms. *J. Exp. Med.,* **91**, 197 (1950).

7. H. Noll, H. Bloch, J. Asselineau, and E. Lederer, The chemical structure of the cord factor of *Mycobacterium tuberculosis, Biochim. Biophys. Acta,* **20**, 299 (1956).

8. T. Ioneda, E. Lederer, and J. Rozanis, Sur la structure de diesters de tréhalose (cord factors) produits par *Nocardia asteroides* et *N. rhodochrous. Chem. Phys. Lipids,* **4**, 375 (1970).

9. M. T. Pommier and G. Michel, Glycolipides de *Nocardiae.* Isolement et caractérisation de mononocardomycolates et de dinocardomycolates de tréhalose dans une souche de *Nocardia caviae. Chem. Phys. Lipids,* **24**, 149 (1979).

10. T. Ioneda, M. Lenz, and J. Pudles, Chemical constitution of a glycolipid from *C. diphtheriae* P. W. 8. *Biochem. Biophys. Res. Commun.,* **13**, 110 (1963).

11. A. Bekierkunst, Acute granulomatous response produced in mice by trehalose-6,6'-dimycolate. *J. Bacteriol.,* **96**, 958 (1968).

12. I. Azuma, S. Kishimoto, Y. Yamamura, and J. F. Petit, Adjuvanticity of mycobacterial cell walls. *Jap. J. Microbiol.,* **15**, 193 (1971).

13. B. Zbar, E. Ribi, T. Meyer, I. Azuma, and H. J. Rapp, Immunotherapy of cancer: Regression of established intradermal tumors after intralesional injection of mycobacterial cell walls attached to oil droplets. *J. Natl. Cancer Inst.,* **52**, 1571 (1974).

14. J. F. Petit and E. Lederer, Structure and immunostimulant properties of mycobacterial cell walls. In R. Y. Stanier, H. J. Rogers, and J. D. Ward, Eds., *Symposia of the Society for General Microbiology Number XXVIII. Relations Between Structure and Function in the Prokaryotic Cell,* Cambridge University, Cambridge, UK 1978, p. 177.

15. A. Adam, R. Ciorbaru, J. F. Petit, and E. Lederer, Isolation and properties of a macromolecular water soluble immunoadjuvant fraction from the cell wall of *Mycobacterium smegmatis. Proc. Natl. Acad. Sci. (USA),* **69**, 851 (1972).

16. L. Chedid, M. Parant, R. H. Gustafson, and F. M. Berger, Biological studies of a nontoxic, watersoluble immunoadjuvant from mycobacterial cell walls. *Proc. Natl. Acad. Sci. (USA),* **69**, 855 (1972).

17. A. Adam, R. Ciorbaru, F. Ellouz, J. F. Petit, and E. Lederer, Adjuvant activity of monomeric bacterial cell wall peptidoglycan. *Biochem. Biophys. Res. Commun.,* **56**, 561 (1974).

18. F. Ellouz, A. Adam, R. Ciorbaru, and E. Lederer, Minimal structural requirements for adjuvant activity of bacterial peptidoglycan derivatives. *Biochem. Biophys. Res. Commun.,* **59**, 1317 (1974).

19. C. Merser, P. Sinäy, and A. Adam, Total synthesis and adjuvant activity of bacterial peptidoglycan derivatives, *Biochem. Biophys. Res. Commun.,* **66**, 1316 (1975).

20. L. Chedid, F. Audibert, and A. G. Johnson, Biological activities of muramyl dipeptide, a synthetic glycopeptide analogous to bacterial immunoregulating agents. *Prog. Allergy,* **25**, 63 (1978).

21. P. Dukor, L. Tarcsay, and G. Baschang, Immunostimulants. *Annu. Rep. Med. Chem.* **14**, 146 (1979).

22. D. E. S. Stewart-Tull, The immunological activities of bacterial peptidoglycans. *Annu. Rev. Microbiol.,* **34**, 311 (1980).

23. M. Parant, Biologic properties of a new synthetic adjuvant, muramyl dipeptide (MDP). *Springer Semin. Immunopathol.,* **2**, 101 (1979).

24. E. Lederer, Synthetic immunostimulants derived from the bacterial cell wall. *J. Med. Chem.,* **23**, 819 (1980).

25. E. Lederer, Immunostimulation. Recent progress in the study of natural and synthetic immunomodulators derived from the bacterial cell wall. In M. Fougereau, and J. Dausset, Eds., *Immunology 80,* Academic, London, 1980, p. 1194.

26. P. Lefrancier and E. Lederer, Chemistry of synthetic immunomodulant muramyl peptides. In W. Herz and O. Grisebach, Eds., *Progress in the Chemistry of Organic Natural Products,* Vol. 40, Springer Verlag, Vienna, 1981, p. 1.

27. A. Adam, M. Devys, V. Souvannavong, P. Lefrancier, J. Choay, and E. Lederer, Correlation of structure and adjuvant activity of *N*-acetyl muramyl-L-alanyl-D-isoglutamine (MDP), its derivatives and analogues. Anti-adjuvant and competition properties of stereoisomers. *Biochem. Biophys. Res. Commun.,* **72**, 339 (1976).

28. M. Tsujimoto, F. Kinoshita, T. Okunaga, S. Kotani, S. Kusumoto, K. Yamamoto, and T. Shiba, Higher immunoadjuvant activities of *N*-acetyl-β-D-glucosaminyl-(1-4)-*N*-acetyl-muramyl-L-alanyl-D-isoglutamine in comparison with *N*-acetylmuramyl-L-alanyl-D-isoglutamine. *Microbiol. Immunol.,* **23**, 933 (1979).

29. P. L. Durette, E. P. Meitzner, and T. Y. Shen, Synthesis of *O*-(2-acetamido-2-deoxy-β-D-glucosyl)-(1-4)-*N*-acetylmuramoyl-L-alanyl-D-isoglutamine, the repeating disaccharide-dipeptide unit of the bacterial cell-wall peptidoglycan. *Carbohydr. Res.,* **77**, C1 (1979).

30. T. Koga, S. Sakamoto, K. Onoue, S. Kotani, and A. Sumiyoshi, Efficient induction of collagen arthritis by the use of a synthetic muramyl dipeptide. *Arthr. Rheumat.,* **23**, 993 (1980).

31. J. C. Drapier, G. Lemaire, J. P. Tenu, and J. F. Petit, Biosynthesis and secretion of plasminogen activator by thioglycollate-elicited macrophages. In J. G. Kaplan, Ed., *The Molecular Basis of Immune Cell Function,* Elsevier, Amsterdam, 1979, p. 458.

32. C. A. McLaughlin, S. M. Schwartzman, B. L. Horner, G. H. Jones, J. G. Moffatt, J. J. Nestor, Jr., and D. Tegg, Regression of tumors in guinea pigs after treatment with synthetic muramyl dipeptides and trehalose dimycolate. *Science,* **208**, 415 (1980).

33. A. Adam, M. Devys, V. Souvannavong, P. Lefrancier, J. Choay, and E. Lederer, Correlation of structure and adjuvant activity of *N*-acetyl-muramyl-Lalanyl-D-isoglutamine (MDP), its derivatives and analogues. Anti-adjuvant and competition properties of stereoisomers. *Biochem. Biophys. Res. Commun.,* **72**, 339 (1976).

34. L. Chedid, F. Audibert, P. Lefrancier, J. Choay, and E. Lederer, Modulation of the immune response by a synthetic adjuvant and analogs. *Proc. Natl. Acad. Sci. (USA),* **73**, 2472 (1976).

35. I. Azuma, K. Sugimura, T. Taniyama, M. Yamawaki, Y. Yamamura, S. Kusumoto, S. Okada, and T. Shiba, Adjuvant activity of mycobacterial fractions: Immunological properties of synthetic *N*-acetyl-muramyl dipeptide and the related compounds. *Infect. Immun.,* **14**, 18 (1976).

36. R. G. White, L. Bernstock, R. G. Johns, and E. Lederer, The influence of components of *Mycobacterium tuberculosis* and other mycobacteria upon antibody production to ovalbumin. *Immunology,* **1**, 54 (1958).

37. I. Azuma, K. Sugimura, M. Yamawaki, M. Uemiya, S. Kusumoto, S. Okada, T. Shiba, and Y. Yamamura, Adjuvant activity of synthetic 6-O-"mycoloyl"-N-acetylmuramyl-L-alanyl-D-isoglutamine and related compounds. *Infect. Immun.,* **20,** 600 (1978).

38. S. Kusumoto, M. Inage, T. Shiba, I. Azuma, and Y. Yamamura, Synthesis of long chain fatty acid esters of N-acetylmuramyl-L-alanyl-D-isoglutamine in relation to antitumor activity. *Tetrahedron Lett.,* **49,** 4899 (1978).

39. T. Shiba, S. Okada, S. Kusumoto, I. Azuma, and Y. Yamamura, Synthesis of 6-O-mycoloyl-N-acetylmuramyl-L-alanyl-D-isoglutamine with antitumor activity. *Bull. Chem. Soc. Jap.,* **51,** 3307 (1978).

40. M. Uemiya, I. Saiki, T. Kusama, I. Azuma, and Y. Yamamura, Adjuvant activity of mycoloyl derivatives of N-acetylmuramyl-L-alanyl-D-isoglutamine in mice and guinea pigs. *Microbiol. Immunol.,* **23,** 821 (1979).

41. S. Kobayashi, T. Fukuda, H. Yukimasa, I. Imada, M. Fujino, I. Azuma, and Y. Yamamura, Synthesis of lipophilic muramyl dipeptide derivatives via O-aminoacyl intermediates. *Bull. Chem. Soc. Jap.,* **53,** 2917 (1980).

42. P. Lefrancier, M. Petitou, M. Level, M. Derrien, J. Choay, and E. Lederer, Synthesis of N-acetyl-muramyl-L-alanyl-D-glutamic- α -amide (MDP) or - α -methyl ester derivatives, bearing a lipophilic group at the C-terminal peptide end. *Internatl. J. Pep. Prot. Res.,* **14,** 437 (1979).

43. M. A. Parant, F. M. Audibert, L. A. Chedid, M. R. Level, P. L. Lefrancier, J. P. Choay, and E. Lederer, Immunostimulant activities of a lipophilic muramyl dipeptide derivative and of desmuramyl peptidolipid analogs. *Infect. Immun.,* **27,** 825 (1980).

44. D. Migliore-Samour, J. Bouchaudon, F. Floc'h, A. Zerial, L. Ninet, G. H. Werner, and P. Jollès, A short lipopeptide, representative of a new family of immunological adjuvants devoid of sugar. *Life Sci.,* **26,** 883 (1980).

45. K. Masek, M. Zaoral, J. Jezek, and V. Krchnak, Structure specificity of some immunoadjuvant synthetic glycopeptides. *Experientia,* **35,** 1397 (1979).

46. F. Audibert, B. Heymer, C. Gros, K. H. Schleifer, P. H. Seidl, and L. Chedid, Absence of binding of MDP, a synthetic immunoadjuvant, to anti-peptidoglycan antibodies. *J. Immunol.,* **121,** 1219 (1978).

47. M. Parant, F. Parant, L. Chedid, A. Yapo, J. F. Petit, and E. Lederer, Fate of the synthetic immunoadjuvant, muramyl dipeptide (^{14}C-labelled) in the mouse. *Internatl. J. Immunopharmacol.,* **1,** 35 (1979).

48. M. Parant, C. Damais, F. Audibert, F. Parant, L. Chedid, E. Sache, P. Lefrancier, J. Choay, and E. Lederer: *In vivo* and *in vitro* stimulation of nonspecific immunity by the β -D- ρ -aminophenyl glycoside of N-acetyl-muramyl-L-alanyl-D-isoglutamine (MDP) and an oligomer prepared by cross-linking with glutaraldehyde. *J. Infect. Dis.,* **138,** 378 (1978).

49. L. Chedid, M. Parant, F. Parant, F. Audibert, P. Lefrancier, J. Choay, and M. Sela, Enhancement of certain biological activities of muramyl dipeptide derivatives after conjugation to a multi-poly (DL-alanyl)—poly(L-lysine) carrier. *Proc. Natl. Acad. Sci. (USA),* **76,** 6557 (1979).

50. F. Audibert, L. Chedid, P. Lefrancier, and J. Choay, Distinctive adjuvanticity of synthetic analogs of mycobacterial water-soluble components. *Cell. Immunol.,* **21,** 243 (1976).

51. L. Chedid and F. Audibert, Activity in saline of chemically well defined non-toxic bacterial adjuvants. In P. A. Miescher, Ed., *Immunopathology, VIIth International Symposium,* Schwabe, Basel, 1976, p. 382.

52. F. Audibert, L. Chedid, and C. Hannoun, Augmentation de la réponse immunitaire au vaccin grippal par un glycopeptide synthétique adjuvant (N-acétyl muramyl-L-alanyl-D-isoglutamine). *C. R. Acad. Sci. (Paris),* **285,** (Series D), 467 (1977).

53. R. G. Webster, W. P. Glezen, C. Hannoun, and W. G. Laver, Potentiation of the immune response to influenza virus subunit vaccines. *J. Immunol.,* **119,** 2073 (1977).

54. E. Mozes, M. Sela and L. Chedid: Efficient genetically controlled formation of antibody to a synthetic antigen (poly (L-Tyr, L-Glu)-poly(DL-A1a)-poly(L-Lys) covalently bound to a synthetic adjuvant (N-acetylmuramyl-L-alanyl-D-isoglutamine). *Proc. Natl. Acad. Sci. (USA)*, **77**, 4933 (1980).

55. R. Arnon, M. Sela, M. Parant, and L. Chedid, Anti-viral response elicited by a completely synthetic antigen with built-in adjuvanticity. *Proc. Natl. Acad. Sci. (USA)*, **77**, 6769 (1980).

56. R. T. Reese, W. Trager, J. B. Jensen, D. A. Miller, and R. Tantravahi, Immunization against malaria with antigen from *Plasmodium falciparum* cultivated *in vitro*. *Proc. Natl. Acad. Sci. (USA)*, **75**, 5665 (1978).

57. G. H. Mitchell, W. H. G. Richards, A. Voller, F. M. Dietrich, and P. Dukor, Nor-MDP, saponin, corynebacteria, and pertussis organisms as immunological adjuvants in experimental malaria vaccination of macaques. **Bull. WHO, 57,** 189 (1979).

58. W. A. Siddiqui, D. W. Taylor, S. C. Kan, K. Kramer, S. M. Richmond-Crum, S. Kotani, T. Shiba, and S. Kusumoto, Vaccination of experimental monkeys against *Plasmodium falciparum:* A possible safe adjuvant. *Science*, **201**, 1237 (1978).

59. C. Carelli, F. Audibert, and L. Chedid, Persistent enhancement of cell-mediated and antibody immune responses after administration of MDP derivatives with antigen in metabolizable oil *Infect. Immun.*, **33**, 312 (1981).

60. C. Leclerc, D. Juy, E. Bourgeois, and L. Chedid, *In vivo* regulation of humoral and cellular immune responses of mice by a synthetic adjuvant, N-acetyl-muramyl-L-alanyl-D-isoglutamine, muramyl dipeptide for MDP. *Cell. Immunol.*, **45**, 199 (1979).

61. V. Souvannavong and A. Adam, Opposite effects of the synthetic adjuvant N-acetyl-muramyl-L-alanyl D-isoglutamine on the immune response in mice depending on experimental conditions. *Eur. J. Immunol.*, **10**, 654 (1980).

62. T. Kishimoto, Y. Hirai, K. Nakanishi, I. Azuma, A. Nagamatsu, and Y. Yamamura, Regulation of antibody response in different immunoglobulin classes. VI. Selective suppression of IgE response by administration of antigen-conjugated muramylpeptides. *J. Immunol.*, **123**, 2709 (1979).

63. L. Chedid, M. Parant, F. Parant, P. Lefrancier, J. Choay, and E. Lederer, Enhancement of non-specific immunity to *Klebsiella pneumoniae* infection by a synthetic immunoadjuvant (N-acetyl-muramyl-L-alanyl-D-isoglutamine) and several analogs. *Proc. Natl. Acad. Sci. (USA)*, **74**, 2089 (1977).

64. M. Parant, F. Parant, and L. Chedid, Enhancement of the neonate's non-specific immunity to *Klebsiella* infection by muramyl dipeptide, a synthetic immunoadjuvant. *Proc. Natl. Acad. Sci. (USA)*, **75**, 3395 (1978).

65. F. Kierszenbaum and R. W. Ferraresi, Enhancement of host resistance against *Trypanosoma cruzi* infection by the immunoregulatory agent muramyl dipeptide. *Infect. Immun.*, **25**, 273 (1979).

66. J. Tribouley, J. Tribouley-Duret, and M. Appriou, Influence du muramyl dipeptide (MDP) sur la résistance du Rat vis-à-vis de *Schistosoma mansoni*. *C. R. Soc. Biol.*, **173**, 1046 (1979).

67. M. Parant, G. Riveau, F. Parant, C. A. Dinarello, S. M. Wolff, and L. Chedid: Effect of indomethacin on increased resistance to infection and on febrile responses induced by muramyl dipeptide. *J. Infect. Dis.*, **142**, 708 (1980).

68. M. Sackmann and F. M. Dietrich, The effect of normuramyldipeptide, a synthetic immunostimulant, on host defence mechanisms and efficacy of antibiotics in immunosuppressed mice. Paper presented at International Symposium on Infections in the Immunocompromised Host, Veldhoven (Eindhoven), The Netherlands, June 1–5, 1980.

69. S. Kotani, Y. Watanabe, T. Shimono, K. Harada, T. Shiba, S. Kusumoto, K. Yokogawa, and M. Taniguchi, Correlation between the immunoadjuvant activities and pyrogenicities of synthetic N-acetyl-muramyl peptides or -amino acids. *Biken J.*, **19**, 9 (1976).

70. C. A. Dinarello, R. J. Elin, L. Chedid, and S. M. Wolff, The pyrogenicity of the synthetic adjuvant muramyl dipeptide and two structural analogues. *J. Infect. Dis.*, **138**, 760 (1978).

71. J. Rotta, M. Rye, K. Masek, and M. Zaoral, Biological activity of synthetic subunits of Streptococcus peptidoglycan. I. Pyrogenic and thrombocytolytic activity. *Exp. Cell. Biol.,* **47,** 258 (1979).

72. L. Chedid, M. Parant, and G. Riveau, Immunopharmacological activities of MDP after chemical modification or association with indomethacin. In D. R. Webb, Ed., *Pharmacology of the Reticuloendothelial System,* Dekker, New York (in press).

73. S. Kotani, K. Harada, T. Kitaura, T. Shiba, S. Kusumoto, M. Inage, K. Yokogawa, S. Kawata, and A. Inoue, Liberation of serotonin in rabbit platelets by various bacterial cell walls, a water soluble cell wall fragment and synthetic 6-0-mycoloyl N-acetyl muramyl tetrapeptide. *Internatl. J. Immunopharmacol.,* **2,** 213 (1980).

74. E. E. Ribi, J. L. Cantrell, K. B. Von Eschen, and S. M. Schwartzman, Enhancement of endotoxic shock by N-acetylmuramyl-L-alanyl-(L-seryl)-D-isoglutamine (muramyl dipeptide). *Cancer Res.,* **39,** 4756 (1979).

75. C. Asselineau and J. Asselineau, Trehalose containing glycolipids, *Progr. Chem. Fats Other Lipids,* **16,** 59 (1978).

76. P. J. Brennan and M. B. Goren, Mycobacterial glycolipids as bacterial antigens. *Biochem. Soc. Transact.,* **5,** 1687 (1977).

77. E. Lederer, Cord factor and related trehalose esters, *Chem. Phys. Lipids,* **16,** 91 (1976).

78. E. Lederer, Cord factor and related synthetic trehalose diesters, *Springer Semin. Immunopathol.,* **2,** 133 (1979).

79. A. Bekierkunst, I. S. Levij, E. Yarkoni, E. Vilkas, A. Adam, and E. Lederer, Granuloma formation induced in mice by chemically defined mycobacterial fractions. *J. Bacteriol.,* **100,** 95 (1969).

80. A. Bekierkunst, E. Yarkoni, I. Flechner, S. Morecki, E. Vilkas, and E. Lederer, Immune response to sheep red blood cells in mice pretreated with mycobacterial fractions. *Infect. Immun.,* **4,** 256 (1971).

81. R. Saito, S. Nagao, M. Takamoto, K. Sugiyama, M. Takamoto, K. Sugiyama, and A. Tanaka, Adjuvanticity (immunity-inducing property) of cord factor in mice and rats. *Infect. Immun.,* **16,** 725 (1977).

82. M. Parant, F. Audibert, F. Parant, L. Chedid, E. Soler, J. Polonsky, and E. Lederer, Non-specific immunostimulant activities of synthetic trehalose-6,6'-diesters (lower homologs of cord factor). *Infect. Immun.,* **20,** 12 (1978).

83. K. N. Masihi, W. Brehmer, and H. Werner, The effects of toxoplasma cell fractions and mycobacterial immunostimulants against virulent *Toxoplasma gondii* in mice. *Zbl. Bakt. Hyg. I. Abt. Orig. A,* **245,** 377 (1979).

84. E. Yarkoni and A. Bekierkunst, Nonspecific resistance against infection with *Salmonella typhi* and *S. typhimurium* induced in mice by cord factor (trehalose 6,6'-dimycolate) and its analogues. *Infect. Immun.,* **14,** 1125 (1976).

85. E. E. Ribi, R. L. Anacker, W. R. Barclay, W. Brehmer, S. C. Harris, W. R. Leif, and J. Simmons, Efficacy of mycobacterial cell walls as a vaccine against airborne tuberculosis in the rhesus monkey, *J. Infect. Dis.,* **123,** 527 (1971).

86. M. Parant, F. Parant, L. Chedid, J. C. Drapier, J. F. Petit, J. Wietzerbin, and E. Lederer, Enhancement of non-specific immunity to bacterial infection by cord factor (6,6'-trehalose dimycolate). *J. Infect. Dis.,* **135,** 771 (1977).

87. I. A. Clark, Protection of mice against *Babesia microti* with CF, COAM, zymosan, glucan, *Salmonella* and *Listeria*. *Parasite Immunol.,* **1,** 179 (1979).

88. G. R. Olds, L. Chedid, E. Lederer, and A. F. Mahmoud, Introduction of resistance to *Schistosoma mansoni* by natural cord factor and synthetic lower homologs. *J. Infect. Dis.,* **141,** 473 (1980).

89. R. Saito, A. Tanaka, K. Sugiyama, and M. Kato, Cord factor not toxic in rat. *Am. Rev. Resp. Dis.* **112,** 578 (1975).

90. R. Yarkoni, H. J. Rapp, J. Polonsky, and E. Lederer, Immunotherapy with an intralesion-ally administered synthetic cord factor analogue. *Internatl. J. Cancer,* **22,** 564 (1978).

91. E. Suter and E. M. Kirsanow, Hyperreactivity to endotoxin in mice infected with myco-bacteria. Induction and elicitation of the reactions. *Immunology,* **4,** 354 (1961).

92. E. Yarkoni, M. S. Meltzer, and H. J. Rapp, Failure of trehalose-6,6′-dimycolate (P₃ or cord factor) to enhance endotoxin lethality in mice. *Infect. Immun.,* **14,** 1375 (1976).

93. E. Yarkoni and H. J. Rapp, Toxicity of emulsified trehalose-6,6′-dimycolate (cord factor) in mice depends on the size distribution of the mineral oil droplets, *Infect. Immun.,* **20,** 856 (1978).

94. I. Azuma, K. Sugimura, M. Yamawaki, M. Uemiya, S. Kusumoto, S. Okada, T. Shiba, and Y. Yamamura, Adjuvant activity of synthetic 6-*O*-"mycoloyl"-*N*-acetylmuramyl-L-alanyl-D-isoglutamine and related compounds. *Infect. Immun.,* **20,** 600 (1978).

95. M. Uemiya, K. Sugimura, T. Kusama, I. Saiki, M. Yamawaki, I. Azuma, and Y. Yama-mura, Adjuvant activity of 6-*O*-mycoloyl derivatives of *N*-acetyl-muramyl-L-seryl-D-iso-glutamine and related compounds in mice and guinea pigs. *Infect. Immun.,* **24,** 83 (1979).

96. I. Azuma, M. Yamawaki, M. Uemiya, I. Saiki, Y. Panio, S. Kobayashi, T. Fukuda, I. Imada, and Y. Yamamura, Adjuvant and antitumor activities of quinonyl-*N*-acetyl-mur-amyl dipeptides. *Gann,* **76,** 847 (1979).

97. I. J. Fidler, S. Sone, W. E. Fogler, and Z. L. Barnes, Eradication of spontaneous metastases and activation of alveolar macrophages by intravenous injection of liposomes containing muramyl dipeptide. *Proc. Natl. Acad. Sci. (USA),* **78,** 1680 (1981).

98. R. Baumal, A. Marks, J. Mahoney, and A. Bose, Induction of cytotoxic factors by im-munization of mice with Freund's adjuvant component. *Cancer Res.,* **40,** 1630 (1980).

99. A. Bekierkunst, I. S. Levij, E. Yarkoni, E. Vilkas, and E. Lederer, Suppression of urethan induced lung adenomas in mice treated with trehalose-6,6′-dimycolate (cord factor) and living Bacillus Calmette Guérin. *Science,* **174,** 1240 (1971).

100. E. Yarkoni, A. Bekierkunst, J. Asselineau, R. Toubiana, M. J. Toubiana, and E. Lederer, Suppression of growth of Ehrlich ascites tumour cells in mice pretreated with synthetic analogs of trehalose-6,6′-dimycolate (cord factor). *J. Natl. Cancer Inst.,* **51,** 717 (1973).

101. C. Leclerc, A. Lamensans, L. Chedid, J. C. Drapier, J. F. Petit, J. Wietzerbin, and E. Lederer, Non-specific immunoprevention of L1210 leukemia by cord factor (6,6′-dimyco-late of trehalose) administered in a metabolizable oil. *Cancer Immunol. Immunother.,* **1,** 227 (1976).

102. E. Yarkoni and H. J. Rapp, Granuloma formation in lungs of mice after intravenous administration of emulsified trehalose-6,6′-dimycolate (cord factor): Reaction intensity depends on size distribution of the oil droplets. *Infect. Immun.,* **18,** 552 (1977).

103. E. Yarkoni and H. J. Rapp, Tumor regression after intralesional injection of mycobacterial components emulsified in 2,6,10,15,19,23-hexamethyl-2,6,10,14,18,22-tetracosahexaene (squalene), 2,6,10,15,19,23-hexamethyltetracosane (squalane), peanut oil, or mineral oil. *Cancer Res.,* **39,** 1518 (1979).

104. M. B. Goren, O. Brokl, P. Roller, E. M. Fales, and B. C. Das, Sulfatides of *Mycobac-terium tuberculosis,* the structure of the principal sulfatide (SL-I). *Biochemistry,* **15,** 2728 (1976).

105. E. Yarkoni, M. B. Goren, and H. J. Rapp, Effect of sulfolipid I on trehalose 6-6′-dimyco-late (cord factor) toxicity and antitumour activity. *Infect. Immun.,* **24,** 586 (1979).

106. M. V. Pimm, R. W. Baldwin, J. Polonsky, and E. Lederer, Immunotherapy of an ascitic rat hepatoma with cord factor (trehalose-6,6′-dimycolate) and synthetic analogues. *Inter-natl. J. Cancer,* **24,** 780 (1979).

107. M. V. Pimm, R. W. Baldwin, and E. Lederer, Suppression of an ascitic rat hepatoma with cord factor and Nocardia cell wall skeleton in squalene emulsion. *Eur. J. Cancer,* **16,** 1645 (1980).

108. S. Sukumar, J. T. Hunter, E. Yarkoni, H. J. Rapp, B. Zbar, and E. Lederer, Efficacy of mycobacterial components in the immunotherapy of mice with pulmonary tumor deposits. *Cancer Immunol. Immunother.* **11**, 125 (1981).

109. A. Bekierkunst, L. Wang, R. Toubiana, and E. Lederer, Immunotherapy of cancer with non-living BCG and fractions derived from mycobacteria: role of cord factor (trehalose-6,6′-dimycolate) in tumour regression. *Infect. Immun.*, **10**, 1044 (1974).

110. A. Bekierkunst, Immunotherapy of cancer with nonliving mycobacteria and cord factor (trehalose-6,6′-dimycolate) in aqueous medium. *J. Natl. Cancer Inst.*, **57**, 963 (1976).

111. T. J. Meyer, E. E. Ribi, I. Azuma, and B. Zbar, Biologically active components from mycobacterial cell walls. II. Suppression and regression of strain-2 guinea pig hepatoma. *J. Natl. Cancer Inst.*, **52**, 103 (1974).

112. M. T. Kelly, C. A. McLaughlin, and E. E. Ribi, Eradication of microscopic lymph node metastases of the guinea pig line-10 tumor after intradermal injection of endotoxin plus mycobacterial components. *Cancer Immunol. Immunother.*, **4**, 29 (1976).

113. R. Toubiana, E. Ribi, C. McLaughlin, and S. M. Strain, The effect of synthetic and naturally occurring trehalose fatty acid esters in tumor regression. *Cancer Immunol. Immunother.*, **2**, 189 (1977).

114. E. Yarkoni and H. J. Rapp, Immunotherapy of a guinea pig hepatoma with mycobacterial vaccines: Comparison of BCG cell walls and cell wall skeletons. *Infect. Immun.*, **21**, 1029 (1978).

115. G. Vosika, J. R. Schmidtke, A. Goldman, E. Ribi, R. Parker, and G. R. Gray, Intralesional immunotherapy of malignant melanoma with *M. smegmatis* cell wall skeleton combined with trehalose dimycolate (P₃), *Cancer*, **44**, 495 (1979).

116. G. Vosika, J. Schmidtke, A. Goldman, R. Parker, E. Ribi, and G. R. Gray, Phase I–II study of intralesional immunotherapy with oil-attached *M. smegmatis* cell wall skeleton and trehalose dimycolate. *Cancer Immunol. Immunother.*, **6**, 135 (1979).

117. G. Vosika, J. R. Schmidtke, A. Goldman, R. Parker, E. Ribi, and G. R. Gray, Phase I study of intradermal immunotherapy with oil-attached *M. smegmatis* cell wall skeleton and trehalose dimycolate. *Cancer Immunol. Immunother.*, **4**, 221 (1980).

118. H. A. Cohen and A. Bekierkunst, Treatment of *Mycosis fungoides* with heat-killed BCG and cord factor. *Dermatologica*, **158**, 104 (1979).

119. E. Yarkoni, E. Lederer, and H. J. Rapp, Immunotherapy of experimental cancer with a mixture of synthetic muramyl dipeptide and trehalose dimycolate. *Infect. Immun.* **32**, 273 (1981).

120. E. E. Ribi, K. Takayama, K. Milner, G. R. Gray, M. B. Goren, R. Parker, C. McLaughlin, and M. Kelly, Regression of tumours by an endotoxin combined with trehalose mycolates of differing structure. *Cancer Immunol. Immunother.*, **1**, 265 (1976).

121. C. A. McLaughlin, S. M. Strain, M. D. Bickel, M. B. Goren, I. Azuma, K. Milner, J. L. Cantrell, and E. E. Ribi, Regression of line-10 hepatocellular carcinomas following treatment with water-soluble, microbial extracts combined with trehalose or arabinose mycolates. *Cancer Immunol. Immunother.*, **4**, 61 (1978).

122. E. E. Ribi, R. Toubiana, S. M. Strain, K. C. Milner, C. McLaughlin, J. Cantrell, I. Azuma, B. C. Das, and R. Parker, Further studies on the structural requirements of agents for immunotherapy of the guinea pig line-10 tumour. *Cancer Immunol. Immunother.*, **3** 171 (1978).

123. E. Ribi, R. Parker, S. M. Strain, Y. Mizuno, A. Nowotny, K. B. von Eschen, J. L. Cantrell, C. A. McLaughlin, K. M. Hwang, and M. B. Goren, Peptides as requirement for immunotherapy of the guinea pig line 10 tumor with endotoxins. *Cancer Immunol. Immunother.*, **7**, 43 (1979).

124. E. Yarkoni and H. J. Rapp, Influence of oil and Tween concentrations on enhanced endotoxin lethality in mice pretreated with emulsified trehalose-6,6′-dimycolate (cord factor). *Infect. Immun.*, **24**, 571 (1979).

125. M. Février, J. L. Birrien, C. Leclerc, L. Chedid, and P. Liacopoulos, The macrophage, target cell of the synthetic adjuvant muramyl dipeptide. *Eur. J. Immunol.*, **8**, 558 (1978).

126. T. Taniyama and H. T. Holden, Direct augmentation of cytolytic activity of tumor-derived macrophages and macrophage cell lines by muramyl dipeptide. *Cell. Immunol.*, **48**, 369 (1979)

127. M. J. Pabst and R. B. Johnston, Increased production of superoxide anion by macrophages exposed *in vitro* to muramyl dipeptide or lipopolysaccharide. *J. Exp. Med.*, **151**, 101 (1980).

128. S. M. Wahl, L. M. Wahl, J. B. McCarthy, L. Chedid, and S. E. Mergenhagen, Macrophage activation by mycobacterial water-soluble components and synthetic muramyl dipeptide. *J. Immunol.*, **122**, 2226 (1979).

129. A. Adam, V. Souvannavong, and E. Lederer, Nonspecific MIF-like activity induced by the synthetic immunoadjuvant: *N*-Acetylmuramyl-L-alanyl-D-isoglutamine (MDP), *Biochem. Biophys. Res. Commun.*, **85**, 684 (1978).

130. S. Nagao, A. Tanaka, Y. Yamamoto, T. Koga, K. Onoue, T. Shiba, K. Kusumoto, and S. Kotani, Inhibition of macrophage migration by muramyl peptides. *Infect. Immun.*, **24**, 308 (1979).

131. D. Juy and L. Chedid: Comparison between macrophage activation and enhancement of non-specific resistance to tumors by mycobacterial immunoadjuvants. *Proc. Natl. Acad. Sci. (USA)*, **72**, 4105 (1975).

132. J. P. Tenu, E. Lederer, and J. F. Petit, Stimulation of thymocyte mitogenic protein secretion and of cytostatic activity of mouse peritoneal macrophages by trehalose dimycolate and muramyl dipeptide. *Eur. J. Immunol.*, **10**, 647 (1980).

133. S. Sone and I. J. Fidler, Synergistic activation by lymphokines and muramyl dipeptide of tumoricidal properties in rat alveolar macrophages. *J. Immunol.*, **125**, 2454 (1980).

134. S. Sone and I. J. Fidler, *In vitro* activation of tumoricidal properties in rat alveolar macrophages by synthetic muramyl dipeptide encapsulated in liposomes. *Cell. Immunol.*, **57**, 42 (1981).

135. M. Kato and J. Asselineau, Chemical structure and biochemical activity of cord factor analogs 6,6'-dimycoloyl sucrose and methyl 6-mycoloyl-α-D-glucoside. *Eur. J. Biochem.*, **22**, 364 (1971).

136. M. Kato, T. Tamura, G. Silve, and J. Asselineau, Chemical structure and biochemical activity of cord factors analogs. A comparative study of esters of methyl glucoside and non-hydroxylated fatty acids. *Eur. J. Biochem.*, **87**, 497 (1978).

137. G. Lanéelle and J. Tocanne, Evidence for penetration in liposomes and in mitochondrial membrances of a fluorescent analogue of cord factor. *Eur. J. Biochem.*, **109**, 177 (1980).

138. E. Durand, M. Welby, G. Lanéelle, and J. F. Tocanne, Phase behaviour of cord factor and related bacterial glycolipid toxins. A monolayer study. *Eur. J. Biochem.*, **93**, 103 (1978).

139. E. Durand, M. Gillois, J. F. Tocanne, and G. Lanéelle, Property and activity of mycoloyl esters of methyl glucoside and trehalose. Effect on mitochondrial oxidative phosphorylation related to organization of suspensions and to acyl-chain structures, *Eur. J. Biochem.*, **94**, 109 (1979).

140. E. Yarkoni, H. J. Rapp, J. Polonsky, J. Varenne, and E. Lederer, Regression of a murine fibrosarcoma after intralesional injection of a synthetic C_{39} glycolipid related to cord factor. *Infect. Immun.*, **26**, 462 (1979).

141. U. H. Behling, B. Campbell, Chung-Ming Chang, C. Rumpf, and A. Nowotny, Synthetic glycolipid adjuvants. *J. Immunol.*, **117**, 847 (1976).

142. M. M. Ponpipom, R. L. Bugianesi, T. Y. Shen, and A. Friedman, Glycolipids as potential immunologic adjuvants. *J. Med. Chem.*, **23**, 1184 (1980).

143. E. Yarkoni, L. Wang, and A. Bekierkunst, Stimulation of macrophages by cord factor and by heat-killed and living BCG. *Infect. Immun.*, **16**, 1 (1977).

144. I. Ofek and A. Bekierkunst, Chemotactic responses of leukocytes to cord factor (trehalose-6,6′-dimycolate). *J. Natl. Cancer Inst.,* **57**, 1379 (1976).

145. M. T. Kelly, Plasma-dependent chemotaxis of macrophages towards BCG cell walls and the mycobacterial glycolipid P3. *Infect. Immun.,* **15**, 180 (1977).

146. V. D. Ramanathan, J. Curtis, and J. L. Turk, Activation of the alternative pathway of complement by mycobacteria and cord factor. *Infect. Immun.,* **29**, 30 (1980).

5

Thymosins and Other Hormone-Like Factors of the Thymus Gland

ALLAN L. GOLDSTEIN
TERESA L. K. LOW
GARY B. THURMAN
MARION ZATZ
NICHOLAS R. HALL
JOHN E. McCLURE
SHU-KUANG HU
RICHARD S. SCHULOF

Department of Biochemistry and Department of Medicine
The George Washington University School of Medicine and Health Sciences
Washington, D.C.

This work was supported in part by grants from the National Cancer Institute, CA 24974, CA 29943; The National Institute of Aging, AG 01531; and Hoffmann-La Roche, Inc.

1. INTRODUCTION

It is now well established that a functioning thymus gland is an essential requirement for the normal development and maintenance of cell-mediated (T-cell) immunity. The thymus is responsible for the normal maturation of many different subclasses of T lymphocytes, including various effector cell and immunoregulatory (i.e., helper or suppressor) T-cell subpopulations. During the past decade the endocrine role of the thymus gland has been elucidated. The thymus is now believed to exert its influence by releasing humoral agents that act *in situ* and at distant target tissue sites (e.g., peripheral lymphoid tissues) through the blood. A number of laboratories have succeeded in isolating and purifying factors with thymic hormonelike activity from both thymus tissue and serum. The best characterized fractions are thymosin fraction 5, thymosin α_1, thymosin β_4, thymosin α_7, thymopoietin II (TP), thymic humoral factor (THF), and *facteur thymique serique* (thymic serum factor) (FTS). Several of these peptides have now been purified to homogeneity, sequenced, chemically synthesized, and, in the case of thymosin α_1, biologically synthesized with the use of recombinant DNA procedures.

Since patients with neoplastic disease frequently manifest abnormalities in both T-cell number and function, agents that restore normal T-cell physiology have been sought to serve as adjunctive measures to conventional treatment modalities. Such agents also have potential in helping to reverse the significant immunosuppressive effects of chemotherapy and radiation therapy. The importance of defined thymic hormones as modifying agents of host T-cell function has been established in studies with children receiving thymosin fraction 5 for a variety of primary immunodeficiency diseases. A logical sequel to such investigations has been to utilize thymic hormones in an attempt to restore immune competence in patients with neoplastic disorders. To date, more than 300 cancer patients have been treated with thymosin fraction 5 or thymosin α_1 by Phase I or II protocols, and numerous other studies are currently in progress.

In this chapter we review the pertinent historical background that has provided the physiological basis for therapeutic trials with thymosin and the other thymic hormones. In addition, we summarize the increasingly complex nomenclature and characteristics of the well-defined thymic hormones. Finally, we review the results of therapeutic studies with thymosin in patients with immunodeficiency and autoimmune and neoplastic diseases and discuss the prospectives for further investigation.

2. HISTORICAL BACKGROUND: THYMOSIN AND THE ENDOCRINE THYMUS

The rapidity with which interest in the thymus and thymic hormones has expanded in the last decade is reflected by the publication of several volumes, symposia, and current reviews on the subject of the thymus and its hormones (1–11). As a result of many investigations, it is now generally believed that all the classical criteria for categorizing the thymus as an endocrine organ have been satisfied. These include the observations that (1) extirpation of the thymus in neonatal or adult animals results in specific immune system defects, (2) thymic grafts ameliorate the consequences of thymectomy, (3) the reconstitutive effects of thymus grafting could be replaced to a great extent by the administration of cell-free organ extracts, (4) purified, well-characterized and synthesized products exhibited activity identical to crude thymic extracts, (5) biological activity characteristic of thymic products was detected circulating in blood, and (6) such serum activity could no longer be identified following extirpation of the thymus but could be reconstituted by thymus grafting or by parenteral injections of thymic extracts. Each of these aspects of thymus physiology is more fully reviewed in the following sections.

2.1. Neonatal Thymectomy Studies

The important role of the thymus in the development of immunologic responsiveness was elucidated from observations in animals thymectomized in the perinatal period (12,13). Such animals exhibited severe defects, including a depletion of lymphocytes in the blood, lymph nodes, and spleen and impaired immune responses to environmental pathogens. They developed a typical wasting syndrome that was characterized by slowing of growth and premature mortality. Immunologically, the animals were defective in the ability to reject foreign grafts and to manifest delayed type hypersensitivity skin tests. Their lymphocytes exhibited deficient graft-versus-host responses and impaired blastogenesis in response to T-cell mitogens such as phytohemagglutinin (PHA) or concanavalin A (Con A) or to allogeneic cells in mixed leukocyte cultures (MLC). The immune defects resulting from neonatal thymectomy resembled those found in congenitally athymic (nude) mice and in patients with the DiGeorge syndrome.

2.2. Thymus Grafting and Thymic Extract Replacement Studies

A possible endocrine role for the thymus was first considered when it was demonstrated that the implantation of a single thymus gland in subcutaneous or intraperitoneal sites could almost completely prevent the wasting disease, lymphocyte abnormalities, and immunologic deficiencies otherwise seen in neonatally thymectomized animals (14). Similar results were obtained by using thymus tissue (15) as well as a nonlymphoid epithelial thymoma (16), transplanted within cell-impermeable millipore diffusion chambers. These observations led several investigators to explore the immune restorative properties of crude extracts from animal (e.g., mouse, rat, calf) thymus glands. The most thoroughly studied extract was termed *thymosin* by Drs. Allan L. Goldstein and Abraham White. These investigators and their colleagues have shown that when administered to neonatally thymectomized mice, partially purified bovine thymosin (1) reduced the incidence of wasting and death (17), (2) stimulated lymphocytopoiesis (18,19), and (3) restored cell-mediated immunity such as the ability to reject skin allografts (19,20). Thus it was demonstrated that extractable agents originating in thymic tissue were capable of promoting the maturation of immune competence.

It has remained for subsequent studies to identify the thymic epithelial cells as the sites of synthesis and secretion of the thymic hormones. This conclusion was reached as a result of tissue culture experiments (see subsection on thymic epithelial supernatants in Section 3.5) and by demonstrating the presence of secretory granules (21–23) and various thymic hormones (23–27), such as thymosin α_1 (26), within epithelial cells.

2.3. Thymectomy in the Adult

The important role of the thymus gland in the maintenance of immune competence in the adult has only recently become appreciated. Since functionally mature peripheral blood T lymphocytes exhibit a relatively long life-span (28, 29) (6 to 9 months in rodents), the gross effects of adult thymectomy do not become readily apparent until many months following the surgery (30,31). Adult thymectomized mice have been shown to exhibit a gradual decrease in T-cell number and function. For example, a decrease in lymphocyte proliferative responses to PHA become apparent beginning at 12 to 24 weeks following adult thymectomy (32). However, the development of more sensitive immunologic techniques allowed for the recognition of many changes in the immune system shortly after adult thymectomy (33).

In 1971 Bach and colleagues (34) reported that one of the earliest changes in mice, which occurred 2 weeks following adult thymectomy, was the loss of azathioprine-sensitive E-rosette-forming spleen cells (T cells). These investigators also demonstrated that the population of azathioprine-sensitive T cells could be restored after a short term of *in vitro* incubation of spleen cells with various thymic factors, including thymosin (35). Their system has subsequently been utilized to follow the purification of several different thymic preparations and has been adapted to study circulating thymic hormone activity in the blood (36).

2.4. Circulating Thymic Hormone Activity

Using the rosette-azathioprine assay system described in Section 2.3, Bach and Dardenne were the first to demonstrate the presence in serum of biological activity analogous to that of thymosin (5,6,35,36). Sera from animals and humans exhibited similar activity, but such activity was lacking in samples from nude mice and adult thymectomized mice. Kinetic studies in mice revealed that serum activity disappeared within several hours after thymectomy and could be reconstituted by thymus transplantation but not after thymocyte administration or lymph node grafting.

Two other biological assays capable of measuring serum thymic hormone-like activity have recently been developed. The bioassay of Twomey and colleagues (37,47) uses thymopoietin as a standard and measures the induction of the thymus-derived antigen (Thy 1.2) on null mouse lymphocytes obtained from the spleens of nude mice. The assay by Astaldi et al. (38) measures the capacity of serum samples to increase cyclic AMP synthesis in murine thymocytes. The three different assays have been shown to be comparable in that all of them demonstrate a progressive loss of serum thymic hormone activity with age or following thymectomy (39–41). However, since several different thymic products exert similar biological activity, the assays cannot be used to identify the presence of any specific hormone. Indeed, it is not known at present whether the three methods detect identical or related substances.

In humans serum thymic hormone activity begins to decrease at puberty and reaches its lowest levels during the fifth and sixth decades of life (42). The age-related decrease in serum activity probably reflects the gradual involution of the thymus gland and precedes the well-documented deterioration of immune competence with age (42). However, the association between decreasing thymus gland activity and the increasing incidence of autoimmune disorders and cancer in the aged population provides a rational basis for the therapeutic use of thymic hormones in such individuals.

Clinical studies with these three assays have shown that serum thymic hormone levels are decreased in immunodeficiency diseases, such as the DiGeorge syndrome (41) and in systemic lupus erythematosus (43), Hodgkins disease (44), and childhood asthma (45). Levels are increased in rheumatoid arthritis (43), mycosis fungoides (46), and in older patients with chronic mucocutaneous candidiasis (48). Radioimmunoassays (42, 49–51) and radioreceptor assays (52) for several of the better characterized thymic hormones are in various stages of development, and it is hoped that the availability of more specific and sensitive methods will help to better define the role of the various hormones in health and disease.

3. THYMIC HORMONES: NOMENCLATURE AND PROPERTIES OF FACTORS PREPARED FROM THYMIC TISSUE

Classical endocrinology has taught us that an endocrine gland may either secrete a single hormone or be capable of synthesizing and secreting several hormones differing in chemical structure and biological activity. The thymus appears to be a member of this second category, inasmuch as several biochemically distinct hormonelike products have been prepared from this tissue. In some instances these different fractions resemble one another in their biological effects; in other cases the purified products exhibit only certain of the established biological actions that have been attributed to the endocrine functions of the thymic gland.

The most critical criterion for acceptance of any putative endocrine product as a hormone is its ability to replace specific functions of the extirpated or absent gland in experimental conditions. For the thymus, the agent in question should exhibit activity in one of the following biological models:

1. Absolute requirements include amelioration of immunological impairment in:
   a. The neonatally thymectomized animal.
   b. The adult thymectomized, immunosuppressed animal.
   c. The congenitally athymic mouse.
2. Supportive evidence:
   a. Enhancement of immunologic responses evaluated in a variety of *in vitro* and *in vivo* assays reflecting activities of T cells.
   b. Synthesized in the thymus of nonlymphoid cells.
   c. Binds to receptors on specific lymphoid precursor cells.

It should be stressed that these criteria are not satisfied by other nonspecific immune enhancing agents, such as levamisole, BCG, and interferon. As discussed in detail in other chapters of this book, although these agents clearly enhance many immunologic parameters, they do not mimic the role of an *in situ* thymus gland.

It is clear from what follows that there are a multitude of distinct, biologically active agents obtained from the thymus that have overlapping effects on the lymphoid system. It is unlikely that all these agents are thymic hormones. Rather, some of these compounds may be lymphoid products that nonspecifically activate lymphocytes and mimic the thymic hormones. Our task is to define the true thymic hormones and those lymphocyte precursors that are uniquely dependent on these true thymic hormones for initiation of their maturational sequence.

A number of factors with thymic hormonelike activity have been prepared from thymus tissue and blood; these preparations are in various stages of characterization. Among the preparations, thymosin fraction 5, thymopoietin II, THF, and FTS are the most thoroughly studied and best characterized. Thymosin fraction 5 has been found to contain a number of active peptides with molecular weights ranging from 1000 to 15,000. Several thymosin peptides have now been purified to homogeneity. To date, four thymic hormones have been sequenced: thymosin α_1 [molecular weight (MW) 3108]; thymosin β_4 (MW 4982); thymopoietin II (MW 5562); and FTS (MW 857). These thymic peptides appear to be chemically unrelated.

The demonstration that several different agents are produced by the thymus immediately raises the question of whether any single thymic hormone can elicit all the potential biological functions of the thymus gland or whether each hormone acts to regulate specific, selective aspects of T-cell differentiation. This last possibility would explain why diverse products have been reported to have thymic hormonelike activity and may also have some significance for the future in regard to developing more precise practical application of these substances for the specific amelioration of various types of impaired immunologic states in a number of clinical conditions.

In Sections 3 and 4 we consider the chemistry and biology of purified factors isolated from thymic tissue and purified factors with thymic hormonelike activity isolated from blood. The discussion includes a summary of the biochemical and immunologic properties of the isolated products. We categorize a product as a thymic hormone if it has been isolated from thymus tissue and if it exhibits biological effects that have been established as characteristic of the gland. Alternatively, a preparation with thymic hormonelike activity might be present in nonthymic tissue (e.g., blood) either as a *de novo* secretory product from the thymus and/or as a fraction derived from chemical alterations that have occurred either in the gland of origin or subsequent to its entrance into the circulation. In the latter case, in the absence of evidence that the putative hormone can be identified as a constituent of the thymus, its biological actions should at least resemble those of extracts of the gland itself.

3.1. Thymosin and Its Component Polypeptides

The thymosin studies (see Section 2.2), initiated at the Albert Einstein College of Medicine in New York by Drs. Abraham White and Allan L. Goldstein, have contributed to the elucidation of the endocrine function of the thymus (7–11, 17–20, 53–84). In addition, thymosin fraction 5 was the first well-defined thymic preparation to be used in patients with primary immunodeficiency diseases (67,68,70, 73–77), autoimmune diseases (78), and advanced malignancies (69,72, 79–84).

Thymosin Fractions 5 and 5A.   Thymosin fraction 5 is prepared from calf thymus, as described by Hooper et al. (55). The crude thymus extract is purified by a heat step, acetone precipitation, and fractionation with ammonium sulfate. The 25 to 50% ammonium sulfate precipitate is further subjected to ultrafiltration in Amicon DC-2 hollow fiber system to yield fraction 5. The 50 to 95% ammonium sulfate cut is also collected and processed through DC-2 and Sephadex G-25 to yield fraction 5A (57). Fraction 5 contains at least 30 different polypeptides and exhibits activity in each of the several different assays employed to monitor the thymosin purification (Table 1). Fraction 5A similarly contains multiple components.

Nomenclature of Thymosin Polypeptides.   Analytical isoelectric focusing of thymosin fraction 5 has revealed the presence of a number of components in the preparation. A nomenclature, based on the isoelectric focusing pattern of thymosin fraction 5 in the pH range of 3.5 to 9.5, has been described (57) and is illustrated in Figure 1. The separated polypeptides are divided into three regions: the α region consists of polypeptides with isoelectric points below 5.0; the β region, 5.0 to 7.0; and the γ region, above 7.0. The subscript numbers α_1, α_2, β_1, β_2, and so on are used to identify the polypeptides from each region as they are isolated. The purified polypeptides are tested in various assay systems to study their biological efficacy, and the active polypeptides are then given the prefix "thymosin"; the components that are inactive and are believed not to be involved specifically in controlling T-cell maturation and

TABLE 1. Some Biological Properties of Thymosin Fraction 5 and Its Component Polypeptides[a]

Thymosin fraction 5

In vitro enhancement of

Number of azathioprine-sensitive E-rosette-forming spleen cells from adult thymectomized mice

Appearance of phenotypic T-cell markers on mouse spleen and bone marrow cells

Responsivity to mitogens

Mixed lymphocyte reaction

Conversion of bone marrow cells into cells reactive in the graft-versus-host reaction *in vivo*

Production of suppressor T-cells

Production of macrophage inhibitory factor.

Production of antibody to sheep erythrocytes by spleen cells of normal and thymectomized mice

Intracellular cyclic GMP levels of mouse spleen cells

Terminal deoxynucleotidyl transferase (TdT) activity

Specific antibody production to tetanous, meningococcal and gonococcal antigens

LRF and LH

In vivo enhancement of

Lymphocytopoiesis in normal, germ-free, adrenalectomized, neonatally thymectomized, athymic mice

Rate of allograft rejection in normal and neonatally thymectomized mice

Resistance to progressive growth of Moloney virus-induced sarcoma in normal mice

Mixed lymphocyte reaction (*in vivo − in vitro*) by lymphoid cells from normal or neonatally thymectomized mice

Lymphoid cell response to mitogens (*in vivo − in vitro*) by cells of normal and athymic mice

Resistance to growth of allogeneic and xenogeneic tumors in athymic mice

Delay of abnormal thymocyte differentiation (loss of suppressor function) in NZB mice

Antibody production to sheep erythrocytes (*in vivo + in vitro*)

Survival in tumor-bearing mice (in conjunction with chemotherapy)

Interferon production following viral challenge

LH

Thymosin α_1

In vitro enhancement of

Numbers of E-RFCs in cancer patients

Percentage of autologous RFCs in cancer patients

Secondary T-cell dependent IgG, IgM, and IgA antibody responses

Percentage of macrophage inhibitory factor (MIF)

TABLE 1.   (Continued)

Expression of Thy 1.2 and Lyt 1,2,3 positive cells

T-cell dependent specific antibody production

Helper T cell activity

TdT$^+$ cells in the bone marrow and spleen (at high concentrations of thymosin α_1)

In vitro suppression of

TdT activity in murine thymocytes at low concentrations

Elevated T_γ/T_μ ratios in peripheral blood of cancer patients

In vivo enhancement of

Lymphoid cell responses to mitogens (*in vivo* + *in vitro*)

Lymphotoxin production (*in vivo* + *in vitro*)

Survival in tumor-bearing mice

Thymosin α_7

In vitro enhancement of

Suppressor T cells

Expression of Lyt 1,2,3 positive cells

Thymosin β_3 and β_4

In vitro and *in vivo* induction of TdT in separated bone marrow cells from normal or
athymic mice

In vivo induction of TdT levels in thymocytes of immunosuppressed mice

In vivo reconstitution of immune responses in immunosuppressed mice

In vitro induction of LRF and LH

^{a}See subsections on animal and human studies of thymosin biology in Sections 3.1 of the text.

function are given the prefix "polypeptide." For comparative purposes, the
location of FTS, thymopoietin, and THF on the gel and their isoelectric points
are included. It has been reported that trace amounts of FTS (85) and thymopoietin (49,86) are found in thymosin fraction 5. In the case of FTS we have
indeed found that there are, as measured by radioimmunoassay (RIA), trace
amounts of FTS-like material in thymosin fraction 5. However, the levels are
about the same as found in fraction 5 preparations isolated from calf spleen,
liver, or kidney. As summarized in Table 1, the various thymosin polypeptides
have been shown to exhibit a wide range of activities in several different assays
that assess T-cell function in mice.

Thymosin α_1.   The first thymosin polypeptide isolated from the highly
acidic region of bovine fraction 5 has been termed *thymosin α_1*. This peptide
is highly active in several bioassays (Table 1). Thymosin α_1 was isolated from
fraction 5 by ion-exchange chromatography on CM-cellulose and DEAE-cellu-

Isoelectric Focusing of Thymosin Fraction 5
in LKB PAGplate (pH3.5-9.5)

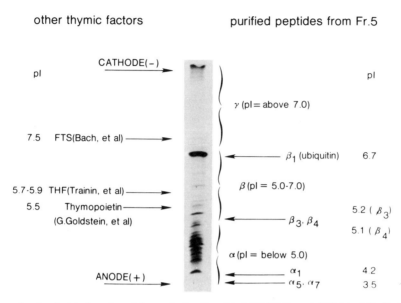

Figure 1. Isoelectric focusing of thymosin fraction 5 in LKB PAG$_{plate}$ (pH 3.5 to 9.5). Purified thymosin peptides from the α, β, and γ regions are identified. The isoelectric points of of several other well-characterized thymic factors are illustrated for comparison.

lose, as well as gel filtration on Sephadex G-75 (56,57). The yield of thymosin α_1 from fraction 5 is about 0.6%. Thymosin α_1 is a polypeptide consisting of 28 amino acid residues with a molecular weight of 3108. The complete amino acid sequence (58) of this peptide is shown in Figure 2. The amino terminus of thymosin α_1 is blocked by an acetyl group.

Comparison of the sequence of thymosin α_1 with the published sequence of other factors (see Figure 2) such as thymopoietin II (87) and FTS (88) reveals no homology. Computer analysis of the sequence of α_1 has established that α_1 bears very little homology to any of the 957 protein sequences that have been published to date (58).

Freire and co-workers (89) at the Roche Institute for Molecular Biology have performed experiments to determine whether some of the reported thymic hormones are actually synthesized in the thymus gland. The translation of messenger RNA isolated from calf thymus was carried out in the cell-free wheat germ system. The radioactive products that were immunoprecipitable with antisera against thymosin fractions were analyzed and found to be identical to those expected for tryptic peptides from thymosin α_1. The results suggested that thymosin α_1 was indeed synthesized in the thymus. Furthermore,

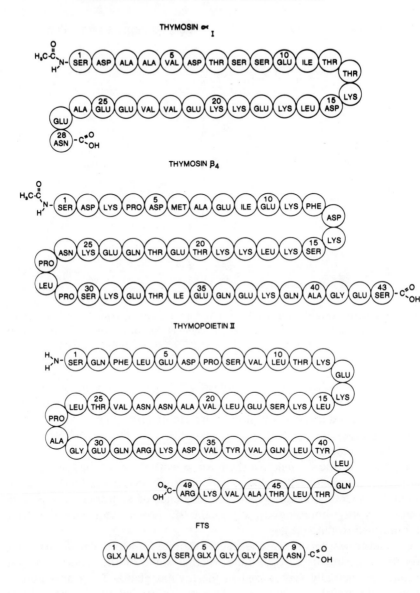

Figure 2. Sequence analysis of purified thymic factors: thymosin α_1; thymosin β_4; thymopoietin II; and FTS.

α_1 was probably synthesized as a longer peptide chain of 16,000 daltons and was processed (or degraded) to form the peptide detected in preparations isolated from the thymus.

Thymosin α_1 has been chemically synthesized by Wang and co-workers by both solution synthesis (90) and solid-phase (91) procedures. The purified material migrates as a single band on acrylamide gel isoelectric focusing (pH 3.5 to 9.5) and on high-voltage silica gel thin-layer electrophoresis (pH 1.9 and 5.6) indistinguishable from the natural thymosin α_1. The synthetic α_1, prepared by Wang et al. (90), has been tested in several biological assays and appears to have activity similar to the natural material. More recently a modified procedure for chemical synthesis of thymosin α_1 has been reported by Birr et al. (92) and for solid phase by Folkers (93).

Most recently Wetzel et al. (94) have reported the isolation and complete chemical characterization of a N^α-desacetyl thymosin α_1 utilizing recombinant DNA procedures. In this most important new development the gene for thymosin α_1 was synthesized, inserted into a plasmid, and cloned in a strain of *Escherichia coli,* as illustrated in Figure 3. The structure of the N^α-desacetyl thymosin α_1 was confirmed by sequence analysis, and the molecule was found to be biologically active *in vitro.*

To evaluate the species variation of the thymosin polypeptides, thymosin fraction 5 has been prepared from thymus tissues of different species, including human, pig, sheep, chinchilla, and mouse. The human thymus tissue was obtained from tissue excised during open heart surgery and from selected autopsies (8). Thymosin α_1 from several animal species has been prepared from fraction 5 by using a modification of the extraction and fractionation procedures developed for the isolation of bovine α_1. Human (8), porcine (95), and ovine thymosin α_1 (95) have also been partially sequenced. From the results obtained, these substances appear to have a sequence identical to that of bovine thymosin α_1.

Thymosins α_5 and α_7. Both partially purified peptides were isolated from fraction 5 by ion-exchange chromatography on CM-cellulose and DEAE-cellulose and gel filtration on Sephadex G-75 (Low, T. L. K., and Goldstein, A. L., unpublished). They are highly acidic with isoelectric points around 3.5 and are free of carbohydrate and lipid. Thymosin α_5 has a molecular weight of approximately 3000 and thymosin α_7 of approximately 2200.

Thymosins β_3 and β_4. Both preparations were isolated from fraction 5A by chromatography on DEAE-cellulose and gel filtration on Sephadex G-75 (96). They were found to induce terminal deoxynucleotidyl transferase positive cells in several different model systems (Table 1). Thymosin β_3 has an isoelectric point of 5.2 and a molecular weight of approximately 5500. Thymosin β_4 has an isoelectric point of 5.1 and a molecular weight of 4982. Both peptides share an identical sequence through most of their amino-terminal part and differ in the carboxyl-terminal ends. As illustrated in Figure 2, the sequence of

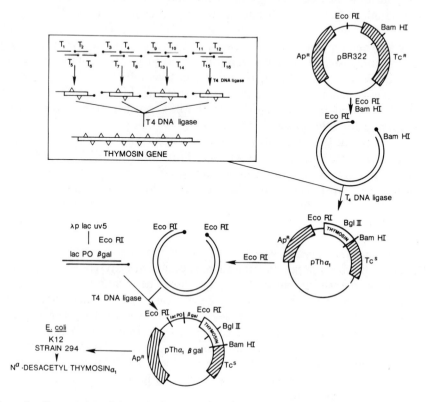

Figure 3. Construction of the gene plasmid for N^α-desacetyl thymosin α_1. The primary sequence of the gene was accomplished by using preferred prokaryotic codons with elimination of codons with multiple specificity and minimization of AT or GC regions. The gene was ligated into plasmids and placed under lac operon control and expressed as part of a β-galactosidase chimeric protein.

thymosin β_4 has been established (96). A computer search of the sequence of thymosin β_4 against other protein sequences published to date for possible sequence homology has been conducted (personal communication through the National Biomedical Research Foundation, Georgetown University Medical Center, Washington D.C., 20007). The results do not indicate a statistically significant relationship of thymosin β_4 to any other sequenced protein currently stored in the data bank.

Polypeptide β_1. The most predominant band on isoelectric focusing of thymosin fraction 5 is polypeptide β_1 (see Figure 1). This peptide was isolated from fraction 5A by chromatography on DEAE-cellulose and gel filtration on Sephadex G-75 (57). The amino acid sequence of β_1 has been determined (58). It is composed of 74 amino acid residues with a molecular weight of 8451 and an isoelectric point of 6.7. It is believed that this peptide is not involved in thymic hormone action based on the observation that this peptide was not active in any of our assay systems. The sequence of β_1 was found to be identical to ubiquitin (97) and a portion of protein A24, a nuclear chromosomal protein (98). It has been postulated that ubiquitin is a degradative product of A24 (99).

Biology of Thymosins: Studies in Animals (Table 1).   Thymosin preparations have been found to be effective in partially or fully inducing and maintaining immune function in a variety of normal and immunodeficient animal models (17–19, 59–65, 100–121). Thymosin treatment has been shown to increase the survival of neonatally thymectomized mice (17,20), accelerate skin graft rejection (19,60,63), restore graft-versus-host reactivity (59), and accelerate development of immune functions in newborn mice (17,20,59). Thymosin affects the responsivity of lymphocytes from nude (102,107,108,113), normal (108–110, 113), and tumor-bearing mice and from rats (103,104,111,112) and causes immature lymphoid cells to acquire distinctive T-cell surface antigens (65, 113–115).

Several animal model systems have been utilized to assess the influence of thymosin administration on the development of the immune perturbations normally associated with old age and autoimmune disorders. Thymosin treatment of NZB mice reconstituted suppressor cell and other T-cell functions and temporarily induced remissions in the autoimmune disease that such animals develop (116,117,122). Administration of thymosin to casein-treated mice reduced the incidence of amyloidosis (118). In aged mice thymosin administration significantly increased hemagglutinin responses (119); the *in vitro* incubation of lymphocytes from aging thymectomized rats with thymosin corrected their cell cycle growth characteristics to those seen in cells from young animals (120).

Recent experimental approaches utilizing thymosin have shown its effectiveness in inducing the differentiation of specific subclasses of T lymphocytes (killer, helper, and suppressor cells) (99,108, 111–113, 118,119,122) and have shown that specific purified thymosin peptides isolated from thymosin fraction 5 can induce certain markers (TdT, Thy-1, and Lyt) and functional expressions of lymphocyte maturation (65,101,110, 113–115, 118,123,124). For example, thymosin fraction 5 and thymosin polypeptides β_3 and β_4 have been shown to induce TdT activity *in vitro* and *in vivo* in precursor cells from normal and nude mice (102, 126–128). On the other hand, thymosin α_1, a potent inducer of helper T cells (129), appears to decrease TdT expression in thymocytes when used at low concentrations (130) and induce TdT expression at high concentrations (128). Such results have indicated that the individual thymosin polypeptides probably act at different steps in promoting the differentiation of precursor cells into functionally mature thymocytes. The thymosin peptides β_3 and β_4 appear to act before the prothymocyte stage, whereas α_1 appears to act at both early and late stages of thymocyte maturation. The present working model for the proposed role of the various thymosin polypeptides in T-cell maturation is shown in Figure 4.

Biology of Thymosins: Studies in Humans.   Many studies have documented that the *in vitro* incubation of thymosin with peripheral blood lymphocytes (PBL) from patients with a number of different disorders results in a significant enhancement of both T-cell number and functions. Thymosin-induced augmentation of E-rosette-forming cells (E-RFC) has proven to be a useful diagnostic assay for identifying patients who may respond to thymosin therapy *in vivo* based on their capacity to respond to thymosin *in vitro*. Thymosin increases both the percent and the absolute number of E rosettes formed by PBL from patients with primary immunodeficiencies (69,70, 72–76), cancer (79–84, 131–135), allergies (136), asthma (137), severe burns (138), viral infections (139), liver disease (140), tuberculosis (141), kwashiorkor (142), systemic lupus erythematosus, and rheumatoid arthritis (125,143) and in aged normal individuals (144). Thymosin α_1 is up to 100 times as active as fraction 5 in increasing

PROPOSED ROLE OF THYMOSIN PEPTIDES IN T-CELL MATURATION

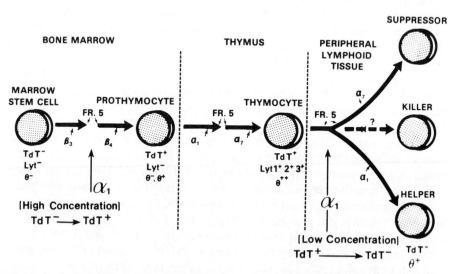

Figure 4.   Proposed role of thymosin peptides in T-cell maturation. Thymosins β_3 and β_4 promote early stem cell differentiation to the prothymocyte stage. Thymosin α_1 promotes both early and late steps of T-cell differentiation. Thymosin α_7 is associated with the generation of functionally mature suppressor T cells and α_1 with the generation of helper T cells.

the percentage and the absolute numbers of T-cell rosettes (145). Thymosin does not exhibit a marked effect on E-RFC of most normal individuals or of patients with initial T-cell levels within the normal range. An example of the correlation between *in vitro* response and *in vivo* (thymosin-induced) increase in E-RFC from 27 cancer patients is shown in Table 2 (68). In a larger study of 388 patients with head and neck, mediastinal, and pelvic malignancies and of 277 normal adults, the *in vitro* response to thymosin correlated inversely with initial T-cell levels for each group, including the normal individuals (135). Following radiation therapy, PBL from patients with mediastinal malignancies exhibited the most significant increase in E-RFC following thymosin injection. It was suggested that mediastinal radiation had resulted in specific impairment of thymus gland function in such individuals, thus leading to greater numbers of circulating thymosin-sensitive precursor cells (135).

In normal adults putative stem cells express E-rosette receptors following incubation with thymosin fraction 5 (146). Peripheral blood null lymphoid cells isolated by bovine serum albumin density gradients (147) or by nylon column filtration and E-rosette depletion (148) can be induced to become E-RFC after *in vitro* exposure to thymosin. No changes in B cells, monocytes, or in Fc or C_3 receptor-bearing cells could be documented. Therefore, thymosin appears to act selectively on T-cell precursors. The thymosin-induced T cells exhibit enhanced responsiveness to phytohemagglutinin (PHA) and to allogeneic cells (MLC) (146). It is noteworthy that PBL from patients with severe combined immunodeficiency diseases do not respond to thymosin *in vitro* (149). Such patients are believed to lack a population of thymosin-responsive stem cells.

In vitro thymosin treatment has been shown to significantly alter the proportions of several different subsets of T cells in cancer patients. A subpopulation of human T cells representing approximately 26% of the lymphocyte pool of healthy individuals is able to bind autologous red blood cells (ARBC) and are called *autologous rosette-forming cells* (150). In cancer patients this population of T cells is significantly reduced (151). Recently it has been shown (152) that a short-term incubation with thymosin α_1 produced a significant and constant increase in ARBC percentages in cancer patients with solid tumors.

TABLE 2.   E Rosettes (ER) in 27 Cancer Patients

Prethymosin (*In Vitro*)		Postthymosin (*In Vivo*)	
Initial ER	Responders[a]	Initial ER	Responders[b]
< 45%	8/10 (80%)	< 45%	8/9[c] (89%)
> 45%	2/17 (12%)	> 45%	8/17 (47%)

[a] Show a significant increase in peripheral blood E-RFCs after incubation with thymosin *in vitro*.

[b] Show a significant increase in peripheral blood E-RFCs following thymosin injection.

[c] One patient evaluated but not treated with thymosin (68).

Several other functional subclasses of human T cells have been identified with the use of either serologic techniques (which employ monoclonal hybridoma-produced antibodies) or by identifying specific surface receptors for the Fc portions of immunoglobulins (153).

It has been reported that there are distinct subsets of T cells that possess specific receptors for the Fc portion of IgG or IgM and are called $T\gamma$ and $T\mu$ cells, respectively (153). Chretien et al. (154) have recently analyzed the effects of short-term *in vitro* incubation of thymosin α_1 on the proportions of $T\gamma$ and $T\mu$ cells in the peripheral blood of normal individuals and cancer patients. Thymosin α_1 had no effect on the $T\gamma/T\mu$ ratios in normal individuals. However, $T\gamma$ proportions are generally elevated in cancer patients, resulting in elevated $T\gamma/T\mu$ ratios. Short-term incubation with thymosin α_1 had a significant effect of lowering $T\gamma/T\mu$ ratios to normal levels.

Most recently, Lowell et al. (155), using a solid-phase RIA to detect *in vitro* secretion by human peripheral blood lymphocytes (PBL) of IgG, IgM, IgA directed against specific bacterial antigens, found that thymosin fraction 5 and thymosin α_1 stimulate secretion of antibacterial antibodies *in vitro*. When PBL—obtained from individuals who had been immunized with tetanus toxoid (TT), group C meningococcal polysaccharide (Mgc) and/or gonococcal pilus (GP) vaccines—were cultured with pokeweed mitogen (PWM), addition of either thymosin fraction 5 or synthetic thymosin α_1 markedly enhanced the secretion of specific anti-TT, anti-Mgc, and/or anti-GP antibodies. The total amount of polyclonal antibody secreted, however, was not necessarily enhanced and was often suppressed. Thymosin also stimulated specific antibody secretion by PBL, which had been highly depleted of mature T cells. In the absence of the B-cell activator PWM, when PBL could not secrete antibodies, thymosin was ineffective. These results support the concept that thymosin can potentiate the development of functional specific helper T cells among human PBL.

3.2. Thymopoietin

Isolation and Chemical Characterization of Thymopoietin. Thymopoietin (initially termed *thymin*) was first isolated by Dr. G. Goldstein (156–158). The preparation of this peptide resulted from experimental studies related to the human disease myasthenia gravis. This disease is characterized by a deficit in neuromuscular transmission and thymic malfunction. On the basis of a biological assay measuring impairment of neuromuscular transmission, thymopoietin was first isolated by following its capacity to induce blockage such as is seen in patients with myasthenia gravis. This thymic factor can also induce differentiation of bone marrow cells into mature T cells *in vitro* and hence has been claimed to be a putative thymic hormone (159). The purification procedures include homogenization, a heat step, two passages on Sepha dex G-50, and fractionation on hydroxyapatite and QAE-Sephadex columns. The yield is approximately 1 mg/kg of tissue. The two isopeptides, thymopoietin I and II, are apparently related by peptide mapping and immunologic cross-reactions. Thymopoietin II has a molecular weight of 5562 daltons and a pI of 5.5. The sequence of the molecule has been delineated (Figure 2) (87).

Goldstein changed the nomenclature of his preparations to avoid confusion with the pyrimidine base, thymine, and designated his product as thymopoietins I and II in view of their apparent capacity to stimulate the maturation of lymphoid tissue (158). The two preparations appeared to be closely related polypeptides since they were immunologically cross-reactive and had indistinguishable biological activities. This close relationship was confirmed when it was shown that thymopoietins I and II differed by only two residues (87). Since these substitutions do not affect the biological activity of thymopoietin, Goldstein (157) has suggested that the two thymopoietins probably represent isohormonal variations.

Goldstein and his colleagues initiated studies to determine whether their fractions might induce the expression of various T-cell antigens in normal bone marrow cells. These studies led to the purification of a third polypeptide, which initially was thought to be the precursor of thymopoietin. This molecule was termed *ubiquitin* because of its wide distribution in nature in tissues other than the thymus (97). The amino acid sequences of all of these molecules have been established (87,97). Recently Fugino et al. (160) reported the synthesis of the entire 49 amino acid chain of thymopoietin II and established that the product had biological activity similar to native thymopoietin II.

A tridecapeptide fragment of thymopoietin, corresponding to residues 29 through 41, was synthesized by solid-phase methodology and was shown to have the biological activity of 3% of the parental activity of the entire molecule (161). In addition, biologically active pentapeptide, Arg-Lys-Asp-Val-Tyr, corresponding to residues 32 through 36 of the 49 amino acid sequence of thymopoietin (162) has been synthesized.

Comparisons of the available data suggest that thymopoietins I and II are distinct from other thymic factors. At the present time there is no evidence of homology of thymopoietins I or II with any of the established structures of the polypeptides in calf thymosin fraction 5. However, as described previously, the sequence of ubiquitin appears to be identical with that of a peptide isolated from thymosin fraction 5 by Low et al. (57,58) and termed polypeptide β_1. Polypeptide β_1 and ubiquitin are the N-terminal 74 amino acids of A24, a nonhistone chromosomal protein (97–99).

Biology of Thymopoietin. In view of the close similarities in chemical properties of thymopoietins I and II, the biological data reported for these polypeptides have generally been obtained with thymopoietin II (163–165). These data and some of the biologic properties of thymopoietin are as follows (156–159, 161,162,164,165, 218–223):

1. Activities *in vitro:*
   a. Induction of differentiation of murine prothymocytes to thymo-cytes, as detected by cell surface makers (e.g., Thy 1, TL, Lyt 1,2,3) and functional characteristics (e.g., responsiveness to T-cell mito-gens).
   b. Increase in intracellular cAMP concentration in thymocytes.
   c. Increase in intracellular cGMP synthesis in fractionated lympho-cytes.
   d. Enhancement of lymphoid cell transcription and translation of DNA.
   e. Inhibition of early stage of B-cell differentiation.
   f. Induction of a late stage of B-cell differentiation.
   g. Induction of complement receptor on human granulocytes.
   h. Increase in the proportions of Tγ cells in the blood of normal donors.
   i. Induction of E-RFC from human bone marrow precursor cells.

2. Activities *in vivo:*
   a. Impairment of neuromuscular transmission in the mouse and rat.
   b. Induction of prothymocytes of nude mice with appearance of cells with TL^+ Thy 1^+ phenotypes in the spleen and TL^- Thy 1^+ in lymph nodes.
   c. Delay the onset and reduce the severity of autoimmune hemolytic anemia in NZB mice.
   d. Enhance the lower than normal mixed lymphocyte reactivity of lymph node cells of NZB mice with established autoimmune disease.
   e. Enhance the reduced T-cell-dependent antibody responses of aged mice.

Recently the biological activities of the pentapeptide representing residues 32 to 36 of thympoietin (designated TP-5) have been studied in a model de-signed to examine whether the thymus gland or its products can ameliorate or prevent the immune deficiencies that accompany aging (164). Spleen cells from aged mice exposed either *in vitro* or *in vivo* to the synthetic TP-5 showed par-tial restoration of the number of antibody-forming plaque cells and high-affinity plaque-forming cells to the antigen dinitrophenylated bovine gamma globulin. The data indicated that TP-5 may enhance the capacity of aged mice to retain, in part, their immune function.

3.3. Thymic Humoral Factor (THF)

Isolation and Chemical Characterization of THF.   The thymic hormone research being pursued in the laboratory of Dr. N. Trainin at the Weizmann Institute of Science in Rehovot, Israel, partially developed from the early observations made while Trainin was at the National Cancer Institute (166,167). These studies demonstrated that thymus tissue in millipore chambers im-planted into neonatally thymectomized mice led to the restoration of specific immunologic competence in these animals. Subsequently, Trainin and his colleagues pursued these observations by preparing cell-free extracts that conferred immune competence to spleen cells from neonatally thymectomized mice *in vitro*. The initial bioassay was an *in vitro* model of the graft-versus-host reaction. In this assay the immunocompetence of isolated lymphoid cell populations was assessed by the ability of these populations to induce an increase in weight or size of an allogeneic spleen explant. It was observed that spleen cells from neonatally thymectomized mice did not achieve this competence unless they were previously exposed to the thymic extracts.

The initial product was generally obtained from calf thymus, but syngeneic mouse extracts were also shown to be active in this assay. The method used for the isolation of purified THF involved prolonged dialysis of crude thymic homogenates against cold distilled water. More recently the further purification of THF to homogeneity has been achieved (168,169). The procedure involves successive chromatographic steps on Sephadex G-10 and G-25 and DEAE-Sephadex A-25. The homogeneity of THF has been established by isoelectric focusing on polyacrylamide gels. The isoelectric point of THF is 5.6. The amino acid composition of purified THF is shown in Table 3. On the basis of leucine as unity, the minimal weight is 3220.

There is no apparent relationship between the composition of THF and thymosin α_1. Data for the amino acid sequence of THF are awaited with interest. These data will establish the relationship, if any, to other thymic peptides that have been isolated and sequenced.

Biology of THF.   Until recently the extensive *in vitro* and *in vivo* biological data reported for thymic humoral factor (THF) were obtained with a relatively crude fraction prepared from calf thymus. Although much of the extensive biological data obtained with the earlier, relatively impure thymic fraction (see the following list) have not been reassessed with the homogenous THF, a few

TABLE 3.   Amino Acid Composition of THF

Amino Acid Residue	Number of Residues (Leucine = 1)
Aspartic acid	4
Threonine	1
Serine	5
Glutamic acid	8
Proline	2
Glycine	5
Alanine	2
Leucine	1
Lysine	1
Arginine	2
	31

Source: Kook et al. (167).

of these assays have been repeated with the homogeneous product. The following list presents a summary of some of the biological properties of THF (3,167, 207–213, 224–228):

1. Restoration of the ability of spleen cells from neonatally thymectomized mice, incubated with THF *in vitro,* to participate in an *in vitro* graft-versus-host reaction.

2. Increase of the *in vitro* survival of thymocytes incubated in the presence of hydrocortisone.

3. Enhancement of ability of normal spleen cells to respond to PHA and Con A.

4. Enhancement of elicitation of a mixed lymphocyte reaction by spleen cells from neonatally thymectomized mice incubated *in vitro* with THF or by spleen cells from neonatally thymectomized mice treated *in vivo* with THF.

5. Restoration of ability of neonatally thymectomized mice to reject an allogeneic skin graft or an inoculum of allogeneic fibrosarcoma cells.

6. Restoration of ability of spleen cells from neonatally thymectomized donors to induce an *in vivo* graft-versus-host reaction.

7. Restoration of capacity of T cells from thymectomized donors to differentiate into cytotoxic cells.

8. Promotion of T-cell helper function in thymus-deprived mice.

9. Inhibition of generation of effector cells *in vitro* during the sensitization phase of cell-mediated cytotoxic activity.

10. Enhancement *in vitro* of the synthesis of cyclic AMP by mouse thymocytes.

11. Enhancement of the intracellular spleen cell concentration of cyclic AMP of spleen cells from neonatally thymectomized mice treated *in vivo* with THF.

12. *In vitro* enhancement of human T-cell rosettes, LMIF production, and graft-versus-host responses by PBL from patients with immunodeficiency and autoimmune and infectious diseases.

13. Enhancement of intracellular cyclic AMP levels in human umbilical cord blood lymphocytes.

3.4. Thymosin Fraction 5-Like Preparations

Thymic Factor (TFX).   The role of immunologic mechanisms in the pathogenesis of leukemia and their effects on the course of the disease have been a subject of study by Aleksandrowicz and his colleagues in Poland since 1948 (170). In view of later observations indicating the involvement of the thymus in hematopoiesis, Aleksandrowicz's institute initiated studies during the period of 1972 to 1974 with the goal of stimulating host immunologic mechanisms. In initial efforts thymus fragments taken from myasthenia gravis patients were transplanted into selected patients with leukemia and Hodgkin's disease. The appearance of immunologic enhancement a short time after the thymus transplant led the group in Krakow to begin work in 1973 on the clinical usefulness of calf thymus extract.

In the early studies an aqueous extract of calf thymus tissue, termed TFX, was employed. Evidence that the administration of TFX resulted in enhancement of humoral and cell-mediated immunity (171,172) led to attempts by Aleksandrowicz, Skotnicki, and their colleagues to purify the crude aqueous preparations of TFX.

Skotnicki has recently published (173) a procedure that resulted in a highly purified TFX. The aqueous extract of thymus glands from 5- to 7-week-old calves was subjected to $(NH_4)_2SO_4$ fractionation, ion-exchange chromatography, and precipitation with ethyl alcohol. The insoluble fraction was shown to be a protein that was homogeneous on polyacrylamide gel electrophoresis. The isolated molecule was free of lipid, carbohydrate, and nucleotide. Electrophoresis with 0.1% SDS at pH 6.8 indicated a molecular weight of approximately 4200. The amino acid composition of TFX is presented in Table 4.

Comparisons of the amino acid composition of TFX, thymosin α_1, thymopoietin, and THF show no evident similarity among these various preparations. In the absence of sequence analysis of TFX, the data available cannot

TABLE 4.   Amino Acid Composition of TFX

Amino Acid	nmole/100 nmole of Protein
Aspartic acid	7.0
Threonine	4.2
Serine	4.1
Glutamic acid	11.4
Proline	11.9
Glycine	25.7
Alanine	8.0
Valine	3.2
Methionine	1.0
Isoleucine	3.9
Leucine	5.3
Tyrosine	1.2
Phenylalanine	1.8
Histidine	1.2
Lysine	5.2
Arginine	4.9
	100.0

Source: Skotnicki (173).

as yet contribute to clarification of the question regarding its possible chemical relationship to the other putative thymic hormones.

Biology of TFX.   The biological activities of the calf thymic product TFX (both the earlier preparations and the reported homogeneous product) have been studied by *in vitro* and *in vivo* assays (174). Some of the more significant activities that have been described are included in the following list (173,174):

1. Activities *in vitro:*
   a. Restoration of the azathioprine sensitivity of spleen rosette-forming cells from adult thymectomized mice.
   b. Increased rosette formation by human cord blood lymphocytes.
   c. Increased levels of intracellular cAMP and protein kinase of blood lymphocytes of patients with chronic lymphocytic leukemia.
2. Activities *in vivo:*
   a. Enhanced response to mitogens of lymph node cells from mice treated *in vivo* with TFX.
   b. Increased survival of mice exposed to γ radiation with an increase in the LD_{50} dose.
   c. Increase in number of blood T lymphocytes and return of delayed hypersensitivity (human).

Thymostimulin (TS).   Falchetti and his colleagues in Italy have modified the procedure of Hooper et al. (55) and have prepared a thymosin fraction 5-like preparation from calf thymus tissue that they designated TP-1 (175). They have changed the name of this preparation to *thymostimulin* (TS) (176). Their procedure for purification is given briefly in the paragraphs that follow.

Calf thymus tissue is first minced and extracted with ammonium acetate. This extract is then treated with ammonium sulfate. The precipitate is dissolved in water and then subjected to ultrafiltration on an Amicon PM-10 membrane, and the filtrate is desalted on Sephadex G-25 and gel filtered on Sephadex G-50. The fractions used show, on electrophoresis on polyacrylamide gels at pH 8.6, two main characteristic bands with an Rf of 0.22 and 0.42.

This fraction has been reported to have a number of similar biological properties to thymosin fraction 5 on human cells *in vitro* (177) and *in vivo* (176).

Biology of TS.   Thymostimulin has been reported to induce markers and specific functions of T lymphocytes in both immunodepressed animals (175) and immunodeficient patients (176,178). Tovo et al. (178) have reported that in children with malignancies and compromised immune responses to herpes virus infections, treatment with TS resulted in dramatic clinical responses and that infections cleared before any improvement in cell-mediated immunity could be determined (178). More recently, it has been found that TS stimulates interferon production in mice following challenge with poly I:poly C (179).

Porcine and Calf Thymic Preparations.   The isolation of thymosin fraction 5-like preparations has been prepared in China by Jin et al. (180) by using porcine thymus and by Liu et al. (181) with the use of calf thymus. A modified E-rosette assay has been used to follow purification of these fractions. Several of the components in the porcine thymic preparations have been further purified.

The isolation procedure for the porcine preparation is briefly as follows. The crude extract of pig thymus is partially denatured by heat, followed by ammonium sulfate fractionation and finally purified by DEAE-cellulose chromatography. This partially purified thymic hormone preparation is free from carbohydrates and nucleotides and contains at least eight or nine protein components, with molecular weight ranging from 9000 to 68,000. The pH range of their isoelectric points is 5.0 to 7.5.

The porcine thymic hormone fraction 5 thus prepared exhibits very high biological activity, as shown by a microrosette assay. Data reported showed that this thymic preparation was active at 0.1 μg per 100,000 to 200,000 lymphocytes in inducing the maturation of T-cell populations (180).

Biology of Porcine and Calf Thymic Preparations.   There are only limited reports of the biological activity with both of these preparations in the literature to date. Of interest is a recent report describing the clinical effects of the calf preparations in patients with opportunistic infections (182). Most of the patients were reported to have serious opportunistic infections, including encephalomyelitis, hepatitis, herpes zoster, and fungal infections associated with immunosuppressed states secondary to cancer. Recently an additional 20 patients with assorted opportunistic infections have been treated, of which 17 have had significant clinical improvement (S.-L. Liu, personal communication).

It has been reported that the porcine thymic hormone may be useful in the treatment of primary immunodeficiency, autoimmune disorders, certain neoplastic diseases and various bacterial viral and fungal infections (180). Treatment of some patients with the porcine thymic hormone 4 mg/day, 3 times/week i.m. for periods of 1 to 3 months has resulted in increases in T-cell percentages (180).

3.5.   Other Thymic Factors

Homeostatic Thymic Hormone (HTH).   Some of the earliest studies of the activity of a cell-free thymic extract were those by Comsa (183). This investigator described the presence in thymic extracts of a fraction that showed antagonistic effects toward thyroxin in normal and hypophysectomized rats and towards a number of other hypophyseal hormones, including adrenocorticotropic hormone, thyrotropic hormone, and the gonadotropins. In contrast to these antagonistic effects, HTH had a synergistic effect with growth hormone. Pertinent to our present considerations of the chemistry of thymic fractions was the report by Comsa (184) that HTH restored antibody production in thymectomized guinea pigs and delayed hypersensitivity in thymectomized rats.

A description of the preparation of HTH from calf thymus has been published (185). The product is apparently a homogeneous glycopeptide with a molecular weight between 1800 and 2500. The final product was shown to mimic the biological activities of the earlier less purified preparations. The composition and sequence of HTH are awaited with interest, particularly since this molecule appears to be the only described thymic hormone-like product in which carbohydrate is present.

The glycopeptide isolated by Comsa and his co-workers (185) has been studied extensively with regard to its biological activities, particularly those that are interrelated to the actions of other endocrine glands. The activity of this product in immunologic phenomena has also been documented. Some of the more significant biological properties are summarized in the following list (184,185):

1. Suppression of deleterious consequences of thymectomy in young (12- to 16-day-old) guinea pigs (e.g., restoration of weight gain and ability to produce antibodies).

2. Restoration of delayed hypersensitivity of thymectomized rats.

3. Positive chemotactic influence on lymphocytes of male rats.

4. Antagonists with adrenocorticotropic, thyrotropic, and gonadotropic hormone action; synergistic with growth hormone.

5. Diminution of the radiation syndrome in guinea pigs.

Lymphocytopoietic Factors (LSH$_h$ and LSH$_r$).   Two protein components have been isolated from bovine thymus by Luckey and his colleagues (186) that have known activity in promoting immune competence when injected into neonatal mice. In these investigations three separate assays were used to follow the biological activity. One utilized the lymphocyte:polymorphonuclear cell ratio in the blood of newborn mice, with assessment of alterations in this ratio following administration of a fraction from bovine thymus. Although this assay did not measure lymphocytopoiesis directly, it was useful in the initial studies. Of the fractions evaluated, two homogenous proteins were obtained, one of which was designated as LSH$_r$ and the other as LSH$_h$. These two proteins had molecular weights of 80,000 and 15,000, respectively. The protein LSH$_r$ was described as heat stable and LSH$_h$ as heat labile. The products were free of carbohydrate. Both proteins appeared to have lymphocytopoietic activity in the neonatal mouse assay. The amino acid composition of LSH$_r$ is presented in Table 5.

Further physical and chemical characterization of LSH$_h$ and LSH$_r$, especially the establishment of the sequence of each of these two substances, will be

TABLE 5. Amino Acid Composition of LSH$_r$

Amino Acid	Percent	Amino Acid	Percent
Alanine	6.14	Lysine	5.94
Arginine	5.72	Methionine	1.22
Aspartic acid	9.70	Phenylalanine	5.97
Cysteine-cystine	1.38	Proline	6.06
Glutamic acid	16.65	Serine	5.68
Glycine	2.55	Threonine	5.37
Histidine	4.46	Tryptophan	Present
Isoleucine	2.72	Tyrosine	4.21
Leucine	10.34	Valine	5.95

Source: Luckey et al. (186)

beneficial in the further clarification of the relationship of these two products to the other postulated thymic hormones.

At the present time the published biological data of the two lymphocytopoietic factors described by Luckey and his associates are relatively limited. In newborn mice both preparations enhanced antibody production to sheep erythrocytes and induced an increase in the ratio of blood lymphocytes to polymorphonuclear cells.

Hypocalcemic and Lymphocytopoietic Substances (TP₁ and TP₂).   In 1944 Ogata and Ito (187) reported that a fraction from calf thymus tissue lowered serum calcium in rabbits. Since that initial observation Mizutani and his colleagues (188) have continued their studies of the hypocalcemic substance from the thymus. With the development of knowledge of the important role of the thymus in immune reactions, these investigators turned their attention to the purification and characterization of their fractions, utilizing both a hypocalcemic and a lymphocyte-stimulatory assay. Two hypocalcemic factors were isolated from two bovine thymus glands, TP₁ and TP₂. These factors appear to be homogeneous on the basis of analytical gel electrophoresis (189).

The biological activities of the two factors prepared from thymic tissue by Mizutani and his associates (188,190) have been shown to include hypocalcemic activity in normal rabbits, enhanced production of antibody to sheep erythrocytes in neonatal mice, and a relative lymphocytosis utilizing the method of Luckey and his associates mentioned previously.

Thymic Epithelial Supernatants.   Several laboratories have reported the presence of thymic hormonelike activity in the cell-free supernatant of cultures of thymic epithelial cells. The most extensive biological studies of such preparations are those from the laboratories of Kater et al. (25) on human thymus epithelium conditioned media (HTEM) and of Kruisbek et al. (191) on thymic epithelial supernatant (TES).

Both HTEM and TES are relatively crude preparations obtained from thymic epithelial cells and have been tested in a variety of assays showing biological activity generally accepted as characteristic of other thymic extracts. For example, when added to cultures of thymocytes, HTEM and TES augment the proliferative responses of these cells to PHA or Con A (25,192). The increased mitogen responsiveness is, at least partially, due to an increase in the number of responsive cells. In addition, the data suggest that the target cells for HTEM and TES are cortisone-sensitive thymocytes and that TES has little effect on mitogen-stimulated spleen and lymph node cultures. Other *in vitro* studies of the activities of TES have demonstrated a stimulatory effect of the fraction on mixed lymphocyte reactivity and on antibody production to sheep erythrocytes by spleen cells from nude mice. The biochemical properties of the factor or factors responsible for the biological effects of HTEM and TES await characterization.

Thymic Polypeptide Preparation (TP).   Since 1949 investigators at the Institute of Endocrinology of the Academy of Medical Sciences in Bucharest, Rumania have been examining the chemistry and biological properties of an aqueous extract prepared from a lipid-free powder of fresh calf thymus. This fraction was designated TP, a thymic polypeptide preparation (193).

On electrophoretic analysis with the then available Tiselius apparatus, the pattern obtained suggested a single product. However, chemical analysis, although indicating the absence of proteins, revealed the presence of amino acids and low-molecular-weight polypeptides. Paper chromatography of the extract gave 13 spots, which on comparison with standards confirmed the presence of amino acids in addition to the polypeptides. This relatively crude extract could be heated to boiling without any apparent loss of biological activity. A similar polypeptide extract was derived from horse embryo thymus obtained at the seventh month of gestation.

The biological properties of the thymic polypeptide preparation described by Milcu and Potop (194) have been studied in some detail. In the majority of these assays the experimental model involved the use of thymectomized animals. Some of the reported biological properties of TP extract are as follows (194):

1. Simulation of Ca^{2+} and PO_4^{3-} deposition in bones of normal rabbits and in rabbits previously subjected to x-irradiation of the thymus.

2. Elevation of serum calcium concentration and decrease in serum inorganic phosphate.

3. Restoration to normal of the depressed liver catalase activity and blood hemoglobin levels of thymectomized rats.

4. Increased synthesis and metabolism of nucleic acids and proteins in the livers of thymectomized rats.

5. Alterations in carbohydrate metabolism (viz., stimulation in liver in

glycogen synthesis, glucose-6-phosphatase, and fructose 1,6-bisphosphatase activities and ATP synthesis).

6. Antiproliferative action on KB tumor cells *in vitro.*

7. Inhibition of growth of tumors induced in rats by methylcholanthrene or dimethylaminoazobenzene.

8. Decrease in hemagglutination titers in lung cell suspensions of mice inoculated with influenza virus.

9. Stimulation of antibody synthesis in immunized, x-irradiated rabbits and in normal rats inoculated with A_2 influenza vaccine.

10. Increased survival in mice inoculated with *Salmonella enteritidis.*

Nonpolar Extracts: Thymosterin. Experiments of Milcu and Potop et al. in 1961 (194,195) described a total lipid extract of the thymus, which, when administered to rats bearing a methylcholanthrene-induced tumor, exhibited significant antitumor activity. Subsequently, purification of this lipid extract was achieved, beginning with lyophilized frozen minced thymus and extraction of the tissue with acetone. Repeated extraction with acetone and with ethyl ether yielded a dry residue on evaporation of the extract *in vacuo.* This fraction was termed the *total lipid extract.*

By the use of selective organic solvent fractionation, four lipid-containing fractions were isolated from calf thymus. One of these, termed *fraction B,* was then separated into three fractions by standard procedures for separating blood steroids. A fraction designated as IIB had significant antitumor activity and on analysis by gas chromatography, contained a high proportion of saturated fatty acids, particularly palmitic and stearic acids and also significant amounts of oleic acid. This fraction was also relatively rich in cholesterol (approximately 58 mg/g fraction).

Fraction IIB was further purified by silica gel chromatography and thin-layer chromatography to yield subfractions designated as IIB_2, IIB_3, and IIB_4. *In vitro* assay of these fractions with the use of KB tumor cell cultures suggested antiproliferative activity in each fraction; however, fraction IIB_3 was distinctly the most active.

Infrared spectroscopy of fraction IIB_3 revealed the presence of a steroid nucleus, as well as 12_a-acetoxy-11 ketones. Further purification of fraction IIB_3 led to the isolation of a compound designated as factor S, which had significant *in vitro* antiproliferative activity. Examination of the structure of the pure factor S indicated a C_{28} steroid with methyl groups at C-21 and C-28. The infrared spectrum also showed the presence of a hydroxyl group bound to the steroid nucleus and either a ketone or an acetate carbonyl in the molecule with the suggestion that the ester was a methyl ester. In view of the structure, the molecule was named *thymosterin.*

Potop and her colleagues have presented data for the biological activity of purified thymosterin (factor S) (196,197). This product was reported to have anti-proliferative action on KB tumor cells in culture (198). The inhibition of proliferation was accompanied by decreases in a number of intracellular enzymes. These investigators have also reported that their nonpolar fraction from thymic tissue effectively repaired the specifically altered metabolism of normal or thymectomized tumor-bearing or x-irradiated animals and enhanced immunologic responsivity, blood hemoglobin, and lymphocyte numbers in neonatal animals (195,197).

4.   THYMIC HORMONE-LIKE FACTORS ISOLATED FROM BLOOD

4.1.   FTS from Pig Serum

Isolation and Chemical Characterization of FTS.   In the course of early interest in assessing the immunologic status and the relative likelihood of kidney rejection in patients with renal transplants, Bach and his colleagues (5,6) developed the azathioprine-rosette assay (see Section 2.4) that detected thymic hormonelike activity in the serum of animals and humans. Although several different thymic extracts were active in their system, these investigators set out to isolate the active agent directly from serum (5,6,9,88, 199–201). Porcine blood was chosen as the starting material, and purification steps included ultrafiltration procedures, Sephadex G-25, and carboxymethyl-cellulose column chromatography. The active factor, FTS, has a molecular weight of 847. It has been characterized as a nonapeptide with the following amino acid sequence:

< Glu-Ala-Lys-Ser-Gln-Gly-Gly-Ser-Asn

From an initial 15 liters of normal pig serum containing 1200 g of total protein, the yield of FTS was 3 μg. The biological activity of the purified product was increased 100,000-fold. The synthesis of FTS has been achieved and the synthetic and isolated natural FTS exhibit comparable biological activities (85,200,201) in those *in vitro* and *in vivo* assays in which they were compared.

Recently, Bach and his colleagues (50), utilizing a RIA for the evaluation of serum FTS levels, have reported the presence of FTS in pig thymic tissue. The latter was at least 10 times higher than pig serum in the concentration of FTS. Facteur thymique serique appears to differ chemically from each of the other well-characterized thymic factors (Figure 2). However, Bach has recently detected trace amounts of FTS in calf thymosin fraction 5 as assessed by RIA (J. F. Bach, personal communication) and has isolated the peptide by chromatographic procedures. This suggests that FTS, or a precursor product, derives from the thymus. However, it should be noted that trace amounts of FTS present in thymosin fraction 5 are similar to those found in highly purified bovine serum albumin (unpublished observations).

Biology of FTS.   The principal biological effects of FTS are summarized in the following list (5,6,9,201,229,230):

1. Stimulation of expression *in vitro* of selected T-cell specific antigens on murine bone marrow and on spleen rosette-forming cells *in vivo* following injection of FTS into either adult thymectomized or athymic, nude mice.

2. Restoration of responsiveness of spleen cells of adult thymectomized rats and NZB mice to mitogens (PHA and Con A) after *in vivo* administration of FTS.

3. Restoration of the capacity of adult thymectomized mice to generate cytotoxic lymphoid cells following treatment *in vivo*.

4. Restoration of capacity of thymectomized, irradiated mice to restrain growth of a Moloney virus-induced sarcoma following treatment with FTS.

5. Enhancement of the generation of effector cytotoxic T cells both *in vitro* and *in vivo*.

6. Inhibition of antibody production in NZB mice challenged with a thymic-independent antigen, such as polyvinyl pyrrolidone.

7. Inhibition of contact sensitivity in normal mice.

8. Delay of allogeneic skin graft rejection in adult mice believed secondary to generation of *suppressor* T cells.

9. Prevention of the appearance of autoimmune hemolytic anemia and Sjogren syndrome in NZB mice.

10. With high doses an increase in anti-DNA antibody production and in incidence of glomerulonephritis in B/W mice.

11. Induction of the transformation of cortisone-sensitive thymocytes into cortisone-resistant thymocytes.

12. *In vitro* inhibition of dexamethasone uptake by thymocytes.

13. Induction of E-RFC *in vitro* from human bone marrow stem cells.

14. Decrease in TdT activity in BSA gradient spearated human bone marrow cells.

15. Enhancement of contact sensitivity to DNFB in adult thymectomized mice.

Facteur thymique serique exhibits activity both *in vitro* and *in vivo* that is characteristic of thymic hormones. Of some interest is the increase in anti-DNA antibody production and increase in glomerulonephritis in B/W mice. This was seen after administration of a relatively high pharmacological dose of FTS, suggesting a decrease in suppressor cell function at this high dose.

4.2. Protein Fraction From Human Plasma

Isolation of Protein Fraction From Human Plasma.   The demonstration of thymic hormonelike activity in human blood (5,38) led White and his colleagues to isolate an active component from human plasma that stimulated azathioprine-sensitive rosettes (202).

Gel filtration of fresh human serum on Sephadex G-150 revealed that approximately 95% of the total azathioprine-sensitive spleen cell rosette assay activity was present in a fraction that coincided with the albumin and prealbumin peak. On the basis of this latter observation, Burton et al. (202) developed a procedure for the isolation of a serum thymic hormonelike factor using Fraction IV of pooled human plasma as starting material. Purification included $(NH_4)_2SO_4$ fractionation, G-150 Sephadex column chromatography, and preparative gel electrophoresis. Fraction 4, the final product, behaved as a homogeneous protein on analytical polyacrylamide gel electrophoresis. The mobility of this fraction and its amino acid composition were identical with preparations of authentic prealbumin (202). The homogeneous protein obtained from pooled human plasma exhibited a molecular weight of 57,700 ± 300. Electrophoresis of fraction 4 in SDS gels indicated that the molecule consisted of four subunits of identical size, analogous to prealbumin.

Immunodiffusion experiments against prealbumin antiserum with fraction 4 and with a commercially obtained prealbumin resulted in the formation of single confluent precipitant arcs. Amino terminal end group analysis showed glycine as the only amino terminal residue in fraction 4 and in authentic prealbumin. These results suggest that the active agent is, indeed, the prealbumin protein. Assessment of the activity of fraction 4 by the *in vivo* assay developed by Bach (5,6) indicated that 2 μg administered intraperitoneally for 3 days could reconstitute the population of azathioprine-sensitive spleen cells.

It should be emphasized that, to the present time, there is no evidence of a chemical relationship of prealbumin to either the FTS (88) of Bach nonapeptide or to the thymus-dependent human serum factor (SF) described by Astaldi and his colleagues (see Section 4.3). The *in vitro* activity of the synthetic FTS reported by Burton et al. (202) is distinctly less than that described by Bach and his associates (201). However, until each synthetic product prepared in the two laboratories is compared by each of the two groups, and preferably at the same time with isolated FTS, it is premature to draw conclusions regarding the possible relationships of the two blood products.

Biology of Protein Fraction from Human Plasma.   The partially purified fraction from human plasma described by Burton et al. (202) has been subjected to several assays in normal and in neonatally thymectomized mice. The results of such assays are summarized in the following list (202)*:

1.   Increase in numbers of azathioprine-sensitive E-rosette forming spleen cells from adult thymectomized mice following either *in vitro* incuba-

*Unpublished results obtained also by Iden, Burton, and White; Segal and White; Mihich, Leung, and White; and Mihich, Ehrke and White.

tion of cells with the fraction or injection of the latter followed by *in vitro* assay.

2. Enhanced survival of neonatally thymectomized mice.
3. Enhanced ability of neonatally thymectomized mice to reject an allogeneic skin graft.
4. Increase in numbers of sheep erythrocyte plaque-forming cells (IgM antibody) *in vitro* by spleen cells from neonatally thymectomized mice treated *in vivo* with the blood fraction.
5. Enhanced mixed lymphocyte reaction of mouse spleen cells incubated with the blood fraction.
6. Decrease in rate of growth of a slow-growing, mammary adenocarcinoma and enhanced survival of DBA/2 female mice when the mice are treated *in vivo* with blood fraction prior to tumor transplantation.

4.3. Thymus-Dependent Human Serum Factor (SF)

Astaldi and his colleagues (38) demonstrated the presence in human serum of a thymus-dependent factor that they designated as SF. This factor was characterized by its ability to increase the intracellular cAMP level of human and mouse thymocytes when the cells were incubated with aliquots of human serum. The target cell for SF was restricted to thymocytes; no effect was observed with normal human peripheral blood lymphocytes, or other lymphoid and nonlymphoid cells.

The stimulation of synthesis of cAMP by SF was no longer observed when normal mouse thymocytes were depleted of hydrocortisone-sensitive cells (203). Furthermore, incubation of thymocytes with SF increased the population of hydrocortisone-resistant cells (204,205). The data were interpreted as indicating that SF acts on hydrocortisone-sensitive cells, increasing their intracellular cAMP and inducing their transformation to hydrocortisone-resistant cells.

The thymic origin of SF is inferred from the following observations. Serum factor was present in the sera of normal donors, declining progressively after the age of 30. It was not detectable in thymectomized, human donors or in patients with thymus-dependent immunodeficiency diseases. Serum factor activity appears to be due to a peptide of molecular weight 500 (Astaldi et al., personal communication) that is distinct from the other serum factors. Most recently, Astaldi, using a modified fractionation scheme, has established that the serum fraction responsible for stimulating cAMP is adenosine (personal communication). Moreover, he has found that adenosine levels in the blood decrease after thymectomy. It is not yet clear whether the immunologic reconstitution seen with the partially purified SF is also due to adenosine.

5. THYMIC HORMONES: SUMMARY

It should be evident from the preceding discussion that a great multiplicity of apparently unique thymic factors exist that are capable of promoting thymus-dependent immune responses. Although the precise relationships among the various factors are still not defined, a number of generalizations can be made:

1. Thymic factors can induce the rapid appearance *in vitro* of murine surface T-cell differentiation antigens (e.g., Thy 1, Lyt 1,2,3) from precursor cells devoid of such surface markers.

2. Thymic factors tend to increase the proportions and absolute numbers of human E-RFCs *in vitro*. Such an effect is observed with normal precursor (e.g., bone marrow) cell populations, as well as with peripheral blood lymphoid cells from patients with a variety of primary and secondary immunodeficiencies, including cancer. The magnitude of the effect correlates inversely with initial T-cell levels.

3. Thymic factors can affect the expression of TdT by T-cell precursor cells. However, the levels of this enzyme may be either augmented or depressed, depending on which stage of differentiation is affected.

4. Some of the well-defined factors, such as the thymosins, THF, FTS, and thymopoietin, exhibit a wide range of immune restorative properties *in vivo* in various animal models. The interpretation of such studies is often difficult because of the multiple influences of these agents on various immunoregulatory (e.g., helper, suppressor) subsets of T cells.

Several words of caution are necessary regarding these generalizations. It does not necessarily follow that if an agent can induce T-cell surface characteristics *in vitro,* it will also result in significant alterations of immune functions *in vivo.* Furthermore, we cannot assume that positive results in animal systems will accurately reflect the therapeutic effectiveness of thymic hormones in humans. Nevertheless, the experimental data documenting the role of thymic factors in augmenting immune function has provided the rationale for clinical trials with such agents.

6. CLINICAL TRIALS WITH THYMOSIN

To the present time, most clinical studies of thymic preparations have been reported with three products, namely, bovine thymosin fraction 5 (66,84,149, 206), thymic humoral factor (207–213), and several thymosin fraction 5-like preparations, such as TS (175,176), porcine (180), and bovine (181) thymic preparations studied in China and TFX (170–174). Thymosin fraction 5 has been utilized in the largest number of clinical trials to date. This fraction has been chosen for therapeutic studies because it contains a number of different biologically active polypeptides. It is also apparent that thymosin injections in humans and animals result in detectable serum thymic hormone activity as measured in the assays of Bach (34) and Astaldi (71).

Most of the reported thymic hormone trials in patients with a variety of disorders cannot be critically evaluated at present since either the number of treated patients with a clinical syndrome was too small to permit proper statistical analysis of the findings or subjects receiving placebo were not included. Nonetheless, thymic hormone replacement therapy is proving to be of significant benefit in treating children with primary immunodeficiency diseases. Clinical trials with thymosin, now entering their seventh year, have resulted in significant improvements in T-cell numbers and function, decreased infections, increased weight gain, and overall clinical improvement (66–77).

In cancer patients Phase I toxicity studies and a limited number of Phase II trials in patients with advanced disease have been carried out over the past 5 years. Thymosin appears to be relatively nontoxic and to induce increased T-cell numbers and function. The recent positive Phase II trials of Chretien and colleagues (81–83) in patients with oat cell carcinoma of the lung have provided the stimulus for further therapeutic investigations using thymosin and other thymic factors in cancer patients. In Sections 6.1 through 6.3 we review results of the initial clinical trials with thymosin. This discussion serves to illustrate the potential *in vivo* effects of thymic factors on human disease.

6.1. Immunodeficient Patients

Over 80 children have received thymosin fraction 5 for a variety of primary immunodeficiency diseases (66–75). These patients have been treated with injections of thymosin up to 400 mg/m² for periods of over 6 years (usually daily for two to four weeks, then once per week). Most of the patients have received 60 mg/m² thymosin by subcutaneous injection. There has been no evidence of liver, kidney, or bone marrow toxicity in this group due to thymosin administration. There was a close correlation between the number of patients who responded *in vitro* in the E-rosette assay and those patients who have responded *in vivo* with increased absolute T-cell numbers and clinical improvement.

In a more recent study of 17 immunodeficient patients in whom other forms of therapy were either unsuccessful or could not be utilized, Wara and Ammann have reported significant clinical improvement in patients with a number of thymic-dependent immunodeficiency diseases treated with thymosin (70). The patients all had *in vitro* evidence of enhanced E-RFC percentages following incubation with thymosin fraction 5 and/or enhanced lymphocyte function as assayed in MLC.

In a follow-up report of the work of Barrett et al. (72), Wara et al. (73) have correlated changes in MLC reactivity *in vivo* following thymosin therapy with pretherapy enhancement of MLC reactivity by *in vitro* thymosin incubation in a group of 18 patients. In this retrospective analysis they found that pretherapy lymphocyte incubation with thymosin *in vitro* resulted in greater than 119% enhancement of MLC reactivity in those patients who had normal MLC reactivity after therapy. Conversely, in those patients who did not develop normal MLC responses after therapy, pretherapy lymphocyte incubation with thymosin resulted in 7 to 99% enhancement of MLC reactivity. Wara et al. (73) observed that if the criteria for a positive enhancement *in vitro* is greater than 100%, six of eight patients positive *in vitro* response correlated with subsequent response to therapy. Thus it is possible that pretherapy augmentation of MLC with thymosin can be used as an indicator of the *in vivo* efficacy of thymosin to enhance the aspect of T-cell function. A prospective study in larger numbers of patients is necessary to better define "significant" percent enhancement of MLC reactivity with thymosin incubation.

In a subsequent study Barrett et al. (72) observed that T-cell numbers were increased to normal with thymosin *in vitro* in three of five DiGeorge patients. When thymosin was given *in vivo,* the same three patients responded by an improvement in T-cell numbers and function. Similarly, in a single case report, Sharp and Peterson (74) reported a significant improvement of cellular immunity in a DiGeorge patient treated with thymosin fraction 5.

In one patient with thymic hypoplasia and nucleoside phosphorylase deficiency treated for 9 months with thymosin at a dose of 1 mg/kg, Ammann et al. (76) reported an increase in the percentage of E-rosettes and the total number of T cells and a return of the PHA and MLC response to greater than 50% of normal control values. However, with the development of systemic type 1 reactions following thymosin administration, therapy was discontinued. Immunologic studies returned to previous abnormal values.

Most recently in a case report by Rubenstein et al. (77) in a patient with adenosine deaminase deficiency and combined immunodeficiency it was found that thymosin therapy improved the clinical course of the disease when given with red-cell transfusions. The *in vivo* improvement in cell-mediated immunity correlated with the *in vitro* response to thymosin.

6.2. Autoimmune Disorders

Lavastida and Daniels (78) (University of Texas Medical Branch, Galveston) have conducted a small Phase I trial in patients with autoimmune disease. To date, five patients with autoimmune diseases have been treated with thymosin fraction 5 for periods ranging from 4 to 16 months (78). Four of the patients had systemic lupus erythematosus (SLE), and the fifth had rheumatoid arthritis (RA).

As indicated in Table 6 during thymosin, significant changes were seen in peripheral blood T-cell and null-cell percentages and a major decrease in a cytotoxic serum factor that is present in many patients with autoimmune diseases. This heterologous factor causes the lysis of murine thymocytes in the presence of complement. On the basis of these encouraging findings, a Phase

TABLE 6.   Changes in Lymphocyte Subpopulations and Decreased Serum Cytotoxicity Following *in vivo* Administration of Thymosin in Patients with Autoimmune Diseases[a]

Disease	Patient	Percent T cells		Percent Null cells		Percent B cells		Percent Cytotoxicity[b]	
		Pre-Rx	Rx	Pre-Rx	Rx	Pre-Rx	Rx	Pre-Rx	Rx
SLE	AB	31	67	58	9	11	24	27	0
SLE	ML	49	51 to 71	N/D	0	N/D	29	10	0
SLE	JAR	24[a]	71	60[a]	12	16[a]	17	76	0
RA and SS	JW	45	68	17	0	38	33	57	0
SLE	EH	37[a]	52 to 62	48[a]	36	15[a]	12	18	0

Source: Lavastida and Daniels (78).

[a] Early treatment (Rx).

[b] Normal values = 0 to 10%. Capacity of patients serum to lyse murine thymocytes in the presence of complement.

[c] SS: Sjogren syndrome.

II randomized trial is planned by Daniels to determine the efficacy of thymosin therapy in SLE.

Although the mechanism of immune reconstitution with thymosin fraction 5 in patients with rheumatoid diseases is not as yet defined, it may be related to induction of a subpopulation of thymosin-activated suppressor or regulator T cells. Such a population of cells can be induced *in vitro* by incubation of PBL with thymosin or cultured thymic epithelium (214).

6.3.   Phase I and Phase II Cancer Trials

More than 200 cancer patients have been treated according to Phase I or Phase II protocols. Cancer patients have been treated for periods of up to 4 years. As with pediatric patients, no major side effects have been seen in the majority of patients treated with thymosin fraction 5. In addition, Dr. A. Ommaya (National Institute of Neurological Diseases) and P. Chretien (National Cancer Institute) have just completed a small Phase I trial in patients with brain tumors using synthetic thymosin α_1 prepared by Hoffmann-La Roche (Nutley, N.J.). Fourteen patients with anaplastic gliomas who had received surgical and radiation treatments with and without concurrent intratumoral 8-azaguanine therapy, were entered into a Phase I trial testing thymosin α_1 versus thymosin fraction 5. Three patients received fraction 5 at 60 mg/m² subcutaneously twice weekly for 4 weeks; four patients received α_1 at 900 μg/m²; five patients received α_1 at 600 μg/m²; and two patients received α_1 at 300 μg/m² for the same duration. Total T cells, the change in percent T cells after incubation with *in vitro* thymosin (ΔT), and routine neurologic, hematologic, and cardiopulmonary monitoring were undertaken for 2 weeks pretreatment, during the 4 weeks of treatment, and for 4 weeks posttreatment. The patients were divided into two groups, a clinically deteriorating and a clinically stable group. Mean ΔT values were then compared for the pre-, during, and posttreatment groups. Pre- and post-ΔT values were significantly different in both groups at the $p < .025$ level, a difference that did not appear until after the treatment was completed. There were no significant differences between the ΔT values of the two groups at the pre-, during, and posttreatment periods, although the clinically stable group showed a more dramatic difference between the pre- and posttreatment ΔT values. No clinical or hematologic toxic effects were noted in any of the patients receiving α_1 during the trial.

The need for proper immune evaluation prior to thymosin-containing chemoimmunotherapy was established by Patt et al. (215) in a small, nonrandomized study of patients with Stage IIIB melanoma. Twenty-eight patients were immunologically evaluated and then treated with thymosin fraction 5, plus either BCG alone or BCG with DTIC. Immune competence was assessed by delayed-type-hypersensitivity (DTH) skin testing, enumeration of E-RFC in the blood, and assessment of PBL proliferative responses to PHA and Con A.

Thymosin treatment consisted of various schedules using subcutaneous injections of either a low dose (4 mg/m^2) or a high dose (40 mg/m^2) of the hormone. These investigators found that immunocompetent melanoma patients treated with high-dose thymosin plus BCG relapsed earlier than those treated with low-dose thymosin and BCG. However, high-dose thymosin treatment significantly improved the disease-free survival of the immunoincompetent patient group, whereas low-dose thymosin was not detrimental to this group. This investigation appeared to confirm the numerous *in vitro* studies with thymosin (see subsection on thymosin biology studies in humans in Section 3.1), which had suggested that immunoincompetent cancer patients were the ones most likely to benefit therapeutically from high-dose thymosin administration (68).

The first randomized Phase II trials of thymosin were designed by Dr. Paul Chretien, Associate Chief of Surgery and Head of Tumor Immunology at the NCI, and carried out by Dr. Martin Cohen and his colleagues at the Washington VA Hospital. The trial was a three-arm study in 55 patients with oat cell carcinoma of the lung. Carried out from February 1976 to January 1977, chemotherapy included 6 weeks of an intensive phase using a regimen comprised of cytoxan, methotrexate, and CCNU, followed by a 6-week course of less intensive chemotherapy consisting of vincristine, adriamycin, and procarbazine. Surviving patients received one or two courses of maintenance chemotherapy with the use of alternating combinations of these drugs and/or several other agents. All patients were randomized to receive subcutaneous injection of thymosin fraction 5 to 60 mg/m^2, thymosin fraction 5, 20mg/m^2, or placebo twice weekly during the first 6 weeks of intensive chemotherapy. The results of this trial have recently been reported (81–83) and are illustrated in Figure 5. Overall tumor response did not differ significantly among the

THYMOSIN IN CONJUNCTION WITH CHEMOTHERAPY IN PATIENTS WITH SMALL CELL BRONCHOGENIC CARCINOMA:

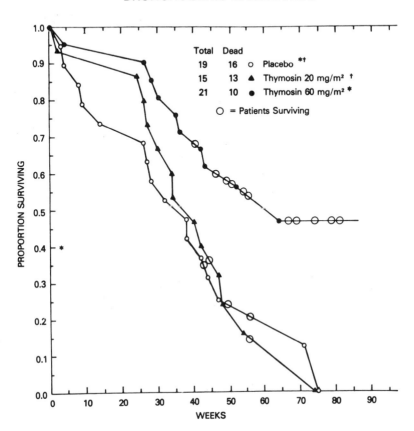

Figure 5. Thymosin, in chemotherapy of cancer patients [after Cohen et al. (81) and Chretien et al. (206)]. Survival kinetics of oat cell carcinoma patients given 60 mg/m² of thymosin (O) and 20 mg/m² of thymosin 5 (△) twice weekly subcutaneously during the first 6 weeks of intensive chemotherapy. Thymosin increased median survival from 240 days to more than 450 days.

three treatment groups. However, thymosin (60 mg/m²) significantly prolonged survival in patients who had eradication of all detectable disease by chemotherapy (median survival chemotherapy plus placebo 240 days, versus 450 days for chemotherapy plus thymosin at 60 mg/m²). The median survival is now over 500 days. Six of the original 21 patients in the high-dose thymosin group were alive and tumor free at over 2 years (M. Cohen, personal communication).

As indicated in Tables 7 and 8, prolonged survival of the lung cancer patients was found to correlate directly with initial low levels of T cells and low

TABLE 7.   Relationship Between Pretreatment Total T Cells and Survival in Lung Cancer Patients Receiving Thymosin

| Local T-cell Level | Median Survival in Days[a] | | Comparison Between Treatment Groups by Life-Table Analysis (Genan's Test) |
	Chemotherapy and Thymosin 60 mg/m²	Chemotherapy Alone	
High: > 775/mm³	350 (9)	285 (11)	$p = .28$ (one-sided)
Low: < 775/mm³	405 (12)	180 (8)	$p = .006$ (one-sided)

Source: Chretien et al. (206).

[a] Number of patients given in parentheses.

levels of α_2HS glycoproteins (82,83). The patients who benefited most from thymosin were those with relatively low immune reactivity. Hence this study was interpreted to indicate that whereas thymosin had no detectable direct antitumor effect, it may have ameliorated the immune defects due to the tumor or induced by the chemotherapy.

Although more effective chemotherapy regimens will no doubt subsequently be developed for small-cell lung cancers (216), this lung cancer trial with thymosin was the first positive controlled trial involving a thymic hormone preparation or, for that matter, any biological modifier in oat cell carcinoma. This study has provided the stimulus for several other Phase II trials utilizing thymosin and other thymic factors as adjuncts to conventional chemotherapy. These ongoing trials include the following:

1.   *Squamous Cell Carinoma of the Head, Neck, and Esophagus.*   This study, directed by Dr. William M. Wara at the University of California Medical Center in San Francisco, is a randomized schedule with and without thymosin fraction 5 as an adjunct to conventional radiotherapy (217). As of January 1, 1980, 55 head, neck, and esophageal cancer patients have been entered on the thymosin protocol. To date, after 18 months of entering, using a Kap-

TABLE 8.   Relationship Between Pretreatment Serum α-HS-Glycoprotein Levels and Survival

| α_2-HS-Glycoprotein | Median Survival in Days[a] | | Comparison Between Treatment Groups by Life-Table Analysis (Genan's Test) |
	Chemotherapy and Thymosin 60 mg/m²	Chemotherapy Alone	
High: > 60.5 mg/dl	300 (10)[b]	262 (11)	$p = .17$ (one-sided)
Low: < 60.5 mg/dl	495 (10)	180 (8)	$p = .039$ (one-sided)

Source: Chretien et al. (206).

[a] Number of patients given in parentheses.

lan-Meier curve for disease-free interval, there appears to be no significant difference ($p < .07$) in the disease-free interval (Wara, personal communication) in both groups. This is the point in time when recurrences become evident, especially in the head and neck cancer patients treated with radiation or surgery alone. Of interest is the tend of fewer relapses in the thymosin-treated group in comparison to patients receiving placebo (Wara, personal communication). Therefore, further follow-up will be necessary to determine the efficacy of thymosin therapy in this group of patients.

2. *Oat Cell Lung Carcinoma.* This study, at Memorial Sloan-Kettering Hospital, New York City, was begun on June 1, 1979. It is planned to enter 80 patients into this study in a randomized treatment schedule with and without thymosin, as an adjunct to conventional chemotherapy and radiotherapy.

3. *Lung Carcinoma.* This is a pilot study at the University of Maryland Medical School. It was started on July 5, 1979, with a total of 20 patients. It is a comparison of thymosin fraction 5 and thymosin α_1 in Phase I testing.

4. *Oat Cell Lung Carcinoma.* This study is being conducted at the University of South Carolina Medical School in Columbia. It will be double-blind, randomized thymosin versus placebo trial. It is planned to enter 120 patients into this study, which was started in August 1979.

7. FUTURE PROSPECTS FOR THYMIC HORMONES IN TREATMENT OF CANCER AND IMMUNODEFICIENCY DISEASES

The ultimate significance of the thymosins and other thymic factors in cancer treatment should be in providing a means of safely augmenting specific T lymphocyte functions in patients with diminished thymic-dependent immunity. In anergic cancer patients, the thymic hormones may be of importance as an adjunct to conventional treatments by increasing T-cell function in response not only to tumor cells, but also to pathogens, thus reducing the high incidence of infection that often accompanies cancer treatments.

The positive clinical trials to date with thymosin fraction 5 in children with immunodeficiency diseases, the positive oat cell trial of Chretien and his colleagues, and the positive studies reported with THF and several thymosin fraction 5-like preparations offer a strong rationale for rapidly confirming the clinical studies and expanding the basic research programs with the goal of purifying, further characterizing, and increasing the availability of the various thymic factors. Confirmatory clinical trials with the use of thymosin fraction 5 in lung cancer patients are already in progress in several centers. The clinical studies are being conducted at institutions that are equipped with facilities for performing detailed immunologic profiles on the patients being treated. In the completed oat cell and melanoma trials such assays appeared to identify the patients that benefited most from thymosin.

Several pharmaceutical companies have standardized and scaled up the procedures for increased production of thymic factors such as thymosin fraction

5. However, further clinical assessment is needed of the synthetic thymosins and thymosinlike polypeptides (e.g., thymosin α_1, thymosin β_4, thymopoietin, FTS). The availability of active agents that can be synthesized in the laboratory will circumvent the technical problems associated with the isolation of various thymic hormones from bulk quantities of thymus tissue or serum.

It will also be important to develop experimental animal tumor models that can be used to explore the efficacy of administering thymic hormones by various routes (locally, systemically and perhaps even orally) and in combination with other biological response modifiers, such as lymphokines, adjuvants, or interferons, or with tumor cell antigens. It is to be anticipated that over the next decade well-planned clinical trials will help to determine the optimal conditions for employing thymic hormones as a therapeutic modality in the treatment of cancer.

REFERENCES

1. A. L. Goldstein, A. Asanuma, and A. White, The thymus as an endocrine gland: Properties of thymosin, a new thymic hormone. *Rec. Progr. Horm. Res., 26*, 505 (1970).

2. H. Friedman, Thymic factors in immunity. *Ann. N. Y. Acad. Sci., Vol. 249*, (1975).

3. N. Trainin, Thymic hormones and the immune response. *Physiol. Rev., 54*, 272 (1974).

4. A. White and A. L. Goldstein, The endocrine role of the thymus and its hormone, thymosin, in the regulation of the growth and maturation of host immunological competence. *Adv. Metab. Disorders, 8*, 359 (1974).

5. J. F. Bach and C. Carnaud, Thymic factors. *Progr. Allergy, 21*, 418 (1976).

6. J. F. Bach, Thymic hormones: Biochemistry, biological and clinical activities. *Annu. Rev. Pharmacol. Toxicol., 17*, 281 (1977).

7. A. L. Goldstein, G. B. Thurman, T. L. K. Low, J. L. Rossio, and G. E. Trivers, Hormonal influences on the reticuloendothelial system: Current status of the role of thymosin in the regulation and modulation of immunity. *J. Reticuloendotherl. Soc., 23*, 253 (1978).

8. T. L. K. Low and A. L. Goldstein, Structure and Function of Thymosin and Other Thymic Factors. In R. Silber, J. Lobuc, and A. S. Gordon, Eds., *The Year In Hematology,* Plenum, New York, 1978, p. 281.

9. J. F. Bach, Thymic hormones. *J. Pharmacol., 1*, 277 (1979).

10. G. E. Trivers and A. L. Goldstein, The Endocrine Thymus: A role for Thymosin and Other Thymic Factors in Cancer Immunity and Therapy. In J. J. Marchalonis, Michael G. Hanna, and I. J. Fidler, Eds., *Cancer Biology Reviews,* Vol. 1, Dekker, New York, 1980, p. 49.

11. A. White, The thymus as an endocrine gland: Chemistry and biological actions of products with thymic hormone-like activity. In G. Litwack, Ed., *Biochemical Actions of Hormones,* Vol. VII, Academic, New York, pp. 1–46 1981.

12. J. F. A. P. Miller, Immunological function of the thymus. *Lancet, 2*, 748 (1961).

13. R. A. Good and A. E. Gabrielson, Eds., *The Thymus in Immunobiology: Structure, Function and Role in Disease,* Hoeber-Harper, New York, 1964.

14. J. F. A. P. Miller, Role of the thymus in transplantation immunity. *Ann. N. Y. Acad. Sci., 99*, 340 (1962).

15. R. N. Levey, N. Trainin, and L. W. Law, Evidence for function of thymic tissue in diffusion chambers implanted in neonatally thymectomized mice. Preliminary report. *J. Natl. Cancer Inst., 31*, 199 (1963).

16. G. Stutman, E. J. Yunis, and R. A. Good, Carcinogen-induced tumors of the thymus. III. Restoration of neonatally thymectomized mice with thymomas in cell-impermeable chambers. *J. Natl. Cancer Inst.*, **43**, 499 (1969).

17. Y. Asanuma, A. L. Goldstein, and A. White, Reduction in the incidence of wasting disease in neonatally thymectomized CBAW mice by the injection of thymosin. *Endocrinology*, **86**, 601 (1970).

18. J. J. Klein, A. L. Goldstein, and A. White, Enhancement of *in vitro* incorporation of labeled precursors into DNA and total protein of mouse lymph nodes after administration of thymic extracts. *Proc. Natl. Acad. Sci. (USA)*, **53**, 812 (1965).

19. M. A. Hardy, A. L. Goldstein, and A. White, Immunologic effects of a purified thymic hormone, thymosin. *Surg. Forum XXIII*, **23**, 305 (1972).

20. A. L. Goldstein, A. Guha, M. M. Zatz, M. Hardy, and A. White, Purification and biological activity of thymosin, a hormone of the thymus gland. *Proc. Natl. Acad. Sci. (USA)*, **69**, 1800 (1972).

21. F. T. Sanel, Ultrastructure of differentiating cells during thymus histiogenesis. *Z. Zellforsch.*, **83**, 8 (1967).

22. S. L. Clark, Thymus experimental clinical studies. *Ciba Found. Symp.*, 3 (1966).

23. B. Mandi and T. Glant, Thymosin producing cells of the thymus. *Nature (New Biol.)*, **246**, 25 (1973).

24. J. G. Van Den Tweel, C. R. Taylor, J. McClure, and A. L. Goldstein, Detection of thymosin in thymic epithelial cells by an immunoperoxide method. *Adv. Exp. Med. Biol.*, **114**, 511 (1979).

25. L. Kater, R. Oosterom, J. E. McClure, and A. L. Goldstein, Presence of thymosin in human thymic epithelium conditioned medium. *Internatl. J. Immunopharmacol.*, 1, 273 (1979).

26. K. Hirokawa and K. Saitoh, Heterogeneity of thymic epithelial cells revealed by localization of thymosin α_1 and various hydrolytic enzymes in human thymus. *Abstr. 4th Internatl. Congr. Immunol.*, **3**, 3.14 (1980).

27. M. C. Dalakas, W. K. Engel, J. E. McClure, and A. L. Goldstein, Thymosin α_1 in Myasthenia gravis. *New Engl. J. Med.*, **302**, 1092 (1980).

28. J. R. Little, G. Brecker, T. R. Bradley, and S. Rose, Determination of lymphocyte turnover by continuous infusion of ³H thymidine. *Blood*, **19**, 236 (1962).

29. K. E. Buckston and M. C. Pike, Chromosome investigations on lymphocytes from irradiated patients. Effect of time in culture. *Nature*, **202**, 714 (1964).

30. D. Metcalf, Delayed effect of thymectomy in adult life on immunological competence. *Nature*, **208**, 1336 (1965).

31. J. F. A. P. Miller, Effect of thymectomy in adult mice on immunological responsiveness. *Nature*, **208**, 1337 (1965).

32. J. M. Johnston and D. B. Wilson, Origin of immunoreactive lymphocytes in rats. *Cell. Immunol.*, **1**, 430 (1970).

33. R. S. Schulof and A. L. Goldstein, Thymosin and the endocrine thymus. *Adv. Int. Med.*, **22**, 128 (1977).

34. J. F. Bach, M. Dardenne, and A. J. S. Davis, Early effect of adult thymectomy. *Nature (New Biol.)*, **231**, 110 (1971).

35. M. Dardenne and J. F. Bach, Studies of thymus products. I. Modification of rosette-forming cells by thymic extracts and determination of the target RFC subpopulation. *Immunology.*, **25**, 343 (1973).

36. J. F. Bach and M. Dardenne, Studies of thymus products. II. Demonstration and characterization of a circulating thymic hormone. *Immunology.*, **25**, 353 (1973).

37. J. J. Twomey, G. Goldstein, V. M. Lewis, P. M. Bealmear, and R. A. Good, Bioassay determinations of thymopoietin and thymic hormone levels in human plasma. *Proc. Natl. Acad. Sci. (USA)*, **74**, 2541 (1971).

38. A. Astaldi, G. C. B. Astaldi, P. Th. Schellekens, and V. P. Eijsvoogel, Thymic factor in human sera demonstrated by a cyclic AMP assay. *Nature*, **260**, 713 (1976).

39. J. F. Bach, M. Dardenne, M. Pejernik, A. Barvis, P. Levasseur, and H. LeBrand, Evidence for a serum factor secreted by the human thymus. *Lancet*, **2**, 1056 (1972).

40. V. Lewis, J. J. Twomey, G. Goldstein, E. Smithwick, S. Pahwa, R. O'Reilly, R. Pawha, R. A. Good, H. Schulte-Wisserman, S. Horowitz, R. Hong, J. Jones, O. Sieber, C. Kirkpatrick, S. Polmer, and P. Bealmear, Circulating thymic hormone activity in congenital immunodeficiency. *Lancet*, **3**, 471 (1977).

41. M. Dardenne and J. F. Bach, Thymic hormone in immunological diseases. In B. Michel, Ed., *Comptes Rendus 5eme Journees Montpellieraines de Pneumologie*, Masson, Paris, 1976, p. 1.

42. A. L. Goldstein, J. A. Hooper, R. S. Schulof, G. H. Cohen, G. B. Thurman, M. C. McDaniel, A. White, and M. Dardenne, Thymosin and the immunopathology of aging. *Fed. Proc.*, **33**, 2053 (1974).

43. J. F. Bach, M. Dardenne, and J. Clot, Evaluation of Serum Thymus Hormone and T-cells in Rheumatoid Arthritis and Systemic Lupus Erythematosus. In J. Sany and J. Clot, Eds., *Immunological Aspects of Rheumatoid Arthritis*, Karger, Basel, 1975, p. 242.

44. R. Schulof, R. Bockman, J. Garofalo, G. Fernandes, S. Cunningham-Rundles, G. Incefy, N. Day, B. Lee, B. Clarkson, R. Good, and S. Gupta, Multivariate analysis of functional T cell defects and circulating serum factors in Hodgkin's disease. *Cancer*, **48**, 964 (1981).

45. E. Garaci, R. Rochetti, V. Oel Gobbo, C. Tramutoli, C. Rinaldi-Garaci, and C. Imperato, Decreased serum thymic factor activity in asthmatic children. *J. Allergy Clin. Immunol.*, **62**, 357 (1978).

46. B. Safai, M. Dardenne, G. S. Incefy, J. F. Bach, and R. A. Good, Circulating thymic factor, facteur thymique serique (FTS) in mycosis fungoides and Sezary syndrome. *Clin. Immunol. Immunopathol.*, **13**, 402 (1979).

47. J. J. Twomey, V. M. Lewis, B. M. Patten, G. Goldstein, and R. A. Good, Myasthenia gravis, thymectomy and serum thymic hormone activity. *Am. J. Med.*, **66**, 639 (1979).

48. C. H. Kirpatrick, L. E. Greenberg, S. W. Chapman, G. Goldstein, V. M. Lewis, and J. J. Twomey, Plasma thymic hormone activity in patients with chronic mucocutaneous candidiasis. *Clin. Exp. Immunol.*, **34**, 311 (1978).

49. G. Goldstein, Radioimmunoassay for thymopoietin. *J. Immunol.*, **117**, 690 (1976).

50. J. F. Bach, J. M. Pleau, M. Dardenne, and M. A. Bach, Thymus dependency and biological significance of Facteur Thymique Serique. In B. Serrou and C. Rosenfeld, Eds., *INSERUM Symposium No. 8*, Elsevier National Holland Biomedical Press, Paris, 1978, p. 279.

51. John E. McClure and A. L. Goldstein, Changes with age in blood levels of thymosin α_1 as measured by radioimmunoassay. *Proc. 4th Internatl. Congr. Immunol.*, **17**, 2.26 (1980).

52. J. M. Pleau, V. Fuentes, J. L. Morgat, and J. F. Bach, Caracterisation d'un receptor specifique du facteur thymique serique dans une lignee lymphocytaire T humaine. *C. R. Acad. Sci.*, **288**, 445 (1979).

53. J. J. Klein, A. L. Goldstein, and A. White, Effects of the thymus lymphocytopoietic factor. *Ann. N. Y. Acad. Sci.*, **135**, 485 (1966).

54. A. L. Goldstein, F. D. Slater, and A. White, Preparation, assay and partial purification of a thymic lymphocytopoietic factor (thymosin). *Proc. Natl. Acad. Sci. (USA)*, **56**, 1010 (1966).

55. J. A. Hooper, M. C. McDaniel, G. B. Thurman, G. H. Cohen, R. S. Schulof, and A. L. Goldstein, Purification and properties of bovine thymosin. *Ann. N. Y. Acad. Sci.,* **249,** 125 (1975).

56. A. L. Goldstein, T. L. K. Low, M. McAdoo, J. McClure, G. B. Thurman, J. L. Rossio, C.-Y. Lai, D. Chang, S.-S. Wang, C. Harvey, A. H. Ramel, and J. Meienhofer, Thymosin α_1: Isolation and sequence analysis of an immunologically active thymic polypeptide. *Proc. Natl. Acad. Sci. (USA),* **74,** 725 (1977).

57. T. L. K. Low, G. B. Thurman, M. McAdoo, J. McClure, J. L. Rossio, P. H. Naylor, and A. L. Goldstein, The chemistry and biology of thymosin. I. Isolation, characterization and biological activites of thymosin α_1 and polypeptide β_1 from calf thymus. *J. Biol. Chem.,* **254,** 981 (1979).

58. T. L. K. Low and A. L. Goldstein, The chemistry and biology of thymosin. II. Amino acid sequence analysis of thymosin α_1 and polypeptide β_1. *J. Biol. Chem.,* **254,** 987 (1979).

59. L. W. Law, A. L. Goldstein, and A. White, Influence of thymosin or immunological competence of lymphoid cells from thymectomized mice. *Nature,* **219,** 1391 (1968).

60. M. A. Hardy, J. Quint, A. L. Goldstein, D. State, and A. White, Effect of thymosin and an antithymosin serum in allograft survival in mice. *Proc. Natl. Acad. Sci. (USA),* **61,** 875 (1968).

61. A. L. Goldstein, S. Banerjee, G. L. Schneebeli, T. F. Dougherty, and A. White, Acceleration of lymphoid tissue regeneration in X-irradiated CBA/W mice by injection of thymosin. *Rad. Res.,* **41,** 579 (1970).

62. M. A. Hardy, J. Quint, A. L. Goldstein, D. State, A. White, and J. R. Battisto, Effects of an antiserum to calf thymosin on lymphoid cells *in vitro. Proc. Soc. Exp. Biol. Med.,* **130,** 214 (1969).

63. A. L. Goldstein, Y. Asanuma, J. R. Battisto, M. A. Hardy, J. Quint, and A. White, Influence of thymosin on cell-mediated and humoral immune responses of normal and immunologically deficient mice. *J. Immunol.,* **104,** 359 (1970).

64. J. F. Bach, M. Dardenne, A. L. Goldstein, A. Guha, and A. White, Appearance of T-cell markers in bone marrow rosette forming cells after incubation with purified thymosin, a thymic hormone. *Proc. Natl. Acad. Sci. (USA),* **68,** 273 (1971).

65. G. H. Cohen, J. A. Hooper, and A. L. Goldstein, Thymosin-induced differentiation of murine thymocytes in allogeneic mixed lymphocyte cultures. *Ann. N. Y. Acad. Sci.,* **249,** 145 (1975).

66. D. W. Wara, A. L. Goldstein, N. Doyle, and A. J. Ammann, Thymosin activity in patients with cellular immunodeficiency. *New Engl. J. Med.,* **292,** 70(M75) (1975).

67. A. L. Goldstein, D. W. Wara, A. J. Ammann, H. Sakai, N. S. Harris, G. B. Thurman, J. A. Hooper, G. H. Cohen, A. S. Goldman, A. S. Costanzi, and M. C. McDaniel, First clinical trial with thymosin: Reconstitution of T cells in patients with cellular immunodeficiency diseases. *Transplant. Proc.,* **7,** 681 (1975).

68. J. L. Rossio and A. L. Goldstein, Immunotherapy of cancer with thymosin. *World Surg.,* **1,** 605 (1977).

69. A. L. Goldstein and J. L. Rossio, Thymosin for immunodeficiency diseases and cancer. *Comp. Therp.,* **4,** 49 (1978).

70. D. W. Wara and A. J. Ammann, Thymosin treatment of children with primary immunodeficiency disease. *Transplant. Proc.,* **10,** 203 (1978).

71. A. Astaldi, G. C. B. Astaldi, P. Wijermans, M. Groeneuond, P. Th. A. Schellikens, and V. P. Eijsvogel, Thymosin-induced human serum factor increasing cyclic AMP. *J. Immunol.,* **119,** 1106 (1978).

72. D. J. Barrett, D. W. Wara, A. J. Ammann, and M. J. Cowan, Thymosin therapy in the DiGeorge Syndrome. *J. Pediatr.,* **97,** 66 (1980).

73. D. W. Wara, D. J. Barrett, A. J. Ammann, and M. J. Cowan, *In vitro* and *in vivo* enhancement of mixed lymphocyte culture reactivity by thymosin in patients with primary immunodeficiency disease. *Ann. N. Y. Acad. Sci.,* **332,** 128 (1980).

74. M. R. Sharp and D. A. Peterson, Improvement of cellular immunodeficiency with thymosin. *Clin. Res.,* **26,** A818 (1978).

75. A. L. Goldstein, G. H. Cohen, J. L. Rossio, G. B. Thurman, C. N. Brown, and J. T. Ulrich, Use of thymosin in the treatment of primary immunodeficiency diseases and cancer. *Med. Clin. Natl. Am.,* **60,** 591 (1976).

76. A. J. Ammann, D. W. Wara, and T. Allen, Immunotherapy and immunopathologic studies in a patient with nucleoside phosphorylase deficiency. *Clin. Immunol. Immunopath.,* **10,** 262 (1978).

77. A. Rubenstein, R. Hirschorn, M. Sicklick, and R. A. Murphy, *In vivo* and *in vitro* effects of thymosin and adenosine deaminase on adenosine-deaminase deficient lymphocytes. *New Engl. J. Med.,* **300,** 387 (1979).

78. M. T. Lavastida and J. C. Daniels, The use of thymosin (fraction 5) in autoimmune disorders: A preliminary report. *Fed. Proc.,* **37,** 1669 (1978).

79. J. J. Constanzi, R. G. Gagliano, D. Loukas, F. Delaney, H. Sakai, N. S. Harris, G. B. Thurman, and A. L. Goldstein, The effect of thymosin in patients with disseminated malignancies, A phase I study. *Cancer,* **40,** 14 (1977).

80. J. J. Costanzi, N. Harris, and A. L. Goldstein, Thymosin in patients with disseminated solid tumors. Phase I and II results. Proceedings of Third Conference on Modulation of Host Resistance in Prevention and Treatment of Neoplasias. In M. A. Chirigos, Ed., *Immune Modulation and Control of Neoplasia by Adjuvant Therapy,* Raven, New York, 1978, p. 373.

81. M. H. Cohen, P. B. Chretien, D. C. Ihle, B. E. Fossicek, R. Makuch, P. A. Bunn, A. V. Johnston, S. E. Shackney, M. J. Matthews, S. O. Lipson, D. E. Kenady, and J. D. Minna, Thymosin fraction 5 and intensive combination chemotherapy prolonging the survival of patients with small cell lung cancer. JAMA, **241** 813 (1979).

82. D. S. Lipson, P. B. Chretien, R. Makuch, D. E. Kenady, and M. H. Cohen, Thymosin immunotherapy in patients with small cell carcinoma of the lung. *Cancer,* **43,** 863 (1979).

83. P. B. Chretien, S. D. Lipson, R. Makuch, D. E. Kenady, M. H. Cohen, and J. D. Minna, Thymosin in cancer patients: *In vitro* effects and correlations with clinical response to thymosin immunotherapy. *Cancer Treat. Rep.,* **62,** 1787 (1978).

84. L. Schafer, J. W. Gutterman, E. M. Hersh, G. M. Mavligit, K. Dandridge, G. Cohen, and A. L. Goldstein, Partial restoration by *in vivo* thymosin of E-rosettes and delayed-type-hypersensitivity reactions in immunodeficient cancer patients. *Cancer Immunol. Immunother.,* **1,** 259 (1976).

85. M. Dardenne, J. C. Monier, J. M. Pleau, and J. F. Bach, Characterization of facteur thymic serique (FTS) in the thymus. *Proc. 4th Internatl. Congr. of Immunol.,* **3,** 3.05 (1980).

86. M. E. Gershwin, W. Kruise, and G. Goldstein, The effect of thymopoietin and ubiquitin on spontaneous immunopathology of New Zealand mice. *J. Rheumatol.* **6,** 610 (1979).

87. D. H. Schlesinger and G. Goldstein, The amino acid sequence of thymopoietin II. *Cell,* **5,** 361 (1975).

88. J. M. Pleau, M. Dardenne, Y. Blouquit, and J. F. Bach, Structural study of circulating thymic factor: A peptide isolated from pig serum II. Amino acid sequence. *J. Biol. Chem.,* **252,** 8045 (1977).

89. M. Freire, O. Crivellaro, C. Isaacs, J. Moschera, and B. L. Horecker, Translation of mRNA from calf thymus in the wheat germ system: Evidence for a precursor of thymosin α_1. *Proc. Natl. Acad. Sci. (USA),* **75,** 6007 (1978).

90. S. S. Wang, I. D. Kulesha, and D. P. Winter, Synthesis of thymosin α_1. *J. Am. Chem. Soc.,* **101,** 253 (1978).

91.   S. S. Wang, R. Makofske, A. E. Bach, and R. B. Merrifield, Solid phase synthesis of thymosin α_1. *Internatl. J. Pept. Protein Res.*, **15**, 1 (1980).

92.   C. Birr and U. Stollenwerk, Synthesis of thymosin α_1, a polypeptide of the thymus. *Angew. Chem.*, **91**, 422 (1979).

93.   K. Folkers, Current advances in biologically active synthetic peptides. Paper presented at 12th Miles International Symposium on Polypeptide Hormones, Baltimore, Md., July 11–13, 1979 (in press).

94.   R. Wetzel, H. L. Heyneker, D. V. Goeddel, P. Jhurani, J. Shapiro, R. Crea, T. L. K. Low, J. E. McClure, and A. L. Goldstein, Production of biologically active N^α-desacetyl thymosin α_1 through expression of a chemically synthesized gene. *Biochemistry*, **19**, 6096 (1980).

95.   T. L. K. Low, S. K. Hu, and A. L. Goldstein, Pharmacological enhancement of immunity: Role of thymosin and the endocrine thymus in the maintenance of immune balance. *Adv. Pharm. Therap.*, **4**, 149 (1978).

96.   T. L. K. Low, S. K. Hu, and A. L. Goldstein, Complete amino acid sequence of bovine thymosin β_4: A thymic hormone that induces terminal deoxynucleotidyl transferase activity in thymocyte populations. *Proc. Natl. Acad. Sci.*, **78**, 1162 (1981).

97.   D. H. Schlesinger, G. Goldstein, and H. D. Niall, The complete amino acid sequence of ubiquitin, an adenylate cyclase stimulating polypeptide probably universal in living cells. *Biochemistry*, **14**, 2214 (1975).

98.   M. O. J. Olson, I. L. Goldknopf, K. A. Guetziw, G. T. James, T. C. Hawkin, C. J. Mays-Rothberg, and H. Busch, The NH_2 and COOH-terminal amino acid sequence of nuclear protein A24. *J. Biol. Chem.*, **251**, 5901 (1976).

99.   L. T. Hunt and M. O. Dayhoff, Amino acid sequence identity of ubiquitin and the non-histone component of nuclear protein A24. *Biochem. Biophys. Res. Commun.*, **74**, 650 (1977).

100.   A. L. Goldstein, G. B. Thurman, G. H. Cohen, and J. A. Hooper, Thymosin: Chemistry, Biology and Clinical Applications. In D. W. van Bekkum, Ed., *The Biological Activity of Thymic Hormones,* Kooyker Scientific Publications, Rotterdam, 1975, p. 173.

101.   G. D. Marshall, T. L. K. Low, G. B. Thurman, and A. L. Goldstein, Recent Advances in Thymosin Research. In B. Serrou and C. Rosenfeld, Eds., *Human Lymphocytes Differentiation. Its Application to Cancer,* INSERM Symposium No. 8, Elsevier/North Holland Biomedical Press, Paris, 1978, p. 271.

102.   N. H. Pazmino, J. H. Ihle, R. N. McEwan, and A. L. Goldstein, Control of differentiation of thymocyte precursors in the bone marrow by thymic hormones. *Cancer Treat. Rep.*, **62**, 1749 (1978).

103.   M. Zisblatt, A. L. Goldstein, F. Lilly, and A. White, Acceleration by thymosin of the development of resistance to murine sarcoma virus-induced tumor in mice. *Proc. Natl. Acad. Sci. (USA)*, **66**, 1170 (1970).

104.   M. A. Hardy, M. Zisblatt, N. Levine, A. L. Goldstein, F. Lilly, and A. White, Reversal by thymosin of increased susceptibility of immunosuppressed mice to Moloney sarcoma virus. *Transplant. Proc.*, **3**, 926 (1971).

105.   A. L. Goldstein, A. Guha, M. L. Howe, and A. White, Ontogenesis of cell-mediated immunity in murine thymocytes and spleen cells and its acceleration by thymosin, a thymic hormone. *J. Immunol.*, **106**, 773 (1971).

106.   M. Zatz, A. White, R. S. Schulof, and A. L. Goldstein, The effect of antithymosin globulin on the recovery of T cells in ATS-treated mice. *Ann. N. Y. Acad. Sci.*, **249**, 499 (1975).

107.   G. B. Thurman, B. B. Silver, J. A. Hooper, B. C. Giovanella, and A. L. Goldstein, *In vitro* mitogenic responses of spleen cells and ultrastructural studies of lymph nodes from nude mice following thymosin administration *in vivo*. In J. Rygaard and C. O. Polvsen, Eds., *Proceedings of First International Workshop on Nude Mice,* Gustav Fischer Verlag, Stuttgart, Germany, 1974, p. 105.

108. G. B. Thurman, A. P. Steinberg, A. Ahmed, D. M. Strong, M. E. Gershwin, and A. L. Goldstein, Thymosin induced increase in mitogenic responsivity of lymphocytes of normal, NZB and nude mice. *Transplant. Proc.,* **7**, 299 (1975).

109. G. H. Cohen and A. L. Goldstein, Mixed Lymphocyte Reaction Bioassay for Thymosin. In D. W. van Bekkum, Ed., *The Biological Activity of Thymic Hormones,* Kooyker Scientific Publications, Rotterdam, 1975, p. 257.

110. A. Ahmed, A. H. Smith, D. M. Wong, G. B. Thurman, A. L. Goldstein, and K. W. Sell, *In vitro* induction of Lyt surface markers on precursor cells incubated with thymosin polypeptides. *Cancer Treat. Rep.,* **62**, 1739 (1978).

111. M. A. Chirigos, *In vitro* and *in vivo* studies with thymosin. In M. A. Chirigos, Ed., *Immune Modulation and Control of Neoplasia by Adjuvant Therapy,* Raven, New York, 1978, p. 305.

112. B. A. Khaw and A. H. Rule, Immunotherapy of the Dunning Leukemia with thymic extracts. *Br. J. Cancer,* **28**, 288 (1973).

113. M. P. Scheid, M. K. Hoffman, K. Komuro, H. Hammerling, E. A. Boyse, G. H. Cohen, J. A. Hooper, R. S. Schulof, and A. L. Goldstein, Differentiation of T cells induced by preparations from thymus and by non-thymic agents, *J. Expt. Med.,* **138**, 1027 (1973).

114. A. Ahmed, A. H. Smith, and K. W. Sell, Maturation of Thymus-Derived Cells under the Influence of Thymosin. In M. A. Chirigos, Ed., *Immune Modulation and Control of Neoplasia by Adjuvant Therapy,* Raven, New York, 1978, p. 293.

115. A. Ahmed, A. H. Smith, K. W. Sell, A. D. Steinberg, M. E. Gershwin, G. B. Thurman, and A. L. Goldstein, Thymic-dependent anti-hapten response in congenitally athymic (nude) mice immunized with DNP-thymosin. *Immunology,* **33**, 757–765 (1977).

116. M. E. Gershwin, A. Ahmed, A. D. Steinberg, G. B. Thurman and A. L. Goldstein, Correction of T cell function by thymosin in New Zealand mice. *J. Immunol.,* **113**, 1068 (1974).

117. N. Talal, M. Dauphinee, R. Philarisetty, and R. Goldblum, Effect of thymosin on thymocyte proliferation and autoimmunity in NZB mice. *Ann. N. Y. Acad. Sci.,* **249**, 438 (1975).

118. M. A. Scheinberg, A. L. Goldstein, and E. S. Cathcart, Thymosin restores T cell function and reduces the incidence of amyloid disease in casein-treated mice. *J. Immunol.,* **115**, 156 (1976).

119. H. R. Strausser, L. A. Bober, R. A. Busci, J. A. Schillcock, and A. L. Goldstein, Stimulation of the hemagglutinin response of aged mice by cell-free lymphoid tissue fractions and bacterial endotoxin. *Exp. Gerontol.,* **6**, 373 (1971).

120. M. P. Dabrowski and A. L. Goldstein, Thymosin induced changes in the cell cycle of lymphocytes from aging and neonatally thymectomized rats. *Immunol. Commun.,* **5**, 695 (1976).

121. G. B. Asherson, M. Sembala, B. Mayhew, and A. L. Goldstein, Adult thymectomy prevention of the appearance of suppressor T cells which depress contact sensitivity to picryl chloride and reversal of adult thymectomy effect by thymus extract. *Eur. J. Immunol.,* **6**, 699 (1976).

122. M. J. Dauphinee, N. Talal, A. L. Goldstein, and A. White, Thymosin corrects the abnormal DNA synthetic response of NZB mouse thymocytes. *Proc. Natl. Acad. Sci. (USA),* **71**, 2637 (1974).

123. G. B. Thurman, J. L. Rossio, and A. L. Goldstein, Thymosin induced enhancement of MIF production by peripheral blood lymphocytes of thymectomized guinea pigs. In D. O. Lucas, Ed., *Regulatory Mechanisms in Lymphocyte Activation,* Academic, New York, 1977, p. 629.

124. T. L. K. Low, G. B. Thurman, C. Chincarini, J. E. McClure, G. D. Marshall, S. K. Hu, and A. L. Goldstein, Current status of thymosin research: Evidence for the existence of a family of thymic factors that control T cell maturation *Ann. N. Y. Acad. Sci.,* **332**, 33 (1979).

125. M. A. Scheinberg, E. S. Cathcart, and A. L. Goldstein, Thymosin-induced reduction of "null cells" in peripheral-blood lymphocytes of patients with systemic lupus erythematosus. *Lancet,* **22,** 424 (1975).

126. N. H. Pazmino, J. N. Ihle, and A. L. Goldstein, Induction *in vivo* and *in vitro* of terminal deoxynucleotidyl transferase by thymosin in bone marrow cells from athymic mice. *J. Exp. Med.,* **147,** 708 (1978).

127. S. K. Hu, T. L. K. Low, and A. L. Goldstein, *In vivo* induction of terminal deoxynucleotidyl transferase (TdT) by thymosin or hydrocrotisone acetate (HCA) treated mice. *Fed. Proc.,* **38,** 1079A (1979).

128. I. Goldschneider, A. Ahmed, F. J. Bollum, and A. L. Goldstein, Induction of terminal deoxynucleotidyl transferase and Lyt antigens with thymosin: Identification of multiple subsets of prothymocytes in mouse bone marrow and spleen. *Proc. Natl. Acad. Sci.,* **78,** 2469 (1981).

129. A. Ahmed, D. M. Wong, G. B. Thurman, T. L. K. Low, A. L. Goldstein, S. J. Sharkis, and I. Goldschneider, T-lymphocyte maturation: Cell surface markers and immune function induced by T-lymphocyte cell-free products and thymosin polypeptides. *Ann. N. Y. Acad. Sci.,* **332,** 81 (1979).

130. S. K. Hu, T. L. K. Low, and A. L. Goldstein, Modulation of terminal deoxynucleotidyl transferase (TdT) *in vitro* by thymosin fraction 5 and purified thymosin α_1 in normal thymocytes. *Fed. Proc.,* **39,** 1133 (1980).

131. D. E. Kenady, P. B. Chretien, C. Potvin, and R. M. Simon, Thymosin reconstitution of T cell deficits *in vitro* in cancer patients. *Cancer,* **39,** 575 (1977).

132. H. Sakai, J. J. Costanzi, D. F. Loukas, R. G. Gagliano, S. E. Ritzmann, and A. L. Goldstein, Thymosin-induced increase in E-rosette-forming capacity of lymphocytes in patients with malignant neoplasms. *Cancer,* **36,** 974 (1975).

133. N. A. Byrom, S. Retsas, A. J. Dean, and J. R. Hobbs, The importance of dose of thymosin for the *in vitro* induction of T lymphocytes from patients with solid tumors. *Clin. Oncol.,* **4,** 25 (1978).

134. N. A. Byrom, M. A. Campbell, A. J. Dean, D. M. Timlin, C. Vollcers, D. C. Bodenhan, J. R. Hobbs. Thymosin-inducible lymphocytes in the peripheral blood of patients with malignant melanoma. *Cancer Treat. Rep.,* **62,** 1769 (1978).

135. D. E. Kenady, P. B. Chretien, C. Potvin, R. M. Simon, J. C. Alexander, and A. L. Goldstein, Effect of thymosin *in vitro* on T cell levels during radiation therapy: Correlations with radiation portal and dose, tumor histology and initial T cell level. *Cancer,* **39,** 642 (1977).

136. N. A. Byrom, R. C. Staughton, M. A. Campbell, D. M. Timlin, M. Chooi, A. M. Lane, P. W. N. Copeman, and J. R. Hobbs, Thymosin inducible "null" cells in atopic eczema. *Br. J. Dermatol.,* **100,** 499 (1978).

137. N. A. Byrom, F. Caballero, M. A. Campbell, M. Chooi, A. M. Lane, K. Hugh-Jones, D. M. Timlin, and J. R. Hobbs, T-cell depletion and thymosin inducibility in asthmatic children. *Clin. Exp. Immunol.,* **31,** 490 (1978).

138. S. Ishizawa, H. Sakai, H. E. Sarles, D. L. Larson, and J. C. Daniels, Effect of thymosin on T-lymphocyte functions in patients with acute thermal burns. *J. Trauma,* **18,** 48 (1978).

139. M. A. Scheinberg, W. R. Blacklow, A. L. Goldstein, T. A. Parrimo, F. B. Rose, and E. S. Cathcart, Influenza: Response of T cell lymphopenia to thymosin. *New Engl. J. Med.,* **294,** 1208 (1976).

140. M. G. Mutchnick and A. L. Goldstein, *In vitro* thymosin effect on T lymphocytes in alcoholic liver disease. *Clin. Immunol. Immunopathol.,* **12,** 271 (1979).

141. M. A. Vladiminsky, V. P. Streltsov, and V. M. Bachmann, *In vitro* restoration by thymosin of T lymphocytes from patient with lung tuberculosis. *Biomed. Exp.,* **29,** 3 (1978).

142. S. O. Olusi, G. B. Thurman, and A. L. Goldstein, Effect of thymosin on T-lymphocyte rosette formation in children with Kwashiorkor. *Clin. Immunol. Immunopathol.,* **15,** 687 (1980).

143. H. Moutsopoulos, K. H. Fye, S. Sawada, M. J. Becker, A. L. Goldstein, and N. Talal, The *in vitro* effect of thymosin on T-lymphocyte rosette formation in rheumatic diseases. *Clin. Exp. Immunol.,* **26,** 563 (1976).

144. J. Rovensky, A. L. Goldstein, P. J. L. Holt, J. Pekarek, and T. Mistina, Thymosin-restored T lymphocyte function in clinically healthy middle-aged subjects. *Casopis, Lekara Ceskych.,* **116,** 1063 (1977).

145. G. B. Thurman, G. D. Marshall, T. L. K. Low, and A. L. Goldstein, Recent developments in the classification and bioassay of thymosin polypeptides. In M. R. Quastel, Ed., *Cell Biology and Immunology of Leukocyte Function,* Academic, New York, 1979, p. 189.

146. S. D. Horowitz and A. L. Goldstein, The *in vitro* induction and differentiation of putative human stem cells by thymosin and agents that affect cyclic AMP. *Clin. Immunol. Immunopathol.,* **9,** 408 (1978).

147. J. Kaplan, Characterization of thymosin-responsive peripheral blood null cells. *Cancer Treat. Rep.,* **62,** 1757 (1978).

148. J. Kaplan and W. D. Peterson, Depletion of human T-lymphocyte antigens (HTLA antigens) on thymosin-inducible T-cell precursors. *Clin. Immunol. Immunopathol.,* **9,** 436 (1978).

149. H. Maahinney, V. F. D. Gleadhill, and S. McCrea, *In vitro* and *in vivo* responses to thymosin in severe combined immunodeficiency. *Clin. Immunol. Immunopathol.,* **14,** 196 (1979).

150. J. Caraux, C. Thierry, and B. Serrou, The binding of autologous erythrocytes by human lymphocytes. *Biomedicine,* **29,** 151 (1978).

151. J. Caraux, C. Thierry, and B. Serrou, Human autologous rosettes and prognostic significance of variations in autologous rosette-forming cells in the peripheral blood of cancer patients. *J. Natl. Cancer Inst.,* **63,** (3), 593 (1979).

152. J. Caraux, A. L. Goldstein, C. Esteve, and B. Serrou, Thymosin α_1 restores depressed binding of autologous erythrocytes by T cells from cancer patients. *Biomedicine* (in press).

153. L. Moretta, M. Ferrarini, and M. D. Cooper, Characterization of human T cell subpopulations as defined by specific receptors for immunoglobulin. *Contemp. Topics. Immunobiol.,* **8,** 19 (1978).

154. P. B. Chretien, R. A. Beveridge, and F. Bistoni, Effect of thymosin μ_1 on Tμ and Tγ cells in cancer patients. (In preparation).

155. G. W. Lowell, L. F. Smith, D. Klein, and W. P. Zollinger, Thymosin stimulates *in vitro* secretional antibacterial antibodies by human peripheral blood lymphocytes. *Proc. 4th Internatl. Congr. Immunol.,* **17,** 2.23 (1980).

156. G. Goldstein and A. Mananaro, Thymin: A thymic polypeptide causing the neuromuscular block of myasthenia gravis. *Ann. N. Y. Acad. Sci.,* **183,** 230 (1971).

157. G. Goldstein, Isolation of bovine thymin: A polypeptide hormone of the thymus. *Nature,* **247,** 11 (1974).

158. G. Goldstein, The isolation of thymopoietin (thymin). *Ann. N. Y. Acad. Sci.,* **249,** 177 (1978).

159. R. S. Basch and G. Goldstein, Induction of T cell differentiation *in vitro* by thymin, a purified polypeptide hormone of the thymus. *Proc. Natl. Acad. Sci. (USA),* **71,** 1474 (1974).

160. M. Fujino, T. Fukada, S. Kawaji, S. Shinagawa, Y. Sugino, and M. Takaoki, Synthesis of the nonatetracontapeptide corresponding to the sequence proposed for thymopoietin II. *Chem. Pharm. Bull.,* **25,** 1486 (1977).

161. D. H. Schlesinger, G. Goldstein, M. P. Scheid, and E. A. Boyse, Chemical synthesis of a peptide fragment of thymopoietin II that induces selective T cell differentiation. *Cell, 5,* 367 (1975).

162. G. Goldstein, M. P. Scheid, E. A. Boyse, D. H. Schlesinger, and J. Van Waunue, A synthetic pentapeptide with biological activity characteristic of the thymic hormone thymopoietin. *Science,* **204,** 1399 (1979).

163. G. Goldstein, Polypeptides regulating lymphocyte differentiation. *Cold Spring Harbor Conf. Cell. Prolif.,* **5,** 455 (1978).

164. M. C. Weksler, J. D. Innes, and G. Goldstein, Immunological studies of aging. IV. The contribution of thymic involution to the immune deficiencies of aging mice and reversal with thymopoietin. *J. Exp. Med.,* **148,** 996 (1978).

165. W. A. Kagan, F. P. Siegal, S. Gupta, G. Goldstein, and R. A. Good, Early stages of human marrow lymphocyte differentiation: Induction *in vitro* by thymopoietin and ubiquitin. *J. Immunol.,* **122,** 686 (1979).

166. R. H. Levey, N. Trainin, and L. W. Law, Evidence for function of thymic tissue in diffusion chambers implanted in neonatally thymectomized mice. Preliminary report. *J. Natl. Cancer Inst.,* **31,** 199 (1963).

167. A. I. Kook, Y. Yakir, and N. Trainin, Isolation and partial chemical characterization of THF, a thymus hormone involved in immune maturation of lymphoid cells. *Cell Immunol.,* **19,** 151 (1975).

168. Y. Yakir, and N. Trainin, Enrichment of *in vitro* and *in vivo* immunological activity of purified fractions of calf thymic hormone. *J. Exp. Med.,* **148,** 71 (1978).

169. N. Trainin, M. Small, D. Zipori, T. Umiel, A. I. Kook, and V. Rotter, Characteristics of THF, a thymic hormone. In D. W. van Bekkum, Ed., *The Biological Activity of Thymic Hormones.* Kooyker Scientific Publications, Rotterdam, 1975, pp. 261–264.

170. J. Aleksandrowicz, G. Turowski, J. Czarnecki, Z. Szmigiel, L. Cybulski, and A. B. Skotnicki, Thymic factor X/TFX/ as a biologically active extract. *Ann. Immunol.,* **7,** 97 (1975).

171. Z. Szmigile, G. Turkowski, W. M. Rzepecki, J. Alexsandrowicz, and A. B. Skotnicki, The effect of myasthenic thymus fragments transplantation on the immune state of patients with proliferative aplastic diseases of the haematopoietic system. *Acta Med. Pol.,* **16,** 61 (1975).

172. W. M. Rzepecki, M. Lukasiewicz, J. Aleksandrowicz, Z. Szmigiel, A. B. Skotnicki, and J. Lisiewicz, Thymus transplantation in leukaemia and malignant lymphogranulomatosis. *Lancet,* **i,** 990 (1976).

173. A. B. Skotnicki, Biologiczna okthwnosc i wlasciwosci fizykochemiczne wyciagu grasiczego TFX. *Pol. Tyg. Lek.,* **28,** 1119 (1978).

174. J. Aleksandrowicz and A. B. Skotnicki, The role of the thymus and thymic humoral factors in immunotherapy of aplastic and proliferative diseases of the hemopoietice system. *Acta Med. Pol.,* **17,** 1 (1976).

175. R. Falchetti, G. Bergesi, A. Eishkof, G. Cafiero, L. Adorini, and L. Caprino, Pharmacological and biological properties of a calf thymus extract (TP-1). *Drugs Exp. Clin. Res.,* **3,** 39 (1977).

176. F. Aiuti, P. Ammirati, M. Fiorilli, R. D'Amelio, F. Franchi, M. Calvani, and L. Businco, Immunologic and clinical investigation on a bovine thymic extract. Therapeutic application in primary immunodeficiency. *Pediatr. Res.,* **13,** 797 (1979).

177. M. G. Bernengo, G. Capella, A. De Matteis, P. A. Tovo, and G. Zina, *In vitro* effect of a calf thymus extract on the peripheral blood lymphocytes of 66 melanoma patients. *Clin. Exp. Immunol.,* **36,** 279 (1979).

178. P. A. Tovo, M. G. Bernengo, L. Cordero di Montezemolo, A. Del Piano, M. Saitta, and P. Nicola, Thymus extract therapy in immunodepressed patients with malignancies and herpes virus infections. *Thymus,* **2,** 41 (1980).

179. A. Pugliese and P. A. Tovo, Potentiation of Poly I:C induced interferon production in mice using a cell thymus extract TP-1. *Thymus,* **1**, 305 (1980).

180. Y. Jin, X. Xu, J. Zhu, Y. Wang, A. Zhu, and H. Zhang, A preliminary study on the isolation, property and function of porcine thymic hormone. *J. Nanking Univ.,* **1**, 115 (1979).

181. S.-L. Liu, C.-S. Hsu, L.-H. Tsuel, K.-C. Yang, and S.-C. Chang, Modification of the purification method and *in vitro* bioassay of thymosin fraction 5. *Acta Biochemica et Biophysica Sinica,* **10**, 413 (1978).

182. S.-L. Liu, Use of calf thymosin fraction 5 in the treatment of 7 cases with acquired immunodeficiency diseases. *Peking Med.,* **1**, 219 (1979).

183. J. Comsa, Thymus substitution and HTH, the homeostatic thymus hormone. In T. D. Luckey, Ed., *Thymic Hormones,* University Park Press, Baltimore, 1973, p. 39.

184. J. Comsa, Consequences of thymectomy upon the leukopoiesis in guinea pigs. *Acta. Endocrinol.,* **26**, 361 (1957).

185. G. Bernardi and J. Comsa, Purification de l'hormone thymique par chromatographie sur colonne. *Experentia,* **21**, 416 (1965).

186. T. D. Luckey, W. G. Robey, and B. J. Campbell, LSH, a lymphocyte-stimulating hormone. In T. D. Luckey, Ed., *Thymic Hormones,* University Park Press, Baltimore, 1973, p. 167.

187. A. Ogato and Y. Ito, Studies on salivary gland hormones. V. Bioassay method based on the hypocalcemic activity in rabbits. *J. Pharm. Soc. Jap.,* **64**, 332 (1944).

188. A. Mizutani, A thymic hypocalcemic component. In T. D. Luckey, Ed., *Thymic Hormones,* University Park Press, Baltimore, 1973, p. 193.

189. A. Mizutani and M. Tanaka, Sequence determination of amino and carboxylterminal residues of hypocalcemic protein TP extracted from bovine thymus glands. *Chem. Pharm. Bull.,* **26**, 2630 (1978).

190. A. Mizutani, I. Suzuki, Y. Matsushita, and K. Hayakawa, Effect of bovine thymic hypocalcemic factor on increasing antibody-producing cells in mice. *Chem. Pharm. Bull.,* **25**, 2156 (1977).

191. A. M. Kruisbek, G. C. B. Astaldi, M. J. Blankwater, L. A. Ziglstra, L. A. Leverb, and A. Astaldi, The *in vitro* effect of a thymic epithelial culture supernatant on mixed lymphocyte reactivity and intracellular cAMP levels of thymocytes and on antibody production of Nu/Nu spleen cells. *Cell. Immunol.,* **35**, 134 (1978).

192. A. M. Kruisbeck, T. C. J. M. Kohose, and J. J. Ziglstra, Increase in T cell mitogen responsiveness in rat thymocytes by thymic epithelial culture supernatants. *Eur. J. Immunol.,* **7**, 375 (1977).

193. S. M. Milcu and N. Simionescu, Rolul sistemului nerves central in desfasurarea hipertrofiei de compensatie a glandei suprarenale le animalele tratate cu extract de timus. *Stud. Cercet. Endocrinol.,* **6**, 535 (1953).

194. S. M. Milcu and I. Potop, Biologic activity of thymic protein extracts. In T. D. Luckey, Ed., *Thymic Hormones,* University Park Press, Baltimore, 1973, p. 97.

195. I. Potop and S. M. Milcu, Isolation, biologic activity and structure of thymic lipids and thymosterin. In T. D. Luckey, Ed., *Thymic Hormones,* University Park Press, Baltimore, 1973, p. 205.

196. S. M. Milcu, I. Potop, R. Peterscu, and E. Ghinea, Effect of thymosterin on lymphocytes *in vitro. Endocrinologie,* **14**, 283 (1976).

197. I. Potop, Structure and properties of thymosterin. *Endocrinologie,* **17**, 2 (1979).

198. S. M. Milcu, I. Potop, R. Petrescu, and E. Ghinea, Effect of thymosterin on desocyribonucleic acid in KB tumor cell cultures *in vitro. Endocrinologie,* **15**, 105 (1977).

199. M. Dardenne, J. M. Pleau, N. K. Man, and J. F. Bach, Structural study of circulating thymic factor, a peptide isolated from pig serum. I. Isolation and purification. *J. Biol. Chem.,* **252**, 8040 (1977).

200. E. Bricas, T. Martinez, D. Blanot, G. Auger, M. Dardenne, J. M. Pleau, and J. F. Bach, The serum thymic factor and its synthesis. In M. Goodman and J. Meienhofer, Eds., Proceedings of the Fifth International Peptide Symposium, Wiley, New York, 1977, p. 564.

201. J. F. Bach, M. A. Bach, D. Blanot, E. Bricus, J. Charreire, M. Dardenne, C. Fournier, and J. M. Pleau, Thymic serum factor. *Bull. Inst. Past.*, **76**, 325 (1978).

202. P. Burton, S. Iden, K. Mitchell, and A. White. Thymic hormone-like restoration by human pre-albumin of azathioprine sensitivity of spleen cells from thymectomized mice. *Proc. Natl. Acad. Sci.* (*USA*), **75**, 823 (1978).

203. G. C. B. Astaldi, A. Astaldi, M. Groenwoud, P. Wijermans, P. T. A. Schellekens, and V. P. Eijsvoogel, Effect of a human serum thymic factor on hydrocortisone-treated thymocytes. *Eur. J. Immunol.*, **7**, 836 (1977).

204. P. Wijermans, G. C. B. Astaldi, A. Facehini, P. T. A. Schellekens, and A. Astaldi, Early events in thymocyte activation. I. Stimulation of protein synthesis by a thymus-dependent human serum factor. *Biochem. Biophys. Res. Commun.*, **86**, 88 (1979).

205. A. Astaldi, G. C. B. Astaldi, P. Wijermans, M. Groenewoud, T. Van Bemael, P. T. A. Schellekens, and V. P. Eijsvoogel, Thymus-dependent serum factor activity on the precursors of mature T cells. In M. R. Quastel, Ed., *Cell Biology and Immunology of Leukocyte Function*, Academic, New York, 1975, p. 221.

206. P. B. Chretien, S. Lipson, R. Makuch, D. Kenady, and M. Cohen, Effects of thymosin *in vitro* in cancer patients and correlation with clinical course after thymosin immunotherapy. *Ann. N. Y. Acad. Sci.*, **332**, 135 (1980).

207. B. Shohat, S. Spitzer, M. Topilsky, and N. Trainin, Immunological profile in sarcoidosis patients. The *in vitro* and *in vivo* effect of thymic humoral factor. *Biomed. Exp.*, **29**, 91 (1978).

208. Z. Dolfin, A. I. Handzel, Y. Altman, T. Hahn, S. Levin, and N. Trainin, *In vitro* effect of thymic humoral factor on human peripheral blood lymphocytes from normal and immunodeficient patients. *Isr. J. Med. Sci.*, **12**, 1259 (1976).

209. Z. T. Handzel, S. Levin, A. Ashkenazi, T. Hahn, Y. Altman, B. Czernohislky, B. Schecter, and N. Trainin, Immune deficiencies of T-system with possible T cell regulatory activity defect. *Isr. J. Med. Sci.*, **13**, 347 (1977).

210. Z. T. Handzel, S. Levin, T. Hahn, Y. Altman, A. Ashkenazi, N. Trainin, and B. Schechter, Infantile partial thymus deficiency: Correction of some *in vitro* T cell functions by THF. *Isr. J. Med. Sci.*, **11**, 1391 (1978).

211. I. Varsano, Y. Danon, L. Jaber, E. Livni, B. Shohat, Y. Yakir, A. Schneyoun, and N. Trainin, Reconstitution of T-cell function in patients with subacute sclerosing periencephalitis treated with thymus humoral factor. *Isr. J. Med. Sci.*, **12**, 1168, (1976).

212. I. Varsano, M. Schofeld, M. Matoth, B. Shohat, T. Englander, V. Rotter, and N. Trainin, Severe disseminated adenovirus infection successfully treated with a thymus humoral factor, THF. *Acta. Paediatr. Scand.*, **66**, 329 (1977).

213. Z. T. Handzel, Z. Dolfin, S. Levin, T. Altman, T. Hahn, N. Trainin, and N. Godot, Effect of thymic humoral factor on cellular immune functions of normal children and of pediatric patients with ataxia telangiectasia and Down's syndrome. *Pediatr. Res.*, **13**, 803, (1979).

214. S. Horowitz, C. O. Borcherding, A. V. Moorthy, R. Chesney, H. Schulte-Wisserman, and R. Hong. Induction of suppressor T cells in systemic lupus erythematosus by thymosin and cultured thymic epithelium. *Science,* **197**, 4307 (1977).

215. Y. Z. Patt, E. M. Hersh, L. A. Schafer, T. L. Smith, M. A. Burgess, J. U. Gutterman, A. L. Goldstein, and G. M. Mavligit, The need for immune evaluations prior to thymosin-containing chemoimmunotherapy for melanoma. *Cancer Immunol. Immunother.*, **7**, 131 (1979).

216. R. B. Livingston, Treatment of small cell carcinoma: Evolution and future directions. *Semin. Oncol.,* **5**, 299 (1978).

217. W. M. Wara, A. J. Ammann, and D. W. Wara, Effect of thymosin and irradiation on immune modulation in head and neck and esophageal cancer patients. *Cancer Treat. Rep.,* **62**, 1775 (1978).

218. G. Goldstein, Lymphocyte differentiations induced by thymopoietin, bursopoietin and ubiquitin. *Symp. Soc. Dev. Biol.,* **35**, 197 (1978).

219. G. Goldstein, M. Scheid, E. A. Boyse, A. Brand, and D. G. Gilmour, Thymopoietin and bursopoietin: Induction signals regulating early lymphocyte differentiation. *Cold Spring Harbor Symp. Quant. Biol.,* **41**, 5 (1977).

220. R. S. Basch and G. Goldstein, Thymopoietin-induced acquisition of responsiveness to T cell mitogens. *Cell. Immunol.,* **20**, 218 (1975).

221. S. Gupta and R. A. Good, Subpopulations of human T lymphocytes II. Effect of thymopoietin, corticosteroids and irradiation. *Cell. Immunol.,* **34**, 10 (1977).

222. G. H. Sunshine, R. S. Basch, R. G. Coffey, K. W. Cohen, G. Goldstein, and J. W. Hadden, Thymopoietin enhances the allogeneic response and cyclic GMP levels of mouse peripheral, thymus-derived lymphocytes. *J. Immunol.,* **120**, 1594 (1978).

223. M. P. Scheid, G. Goldstein, and E. A. Boyse, Differentiation of T cells in nude mice. *Science,* **190**, 4220, (1975).

224. N. Trainin, V. Rotter, Y. Yakir, R. Leve, Z. Handzel, B. Shohat, and R. Zaizov, Biochemical and biological properties of THF in animal and human models. *Ann. N. Y. Acad. Sci.,* **332**, 9 (1979).

225. Y. Yakir, A. I. Kook, M. Schlesinger, and N. Trainin, Effect of thymic humoral factor on intracellular levels of cyclic AMP in human peripheral blood lymphocytes. *Isr. J. Med. Sci.,* **12**, 1191, (1977).

226. C. Carnaud, D. Ilfeld, I. Brook, and N. Trainin, Increased reactivity of mouse spleen cells sensitized *in vitro* against syngeneic tumor cells in the presence of thymic humoral factor. *J. Exp. Med.,* **138**, 1521 (1973).

227. V. Rotter and N. Trainin, Increased mitogenic reactivity of normal spleen cells to T lectins induced by thymus humoral factor (THF). *Cell. Immunol.,* **16**, 413, (1974).

228. V. Rotter, M. Schlesinger, R. Kalderon, and N. Trainin, Response of human lymphocytes to PHA and Con A, dependent on and regulated by THF, a thymic hormone. *J. Immunol.,* **117**, 1927 (1976).

229. D. Erard, J. Charreire, M. T. Auffredou, P. Galanaud, and J. F. Bach, Regulation of contact sensitivity to DNFB in the mouse. Effects of adult thymectomy and thymic factor. *J. Immunol.,* **123**, 1573 (1979).

230. M. A. Bach, Lymphocyte-mediated cytotoxicity: Effects of aging in adult thymectomy and thymic factor. *J. Immunol.,* **119**, 641 (1977).

Immunorestoration by Chemicals

MICHAEL A. CHIRIGOS
The Division of Cancer Treatment
National Cancer Institute, Bethesda, Maryland

MICHAEL J. MASTRANGELO
The Department of Medicine
The Fox Chase Cancer Center
Philadelphia, Pennsylvania

1. INTRODUCTION

The immunologic surveillance of the cancer-bearing host is suppressed by the disease itself and by the cytoreductive therapy required to manage it. The early restoration of host immune function is important for the successful control of cancer, as well as for prevention of life-threatening secondary infectious diseases.

Interest in immunoregulators for use in cancer therapy has led to the discovery of a variety of chemically defined compounds having immunomodulatory properties that have, in turn, been applied to a variety of nonneoplastic diseases, including viral and bacterial infections, immunodeficiency states, and collagen disorders. The availability of several well-defined chemical agents capable of reconstituting and/or stimulating the cellular components of the immune system provides the cancer therapist greater flexibility in developing combined modality treatment regimens.

In this chapter we describe the actions of five chemically defined compounds when examined in a preclinical setting and under clinical conditions.

2. LEVAMISOLE

Tetramisole, the racemic mixture of 2,3,4,6-tetra-hydro-6-phenylimidazo(2, 1-b)thiazole, was introduced as a potent broad-spectrum anthelminthic in 1966 (1). Tetramisole and more recently the levoisomer, levamisole (Figure 1) have been extensively and safely used in veterinary and human medicine (2). The demonstration by Renoux and Renoux (3) that tetramisole augmented the protective effect of a Brucella vaccine in mice triggered extensive investigation of the immunomodulating effects of tetramisole and levamisole. The purpose of this review is to provide background data on the pharmacology, metabolism, mechanism of action, immunologic profile, animal antitumor activity, toxicity,

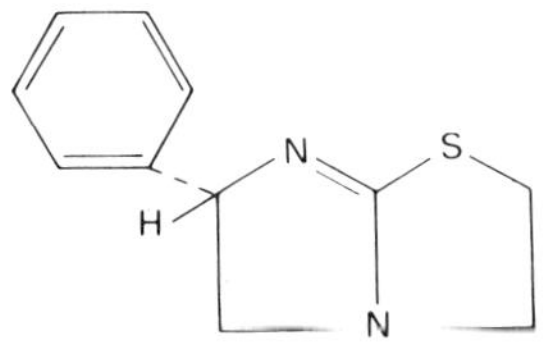

Figure 1. Chemical structure of levamisole (2,3,5,6-tetrahydro-6-phenylimidazo[2,1-b] thiazole).

and clinical antitumor activity. The literature is voluminous but has been extensively reviewed (4–7). Only a brief synopsis of these exhaustive reviews is presented here.

2.1. Pharmacology (8)

Levamisole (MW 240.75) is a stable white crystalline powder. The hydrochloride salt is soluble in most organic solvents. In water it is freely soluble and can hydrolize; the rate of hydrolysis increases with increasing pH or temperature. At a pH of 4 or less, 3 to 18% aqueous solutions of levamisole have remained stable for more than 40 months. Levamisole precipitates at pH 7.5.

2.2. Metabolism (9)

In Animals. Levamisole is well absorbed in several species through the oral, subcutaneous, or intramuscular routes. The plasma half-life of the unchanged drug ranges from 1 to 4 hours.

The drug is widely distributed and can be detected in all tissues and fluids. The highest levels are in the liver and kidney, organs involved in levamisole metabolism.

Levamisole is extensively metabolized and rapidly removed from the body. In rats, less than 1% of the administered radioactive dose remains in the body after 8 days.

There are no obvious species or sex differences in the kinetics of drug metabolism. In rats 46% of the radioactive dose is excreted in the urine and 40% in the feces within 48 hours.

In Humans. As a single oral dose, 150 mg of tritium-labeled levamisole produces a peak plasma level of $0.49 \pm 0.05 \mu g$ of levamisole per milliliter at 2 hours. This is the same concentration as is required *in vitro* for restoring to normal depressed phagocytic and T-lymphocyte function. At the peak level the radioactivity due to unchanged drug is only one-third of the total plasma radioactivity. The plasma half-life of levamisole is 4 hours. There is little difference in peak plasma levels between individuals, indicating that the drug is well absorbed.

Approximately 60% of the administered dose is excreted in the urine by 24 hours (70% by 72 hours). In the same period 4% of the administered radioactivity is excreted through the feces. Only 6% of the urine radioactivity and 4% of the fecal radioactivity are due to unchanged levamisole indicating extensive metabolism.

2.3. Mechanism of Action (5,8, 10–12)

The anthelminthic property of levamisole results from its ability to stimulate autonomic ganglia. It also increases heart rate and strength of contraction.

Levamisole has no direct effect on bacteria, viruses, or fungi. *In vitro* it is not cytotoxic to normal or neoplastic cells.

Levamisole contains an imidazole ring and presumably may function like imidazole in affecting enzymes controlling cyclic nucleotide levels in lymphocytes to affect their function and induce immunoregulation. Thus imidazole and levamisole, which are not themselves mitogenic, elevate cyclic GMP levels in lymphocytes *in vitro* and enhance their proliferative response to mitogens or foreign cells.

2.4. Immunologic Profile of Levamisole

This area has been extensively reviewed by Symoens and Rosenthal (5). Their conclusions are presented in the following subsections.

In Vitro *Test Systems*

Phagocytosis.   Levamisole increased phagocytosis by polymorphonuclear (PMN) cells or macrophages when added to these cells or given to donor animals and humans. The effect was most pronounced on hypofunctional cells from patients and weak or absent on cells from normal donors.

Chemotaxis.   Chemotactic responsiveness of PMN cells and monocytes from patients with defective leukocyte motility could be enhanced by levamisole when added *in vitro* or given *in vivo*.

Migration Inhibition and Lymphokine Production.   Leukocyte migration inhibition in response to antigenic stimulation could be restored when levamisole was administered to anergic patients or added to their cells *in vitro*. The effect of the drug was most pronounced when the antigen used was present in suboptimal concentrations. There was little or no effect in healthy donors with normal skin reactivity or with levamisole alone without antigen. The drug seemed to augment the production of soluble mediators of delayed hypersensitivity by mitogen-stimulated human peripheral lymphocytes *in vitro*. The drug did not induce such a production in the absence of antigen.

Lymphocyte Stimulation.   Levamisole increased nucleic acid or protein synthesis in resting lymphocytes as well as in mitogen, antigen, or allogeneic cell-stimulated T lymphocytes. B-Cell response did not seem to be affected by this agent.

The effects of the drug were most pronounced on hypofunctional cells from old, diseased, or immunosuppressed donors. Following irradiation in humans or cytotoxic treatment in mice, levamisole applied at a critical time was able to restore depressed lymphocyte responsiveness. Administration of levamisole too soon after cytotoxic treatment induced further depression and delayed restoration of the lymphocyte response.

Peripheral, splenic, and thymic T lymphocytes from adult humans or animals seemed to respond to levamisole *in vitro* and *in vivo* under appropriate conditions, although various investigators present contradictory views in this matter. After *in vivo* restoration of lymphocyte responsiveness by levamisole, no further *in vitro* stimulation could be achieved.

Lymphocyte Suppressor Activity.   Human splenocytes and thymocytes incubated with mitogen in the presence of levamisole suppressed the mixed lymphocyte reaction to a significantly higher degree than did cells not exposed to the drug. In contrast, the inhibition of the response of lymphocytes to phytohemagglutinin, which is induced by supernatant fluids of mononuclear cells from anergic patients, was abolished or decreased by levamisole *in vitro*.

Lymphocyte or Macrophage Cytotoxicity.   Lymphocyte cytotoxicity against allogeneic cells was markedly enhanced in the presence of levamisole. The drug effect resulted in more target allogeneic cells killed per lymphocyte. Levamisole exerted its effect either prior to or during sensitization.

In patients with melanoma, levamisole increased the preexisting specific antitumor lymphocyte cytotoxicity, prolonged lymphocyte cytotoxicity induced by a tumor cell vaccine, and even induced lymphocyte cytotoxicity in response to suboptimal and normally ineffective doses of the vaccine. However, such an effect could not be obtained in levamisole-treated mice sensitized with allogeneic cells, syngeneic tumor cells, or allogeneic tumor cells. In the latter cytotoxicity was even decreased. Levamisole failed to restore lymphocyte cytotoxicity in virus-immunosuppressed mice and failed to increase macrophage cytotoxicity in normal mice.

Lymphocyte Counts.   Levamisole restored to normal the number of T cells as determined by the estimation of E-RFCs in patients in whom these numbers were reduced. In those cases where a reduction of T cells was accompanied by increased numbers of Ig-bearing cells, null cells, or EAC-RFCs, a drop in the numbers of B or null cells was observed following levamisole treatment. The increase in T cells and reduction in B or null cells occurred without any significant change in the absolute lymphocyte counts.

Total T- and B-cell counts that were already within the normal range did not change significantly under levamisole therapy, except at very high dose levels. When, after levamisole treatment, E-rosette formation was restored to normal, no further *in vitro* stimulation could be achieved. Preliminary observations suggest that in normals levamisole significantly increases the number of "active" T cells in peripheral blood, as estimated by the modified E-rosette assay of Wybran.

Jerne Plaque Test.   The number of plaque-forming cells (PFC) in the direct (19S) as the indirect (7S) assay was often increased when levamisole was present in the cultures or given to the sensitized donor animals. By itself, however, the drug failed to increase background numbers of PFC. Yet it could partially restore the depression of PFC formation which was induced by cytotoxic agents.

Immunoglobulin Levels and Antibody Formation.   In the vast majority of the animal and human models tested, levamisole had little or no effect on existing serum immunoglobulin levels or on specific antibody production to the particular bacterial, viral, or cellular immunogen.

Interferon.   Levamisole induced the production of interferon by normal human leukocyte cultures. In contrast, no antiviral effect indicative of interferon induction was detected in levamisole-treated mice or in fibroblast cultures to which levamisole was added.

In Vivo Test Systems

Delayed Hypersensitivity.   Skin tests for delayed hypersensitivity to a variety of antigens were frequently restored by levamisole in anergic patients and boosted in subjects whose skin reactivity to antigenic stimulation was reduced. Such observations were made in healthy elderly subjects, cancer patients, leprosy patients, and patients with various other nonmalignant diseases.

Blood Clearance of Colloidal Particles.   The blood clearance of colloidal particles was enhanced by levamisole in cases of a relative deficiency of the reticuloendothelial system as found in aged or cortisone-treated animals, in certain strains of animals, and in diseased humans. Levamisole appeared to restore reticuloendothelial system function rather than to stimulate it above normal functional levels of activity.

Skin Graft Rejection.   No alteration of allogeneic or isogeneic skin graft rejection time was noticed in mice, except at very high doses of levamisole, when rejection time could be shortened.

Graft-Versus-Host Reaction.   The graft-versus-host reaction to splenic cells was increased in mice when the donor or the recipient had been treated with levamisole.

Adjuvant Disease of the Rat.   Levamisole did not influence the primary inflammatory response to the immunization of rats with complete Freund's adjuvant; however, it significantly increased the systemic disease and arthritis induced by this agent.

2.5. Animal Antitumor Effects

As can be seen from Table 1 (taken from reference 7), levamisole does not influence the primary growth and dissemination of tumors.

TABLE 1.   Effect of Levamisole on Primary and/or Metastatic Growth of Various Tumors

Tumor Model	Host	Effect[a]	Reference[b]
P388 leukemia	Mouse	0	62
Moloney LSTRA leukemia	Mouse	0	13
Moloney MCAS-10 leukemia	Mouse	0	15
Moloney lymphoma	Mouse	0	86
Melanoma B16 (s.c. or i.p. route)	Mouse	0	39,62
Madison 109 lung tumor	Mouse	0	62
Meth-A tumor	Mouse	0	49
Sarcoma MO₄	Mouse	0	17
Sarcoma MC-7 and MC-57	Rat	0	58
Walker 256	Rat	0	42
RD-3	Rat	0	86
CELO-virus induced	Hamster	0	86
Spontaneous leukemia in old	Mouse	↓	94
Melanoma B16 (i.v. route)	Mouse	↑↓	39
HSV-1 transformed 14-012-8-1 tumor	Hamster	↓	98
HSV-2 transformed 333-8-9 tumor	Hamster	↓	112
Adenocarcinoma 15091	Mouse	↑	39

[a]0 = no change, decrease (↓) or increase (↑) in tumor growth.

[b]See reference 7 of this chapter for individual references.

Chirigos and Amery (6) have reviewed the animal tumor data regarding the use of levamisole in conjunction with cytoreductive therapy. Mice with systemic lymphosarcoma transplantable ascites (LSTRA) leukemia treated with BCNU had a twofold increase in survival time and a 30% survival rate. Levamisole alone was therapeutically ineffective in that it produced no survivors, but when administered three and 6 days after BCNU treatment, a significant number (90 and 70%, respectively) survived. Delaying treatment with levamisole for 10 days at the 5-mg/kg dose was ineffective. Therapeutic failure could be attributable to the fact that animals treated with BCNU had begun to relapse. However, the therapeutic efficacy of delayed treatment was restored by increasing the dose of levamisole. In a second tumor model, the Lewis lung adenocarcinoma, the effect of MeCCNU plus levamisole was tested. Three parameters were evaluated in this study: effect on life-span, effect on primary tumor weight, and number of lung lesions. Levamisole alone was ineffective in increasing life-span; however, decreases in tumor weight and number of lung lesions were noted. The combined treatment of MeCCNU and levamisole proved more effective than MeCCNU alone, resulting in a significant increase in life-span (30 to 55 days) and decreases in primary tumor weight (6.6 to 5.3 mg) and in the number of lung lesions (18 to 14).

A summary of animal tumor models employing cytoreductive therapy followed by levamisole is presented in Table 2. The results of these studies indi-

TABLE 2.   Effect of Levamisole in Combination with Cytoreductive Therapy

Tumor Model	Host	Cytoreductive Therapy	Effect[d]	Reference
Moloney LSTRA leukemia	Mouse	BCNU, Cyclo[a]	+	18,19
Moloney MCAS-10 leukemia	Mouse	BCNU	+	20
Graffi leukemia	Mouse	BCNU, Cyclo	+	19
Lewis lung carcinoma	Mouse	MeCCNU	+	21
3-MC-induced fibrosarcoma	Mouse	BCNU, Cyclo	+	19
Meth-A tumor	Mouse	Cyclo	+	22
EMT-6	Mouse	Radiation	+	23
KHT fibrosarcoma	Mouse	Radiation	+	23
ADJ-PC5 plasmacytoma	Mouse	ANM[b]	+	24
6C₃HED lymphosarcoma	Mouse	Radiation	0	23
L1210 leukemia	Mouse	Various[c]	0	25
MO4 sarcoma	Mouse	Cyclo	0	26
Epithelioma Spl	Rat	Surgery	0	27

[a]Cyclophosphamide.

[b]Aniline mustard.

[c]Cyclophosphamide, BCNU, 5-fluorouracil, methotrexate, and adriamycin.

[d] + = additive tumor retarding effect and/or increase in survival time; 0 = no additive effect.

cate that levamisole seems to be most effective when used as an adjuvant following cytoreductive therapy.

The dose effect of levamisole was also analyzed to determine if the dose of levamisole, when used singly or combined with cytoreductive therapy, was important. The analysis shown in Tables 3 through 5 are based on a variety of mouse tumor models because there were only fragmentary data for other species. Table 3 shows the results of a comparison between levamisole alone and levamisole as an adjuvant to chemotherapy. When levamisole alone is employed, the 3- to 5-mg/kg dose appears to be critical: a reasonable number of positive responses were attained (9 of 21 compared with a total of 1 of 11

TABLE 3.   Levamisole Alone Versus Levamisole Adjuvant to Cytoreductive Therapy

Levamisole Dose (mg/kg)	Number (%) of Positive Responses	
	Levamisole Alone	Levamisole plus Chemotherapy
1 to 3	0/2 (0)	1/4 (25)
3 to 5	9/21 (42)	21/34 (61)
5 to 10	1/8 (12)	5/11 (45)
> 10	0/1 (0)	3/3 (100)

TABLE 4.   Effect of Levamisole on Transplantable Tumors with Different Growth Rates[a] in Mice

Levamisole Dose (mg/kg)	Number (%) of Positive Responses		
	Slowly Growing	Rapidly Growing	Both
< 1	13/59 (22)	1/35 (2)	14/94 (14)
1 to 3	13/27 (48)	8/97 (8)	21/124 (16)
3 to 5	20/63 (31)	39/161 (24)	59/224 (26)
5 to 10	7/17 (41)	35/80 (31)	32/97 (33)
> 10	6/34 (17)	4/9 (40)	10/43 (23)

[a]Slowly growing tumors, median survival time > 20 days; rapidly growing tumors, median survival time < 20 days.

with other doses). More positive responses were achieved at all the levamisole doses tested when levamisole was combined with chemotherapy than when used alone. Levamisole as an adjuvant treatment appears superior to therapy with levamisole alone.

Another analysis was based on the median survival time of animals with slowly and rapidly growing tumors that received levamisole therapy and/or levamisole adjuvant to cytoreductive therapy (Table 4). Positive results were obtained in 77 of 382 experiments with rapidly growing tumors and 59 of 200 experiments with slowly growing tumors. The greater effect on slowly growing tumors represents a significant difference. In the overall assessment of levamisole dosage, a dose range of 3 to 10 mg/kg appears favorable for both slowly and rapidly growing tumors. Table 5 contains the evaluation of results reported for the effects of levamisole alone and/or as adjuvant therapy on primary tumor growth and metastasis formation. The evaluation indicates that the primary tumor was influenced only marginally (14 of 78 tests). Because relatively few studies were conducted at the 1- to 3-mg/kg and 5- to 10-mg/kg doses of levamisole, no conclusions concerning a dose-response relationship can be drawn.

TABLE 5.   Effect of Levamisole on Metastasizing Transplantable Tumors in Mice

Levamisole Dose (mg/kg)	Number (%) of Positive Responses	
	Primary Tumor	Metastasis Formation
< 1	6/32 (18)	7/32 (21)
1 to 3	1/7 (14)	4/7 (57)
3 to 5	5/34 (14)	16/34 (47)
5 to 10	2/5 (40)	3/5 (60)

2.6. Side Effects

Nonhematologic.   Pinals (13) has reviewed the nonhematologic adverse reactions in 3900 patients (989, rheumatic diseases; 601, other inflammatory diseases; 888, infection disease; 1179, cancer; 243, other diseases) treated with levamisole. These are summarized in Table 6.

The nonhematologic side effects of levamisole include (1) sensorineural reactions, the most common of which is alteration of taste and smell (2) idiosyncratic or allergic reactions, such as a rash and a febrile influenza-like illness, and (3) gastrointestinal symptoms. The sensorineural reactions are seldom of sufficient severity to require discontinuation of treatment. Rash and febrile illness have resulted in withdrawal of levamisole in 7 and 1.5% of cases, respectively, but usually remit spontaneously within a brief interval and are not hazardous except when associated with agranulocytosis. Rash due to levamisole occurs more frequently with rheumatic disease than with other conditions. Gastrointestinal symptoms are mild, quickly reversible, and drug related.

TABLE 6. Adverse Reactions to Levamisole

Type of Reaction[a]	Rheumatic Diseases (989)[b]		Other Diseases (2911)[b]	
	Reaction (%)	Withdrawn (%)	Reaction (%)	Withdrawn (%)
Sensorineural				
Sensory stimulation	6.2	0.5	4.1	0
Hyperalert state	1.8	0	0.9	0
Insomnia	1.4	0	1.2	0
Headache	1.3	0.2	2.0	0
Dizziness	2.9	0	1.1	0
Idiosyncratic				
Rash	14.8	7.0	2.0	0.5
Febrile illness	3.9	1.5	3.1	1.0
Stomatitis	1.9	0.3	0.2	0
Gastrointestinal				
Nausea	5.0	1.3	8.3	0.4
Intolerance	5.7	0.8	4.2	0.4
Anorexia	2.7	0	1.2	0
Vomiting	2.1	0.2	3.8	0
Diarrhea	0.3	0.1	1.4	0

[a]Rare reactions: tremor, vertigo, visual hallucinations, somnolence, confusion, depression, lymphadenopathy, lupuslike reaction, allergic vasculitis, sicca syndrome, increased transaminases, azotemia, proteinuria, polyuria, and angioneurotic edema.

[b]Number of patients evaluated.

Some controlled trials have shown a similar frequency of gastrointestinal symptoms in the placebo group.

Hematologic (14).   When first used as an anthelminthic, levamisole caused no serious hematologic side effects. The first reports of agranulocytosis concerned patients with rheumatoid arthritis who had been treated daily for several months (15). Soon thereafter three fatalities were reported (16–17). In 71 reports in which 1131 rheumatic disease patients received levamisole, 989 patients were screened for side effects, and these were noted in 4.9% of cases. The frequency of hematologic side effects seems much higher in rheumatoid arthritis than in other diseases in which the incidence varies between 0.2% in patients with infectious disease and 2% in patients with cancer.

Mielants and Veys (14) collected data (by questionnaire) on 88 patients with agranulocytosis (selective fall of neutrophils below 20%), 43 patients with leukopenia (leukocytes below 3000/mm^3 but with more than 20% neutrophils), and three patients with thrombocytopenia (platelets less than 50,000/mm^3). Agranulocytosis could not be related to dose or schedule of levamisole, concomitant medications, or the age or sex of the patients. A significant genetic predisposition related to HLA-B27 was noted; B27 was present in 8 of 16 patients with agranulocytosis in whom HLA pattern was studied. This is significantly more than the expected frequency. Rheumatoid arthritis patients who developed agranulocytosis on levamisole usually showed an excellent therapeutic response to the drug. Agranulocytosis on levamisole was always spontaneously reversible on discontinuation of treatment. However, eight fatalities have been reported secondary to intercurrent infection.

The 43 cases of leukopenia differed in that there was no increased prevalence of HLA B27, no bone marrow changes were observed, and agranulocytosis did not develop with continued treatment.

2.7. Clinical Antitumor Effects

Lung Cancer.   In 1972 a cooperative trial of levamisole was initiated by a European group headed by Amery. Two hundred and eleven patients with operable bronchogenic carcinoma (largely squamous cell) were randomized to receive a placebo or levamisole (150 mg/day for 3 consecutive days starting 3 days before surgery and repeated every 2 weeks for 2 years or until relapse). Both groups were comparable in regard to sex, age, skin test reactivity to PPD and DNCB, type of surgery, largest tumor diameter, and regional extent of cancer. Preliminary data were reported in 1975 (28) and the final results were published in 1978 (29). There were no significant differences between the placebo- and levamisole-treated groups regarding number of relapses (50/115 vs. 38/96) and cancer deaths (43/115 vs. 29/96). However, analysis of relapse- and cancer-related death rates with respect to relative dose of levamisole (mg/ kg) showed that "adequately" dosed [≥ 2.3 mg/(kg · day)] patients fared significantly better than did the controls (25 vs. 50% relapses and 15 vs. 44%

deaths, respectively). Further, the data suggest that levamisole diminished hematogenous metastases. These findings require reassessment in a randomized prospective trial in which drug dose is adjusted for weight or body surface area.

Beginning in August 1975 three collaborating centers in the United Kingdom randomly allocated patients with primary operable bronchogenic carcinoma to placebo or levamisole treatment (30). The dose of levamisole was adjusted for body weight (100 mg for patients < 50 kg; 150 mg, 50 to 75 kg; 200 mg, ≥ 75 kg). The schedule of administration was identical to that used by Amery and his colleagues. Of the 135 patients resected before the end of 1976, there were significantly more deaths among those treated with levamisole (16/62) than placebo (5/73) because of an excess of cardiorespiratory deaths 4 to 6 weeks postoperatively. When these cases were eliminated, the levamisole- and placebo-treated groups did not differ in survival (respectively 65 and 68% alive at 60 weeks). These data contradict Amery (31) in that he found no effect on non-tumor deaths. Further, although Anthony et al. (30) attempted to adjust levamisole dose for body size, they were unable to demonstrate a therapeutic benefit for levamisole-treated patients. However, survival data were not analyzed by dose more or less than 2.3 mg/(kg · day).

Wright et al. (32) randomized 136 evaluable patients with resectable non-oat cell carcinoma of the lung to no treatment or intrapleural BCG with or without levamisole (2.5 mg/(kg · day) for 3 days before surgery and for 2 consecutive days each week after surgery for 18 months). With a median follow-up of 446 days, tumors recurred in 25 of 55 (45%) patients treated with intrapleural BCG + levamisole, 12 of 47 (26%) patients treated with intrapleural BCG alone, and 12 of 34 (35%) control patients. Tests of the equality of the recurrence free survival curves for the three treatment groups suggest that the group receiving BCG + levamisole may be doing less well than the other two groups ($p = .067$).

The effects of a combination of levamisole [2.5 mg/(kg · day) for 3 days preoperatively and two 5-day courses postoperatively] and postoperative *C. parvum* were randomly compared to no adjuvant treatment in 38 patients with operable non-small-cell lung cancer by Fox et al. (33). After a brief follow-up, 5 of 21 control patients relapsed, compared with 1 of 17 immunotherapy patients. Definitive conclusions will require more extensive accrual and follow-up.

Breast Cancer.   Rojas and his colleagues (34,35) treated 43 patients with locally advanced breast cancer with radiation using a cobalt source (4000 R to the chest wall and supraclavicular area and 3000 R to the posterior axillary field). After completion of radiation therapy, patients were assigned alternately to either control (23 patients) or levamisole treatment (20 patients, 150 mg/day on 3 consecutive days every other week until progression) groups. The median disease-free interval was 9 months for the control group and 25 months for the treated group ($p < .01$). At 30 months 90% of levamisole-treated patients were alive, compared with 35% of controls. These investigators also demonstrated improvement in DNCB sensitization with levamisole treatment. A larger, prospectively randomized trial is required to confirm these observations.

Several investigators have conducted randomized prospective comparisons of chemotherapy alone or in combination with levamisole in patients with measurable disease. These are summarized in Table 7. Klefstrom et al. (37) and Stephens et al. (38) reported significant improvements in response rate, whereas Paterson et al. (39) failed to show an advantage for levamisole-treated patients. These data are conflicting. Larger cooperative group trials could help to resolve this issue.

Colon Cancer. Verhaegen et al. (40) formed two groups of 30 patients each with operable colorectal cancer "in such a way that they were well comparable for age, sex and Duke's Classification" (A, B1, B2, C). Levamisole (150 mg/day for 3 consecutive days every other week) was started after surgery in one group, and no further treatment was given to the control group. The survival curves for these two groups did not differ significantly until 36 and 39 months (69% for levamisole treatment and 37% for control, $p = < .05$). Benefit was most obvious in patients with Duke's B2 and C colorectal carcinoma to 5-fluorouracil alone or in combination with levamisole. No differences

TABLE 7.   Levamisole in the Treatment of Breast Cancer Patients with Measurable Disease[a]

	Klefstrom (36,37)		
	CMFV	CMFV + L[b]	
CR + PR/total	4/18 (22%)	11/22 (50%)	
	AVC	AVC + L[b]	
CR + PR/total	21/45 (47%)	25/40 (63%)	$p = .03$
Median survival (weeks)	67	105	$p = .05$
	Paterson et al. (38)		
	CMF	CMF + L[c]	
CR + PR/total	18/39 (46%)	18/38 (47%)	
Median survival (months)	NR	21	
	Stephens et al. (39)		
	FAC	FAC + L[d]	
PR/total	8/29 (28%)	17/29 (59%)	$p = < .05$

[a]Abbreviations; L, levamisole; CMFV, cyclophosphamide, methotrexate, fluorouracil, vinblastine; AVC, adriamycin, vincristine, cyclophosphamide; CMF, cyclophosphamide, methotrexate, fluorouracil; FAC, fluorouracil, adriamycin, cyclophosphamide; NR, not reached.

[b]Levamisole dosage was 150 to 200 mg/day for 2 consecutive days each week during 3-week intervals between chemotherapy courses.

[c]Levamisole dosage was 2.5 mg/kg for 2 consecutive days each week while off chemotherapy.

[d]Levamisole dosage was 150 mg/day, days 15, 16, and 17 and 22, 23, and 24 of each chemotherapy cycle.

in disease-free interval or survival were observed between treatment arms. The failure of Borden et al. (41) to confirm the observations of Verhaegen and co-workers (40) may be related to small sample size or the inclusion of 5-fluorouracil in both treatment arms. Alternatively, the positive result of Verhaegen, et al. (40) may be an artifact introduced by the technique used to assemble the treatment and control groups.

Borden et al. (41) randomized 59 patients with recurrent or metastatic colorectal cancer to receive 5-fluorouracil alone or in combination with levamisole. Levamisole-treated patients survived longer (median 17.5 months) than those treated with 5-fluorouracil alone (median 9.8 months) ($p > .05$ to 0.10). Bedikian et al. (42) randomized 39 patients with measurable lesions to either chemotherapy alone (5-fluorouracil + methotrexate or Baker's antifol) or in combination with levamisole. Levamisole did not alter response rates (2/20 vs. 2/19) or median survivals (10.5 vs. 9 months). Both studies include sufficiently small numbers of patients as to preclude definitive conclusions.

Head and Neck Cancer.   One hundred and four evaluable head and neck cancer patients were randomized to receive no further treatment or levamisole (150 mg 3 times/week on alternate weeks for 2 years) following potentially curative surgery (with or without radiation therapy 43–45). Times to recurrence did not differ significantly for these two groups overall. Subset analysis revealed that Stage II patients treated with levamisole were more likely to remain disease free than control patients. Despite the statistical significance of this observation, its validity remains doubtful because this subset consisted of only 19 patients.

Melanoma.   Spitler and Sagebiel (46) conducted a randomized double-blind trial of levamisole (150 mg/day for 3 consecutive days every 2 weeks for 2 years) versus placebo as adjuvant therapy following potentially curative surgery. Patients included 109 who were clinically or histologically Stage I, 90 who were histologically Stage II, and 4 who had remote metastases completely excised. There was no statistically significant difference between the groups regarding disease free interval or survival. The fixed dose of levamisole and the heterogeneous patient population detract from the definitiveness of this negative trial.

Fifty patients with disseminated melanoma refractory to DTIC were given actinomycin-D plus levamisole (150 mg/day for 2 consecutive days each week). An additional 10 patients received levamisole at the higher dose of 200 mg on alternate days. Two complete and two partial remissions were noted (47). The results of this Phase II trial do not differ dramatically from the results achieved with actinomycin-D alone.

Hematologic Malignancies.   Pavlovsky et al. (48) treated two groups of acute lymphoblastic leukemia patients with two consecutive chemotherapy protocols. In the first protocol induction included vincristine and prednisone. Daunomycin was added if remission was not achieved by day 29. For intensification therapy, patients were randomized to receive or not to receive cyclophosphamide and cytosine arabinoside. A second randomization divided maintenance therapy into 6-mercaptopurine plus weekly or twice weekly methotrexate. All patients received intrathecal methotrexate. In the second protocol induction was achieved with vincristine and prednisone in children with white blood cell (WBC) counts less than 20,000. Children with higher WBC counts and adults also received daunomycin. Intensification therapy was cyclophosphamide and cytosine arabinoside in all patients. For the first 6 months of maintenance all patients received 6-mercaptopurine and methotrexate. Subsequently patients were randomized to receive either vincristine plus prednisone alone or sequentially alternating cyclophosphamide and cytosine arabinoside. Again all patients received intrathecal methotrexate. None of these treatment arms proved superior.

One hundred and twenty-three patients who achieved remission on protocol 1 were randomized to receive or not to receive levamisole [120 mg/(m^2 · day)]. The median duration of remission before levamisole was 15 months (range 1 to 34 months). In the second protocol patients were randomized to levamisole immediately after achieving complete remission. The results of levamisole therapy are presented in Table 8. The authors conclude that levamisole used in

TABLE 8.   Therapeutic Efficacy of Levamisole in Hematologic Malignancies

	Chemo	Chemo + Lev	
Acute Lymphocytic Leukemia (48)			
Good-risk patients[a]			
Relapses	53/147	29/146	$p = <.01$
Remission rate (48 months)	52%	69%	
Survival (60 months)	35%	60%	$p = <.0005$
Poor-risk patients[b]			
Relapses	37/61	17/39	$p = $ NS
Remission rate (36 months)	23%	43%	
Survival (48 months)	27%	29%	$p = $ NS
Acute Nonlymphocytic Leukemia (49)			
Evaluable patients	30	27	
Remissions	19	17	
Median remission duration (days)	169	297	$p = $ NS
Median survival responders (days)	360	665	$p = <.05$
Multiple Myeloma (50)			
Evaluable patients	55	58	
Relapses	14	7	
Deaths	11	6	
Median remission duration (weeks)	79	79	

[a]Good risk: age <15 years and WBC <50,000.

[b]Poor risk: age >15 years and/or WBC >50,000.

conjunction with maintenance chemotherapy significantly prolongs remission duration and survival of good risk patients. Although these results are encouraging, the great variability in the time that elapsed between onset of remission and initiation of levamisole treatment in one-third of the patients requires that a confirmatory study be conducted.

Chang et al. (49) treated 60 adult acute nonlymphocytic leukemia patients with daunorubicin and cytosine arabinoside as remission induction and consolidation therapy. Subsequent cytoreductive therapy consisted of escalating doses of methotrexate with citrovorum rescue. Late intensification was accomplished with cytosine arabinoside and thioguanine. The first 30 patients served as controls while the second 30 patients all received levamisole (40 mg/m^2 twice daily for 3 days weekly until relapse) beginning at the second week of induction therapy. The results are presented in Table 8. Enthusiasm for the clinically and statistically significantly improved median survival of the levamisole-treated responders is dampened by the sequential rather than randomized design of this trial.

The Southwest Oncology Group performed a randomized trial of remission induction and maintenance regimens for multiple myeloma (50). The induction compared melphalan plus prednisone with the combination of vincristine, melphalan, cyclophosphamide, and prednisone (VMCP) plus other agents. One hundred fifteen of 345 evaluable patients achieved complete remission (75% tumor regression). These patients were then randomized to maintenance chemotherapy alone (VMCP) or in combination with levamisole. Results are presented in Table 8. Although the medians for remission duration are identical, the remission duration curves differ significantly ($p = .002$).

In summary, levamisole has been included in therapy trials for a wide range of malignancies. However, there is as yet no clear indication of the role of levamisole in the treatment of human cancer. The largest volume of data concerns the use of levamisole as a surgical adjuvant in non-oat cell carcinoma of the lung. The animal data and the results due to Amery (29) suggest that dose is important. Anthony et al. (30) and Wright et al. (32) adjusted dose for body size and in both cases no therapeutic benefit was noted. However, from the data reported by Anthony et al. (30), it is not possible to determine if all or even most of the patients received adequate doses, and Wright et al. (32) did not employ a levamisole-alone arm. Despite these discrepancies, it is clear that at a dose of 2 to 2.5 mg/kg/day, levamisole does not have a major impact on non-oat cell carcinoma of the lung when used as a surgical adjuvant.

The positive trials of Rojas et al. (45) Klefstrom et al. (37), and Stephens et al. (39) in breast cancer and Salmon et al. (50) in multiple myeloma await confirmation. This is a necessary step prior to broader clinical application. Useful activity has also been suggested in leukemia (48,49) and colon (40) and head and neck (45) cancers. Interpretation of the data generated by these latter trials is difficult for various reasons, including small or heterogeneous patient populations, nonrandom design, insufficient follow-up, and retrospective subset search. Further, there have been no definitive negative trials. Interpretation of data from published negative trials is impeded by many of the same problems as those cited previously. In addition, the majority of studies employed an "arbitrary" fixed dose of levamisole.

From the reports available it is tempting to conclude that levamisole will not be of major therapeutic benefit to cancer patients. However, levamisole is simple to administer and by comparison with chemotherapeutic agents is relatively nontoxic. These factors should facilitate the conduct of new clinical trials when proper dose and schedule of administration are more accurately defined. Efforts to determine the optimum biological response modifying dose are under way (51).

3. AZIMEXONE

3.1. Chemistry (52)

The compound BM 12.531 is 2-[2-cyanaziridinyl-(1)]-2-[2-carbamoylaziridinyl-(1)]-propane (prop. INN Azimexone, MW 194)(Figure 2). It is a colorless and odorless crystalline powder. Physiological saline may be used as the solvent by dissolving 100 to 200 mg in 10 ml. The aqueous solution is extremely unstable.

3.2. Pharmacology (53,54)

The acute toxicity is relatively low (LD_{50} in rats: i.p., 2.6 g/kg and orally, 3.1 g/kg; LD_{50} in mice: i.p., 2.3 g/kg and orally, 1.4 g/kg). Azimexone has no alkylating or cytotoxic activities either *in vitro* or *in vivo*. There is little difference in the toxicities on parenteral or oral administration. Investigations with radioactively labeled substances showed that absorption is almost complete. The serum half-life of Azimexone is approximately 6 hours. No pharmacological actions on cardiovascular, renal, or neurologic function could be seen at therapeutic doses in various experimental animals. In the rat there was a dose-dependent increase in the leukocyte count from a dose of 200 mg/kg. Simultaneously there was a fall in the number of erythrocytes. It has not yet been determined whether this action is caused by a toxic or a stimulatory action on the bone marrow.

In a test of tolerance in humans, the dose on intravenous administration was increased stepwise from 20 to 200 mg. Subsequently, multiple doses of 100 or 200 mg ($\geq$ 5 times per 200 mg) were injected within 6 days. There were no clear

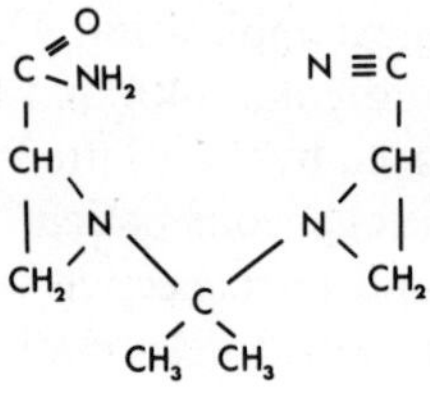

Figure 2. Chemical structure of Azimexone (BM12.531).

indications of side effects that were caused by the administration of Azimexone. Tolerance was good in all cases. In current clinical trials, even higher doses ($\geqslant 500$ mg) have been injected without any reports of relevant side effects.

3.3. Antitumor Activity (53–56)

Antitumor activity could be demonstrated by Azimexone against several mouse tumors (Meth A-sarcoma, Friend virus-induced transplantable leukemia, Ehrlich ascites carcinoma, M109 alveolar carcinoma, L1210, AKR leukemia, Lewis lung carcinoma, and fibrosarcoma), and rat tumors (Walker carcinosarcoma 256 and DS carcinosarcoma). A dose-response relationship was established for Azimexone in Lewis lung carcinoma, AKR leukemia, and fibrosarcoma K-B-23.

Azimexone was evaluated for its capacity to influence the growth of Lewis lung carcinoma at the primary site [subcutaneously (s.c.)] and lung metastases (i.v.). A 10^4 inoculum of cells prepared from the primary tumor site was injected subcutaneously, and Azimexone was administered in a dose of 25 mg/kg i.v. six times at 4-day intervals beginning 1 day following tumor inoculation. Treatment had no effect on growth of the primary s.c. tumor but resulted in a 60% reduction in the number of lung metastases. Similar results were obtained when a 10^4 inoculum of cells, prepared from lung metastatic foci, was injected i.v. An 80% reduction of lung tumor foci was reported.

In the studies of Azimexone treatment in AKR leukemia, four antigenically different types of lymphoma cells were inoculated i.v. into AKR mice. Azimexone was administered i.v. at 25 mg/kg six times at 4-day intervals beginning one day following tumor cell inoculation (Table 9). The data show that Azimexone treatment resulted in significant protection against the development of AKR leukemia. Protection against the nonimmunogenic clone D showed that Azimexone was also active against an antigenically inert tumor.

A dose-response relationship was established for Azimexone in studies relating the take frequency of 10^3 spontaneous AKR leukemia cells injected i.v.

TABLE 9.   Antitumor Effect of Azimexon on AKR Leukemia

Tumor Type (10³ Cells I.V.)	Antigenic Characteristic	Percent Tumor Takes[b]	
		Control	Treated
Spontaneous AKR	Immunogenic[a]	100	50
Clone A	Immunogenic	100	25
Clone B	Immunogenic	100	50
Clone C	Immunogenic	100	50
Clone D	Nonimmunogenic	100	45

[a]Antigenicity determined by antibody formation and formation of cytotoxic cells in AKR mice.

[b]Determined 80 days after tumor challenge.

in relation to the amount of Azimexone per injection and the number of injections. After four, six, or eight injections a clear antitumor effect was established, and the optimum effect was achieved after six injections of 25 mg/kg given at 4-day intervals.

A good therapeutic effect was also reported against K-B-23, a BALB/c fibrosarcoma. Mice were inoculated s.c. with 10^4 K-B-23 tumor cells and received Azimexone, at different doses (from 1 to 60 mg/kg) six times at 4-day intervals. A significant therapeutic effect was achieved within the 15- to 40-mg/kg dose range, with the optimum effect occurring at 25 mg/kg.

The good agreement in the dose-response relationship of Azimexone reported in all three tumor systems was particularly striking. Elevation of the dose beyond a given range tended to weaken the therapeutic effect, although no toxic effects were seen at the higher nontherapeutic doses.

Azimexone was also reported to augment the therapeutic effect of cyclophosphamide on L1210 leukemia. Azimexone administration following cyclophosphamide cytoreductive treatment of mice with systemic leukemia resulted in significant increases in survival time and the percent surviving. This effect could be related to the capacity of Azimexone to act as a lymphocyte restorative agent and/or to its ability to decrease the inherent toxicity of cyclophosphamide.

3.4. Protection Against Cyclophosphamide Toxicity (53, 56–58)

Studies reported concerning the sparing effect of Azimexone on cyclophosphamide toxicity indicate that Azimexone influences acute toxicity. A dose of 320 mg/kg was shown to be 100% lethal in rats; however, administering Azimexone within hours after cyclophosphamide resulted in protecting 25% of the animals from death. At the LD_{50} of 250 mg/kg of cyclophosphamide, additional treatment with Aximexone resulted in 40% protection.

In addition, Azimexone was reported to induce leukocytosis in normal rats. The leukocytosis was found to be dose dependent, and even high doses of Azimexone caused a three- to four-fold increase in the number of leukocytes in the peripheral blood. On examination of the differential cell counts, apart from a slight shift in favor of segmented granulocytes, no other striking change was noted. Of particular significance was the observation that leukopenia induced by cyclophosphamide could be, in most part, reversed by the administration of Azimexone. A rebound of leukocyte count was also reported to occur with cyclic treatment with cyclophosphamide followed by Azimexone treatment. Leukocyte rebound was attained with Azimexone treatment even after five cycles of treatment with cyclophosphamide.

3.5. Protection Against Irradiation (54,55, 57–59)

A therapeutic effect was reported for Azimexone in mice that received total body irradiation ranging from 350 to 650 R. Protection against irradiation lethality was achieved irrespective of whether Azimexone was given before, on the same day, or following irradiation. Irradiation (175 R) reduced the number of leukocytes significantly. When Azimexone was administered three times per week at a dose of 50 mg/kg, a significant increase in the number of leukocytes occurred. When the dose of irradiation was increased to 350 R, a significant compensation of the leukopenia induced by the irradiation could be demonstrated.

The evidence indicates that Azimexone helps to reverse the leukopenia resulting from irradiation or treatment with cytoreductive agents such as cyclophosphamide. Because of the high bone marrow toxicity of such agents, studies were reported on the effect of Azimexone on bone marrow. Results shown in Table 10 indicate that Azimexone was capable of stimulating the proliferation of nucleated bone marrow cells. It was also demonstrated that the addition of Azimexone to bone marrow cells *in vitro* produced an increase in proliferation.

Recently it was reported that treatment of mice with 25 mg/kg Azimexone resulted in an increase in granulocyte-macrophage colony-forming cells (GM-CFC) in spleen and bone marrow after a transient depression in the cell population. Bone marrow monocyte-macrophage colony-forming cells (MM-CFC) increased in 7 days after treatment, whereas splenic MM-CFC were least affected by Azimexone treatment.

3.6. Immunologic Profile

Several studies were reported on the effect of Azimexone on the humoral and cellular immune response and are summarized in Table 11.

3.7. Immunomodulation Against Infection (53,56,66,67)

Two studies were reported concerning Azimexone's immunorestorative properties emphazing microbial infection. Azimexone was used alone or in combination with chloramphenicol in treating an *E. coli* infection. The infective dose was sufficient to kill 85% of the animals. Azimexone alone had no protective effect; however, it was shown to improve the survival rate of mice that

TABLE 10.   Response of Nucleated Bone Marrow Cells in Mouse Femur after 200-R Irradiation and Azimexone Treatment

Treatment	Nucleated Bone Marrow Cells ($\times 10^6$), Days Following Irradiation		
	1	6	8
200 R	10.5 ± 0.4	15.9 ± 0.7	18.6 ± 0.7
200 R + Azimexon	9.9 ± 0.6	21.0 ± 1.5	23.5 ± 0.7
		$p > .05$	$p > .01$
None	25.2 ± 0.9		

TABLE 11.   Summary of Azimexone Effect on Immunologic Responses

	Effect[a]	Reference
Animal Testing		
Delayed-type hypersensitivity	↑	53,55,60
Antibody formation	↑	53,54,60
Lymphocyte stimulation	↑	53
Lymphocyte stimulation (Con A)	↑	53
Phagocytosis	↑	53
Macrophage (tumor cell stasis)	↑	53
Macrophage (tumoricidal)	↑↓	55
Natural killer cell augmentation	↑	62
Human Testing		
T-Cell rosettes	↑	53,63,65
Immunoglobulin	↑	54
Lymphocyte stimulation (PHA)	↑	61,64

[a] ↑ = increased, ↑↓ = variable results.

were treated with subtherapeutic doses of chloramphenicol. Treatment with 40 mg/kg of chloramphenicol alone resulted in a 55% survival, however this survival rate was increased to 90% when Azimexone (24.5 mg/kg) was administered with chloramphenicol.

Protection against a *Candida albicans* infection in immunosuppressed mice was also demonstrated with Azimexone treatment (Table 12). A greater mortality due to infection occurred in the cyclophosphamide-treated animals. The additional treatment with Azimexone apparently reduced the immunosuppressive effects of cyclophosphamide, and the death rate of the treated animals was similar to that of the untreated controls. Similar effects were reported for other organisms such as *Pseudomonas aeruginosa*.

3.8.   Clinical Studies (53,54, 61–65)

Studies on Azimexone demonstrating its sparing effect on cyclophosphamide toxicity, ability to induce leukocytosis and to reconstitute the nucleated cellular components of bone marrow, and low toxicity and side effects in animal studies have prompted human trials to establish its tolerance and effect on cellular components of the immune system.

A study was conducted to determine the influence on the percentage of activated T-lymphocytes in the blood of healthy male and female persons after *in vitro* incubation with various concentrations of Azimexone. In blood samples of 10 of 11 healthy persons, the percentage of activated T-lymphocytes was increased after incubation with various concentrations of Azimexone. The best effect was seen at the 50 μg/ml concentration. No change in the percentage of total T lymphocytes was seen.

**TABLE 12.   Protection Against *Candida Albicans* (219)[a]
in Immunosuppressed Mice**

	Percent Survival on Day			
Treatment[b]	2	4	7	10
None	100	80	65	65
Cyclophosphamide	65	45	30	20
Cyclophosphamide + Azimexone	90	90	75	50

[a]3.1×10^5 spores/mouse.

[b]Azimexone 25 mg/kg p.o. -6, -4, and -2 days before infection; cyclophosphamide
25 mg/kg i.v. -5, -3, and -1 days before infection.

Azimexone tolerance was investigated in 80 cancer patients, some of whom
were given 200 mg i.v. on 5 consecutive days without any side effects attributable to Azimexone. A dose-dependent effect was found influencing the percentage of the activiated T lymphocytes, as measured by the rosette method.
A single 200 mg dose and a 200 mg dose given on 2 consecutive days showed
an elevation of activated T lymphocytes, and five consecutive doses of 200 mg
significantly increased the number of activated T lymphocytes. To test oral
administration, the daily dose was increased stepwise from 1 × 50 mg to 3 ×
100 mg daily. The last dose was administered for 7 days. During this treatment
there was a rise in the active rosette-test-reactive T lymphocytes, especially
when the initial values were low (<30%); thus Azimexone was regarded as
being active when given by the oral route.

Peripheral blood from seven patients with advanced cancer was examined
for response to PHA *in vitro*. They were not undergoing chemotherapy at the
time of the study. The separated lymphocytes were incubated with various
concentrations of Azimexone (0.2 to 10 μg/ml), and the blastogenic response
in the presence or absence of PHA was measured. A dose response was noted,
with the maximum increase of blastogenic response to PHA occurring at the
0.2 μg/ml concentration of Azimexone. Higher doses of Azimexone affected
only some of the lymphocyte cultures, and stimulation was always found to
be lower than that obtained with the 0.2 μg/ml concentration of Azimexone.

Immunoglobulin levels were examined in 10 patients with chronic lymphatic
leukemia who received Azimexone twice weekly at 200 mg per patient intravenously for a period of 6 weeks. No effect was noted on IgA or IgG levels.
The level of IgM was found to be significantly increased during Azimexone
treatment.

An investigation was conducted to assess whether the immunosuppressive
effects of aggressive chemotherapy could be diminished by supportive treatment with Azimexone. After inducing remission in 10 patients with metastatic
breast cancer by combination chemotherapy (cyclophosphamide, methotrexate,
5-fluorouracil, vincristine, and prednisone) given for about 1 year, leukocytes,
T and B lymphocytes, and reactivity of peripheral lymphocytes to different

mitogens were determined at weekly intervals before (eight times), during (eight times while on 100 mg intravenous weekly, then four times while on 400 mg intravenous weekly) and after (four times) treatment with Azimexone. Chemotherapy-induced immunosuppression was markedly diminished during Azimexone administration. A significant increase in the peripheral leukocyte count and mitogen-induced lymphocyte transformation was achieved without any marked influence on the percentage of T and B cells. No severe side-effects of Azimexone were observed.

4. MALEIC ANHYDRIDE-DIVINYL ETHER (MVE)

Maleic anhydride–divinyl ether is a divinyl ether–maleic anhydride copolymer (Figure 3) (also known as *pyran copolymer, DIVEMA,* and *NSC-46015*). The MVE copolymers have been examined extensively for their immunoregulatory capacity. The compounds, which are of various molecular weights, have been reported to possess antitumor activity, regulate T- and B-cell functions, influence macrophage tumoricidal and tumorstasis activity, augment natural killer cell activity, demonstrate antiviral activity, act as adjuvants to tumor cell and viral vaccines, and induce Type I interferon. Many of the early studies were done with pyran copolymers of DIVEMA (NSC-46015), which is a broad-range molecular-weight material. The toxicity associated with this material prompted synthesis of five different narrow-range-molecular-weight MVEs (i.e., MVE-1, 12,500; MVE-2, 15,500, MVE-3, 21,300; MVE-4, 32,000; and MVE-5, 52,600 daltons) in an effort to separate toxic from therapeutic effects. On the basis of several preclinical studies of the 5 MVE compounds, MVE-2 was selected for in depth evaluation and Phase I clinical study. In this section we review studies conducted with both NSC-46015 and MVE-2.

4.1. Pharmacology (68,69)

Several safety evaluation studies were conducted on MVE-2 for support of early clinical trials. The acute toxicologic profile of MVE-2 was examined in mice and rats by the oral [peroral (p.o)], intraperitoneal (i.p.), intramuscular (i.m.) and intravenous (i.v.) routes of administration and in dogs by the intra-

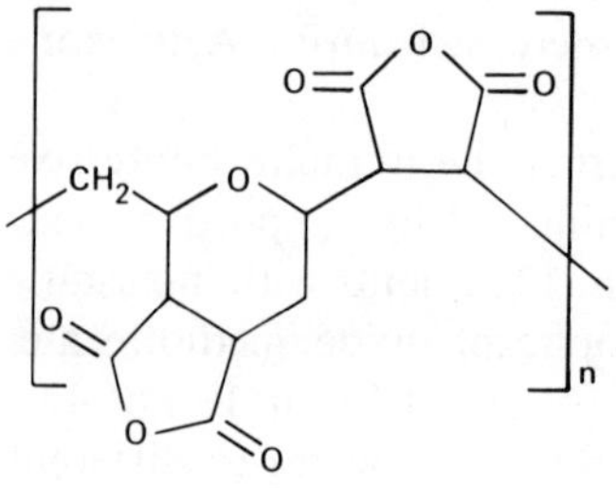

Figure 3. Chemical structure of pyran copolymer (DIVEMA, NSC-46015).

venous route. There were no mortalities or overt toxic symptoms seen in mice or rats when treated p.o., i.p., or i.m. with 1000 mg/kg of MVE-2. A few animals in these groups showed either pale or mottled kidneys when examined at necropsy 14 days after treatment. In some mice treated i.m. enlarged spleens or pale livers were seen. In rats treated i.m. or i.p. there was a loss of body weight and decreased food consumption and on occasion necropsy revealed pale or pitted kidneys. By the i.v. route, the route by which the drug is to be used most frequently at least in initial clinical trials, the LD_{50}s in mice were in the range of 90 to 100 mg/kg, with no difference between males and females. Toxic signs included apnea, spinal flexing, unconsciousness, and hepato-splenomegaly.

In the acute toxicity study in beagle dogs, several doses between 15 and 100 mg/kg were administered intravenously at a constant volume of 1 ml/kg and at a rate of 3 ml/minute. There were no deaths at any of the dose levels tested. Toxic signs were noted at doses of 25 mg/kg and greater. Fifteen mg/kg of MVE-2 was asymptomatic.

In all three species most signs of toxicity occurred during or immediately after dosing and subsided within a few minutes to 30 minutes. In the cases where deaths occurred in the mouse and rat studies, these all occurred immediately after dosing. Signs in the animals basically followed a dose-response relationship, with those seen at the higher dose levels as more severe.

Subacute toxicity studies were conducted in Sprague Dawley rats. Initially MVE-2 was administered by the i.v. route daily for 30 days at doses at 3, 6, and 15 mg/kg per day and biweekly at 15 mg/kg per treatment for 4 weeks. No deaths occurred throughout the study. Some pain was experienced on injection at the high dose. Body weight gain was significantly retarded only in animals treated at the high dose level of 15 mg/kg daily, although there were no adverse effects on food or water consumption in any of the drug-treatment groups. Hematologic, blood coagulation, and clinical chemistry parameters remained within the normal physiologic range.

The liver and spleen were the organs most consistently affected by MVE-2 treatment. Their weights were significantly increased in all male groups receiving daily treatment with MVE-2. Spleen weights were also significantly increased in males dosed twice weekly. Liver and spleen weights were also significantly increased in all treated female groups. No remarkable gross pathology could be attributed to MVE-2 treatment. The only drug related histopathologic change noted was the stimulation of the phagocytic cells of the liver, lymphatic system, and lungs seen at all dose levels.

A subacute toxicity study was also carried out in beagle dogs in which MVE-2 was administered intravenously for 28 consecutive days at doses of 1, 5, and 20 mg/kg · day). No mortalities occurred during this study. Weight gain and food consumption were normal. There were no outstanding effects on hematologic parameters throughout the study. Serum glutamic–oxalacetic transaminase (SGOT), alkaline phosphatase, lactic dehydrogenase (LDH), and cholesterol values seemed to remain elevated. At the medium and high doses, urinary protein was elevated only during the recovery period. Liver and kidney weights were increased in both sexes in the high-dose group and spleen weights were increased in males at the medium and high doses at the end of the dosing period. Only liver weights remained elevated after the 28-day recovery period.

Microscopically, macrophage accumulation was seen in the spleen, liver, kidneys, and regional and systemic lymph nodes in animals in the 5- and 20-mg/kg dose levels at the end of the 28-day dosing period and remained evident in most cases, even after the recovery period. This was an expected finding, based on the known persistent effect of the drug on macrophages. Slight hepatic centrilobular necrosis was seen in recovery males in the high-dose group. Renal tubular degeneration was present in all dogs in the 20-mg/kg dose group, but was rarely seen at lesser doses.

Since MVE-2 should ideally be administered i.v., tests were performed to determine allergic potential, and guinea pigs were sensitized by a single injection of MVE-2 and observed for anaphylacticlike responses after a challenge with MVE-2 administered 2 weeks later. Responses were negative to the lowest dose (1 mg) and highest dose (100 mg), with two of four animals at the 10-mg dose showing minor responses. However, because MVE-2 did not cause the production of detectable anti-MVE-2 antibody in rabbits, it was not considered to be immunogenic.

Because MVE-2 would be administered intravenously, a comprehensive study on the cardiovascular effects was performed in anesthetized mongrel dogs. The 0.1- and 1.0-mg/kg doses caused no measurable effect on arterial blood pressure, heart rate, or respiratory rate. The 10- and 15-mg/kg dose caused severe effects, and the 15-mg/kg dose was fatal in some animals. The decrease in arterial blood pressure was dose related and rapid, in the order of 0.5 to 1.0 minute. At doses of 10 and 15 mg/kg i.v. of MVE-2 a marked tachypnea closely accompanied the depressor effect. Changes in the ECG indicative of myocardial ischemia were seen following the 10- and 15-mg/kg doses.

All the primary effects of MVE-2 could be reversed by intraaortic administration of a 1% calcium chloride solution. The rationale for this antidote was provided by the previously published findings that this polymer complexes with essential cations. Thus it appears that the acute toxic effects of rapid i.v. MVE-2 are those of tetany caused by calcium chelation.

In studies of hematologic parameters in mice injected with 25 mg/kg of MVE-2 the polymer did not markedly alter hemoglobin, erythrocytes, leukocytes, or platelets, nor did MVE-2 affect coagulation factors such as thromboplastin, prothrombin, or fibrinogen. For a further description of the pharmacology and toxicology of MVE-2, the reader is referred to references 68 and 69.

4.2. Antiviral Activity (70–76)

It has been observed that MVE-2 possesses antiviral activity similar to that previously observed with the broad-range-molecular-weight samples (NSC-46015). Some of the results of MVE-2 antiviral activity are shown in Table 13. The antiviral activity exhibited by NSC-46015 and MVE-2 was of a prophy-

TABLE 13.   Antiviral Activity of Pyran Copolymers

Virus Studied	Pyran Copolymer	Effect	Reference
Friend leukemia virus	NSC 46015	+	70
Friend leukemia virus	NSC 46015	+	71
Rauscher leukemia virus	NSC 46015	+	72
Moloney sarcoma virus	NSC 46015	+	73
Encephalomyocarditis	MVE-2	+	74
Herpes simplex 2	MVE-2	+	75

lactic nature. The MVE-2 protective effect was markedly diminished if administered at the same time or after virus inoculation. The mechanism by which MVE-2 exerts its antiviral effect has not been resolved. Two possible mechanisms are interferon induction or macrophage activation. Recent data indicate these two mechanisms may not be mutually exclusive in that interferon has been reported to enhance macrophage virucidal activity.

Pyran copolymer (NSC-46015) was found to be a potent inhibitor of purified DNA polymerase isolated from avian myeloblastosis virus. Unlike other inhibitors, NSC-46015 interacted with the polymerases at a region other than the template site. The inhibitory effect was overcome only by excess enzyme and was not affected by excess template. The observed rate of inhibition by NSC-46015 was shown to vary with the type of polymerase tested. Inhibition was shown with all oncornaviral polymerases (avian myeloblastosis virus, Rauscher leukemia virus, reptilian C-type virus, and PK15 C-type virus), and, to a lesser extent, with mammalian polymerases. However, two of the three bacterial polymerases, by contrast, showed a marked activation.

4.3.   Effect on DNA Synthesis (77)

Pyran copolymer (NSC-46015) was reported to be capable of interacting with the repressed genome of isolated murine liver nuclei in such a way as to allow DNA synthesis to take place when assayed with exogenous bacterial DNA polymerase. This interaction was found to occur immediately and was influenced by the magnesium concentration, pyran concentration, and molecular weight of the pyran. It was found that pyran could reverse the histone-induced inhibition of a pure poly(deoxyadenylate-deoxythymidylate) template primer for DNA synthesis. The results of this study indicate that pyran is able to release the DNA template of murine liver nuclei from restrictions that normally would prevent them from serving as a useful template for DNA synthesis.

4.4.   Antitumor Activity (78–86)

Both MVE-2 and NSC-46015 pyran copolymers have been studied for their primary *in vivo* antitumor activity in a number of animal models. Pyran was

TABLE 14. *In Vivo* Antitumor Effect of Pyran Copolymer (NSC-46015 and MVE-2)

Murine Tumor	Pyran Copolymer	Effect: Increase in Life-Span[a]	Effect: Tumor Inhibition[b]	Reference
MBL-2 leukemia	MVE-2	>30%		78
Mammary CA 16/c	MVE-2	>30%		79
Leukemia L1210	NSC-46015	>20%		80
LSTRA leukemia	NSC-46015	0		81
LSTRA leukemia	MVE-2	0		81
Spontaneous, mammary	MVE-2		67	82
P815 mastocytoma	MVE-2	>20%		74
M109 lung CA	NSC-46015	>70%		83,84,85
B16 melanoma	MVE-2	>20%		86
Lewis lung CA	MVE-2	0		86

[a] Percent increase in life-span over untreated tumor control.
[b] Percent inhibition over untreated tumor control.

reported to be active in five of seven different tumors (Table 14). It was observed that MVE-2 was most effective against the M109 alveolar carcinoma, particularly in its ability to inhibit formation of lung metastases. Of particular interest was its effect on the spontaneous autochthonous murine mammary tumor in CD8F1 mice.

4.5. Pyran Copolymers as Adjuvants to Cytoreductive Therapy (74,78,79,87,88)

The most beneficial effect of the pyran copolymers was found to occur when they were used as supportive therapy following primary cytoreductive treatment (Table 15). Most of the combined treatment modality studies involved chemotherapy. In one study in which MVE-2 was compared to NSC-46015, both agents were found to enhance the therapeutic response following initial treatment with cyclophosphamide. Following surgery, MVE-2 was reported to increase the life-span of mice over other animals that received surgery alone.

In most cases the positive responses attained with MVE-2 against various tumor types occurred when treatment was initiated soon after tumor implantation. Its effectiveness decreased when treatment was delayed, indicating the ability of the pyran copolymers to exert a tumor-retarding effect on a small-tumor burden. This observation was further supported by the responses achieved when the pyran copolymers were employed as a secondary treatment following cytoreductive therapy. The enhanced protection achieved by the combination treatment would indicate that the pyran copolymer was exerting an effect on residual tumor that was initially reduced by the primary cytoreductive therapy.

TABLE 15.   Tumor Response to Combination Treatment with Pyran Copolymer

| Murine Tumor | Combined Modality | | Effect | | |
	Primary[b] Treatment	Pyran Copolymer	Survival (%)	Life-Span[a] (%)	Reference
MCAS-10 leukemia	BCNU	NSC-46015	90	>120	87
LSTRA leukemia	BCNU	NSC-46015	80	> 90	88
Lewis lung cancer	MeCCNU	NSC-46015	—	65	88
Lewis lung cancer	Surgery	MVE-2	—	25	74
MBL-2 leukemia	CY	NSC-46015	50	> 60	79
MBL-2 leukemia	CY	MVE-2	80	> 60	78,79

[a] Percent increase in life-span over control receiving primary treatment alone.

[b] BCNU = 1,3-bis (2-chloroethyl-1-nitrosourea); MeCCNU = 1-(2 chloroethyl)-3-(trans-4-methylcyclohexyl)-1-nitrosourea; CY = cyclophosphamide.

Since the pyran copolymers were not considered to possess cellular antiproliferative activity, the mechanism by which they exerted their tumoricidal and/or tumorstatic effect must be mediated through cellular elements of the immune system.

4.6. Immunotherapy (89)

The concept that macrophages are the effector of tumor cell neutralization was supported by results achieved in a local passive transfer test. In this study mice were immunized by an s.c. inoculation of allogeneic MBL-2 leukemia cells. Randomized groups of normal and tumor-bearing mice received placebo or pyran (NSC-46015) 25 mg/kg i.p. on day 6. Peritoneal exudates (PE) were subsequently harvested on the sixth day (i.e., 12 days from the time of tumor inoculation). Antitumor cytotoxicity *in vivo* was determined by an adoptive transfer type of assay (Winn test) in which MBL-2 tumor cells and PE cells were admixed *in vitro,* and the mixture was then injected subcutaneously into syngeneic mice (Table 16).

TABLE 16.   Local Passive Transfer of Allogeneic Peritoneal Exudate (PE) Cells

Source of PE cells[a]	Median Survival Time (days)	Survival (%)
None	20.0	0
Normal (nontumor)	21.0	0
Pyran treated (nontumor)	26.0	0
Tumor inoculated	23.0	0
Tumor inoculated and pyran treatment	>60.0	90

[a] 2×10^6 PE cells mixed with 10^4 MBL-2 ascites tumor cells and inoculated subcutaneously into C57 B1/6 mice.

The results show that the passive transfer of peritoneal cells from mice treated with pyran or tumor-bearing mice treated with pyran produced a positive Winn test response. The best source of PE macrophage cells was from tumor-bearing mice treated with pyran, resulting in a 90% cure. These results indicate the occurrence of a synergistic reaction between the specific immune response and adjuvant pyran treatment.

4.7. Cellular Elements Affected by Pyran Copolymers

Reticuloendothelial System (68,74,75,90,91).   Mice were treated i.v. with a single injection of 5 to 50 mg/kg of MVE-2. Twenty-four hours later the functional status of the reticuloendothelial system was evaluated by determining the vascular clearance of ^{51}Cr-labeled sheep red blood cells. It was observed that MVE-2 enhanced vascular clearance of the labeled sheep erythrocytes. Uptake of the erythrocytes in liver was unaltered, whereas MVE-2 at a 5- and 25-mg/kg i.v. dose decreased uptake in the spleen, and MVE-2 at 50 mg/kg significantly increased uptake by the lungs. In a similar study MVE-2 at 25 mg/kg was injected into mice i.v., and 24 hours later the functional status of the RES was assessed. At 24 hours the phagocytic index and hepatic phagocytosis were markedly reduced. However, by the third day following treatment MVE-2 produced an enhancement of hepatic phagocytosis and vascular clearance rate that persisted for at least 7 days.

The hepatic involvement in phagocytosis is in keeping with the findings on the tissue distribution of pyran copolymer where liver was found to retain a substantial amount of ^{14}C MVE-2 and/or its metabolites over a 28-day observation period. In order of retention after 28 days, the tissue distribution of MVE-2 and/or its metabolites was: liver, 8%; carcass, 10%; tail, 5.5%; skin, 1.5%; kidneys, 1%; and spleen, 1%.

Macrophage (74,78,84,85,89, 92–100).   The results of several studies implicate macrophage activation as the major mechanism by which pyran copolymers exhibit their effect. Several *in vitro* and *in vivo* studies have demonstrated that macrophages, after exposure to pyran copolymers, are activated and exert a tumoricidal or tumorstatic effect on various tumor cells (Table 17).

Following exposure to the pyran copolymers normal macrophages have been found capable of exerting a tumoricidal or tumorstatic effect on various tumor cell types. The growth of normal cells is not adversely affected by exposure to pyran-activated macrophages. The pyran copolymers alone do not exert any effect on tumor cell growth. Macrophages, harvested from mice treated with pyran copolymers, also exert a tumor killing effect. Present evidence suggests that macrophage recruitment and activation are probably the principal mechanisms responsible for the antitumor activity associated with the administration of pyran copolymers. Intralesional pyran injections led to increased numbers of histiocytes present in the connective tissue surrounding Lewis lung tumors. Moreover, the antitumor activity of pyran injected by the

TABLE 17. Effect of Pyran Copolymers on Macrophage Antitumor Activity

Pyran Copolymer	Tumor Type	Macrophage Source		Reference
		In Vitro[a]	*In Vivo*[b]	
NSC 46015	MBL-2	+	+	92
NSC 46015	M109	+	+	84,85,93
NSC 46015	Lewis lung		+	94
MVE-2	MBL-2	+	+	95,96
MVE-2	M109		+	84
MVE-2	Lewis lung		+	74
MVE-2	mKSA-TU5		+	96
MVE-2	MCA-1		+	96

[a] Macrophages from normal mice incubated *in vitro* with pyran copolymer and tumor cell and reduction of tumor cell growth determined.
[b] Macrophages from mice treated with pyran copolymer incubated *in vitro* with tumor cells and reduction of tumor cell growth determined.

i.p. route against M109 and colon tumor 26 was associated with an increased mobilization and deposit of morphologically activated macrophages at the tumor site. Necrosis was much more extensive in the lesions of pyran-treated animals, and macrophages were intimately associated with necrotic tumor cells in these studies. Whether this mobilization of macrophages is related to the chemo attractant property of pyran for monocytes or to enhancing the immunogenicity of the tumor is yet to be determined.

Although the exact mechanism by which pyran copolymers render macrophages cytotoxic is presently unknown, at least three distinct possibilities exist. Pyran copolymers may activate macrophages by interferon induction because macrophage cultures produce interferon after pyran copolymer treatment *in vitro* and *in vivo* and because antibody-purified fibroblast-derived interferon has been demonstrated to be a potent macrophage activator. Moreover, highly specific anti-interferon globulin has been demonstrated to block the ability of the Type I interferon inducer pyran copolymer to activate macrophages *in vitro,* indicating that endogenous interferon was externalized from the producing cell before induction of the tumoricidal state. Alternatively, pyran may behave as a model gene regulator, binding to nuclear histones and releasing template restriction. It has been reported that ^{14}C-labeled pyran copolymer is rapidly taken up by macrophages; much of this activity can be recovered from isolated nuclei extracted from these cells.

Further evidence for the capacity of pyran copolymer to recruit macrophages was suggested by the study in which it was shown that MVE-2 induced a significant amount of mononuclear cell influx into the peritoneum 6 days following an intraperitoneal injection as well as an increase in nonspecific esterase staining cells. In addition, enhanced migration of esterase staining cells into the peritoneal cavity was accompanied by a marked enhancement of the Fc receptor binding affinity of peritoneal exudate cells from MVE-2-treated animals. Increased binding affinity for Fc indicator cells prepared from increasing dilutions of antibody was seen with macrophages from MVE-2-treated mice. Macrophages from nontreated mice bound poorly to erythrocytes coated with various dilutions of antibody. These results indicate that MVE-2 activated macrophages have a higher density of Fc receptors or receptors that bind more avidly on their surface.

Lysosomal Hydrolases (97).   Injection of pyran copolymer (NSC-46015) into normal mice and mice bearing the M109 Madison lung carcinoma increases serum concentrations of lysozyme, β-glucuronidase, and N-acetyl-β,D-glucosaminidase. The increase in serum lysozyme was not dose dependent. There appeared to be a relationship between pyran copolymer-induced increases in serum lysozyme levels and antitumor effect. Interestingly, the pyran copolymer-stimulated increase in serum lysozyme was not depressed in tumor-bearing mice undergoing MeCCNU chemotherapy.

Effect on Lymphocytes (96, 101–105).   It has been reported that spleen cells from normal mice given pyran copolymer (NSC-46015) showed a 25 to 40 times higher incorporation of ^{3}H-thymidine in the absence of mitogen than did cells from untreated mice. Treatment with pyran copolymer (NSC-46015) results in a transitory increase in both T and B cells in the spleens of normal mice. From indirect immunofluorescent studies, employing anti-B and anti-T sera, T cells were markedly depressed in tumor-bearing mice. In contrast, the T-cell population was significantly higher in tumor-bearing mice treated with pyran copolymer, and the values were near those for normal mice. In similar studies the presence of tumor or pyran treatment did not appear to alter the B-cell population. Studies of the proliferative response to Con A, PHA, and LPS of splenic lymphocytes from tumor-bearing and pyran-treated mice revealed that the tumor-bearing mice usually had T- and B-cell populations lower than those observed for the normal controls. The administration of pyran to tumor-bearing mice resulted in an increase of T cells and a temporary increase in the B-cell population. In tumor-bearing animals pyran appears to reconstitute the depressed T-cell population but has only a transitory effect on the B-cell population.

A subsequent study was conducted to assess the effect of MVE-2 on the lymphocyte subpopulations of M109 tumor-bearing mice that received 500 rads of total body irradiation. By direct immunofluorescence, it was found that the percentage of splenic T lymphocytes was significantly depressed in the irradiated tumor-bearing mice. Mitogenic studies revealed that the T lymphocytes were more depressed in the irradiated tumor-bearing mice than in the corresponding nonirradiated tumor-bearing mice and that MVE was relatively effective in reconstituting the splenic lymphocyte T-cell compartment. The B-cell compartment of the splenic lymphocytes of the irradiated tumor-bearing mice was found to be extremely radiosensitive. With the use of a specific anti-B serum, no B lymphocytes were detected during testing. Blastogenic studies using LPS as the mitogenic probe revealed that the incorporation of ^{3}H-TdR by lymphocytes from irradiated-tumored mice was just slightly higher than background values. Maleic anhydride–divinyl ether proved to be relatively ineffective in reconstituting the splenic B cells of the irradiated tumor-bearing mice.

Effect on Delayed-Type Hypersensitivity (81).   Delayed-type hypersensitivity was studied in male C57B1/6 mice. On day 0, mice were given subcutaneous injections of 1×10^8 sheep red blood cells in the right footpad; MVE-2 at two different concentrations was injected intraperitoneally immediately after the SRBC inoculation. On the fourth day, 1×10^8 SRBC were injected subcutaneously into the left footpad. Twenty-four hours later the thickness of both footpads was measured. It was noted that MVE-2 at both the 5- and 20-mg/kg doses resulted in a significantly enhanced DTH response.

Natural Killer Cell Augmentation (106–108).   The ability of pyran copolymer (NSC-46015) to augment natural killer cell activity against the YAC tumor cell has been confirmed in several studies. In a time-course study with all five MVE compounds (i.e., MVE-1 to MVE-5), the peak of natural killer cell activity occurred on the third day after treatment and was still evident by the sixth day. It was also found that MVE-2 augmented natural killer cell activity against the M109 alveolar carcinoma cell line.

Effect of Pyran Copolymer as an Adjuvant to Tumor Cell Vaccine (80,81).   The five MVE compounds were examined to assess their ability to act as adjuvants to killed L1210 tumor cell vaccine. All five MVE compounds (MVE-1 to MVE-5) were found to strongly potentiate the antitumor immunity stimulated by irradiated L1210 leukemia tumor cells, whereas the vaccine alone was only marginally effective. It was found that MVE-2 alone did not exert any protective effect against live L1210 challenge. The lowest dose tested (10 mg/kg) was found still capable of potentiating the vaccine. This enhanced potentiation by MVE occurred despite the fact that L1210 is a poorly immunogenic tumor requiring multiple vaccinations to achieve a detectable degree of immunity. The immune potentiation demonstrated by MVE was not of a transient nature. A high degree of resistance was still evident on rechallenge 45 days later.

4.8. Clinical Activity

Clinical experience has been largely limited to the original pyran preparation (NSC-46015), which contained polymers of wide-ranging molecular weights. Leavitt et al. (109) treated four patients with viral encephalitis at a dose of 60 mg/kg. Although interferon was induced, there was no therapeutic benefit. The patients did develop a temporary renal failure. Dennis et al. (110) treated four patients with pyran at a dose of 18 mg/kg. Defects in coagulation developed without clinical evidence of bleeding.

Regelson and co-workers (111) have studied pyran in patients with solid tumors. In a Phase I study 29 patients were given daily (median 14 days) 1-hour intravenous infusions at doses ranging from 4 to 16 mg/kg. All patients had fever, chills, and malaise and at doses over 8 mg/kg of thrombocytopenia usually developed. Thirty-three patients with far-advanced solid tumors (median survival 16 days) were incorporated into a Phase II study of daily (median 9 days) infusion pyran therapy at a dose of 12 mg/kg. Malaise, fever, and chills were again noted. Hematologic abnormalities included thrombocytopenia (10) and leukopenia (9). There was one death related to gastrointestinal bleeding. Other toxicities included hypertension and acute central nervous system symptoms. One partial remission was claimed in this group of 33 patients with far-advanced disease.

Excessive toxicity and modest, if any, therapeutic benefit led to a decline in interest in the original pyran preparation. The development of pyran products with more restricted molecular weights has allowed separation of therapeutic and toxic effects. Phase I trials are currently under way with MVE-2, and preliminary data confirm the animal studies in indicating markedly improved safety.

5. ISOPRINOSINE

Isoprinosine (Inosiplex) has been reported to enhance humoral and cellular elements of the immune system. Clinical studies with this agent have been predominantly directed toward its activity as an antiviral agent; its immunomodulating activity is focused on in this review.

5.1. Chemistry (112,113)

Isoprinosine is a compound formed from inosine and the *p*-acetamidobenzoate (PAcBA) salt of *N,N*-dimethylamino-2-propanol (DIP) in a 1:3 molar ratio. Isoprinosine is a white crystalline powder, slightly bitter in taste, soluble in water at room temperature to an extent of 25% (250 mg/ml) and stable in neutral solution. The dosage form commonly administered to humans is 500 mg tablets.

Evidence for interaction of the components (inosine and dimethylammonium isopropanol-*p*-acetamidobenzoate, DIP-PAcBA) to form a complex has been obtained by various techniques, including both synthetic and physicochemical measurements.

5.2. Pharmacology (113–115)

In pharmacologic studies, Isoprinosine has been shown to have minor CNS-depressant properties in mice and cats. No neuromuscular effects were observed. No analgesic, sedative, antipyretic, or anticonvulsive properties were demonstrable. Minimal cardiovascular effects were observed, but no alteration of the effects of histamine, serotonin, or acetylcholine were seen. The pressor action of norepinephrine was potentiated. No immunosuppression or immune toxicity has been found in association with the administration of Isoprinosine. The pharmacokinetics and the metabolism of Isoprinosine were studied by using radiolabeled components in the cat and rhesus monkey and Isoprinosine with double-labeled DIP-PAcBA salt in humans. Of particular importance is the metabolic lability of the inosine moiety of Isoprinosine, the half-life of which is 3 and 50 minutes, respectively, following intravenous and oral administration in rhesus monkeys. More than 90% of the labeled inosine is excreted as allantoin and uric acid. Small amounts of hypoxanthine, xanthine, and adenine are also excreted, whereas less than 5% of the inosine radioactivity enters the purine salvage pathway. The DIP and PAcBA moieties are each converted to one major metabolite, DIP-N-oxide and PAcBA-O-Acyl glucuronide, respectively, both of which appear in substantial quantities in the urine of rhesus monkeys and humans.

In HeLa and primary monkey kidney cell cultures the half-life of the inosine moiety in the medium is slightly less than 2 hours. In both of these tissue culture systems, the sole purine catabolite was hypoxanthine, accounting for all of the metabolized inosine.

5.3. Toxicology (116)

Acute LD_{50} determinations were conducted in male rats, mice, cats, and guinea pigs with a single dose of Isoprinosine by either the p.o., i.v., or i.p. route. Mortality was observed over a 24- to 72-hour time period (Table 18). The LD_{50} values for rodents ranged from 7.5 to 10.0 g/kg by the p.o. route. A similar low degree of toxicity was observed for other species (5.0 g/kg in the cat) and other routes of administration.

Subacute Toxicity.   Isoprinosine was investigated for its subacute toxicity in male and female rats and monkeys during 13 weeks of repeated oral dosing. Dose levels up to 500 mg/(kg · day) failed to reveal any significant toxicologic signs or symptoms.

Two-Year Chronic Toxicity.   In a 2-year chronic toxicity test, male and female rats (DC-Sprague-Dawley) and rhesus monkeys were given 375, 750, or

TABLE 18.   Acute LD_{50} of Isoprinosine (in Milligrams)

Route	Mouse	Rat	Guinea Pig	Cat
Intraperitoneal	4,300	5,000	6,400	
Oral	10,000	7,500		5,000
Intravenous	1,850			

1500 mg/(kg · day) of Isoprinosine in their food. Data obtained on the following parameters revealed no differences between the control animals and animal fed Isoprinosine: food consumption, mortality, hematologic profile, clinical blood chemistry, urinalysis, and gross and microscopic pathology.

Teratology, Fertility, and Reproduction. Studies conducted in Sprague-Dawley rats and albino rabbits failed to demonstrate a teratogenic effect for Isoprinosine. Further, there were no adverse effects on fertility or reproductive performance.

5.4. Immunologic Profile

Lymphocytes (112, 117–121). The several reported effects on the immune system indicate that Isoprinosine functions as an immunostimulator. Isoprinosine was found to augment mitogen-induced proliferation of human peripheral blood lymphocytes *in vitro*. Subsequently, a number of studies have shown that mouse spleen lymphocytes are augmented in their response to a variety of mitogenic and antigenic stimuli (Table 19). No effect on background proliferation has been observed, indicating that the action of Isoprinosine is to potentiate the induction of proliferation by the mitogen. The effects of the drug on mitogen responses appear to occur at the initiation phase. In general, Isoprinosine is most effective in the presence of optimal concentrations of mitogen and under such conditions 1.5- to 3.9-fold mean increases have been observed.

Isoprinosine also induced the appearance of the T-cell-surface marker theta (θ) in prothymocytes, to an extent comparable to that induced by thymopoietin. Prothymocytes isolated from the spleens of nude mice were incubated with inducers of T-cell differentiation such as the thymic hormones. The new appearance of T-cell-surface markers (θ, LY, TL, etc.) characteristic of intrathymic lymphocytes were detected by antisera to these antigens. Isoprinosine induced θ in 10 to 30% of the cells with optimal effects at 1 μg/ml and intermediate activity observed at 0.1 and 10 μg/ml.

TABLE 19.   Lymphocyte Proliferation *in Vitro*

Mitogen	Lymphocyte Source	
	Human Blood	Mouse Spleen
Phytohemagglutinin	+	+
Pokeweed mitogen	+	
Concanavolin A	+	+
Mixed leukocyte culture	+	
Tetanus toxoid	+	
Influenza virus antigen		+
Herpes virus antigen		+

The formation of active T rosettes was augmented by Isoprinosine, whereas stable T rosettes were not affected (120). From *in vitro* studies of Isoprinosine on normal human leukocytes, it was found that the drug significantly increased the percentage of active T rosettes (concentration range 50 to 500 µg/ml) and the percentage of autologous red cell T rosettes (concentration 100 µg/ml). In contrast, Isoprinosine did not modify the percentage of total T rosettes and EAC rosettes.

Suppressor Cells (112,116,122,123). Employing mouse spleen cells, Isoprinosine at concentrations as low as 0.1 µg/ml induced a 35% suppression of the subsequent MLC response. In other studies it was observed that Isoprinosine potentiates Con A-induced suppression; however, investigators were unable to induce suppressor cells in human peripheral blood cells directly when the suppressor blast cells were isolated on albumin gradients. Studies designed to resolve this difference showed that when suppressor cells were not isolated by flotation, Isoprinosine did act to induce suppression, yet when only isolated suppressor blast cells were employed, no such suppressor action was observed. These results indicate that Isoprinosine induces suppressor cells that suppress without undergoing blast transformation. This observation is in keeping with with the observation that Isoprinosine alone does not induce lymphocyte proliferation. Isoprinosine also augments the capacity of Con A to induce suppressor blast cells. The blast cells induced by Con A show greater suppressor action on a per-cell basis. It is not clear whether Isoprinosine in the presence of Con A triggers more suppressor cells to proliferate or enhances the expression of more suppressor function in the same population of cells triggered by Con A alone.

Effects of Isoprinosine have also been observed in other types of immune cells. Leukocyte adherance inhibition was augmented by the drug. Monocyte phagocytosis of yeast was increased, and macrophage function and proliferation were significantly augmented. These effects were found at drug concentrations of only 1 to 10 µg/ml.

Nude Mouse Studies (122). Single injections of Isoprinosine of 0.5 and 5 mg/kg, in athymic nude mice induced (4 days following treatment) 10 and 18% θ-bearing spleen cells, respectively. In addition, treatment of nude mice with 5 mg/kg of Isoprinosine induced a serum factor at 24 hours, thus, in turn, inducing θ bearing cells in 18% of nude spleen cells.

Antibody Formation (121,124,125). Isoprinosine, when tested in the Mishell-Dutton assay, augmented plaque formation to sheep erythrocytes two- to threefold over controls. *In vivo*, Isoprinosine given i.p. at 0.05 to 50 mg/kg at the time of SRBC administration to mice augmented spleen IgM plaque-forming cells two- to threefold. Immunoglobulin-G plaque-forming cells were also found increased two- to threefold at doses between 5 and 50 mg/kg. Oral doses of Isoprinosine (10 to 1000 mg/kg) in the drinking water given with and after antigen achieved similar effects on IgG and IgM plaque-forming cells. In these studies no effects of Isoprinosine were observed on mouse spleen weight, cell yield, or viability.

Tumor Studies (112,119,126)

Adjuvant to Tumor Antigen (119).   A limited series of experiments were conducted to ascertain whether Isoprinosine would act as an adjuvant to killed L1210 Ha leukemia cells. It was seen that the protection given to mice by a previous immunization with 10^6 x-ray-inactivated L1210 Ha leukemia cells against subsequent inocula with live cells of the same compatible tumor was significantly increased if the mice were also given a series of Isoprinosine injections before challenge.

Combined Treatment (119,126).   The effect of Isoprinosine plus cytoreductive therapy (Adriamycin or BCNU) was tested on leukemia-bearing mice. A single or a short sequence of Isoprinosine injections administered to L1210-bearing mice following chemotherapy failed to increase survival time over that obtained with chemotherapy alone. In contrast, a synergistic antitumor effect was reported for Isoprinosine when combined with interferon. Isoprinosine enhanced the antitumor effect of low doses of interferon. After combined treatment, the mean survival time, the tumor incidence, and the final survival rate were significantly increased in mice inoculated with 10^6 Crocker tumor 180/TG cells (purine resistant cell line) when compared with interferon-alone treatment. Isoprinosine alone was ineffective but when combined with interferon treatment increased the median survival time from 45 days (interferon alone) to 64 days (combined treatment).

Allograft (119).   An immunosuppressive effect by Isoprinosine was suggested by studies on the growth of an allogeneic tumor. Normal C_3H (H-2^k) mice resist the transplant of a high number of the incompatable (H-2^d) L1210 Ha leukemia cells. It was observed that C_3H mice inoculated with 10^7 L1210 Ha leukemia cells and treated with Isoprinosine developed a higher number of progressive tumors.

Other Immune Cellular Elements (119).   In studies evaluating the capacity of Isoprinosine to enhance phagocytosis, no significant differences could be detected between control and Isoprinosine-treated hosts when the rate of carbon clearance was measured 1 and 4 days after completion of a 3-day treatment with 0.05 to 50 mg/kg i.p. of Isoprinosine.

Purified peritoneal macrophages obtained 5 days after administration of a similar treatment did not show a significant nonspecific cytotoxic capacity toward lymphoma cells under conditions where cells collected from *C. parvum*-injected mice were highly active, thus suggesting that macrophages were not "activated" by the treatments employed. In view of the important role currently attributed to antibody-dependent cellular cytotoxicity and to natural cytotoxicity as defense mechanisms, these investigators studied the possible effect of Isoprinosine on the functional capacity of K and NK cells. No significant changes with respect to untreated controls were seen in the splenic lymphocytes obtained from mice treated 1 to 5 days earlier with i.p. administration of 0.05 to 50 mg/kg $\times$ 3 of Isoprinosine. These investigators employed YAC lymphoma cells and chicken erythrocytes as targets for NK and K cells.

5.5. Clinical Studies (124, 127–138)

Isoprinosine has been clinically investigated in several viral diseases but has had little evaluation in cancer patients. However, it is worthwhile to review the viral studies in view of Isoprinosine effect on immune responses.

Toxicology. Extensive and rigorous tolerance and safety studies were conducted in healthy human volunteers. Isoprinosine was administered orally for periods of 1 week up to 2 years at doses of 1 to 8 g/day. This resulted in minimal untoward effects, including transient rise in serum and urine uric acid levels and, occasionally, transient nausea associated with the ingestion of a large number of tablets.

Antiviral and Immune Responses. As stated earlier, Isoprinosine has been found to be active in the treatment of several viral diseases. Some of the viral infections for which Isoprinosine has been used include influenza, rhinovirus, herpes simplex, herpes zoster, hepatitis, rubella, viral otitis, and subacute sclerosing panencephalitis. In addition, benefits have resulted from Isoprinosine treatment for patients with immune deficiencies due to aging.

In one double-blind study of volunteers challenged with rhinovirus and treated with either Isoprinosine (4 g/day) or placebo, a 70% lower mean cumulative symptom score was recorded for the Isoprinosine group than for the placebo group. In addition, peripheral blood lymphocytes from the Isoprinosine group 8 days after the start of treatment showed normal response to PHA-induced proliferation compared to pretreatment levels, whereas the placebo group had a 60% decrease in PHA-induced proliferation.

A double-blind placebo-controlled study of Isoprinosine (4 g/day) in influenza A/Victoria-challenged volunteers resulted in a significant increase in influenza-induced lymphocyte proliferation after 3 and 6 days of drug treatment compared to controls and produced a greater increase in lymphocyte cytotoxicity for influenza-infected cells as compared to placebo controls. There was a concurrent reduction in the signs and symptoms of influenza in the drug-treated group compared to the controls and a reduction in virus shedding.

Isoprinosine caused a 138% increase in PHA-induced lymphocyte proliferation in a double-blind placebo-controlled study of 60 herpes simplex patients, whereas the placebo group showed a slight decrease or no change. Lymphotoxin production increased 63% in the Isoprinosine group after 7 days of treatment, whereas a depression of 40% was noted in the placebo group. The Isoprinosine group was reported as showing a 55% cure rate after 7 days of treatment, compared with only a 15% cure rate in the placebo group.

In a multicenter study, Isoprinosine was shown to be able to enhance the chance of survival in subacute sclerosing panencephalitis when compared to historical controls.

The use of Isoprinosine in a multiplicity of other studies of various types of virus infections and immunologic disorders in humans has resulted in variable effects on viral antibody responses, increased mitogen responses, increased lymphotoxin production, increased virus-induced proliferative responses, increased lymphocyte cytotoxicity to viral-infected target cells, increased total rosettes, and increased skin test responses.

6. TUFTSIN

Tuftsin is a naturally occurring peptide that has been reported to perform well-defined biological functions. From studies on the mechanisms of leukokinin stimulation of phagocytosis, it was found that the activity of leukokinin resides in a small peptide fraction. The stimulating agent was determined to be the peptide, tuftsin (139).

Tuftsin, Thr-Lys-Pro-Arg, represents residues 289 through 292 of the heavy chain of gamma globulin (140). Two enzymes are responsible for releasing tuftsin from the carrier leukokinin molecule, tuftsin—endocarboxypeptidase and leukokininase (141). The free tetrapeptide, the only state in which it is biologically active has been shown to stimulate the various functions of granulocytes, monocytes, and macrophages (139,142,143).

6.1. Biological Activity (139)

Tuftsin was reported to stimulate a great number of activities associated with the macrophage and the granulocyte. Some of these activities are motility, phagocytosis, immunogenic function, augmentation of antibody response, tumoricidal and tumoristatic activity toward syngeneic and allogeneic tumor cells *in vivo* and *in vitro,* and bactericidal activity.

6.2. Mechanism of Antitumor Effect (139,142)

Several studies indicate that tuftsin exerts its antitumor effect through activation of the macrophage. By employing the leukemia L1210 cell in *in vitro* and *in vivo* studies, tuftsin was found to activate macrophages to exert tumoricidal activity. *In vitro* exposure of peritoneal macrophages to 10 μg of tuftsin revealed them cytotoxic to L1210 cells. Similar results were reported with a melanoma cell line.

Tuftsin was evaluated *in vivo* for its capacity to retard tumor growth. L1210-bearing mice treated with 0.2 μg of tuftsin per mouse survived for a significantly longer period than did untreated control L1210-bearing mice. The Cloudman S-91 melanoma was also reported to respond to 10 μg/mouse tuftsin treatment. Tuftsin treatment resulted in significant retardation of subcutaneous tumor growth.

Other host immune responses augmented by tuftsin are antibody synthesis and antibody-dependent cellular cytotoxicity. Tuftsin, when injected (20 mg/kg) into mice followed by the injection of a thymus-dependent antigen TNP-KLH, increased antibody formation as determined by splenic plaque formation. Similar results were obtained with a thymus-independent antigen, TNP-lipopolysaccharide.

Tuftsin appears to be a naturally occurring agent that possesses biological response-modifying capacity. It would be an agent of interest for studies in determining its ability to reconstitute or stimulate depressed immunologic functions. Some of the properties of tuftsin that make it a unique immunoregulating agent are:

1. Tuftsin has a carrier or precursor molecule and thus belongs in the category of other known peptide hormones. The carrier parent molecule is leukokinin.

2. There are known specific enzymes that participate in the release of tuftsin from leukokinin: the splenic enzyme tuftsin-endocarboxypeptidase and the phagocyte membrane enzyme leukokininase.

3. There are highly specific receptors to tuftsin that appear to be found only on target phagocytic cells.

4. Tuftsin has been reported to raise the level of cyclic guanylate.

5. Tuftsin activates the phagocytic cell and consequently stimulates all known functions of these cells, such as motility, phagocytosis, augmentation of antibody production, and stimulation of macrophage tumoricidal activity.

REFERENCES

1. D. Thienpont, O. F. J. Vanparijs, A. H. M. Raeymaekers, J. Vandenberk, P. J. A. Demoen, F. T. N. Allewijn, R. P. H. Marsboom, C. J. E. Niemegeers, K. H. L. Schellekens, and P. A. J. Janssen, Tetramasole (R8299): A new potent broad spectrum anthelmintic. *Nature*, **209**, 1084 (1966).

2. P. A. J. Janssen, The Levamisole Story. In E. Jucker, Ed., *Progress in Research,* Vol. 20, Birkhaeuser Verlag, Basel and Stuttgart, 1976, pp. 347–383.

3. G. Renoux and M. Renoux, Effet immunostimulant d'un imidothiazole dans l'immunisation des souris contre l'infection par Brucella abortus. *C. R. Acad. Sci.* (*Paris*), **2720**, 349 (1971).

4. W. K. Amery, F. Spreafico, A. F. Rojas, E. Denissen, and M. A. Chirigos, Adjuvant treatment with levamisole in cancer. A review of experimental and clinical data. *Cancer Treat. Rev.,* **4**, 167 (1977).

5. J. Symoens and M. Rosenthal, Levamisole in the modulation of the immune response. The current experimental and clinical state. *J. Reticuloendothel. Soc.,* **21**, 175 (1977).

6. M. A. Chirigos, and W. K. Amery, Combined levamisole therapy. An overview of its protective effects. In W. D. Terry, Ed., *Immunotherapy of Cancer: Current Status of Trials in Man,* Raven, New York, 1978, pp. 181-195.

7. J. Symoens, Levamisole, an antianergic chemotherapeutic agent. An Overview. In M. A. Chirigos, Ed., *Control of Neoplasia by Modulation of the Immune System,* Vol. 2, Raven, New York, 1977 pp. 1-24.

8. W. L. Donegan, L. R. Heim, G. C. Owens, and D. Sampson, Immunostimulatory effects of levamisole in humans with cancer, *Oncology,* **38,** 168 (1981).

9. J. G. Adams, Pharmacokinetics of levamisole. *J. Rheumatol.,* **5** (Suppl. 4), 137 (1978).

10. G. Goldstein, Mode of action of levamisole, *J. Rheumatol.,* **5** (Suppl. 4), 143 (1978).

11. G. Renoux, and M. Renoux, Roles of the imidazole or thio-moiety on the immunostimulant action of levamisole. In M. A. Chirigos, Ed., *Control of Neoplasia by Modulation of the Immune System,* Vol. 2, Raven, New York, 1977, pp. 67-80.

12. J. Hadden, Levamisole, cyclic nucleotides and immunopharmacology. In M. A. Chirigos, Ed., *Modulation of Host Immune Resistance in the Prevention or Treatment of Induced Neoplasias,* Fogarty International Center Proceedings, No. 28, U.S. Government Printing Office, Washington, D.C., 1977, pp. 353-356.

13. R. S. Pinals, The non-hematologic side effects of levamisole in the treatment of rheumatoid arthritis—A review. *J. Rheumatol.,* **5** (Suppl. 4), 71 (1978).

14. H. Mielants, and E. M. Veys, A study of the hematologic side effects of levamisole in rheumatoid arthritis with recommendations. *J. Rheumatol.,* **5** (Suppl. 4), 77 (1978).

15. M. Rosenthal, U. Trabiet, and W. Muller, Leucocytotoxic effect of levamisole. *Lancet,* **1,** 369 (1976).

16. O. Ruuskanen, M. Remes, and A. L. Makelae, Levamisole and agranulocytosis. *Lancet,* **2,** 958 (1976).

17. R. Clara and J. Germanes, Levamisole and agranulocytosis. *Lancet,* **1,** 42 (1978).

18. M. A. Chirigos, J. W. Pearson, and J. Pryor, Augmentation of chemotherapeutically induced remission of a murine leukemia by a chemical immune-adjuvant. *Cancer Res.,* **33,** 2615 (1973).

19. M. A. Chirigos, J. W. Pearson, and F. S. Fuhrman, Effect of tumor load reduction in successful immunostimulation. *Proc. Am. Assoc. Cancer Res.,* **15,** 16 (1974).

20. M. A. Chirigos, F. S. Fuhrman, and J. Pryor, Prolongation of chemotherapeutically induced remission of a syngeneic murine leukemia by L-2,3,5,6-tetrahydro-6-phenylimidazo [2, 1-b] thiazole hydrochloride. Cancer Res., **35,** 927 (1975).

21. F. Spreafico, A. Vecchi, A. Mantovani, A. Poggi, G. Franchi, A. Anaclerico, and S. Garrantini, Characterization of the immunostimulants levamisole and tetramisole. *Eur. J. Cancer,* **11,** 537 (1975).

22. D. S. Gordon, L. S. Hall, and J. S. McDougal, Levamisole and cytoxan in a murine tumor model: *In vivo* and *in vitro* studies. In M. A. Chirigos, Ed., *Control of Neoplasia by Modulation of the Immune System,* Vol. 2, Raven, New York, 1977, pp. 121-134.

23. C. C. Stewart, C. A. Perez, and B. Hente, Effect of Levamisole in combination with radiotherapy in modifying the growth of murine tumors of differing immunogenicity. In M. A. Chirigos, Ed., *Immune Modulation and Control of Neoplasia by Adjuvant Therapy,* Vol. 7, Raven, New York, 1978, pp. 11-21.

24. M. L. Padarathsingh, J. H. Dean, J. L. McCoy, D. D. Lewis, and J. W. Northing, Restorative effects of Levamisole on cell-mediated immune responses following chemotherapy with aniline mustard in mice bearing ADJ-PC5 plasmacytoma. *Cancer Treat. Rep.,* **11,** 1627 (1978).

25. L. Desplenter and G. Atassi, Influence of tetramisole and its isomers on a chemotherapeutically induced remission of L1210 leukemia. *Jannsen Pharmaceutica, Biological Research Report on Tetramisole, Dexamisole, and Levamisole,* November 1973.

26. M. Debrabander, F. Aerts, and M. Borgus, Effect of levamisole (R12564) in the MO4 tumor system. *Janssen Pharmaceutica Biological Research Report on Levamisole,* October 1973.

27. D. G. Hopper, M. V. Pimm, and R. W. Baldwin, Levamisole treatment of local and metastatic growth of transplanted rat tumours. *Br. J. Cancer,* **32,** 345 (1975).

28. Study Group for Bronchogenic Carcinoma, Immunopotentiation with levamisole in resectable bronchogenic carcinoma: A double-blind controlled trial. *Br. Med. J.,* **3,** 461 (1975).

29. W. K. Avery, Final results of a multicenter placebo-controlled levamisole study of resectable lung cancer. *Cancer Treat. Rep.,* **62,** 1677 (1978).

30. H. M. Anthony, A. J. Mearns, M. K. Mason, D. G. Scott, K. Moghissi, P. B. Deverall, Z. J. Rozycki, and D. A. Watson, Levamisole and surgery in bronchial carcinoma: Increase in deaths from cardiorespiratory failure. *Thorax,* **34,** 4 (1979).

31. W. K. Amery, Randomized levamisole study in resectable lung cancer: 4 year results. In W. D. Terry, Ed., *Proceedings of Second International Conference on Immunotherapy of Cancer,* Bethesda, Md. 4/28-20/80.

32. P. Wright, L. Hill, A. Peterson, R. Anderson, C. Bagley, I. Bernstein, T. Ivey, L. Johnson, E. Morgan, R. Ostenson, and R. Penkham, Adjuvant immunotherapy for lung cancer. In S. E. Jones and S. E. Salmon, Eds., *Adjuvant Therapy of Cancer II,* Grune and Stratton, New York, 1979, pp. 545-552.

33. R. M. Fox, R. L. Woods, M. H. N. Tattersall, and A. Basten, A randomized study of adjuvant immunotherapy with levamisole and Corynebacterium parvum in operable non-small cell lung cancer. *Internatl. J. Rad. Oncol. Biol. Phys.,* **6,** 1043 (1980).

34. A. F. Rojas, E. Mickiewicz, J. N. Feierstein, H. Glait, and A. J. Olivari, Levamisole in advanced human breast cancer. *Lancet,* **1,** 2111 (1976).

35. A. F. Rojas, J. N. Feierstein, H. M. Glait, and A. J. Olivari, Levamisole action in breast cancer. In W. D. Terry and D. Windhorst, Eds., *Immunotherapy of cancer: Present status of trials in man,* Raven, New York, 1978, pp. 635-646.

36. P. Klefstrom, Levamisole in addition to chemotherapy in advanced breast cancer. In H. Rainer, Ed., F. K. Shaltauer Verlag, Stuttgart, 1978, pp. 102-111.

37. P. Klefstrom, P. Holsti, P. Grohn, and E. Heinonen, Combination of levamisole immunotherapy with conventional treatments in breast cancer. In W. D. Terry, Ed., *Proceedings of Second International Conference Immunotherapy of Cancer,* Bethesda, Md., 4/28-30/1980.

38. A. H. G. Paterson, M. Nutting, L. Takats, A. M. Edwards, D. Schinnour, and A. McClillard, Chemoimmunotherapy with levamisole in metastatic breast carcinoma. *Cancer Clin. Trials,* **3,** 5 (1980).

39. E. J. W. Stephens, H. F. Wood, and B. Mason, Levamisole as adjunct to cyclic chemotherapy in end stage mammary carcinoma. In W. D. Terry, Ed., *Proceedings of Second International Conference on Immunotherapy of Cancer,* Bethesda, Md., 4/28-30/1980.

40. H. Verhaegen, J. DeCree, W. DeCock, and M. L. Verhaegen-Declercq, Levamisole therapy in patients with colorectal cancer. In W. D. Terry, Ed., *Proceedings of Second International Conference on Immunotherapy of Cancer,* Bethesda, Md., 4/28-30/80.

41. E. C. Borden, J. Crowley, T. E. Davis, W. H. Wolberg, and D. Groveman, Levamisole: Effects in primary and recurrent colorectal carcinoma. In W. D. Terry, Ed., *Proceedings of Second International Conference on Immunotherapy of Cancer,* Bethesda, Md., 4/28-30/80.

42. A. Y. Bedikian, M. Valdevieso, G. Mavligit, M. A. Burgess, V. Rodreguez, and G. P. Bodey, Sequential chemoimmunotherapy of colorectal cancer. *Cancer,* **42,** 2169 (1978).

43. C. M. Pinsky, H. J. Wanebo, E. Y. Hilal, E. W. Strong, and H. F. Oettgen, Randomized trial of levamisole in patients with squamous cancer of the head and neck. In W. D. Terry, Ed., *Proceedings of Second International Conference on Immunotherapy of Cancer,* Bethesda, Md. 4/28-30/80.

44. H. J. Wanebo, E. Y. Hilal, C. M. Pinsky, E. W. Strong, V. Mike, Y. Hirshaut, and H. F. Oettgen, Randomized trial of levamisole in patients with squamous cancer of the head and neck: A preliminary report. *Cancer Treat. Rep.*, **62**, 1663 (1978).

45. C. M. Pinsky, H. J. Wanebo, E. Y. Hilal, E. W. Strong, and H. F. Oettgen, Randomized trial of levamisole in patients with squamous cancer of head and neck. In W. D. Terry, Ed., *Proceedings of Second International Conference on Immunotherapy of Cancer*, Bethesda, Md., 4/28–30/80.

46. L. E. Spitler and R. Sagebiel, A randomized trial of levamisole versus placebo as adjuvant therapy in malignant melanoma. *New Engl. J. Med.*, **303**, 1143 (1980).

47. S. W. Hall, R. S. Benjamin, U. Lewinski, and G. Mavligit, Actinomycin-D levamisole chemoimmunotherapy of refractory malignant melanoma. *Cancer*, **43**, 1195 (1979).

48. S. Pavlovsky, G. Garay, F. Sackman Muriel, and E. Svarch, Levamisole therapy during maintenance of remission in patients with acute lymphoblastic leukemia. In W. D. Terry, Ed., *Proceedings of Second International Conference on Immunotherapy of Cancer*, Bethesda, Md., 4/28–30/1980.

49. P. Chang, P. H. Wiernik, C. A. Schiffer, and J. L. Lichtenfeld, Levamisole, cytosine arabinoside and daunorubicin therapy of acute nonlymphocytic leukemia. *Proc. Am. Soc. Clin. Oncol.*, **19**, 370 (1978).

50. S. E. Salmon, R. Alexanian, and D. Dixon, Chemoimmunotherapy for multiple myeloma: Effect of levamisole. In W. D. Terry, Ed., *Proceedings of Second International Conference on Immunotherapy of Cancer*, Bethesda, Md., 4/28–30/1980.

51. Y. Hirshaut, H. Kesselheim, C. Pinsky, D. Braun, Jr., H. J. Wanebo, and H. F. Oettgen, Levamisole as an immunoadjuvant: Phase I study and application in breast cancer. *Cancer Treat. Rep.*, **62**, 1693 (1978).

52. V. Bicker, Biochemische and pharmakologische eigenschaften neuer 2-substituierter aziridirie. Beiträge zur experimentellen. *Krebsforschung Fortschr. d. Medizin.*, **96**, 661 (1978).

53. V. Bicker, Immunomodulating effects of BM 12.531 in animals and tolerance in man. *Cancer Treat. Rep.*, **62**, 1987 (1978).

54. V. Bicker, Aziridine dyes: preclinical and clinical Studies. In E. Hersh, M. A. Chirigos, and M. J. Mastrangelo, Eds., *Augmenting Agents in Cancer Therapy*, Vol. 16, Raven, New York, 1981, p. 539.

55. W. A. Stylos, M. A. Chirigos, V. Papademetriou, and L. Lauer, The immunomodulatory effect of BM 12531 (Azimexon) on normal and tumored mice: *In vitro* and *in vivo* studies. *J. Immunopharmacol.*, **2**, 113 (1980).

56. V. Bicker, G. Hebold, A. E. Ziegler, and W. Maus, Animal experiments on the compensation of the immunosuppresive action of cyclophosphamide by BM 12.531. *Exp. Pathol.*, **15**, 49 (1978).

57. V. Bicker, K. D. Friedberg, G. Hebold, and K. Meugel, Reduction of acute toxicity of cyclophosphamide and x-rays by the new immunomodulating compound BM 12.531. *Experientia*, **35**, 1361 (1979).

58. V. Bicker, G. Hebold, and K. D. Friedberg, Reduction of acute toxicity of cyclophosphamide by BM 12.531 (Prop. INN Azimexon). *IRCS Med. Sci.*, **6**, 462 (1978).

59. J. C. Jeng, K. F. McCarthy, M. A. Chirigos, and J. F. Weiss, Effect of Azimexon (BM 12.531) on mouse granulocyte-macrophage and monocyte-macrophage progenitor cells. *Experientia*, **38**, 132 (1982).

60. I. J. Schulz, I. Florentin, C. Bourut, V. Bicker, and G. Mathe, Delayed type hypersensitivity response and humoral antibody formation in mice treated with a new immunostimulant 2-[2-cyanaziridinyl-(1)-2-]2-carbamoylaziridinyl-(1)-propane, BM 12.531. *IRCS Med. Sci.*, **6**, 115 (1978).

61. M. Micksche, M. Colat, and V. Bicker, BM 12.531 (Prop. INN. Azimexon) induced increase in lymphocyte blastogenesis response to PHA. *IRCS Med. Sci.*, **6**, 439 (1979).

62. M. A. Chirigos, V. Papademetriou, A. Bartocci, and E. Read, Immunological and tumor responses to various immunotherapeutic agents. *Internatl. J. Immunopharmacol.,* 3, 329 (1981).

63. D. Boerner, V. Bicker, A. E. Ziegler, V. Stosick, and H. J. Peters, Influence of BM 12.531 (Prop. INN Azimexon) on the lymphocyte transformation and the percentage of active lymphocytes *in vivo* and *in vitro* in man. *Cancer Immunol. Immunother.,* 6, 237 (1979).

64. R. Kreienberg, D. Boerner, J. Melchert, and E. M. Semmel, Reduction of the immuno-suppressive action of chemotherapeutics in patients with mammary carcinoma by Azimexon. *J. Immunopharmacol.* (in press).

65. V. Bicker, G. Hebold, A. E. Ziegler, and V. Haas, Influence of BM 12.531 (Prop. INN Azimexon) on the percentage of activated lymphocytes *in vitro. IRCS Med. Sci.,* 6, 455 (1978).

66. V. Bicker, A. E. Ziegler, and G. Hebold, Synergistic effect of the immunostimulant BM 12.531 (Prop. INN Azimexon) and chloramphenicol on an experimental *Escherichia coli* infection in mice. *IRCS Med. Sci.,* 6, 377 (1978).

67. V. Bicker, A. E. Ziegler, and G. Hebold, Investigations in mice on the potentiation of re-sistance to infection by a new immunostimulant compound. *J. Infect. Dis.,* 139, 389 (1979).

68. R. A. Carrano, F. K. Kinashita, A. R. Imondi, and J. D. Duliucci, MVE-2: Preclinical pharmacology and toxicology. In E. Hersh, M. A. Chirigos, and M. J. Mastrangelo, Eds., *Augmenting Agents in Cancer Therapy,* Vol. 16, Raven, New York, 1981, p. 345.

69. A. E. Munson, K. L. White, and P. C. Klykken, Pharmacology of MVE polymers. In E. Hersh, M. A. Chirigos, and M. J. Mastrangelo, Eds., *Augmenting Agents in Cancer Ther-apy,* Vol. 16, Raven, New York, 1981, p. 329.

70. W. Regelson and O. Foltyn, Prevention and treatment of Friend leukemia virus (FLV) infection by polyanions and phytohemagglutinin, *Proc. Am. Assoc. Cancer Res.,* 7, 58 (1966).

71. T. C. Merigan, Induction of circulating interferon by synthetic anionic polymers of known composition. *Nature (Lond.),* 214, 416 (1967).

72. M. A. Chirigos, W. Turner, J. Pearson, and W. Griffin, Effective antiviral therapy of two murine leukemias with an interferon-inducing synthetic carboxylate copolymer. *In-ternatl. J. Cancer,* 4, 267 (1969).

73. J. W. Pearson, W. Griffin, and M. A. Chirigos, Inhibition of sarcoma and leukemia vi-ruses and a transplantable leukemia by a synthetic interferon inducer. *Proc. Am. Assoc. Cancer Res.,* 10, 269 (1969).

74. P. S. Morahan, D. W. Barnes, and G. E. Munson, Relationship of molecular weight to anti-viral and antitumor activities and toxic effects of maleic anhydride-divinyl ether (MVE) polyanions. *Cancer Treat. Rep.,* 62, 1797 (1978).

75. D. W. Barnes, P. S. Morahan, S. Loveless, and A. E. Munson, The effects of maleic an-hydride-divinyl ether (MVE) copolymers on hepatic microsomal mixed-function oxidases and other biological activities. *J. Pharmacol. Exper. Therapeutics,* 208, 392 (1978).

76. T. S. Papas, T. W. Pry, and M. A. Chirigos, Inhibition of RNA-dependent DNA poly-merase of avian myeloblastosis virus, *Proc. Natl. Acad. Sci., (USA),* 71, 367 (1974).

77. S. J. Mohr, J. G. Massicot, and M. A. Chirigos, Derepression of nuclear template restric-tion for DNA synthesis by the immunostimulator pyran copolymer. *Cancer Res.,* 38, 1610 (1978).

78. M. A. Chirigos, Enhanced antitumor response to combined treatment with maleic vinyl ether. *Exp. Pathol.* (in press).

79. M. A. Chirigos, V. Papademetriou, A. Bartocci, and E. Read, Immunological and tumor responses to various immunotherapeutic agents. In J. Hadden, L. Chedid, P. Mullen, F. Spreafico, Eds., *Advances in Immunopharm.,* Pergamon, Oxford, 1981, p. 217.

80. M. A. Chirigos, W. A. Stylos, R. M. Schultz, and J. R. Fullen, Chemical and biological adjuvants capable of potentiating tumor cell vaccine. *Cancer Res.,* 38, 1085 (1978).

81. M. A. Chirigos and W. A. Stylos, Immunomodulatory effect of various molecular-weight maleic anhydride divinyl ethers and other agents *in vivo*. *Cancer Res.*, **40**, 1967 (1980).

82. R. L. Stolfi and D. S. Martin, Therapeutic activity of maleic anhydride-vinyl ether copolymers against spontaneous autochthonous murine mammary tumors. *Cancer Treat. Rep.*, **62**, 1791 (1978).

83. J. D. Papamathiakis, M. A. Chirigos, and R. M. Schultz, Effect of dose, route, and timing of pyran copolymer therapy against the Madison lung carcinoma. In M. A. Chirigos, Ed., *Immune Modulation and Control of Neoplasia by Adjuvant Therapy*, Raven, New York, 1978, pp. 427–433.

84. N. A. Pavlidis, R. M. Schultz, M. A. Chirigos, and J. Luetzeler, Effect of maleic anhydride-divinyl ether copolymers on experimental M109 metastases and macrophage tumoricidal functions. *Cancer Treat. Rep.*, **62**, 1817 (1978).

85. R. M. Schultz, J. D. Papamatheakis, J. Luetzeler, P. Ruiz, and M. A. Chirigos, Macrophage involvement in the protective effect of pyran copolymer against the Madison lung carcinoma (M109). *Cancer Res.*, **37**, 358 (1977).

86. P. S. Morahan, J. A. Munson, L. G. Baird, A. M. Kaplan, and W. Regelson, Antitumor action of pyran copolymer and tilorone against Lewis lung carcinoma and B16 melanoma. *Cancer Res.*, **34**, 506 (1974).

87. J. W. Pearson, M. A. Chirigos, S. D. Chaparas, and N. A. Sher, Combined drug and immunostimulation therapy against a syngeneic murine leukemia. *J. Natl. Cancer Inst.*, **52**, 463 (1974).

88. S. J. Mohr, M. A. Chirigos, F. S. Fuhrman, and J. W. Pryor, Pyran copolymer as an effective adjuvant to chemotherapy against a murine leukemia and solid tumor. *Cancer Res.*, **35**, 3750 (1975).

89. R. M. Schultz, M. A. Chirigos, and J. D. Papamathiakis, Immunotherapy with allogeneic immune peritoneal cells activated by BCG or pyran copolymer. *Cancer Immunol. Immunother.*, **3**, 183 (1978).

90. W. Regelson, G. Miller, D. S. Breslow, and E. J. Engle, III, The distribution and excretion of ^{14}C tagged pyran copolymer: A synthetic polyanion with RES activity. *Sixth Annual Meeting Reticuloendoethelial Society*, 1969, abstract No. 13, p. 632.

91. J. D. Papamatheakis, R. M. Schultz, M. A. Chirigos and J. G. Massicot, Cell and tissue distribution of ^{14}C labeled pyran copolymer. *Cancer Treat. Rep.*, **62**, 1845 (1978).

92. R. M. Schultz, J. D. Papamatheakis, and M. A. Chirigos, Direct activation *in vitro* of mouse peritoneal macrophages by pyran copolymer (NSC-46015). *Cell. Immunol.*, **29**, 403 (1977).

93. R. M. Schultz, J. D. Papamatheakis, J. Leutzeler, and M. A. Chirigos, Association of macrophage activation with antitumor activity by synthetic and biological agents. *Cancer Res.*, **37**, 3338 (1977).

94. A. M. Kaplan, J. M. Collins, P. S. Morahan, and M. J. Snodgrass, Potential mechanism of macrophage-mediated tumor cell cytotoxicity. *Cancer Treat. Rep.*, **62**, 1823 (1978).

95. J. H. Dean, M. L. Padarathsingh, and L. Keys, Response of murine leukemia to combined BCNU-maleic anhydride-vinyl ether (MVE) adjuvant therapy and correlation with macrophage activation by MVE in the *in vitro* growth inhibition assay. *Cancer Treat. Rep.*, **62**, 1807 (1978).

96. J. H. Dean, M. S. Luster, G. A. Boorman, L. D. Lauer, D. O. Adams, M. L. Padarathsingh, T. R. Jerrells, and A. Mantovani, Macrophage activation by pyran copolymers of graded molecular weight: Approach to quantitative measurement of macrophage activation. In E. Hersh, M. A. Chirigos, and M. J. Mastrangelo, Eds., *Augmenting Agents in Cancer Therapy*, Vol. 16, Raven, New York, 1981, p. 267.

97. A. W. Schrecker, R. M. Schultz, and M. A. Chirigos, Effect of macrophage activation by immunoadjuvants on serum levels of lysosomal hydrolases in mice. *J. Immunopharmacol.*, **1**, 219 (1979).

98. R. P. Harmel and B. Zbar, Tumor suppression by pyran copolymer: Correlation with production of cytotoxic macrophages. *J. Natl. Cancer Inst.,* **54**, 989, (1975).

99. M. J. Snodgrass, P. S. Morahan, and A. M. Kaplan, Histopathology of the host response to Lewis lung carcinoma: Modulation by pyran. *J. Natl. Cancer Inst.,* **55**, 455 (1975).

100. R. M. Schultz and M. A. Chirigos, Selective neutralization by anti-interferon globulin of macrophage activation by L cell interferon, *Brucella abortus* ether extract, salmonella typhimurium lipopolysaccharide, and polyanions. *Cell Immunol.,* **48**, 52 (1979).

101. L. G. Baird and A. M. Kaplan, *In vivo* and *in vitro* mitogenicity of pyran copolymer. *J. Reticuloendothel. Soc.,* **16**, 19a (1974).

102. L. G. Baird, A. M. Kaplan, and W. Regelson, Effects of pyran copolymer on humoral and cellular immunity. *J. Reticuloendothel. Soc.,* **15**, 90 (1974).

103. L. G. Baird, and A. M. Kaplan, Immunoadjuvant activity of pyran copolymers. I. Evidence for direct stimulation of T-lymphocytes and macrophages. *Cell. Immunol.,* **20**, 167 (1975).

104. W. A. Stylos, M. A. Chirigos, C. R. Lengel, and P. J. Lyng, T and B lymphocyte populations of tumor-bearing mice treated with 1,3-bis(chloroethyl)-1-nitrosouria (BCNU) or pyran. *Cancer Immunol. Immunother.,* **5**, 165 (1978).

105. W. A. Stylos, M. A. Chirigos, C. R. Lengel, and J. F. Weiss, Effect of maleic anhydride-vinyl ether on the lymphocyte subpopulations of tumor bearing, irradiated mice. *Cancer Treat. Rep.,* **62**, 1831 (1978).

106. A. Bartocci, V. Papademetriou, and M. A. Chirigos, Enhanced macrophage and natural killer cell antitumor activity by various molecular weight maleic anhydride divinyl ether. *J. Immunopharmacol.,* **2**, 149 (1980).

107. J. Y. Djeu, J. A. Heinbaugh, H. T. Holden, and R. B. Herberman, Augmentation of mouse natural killer cell activity by interferon and interferon inducers, *J. Immunol.,* **122**, 175 (1979).

108. A. Santonni, P. Pucceti, C. Riccardi, R. B. Herberman, and E. Bonmasser, Augmentation of natural killer activity by pyran copolymer in mice. *Internatl. J. Cancer,* **24**, 656 (1979)

109. T. J. Leavitt, T. C. Merigan, and J. M. Freeman, Hemolytic-uremic like syndrome following polycarboxylate interferon induction. Treatment of Dawson's inclusion body encephalitis. *Am. J. Dis. Childh.,* **121**, 43 (1971).

110. L. H. Dennis, A. Angeles, M. Baig, and B. I. Schnider, The effect of pyran polymer on the hemostatic mechanism. American Society Clinical Pharmacology and Chemotherapy. 6th Annual Meeting, 1969, abstract, Chicago, Ill.

111. W. Regelson, B. I. Schnider, J. Colsky, K. B. Olson, J. F. Holland, C. L. Johnston, and L. H. Dennis, Clinical study of the synthetic polyanion pyran copolymer and its role in future clinical trials. In M. A. Chirigos, Ed., *Immune Modulation and Control of Neoplasia by Adjuvant Therapy, Progress in Cancer Research,* Vol. 7, Raven, New York, 1978, p. 469.

112. J. W. Hadden and A. Giner-Sorolla, Isoprinosine and NPT 15392, Modulators of lymphocyte and macrophage development and function. In E. Hersh, M. A. Chirigos, and M. J. Mastrangelo, Eds., *Augmenting Agents in Cancer Therapy,* Vol. 16, Raven, New York, 1981, p. 497.

113. T. Ginsberg, D. G. Streets, and E. Pfadenhouse, Metabolism of the N,N-dimethylamino-2-propanol (DIP) and p-acetamidobenzoic acid (PAcBA) components of isoprinosine in rhesus monkeys. Seventh International Congress of Pharmacology, Paris, 1978, abstract.

114. T. Ginsberg, Urinary excretion of purine metabolites in *Macaca mullatta* following administration of inosine and 1-(dimethylamino)-2-propanol, p-acetamidobenzoate. Fifth International Congress on Pharmacology, 1972, abstract, p. 82.

115. T. Ginsberg, L. N. Simon, and A. J. Glasky, Isoprinosine: Pharmacological and toxicological properties in animals. Seventh International Congress of Pharmacology, Paris, 1978, abstract.

116. L. N. Simon and A. J. Glasky, Isoprinosine: An overview. *Cancer Treat. Rep.,* **62**, 1963 (1978).

117. J. W. Hadden, E. M. Hadden, and R. G. Coffey, Isoprinosine augmentation of phyto-hemagglutinin-induced lymphocyte proliferation. *Infect. Immun.,* **13**, 382 (1976).

118. J. W. Hadden, Effects of Isoprinosine, Levamisole, muramyl dipeptide, and SM 1213 on lymphocyte and macrophage function *in vitro. Cancer Treat. Rep.,* **62**, 1981 (1978).

119. A. Vecchi, M. Sironi, and F. Spreafico, Preliminary characterization in mice of the effect of Isoprinosine on the immune system. *Cancer Treat. Rep.,* **62**, 1975 (1978).

120. J. Wybran, A. Govaerts, and T. Appelboom, Inosiplex, a stimulating agent for normal human T cells and human leukocytes. *J. Immunol.,* **121**, 1184 (1978).

121. G. Renoux, M. Renoux, and J. M. Guillaumin, Isoprinosine as an immunopotentiator. *J. Immunopharmacol.,* **1**, 337 (1979).

122. G. Renoux, M. Renoux, J. M. Guillaumin, and C. Gouzien, Differentiation and regulation of lymphocyte populations: Evidence for immunopotentiator-induced T-cell recruitment. *J. Immunopharmacol.,* **1**, 415 (1979).

123. W. Morin, J. L. Touraine, G. Renoux, and J. W. Hadden, Isoprinosine as an immuno-modulation agent. *Symposium on New Trends in Human Immunology and Cancer Immunotherapy, Montpellier, France* (in press).

124. A. J. Glasky, G. E. Friebertshauser, J. W. Halker, R. A. Settineri, and T. Ginsberg, The role of cell-mediated immunity in the therapeutic action of Isoprinosine on viral disease processes. *Chemotherapy,* **6**, 235 (1977).

125. A. J. Glasky, E. H. Pfadenhauer, R. Settineri, and T. Ginsberg, In H. Meuwissen, Ed., *Combined Immunodeficiency Disease and Adenosine Deaminase Deficiency: A Molecular Defect,* Academic, New York, 1975, pp. 157–179.

126. I. Cerutti, C. Chany, and J. F. Schlumberger, Isoprinosine increases the antitumor action of interferon. *Cancer Treat. Rep.,* **62**, 1971 (1978).

127. L. J. Bradshaw and H. L. Sumner, *In vitro* studies on cell-mediated immunity in patients treated with Inosiplex for herpes virus infection *Ann. N. Y. Acad. Sci.,* **284**, 190 (1977).

128. A. Buge, G. Rancurel, J. Metzger, A. Picard, B. Lesourd, and D. Gardeur, Isoprinosine in treatment of acute viral encephalitis. *Lancet,* **2**, 691 (1979).

129. L. Corey, W. T. Chiang, W. C. Reeves, W. E. Stamm, L. Brewer, and K. K. Holmes, Effect of Isoprinosine on the cellular immune response in initial genital herpes virus infection. *Clin. Res.,* **27**, 41A (1979).

130. T. Ginsberg and A. J. Glasky, Inosiplex: An immunomodulation model for the treatment of viral diseases. *Ann. N. Y. Acad. Sci.,* **284**, 128 (1976).

131. J. W. Hadden, C. Sopez, R. O'Reilly, and E. M. Hadden, Levamisole and inosiplex: Anti-viral agents with immuno-potentiating action, *Ann. N. Y. Acad. Sci.,* **284**, 139 (1976).

132. P. R. Huttenlocher and R. H. Mattson, Isoprinosine in subacute sclerosing panencephalitis, *Neurology,* **29**, 763 (1979).

133. R. H. Mattson, I. T. Lott, and A. J. Fink, Treatment of SSPE with inosiplex: A preliminary report, *Arch. Neurol.,* **32**, 503 (1975).

134. D. M. Pachuta, Y. Togo, R. B. Hornick, Y. Togo, R. B. Harnick, A. R. Schwartz, and S. Tonunaga, Evaluation of isoprinosine in experimental human rhinovirus infection, *Antimicrob. Agents Chemother.,* **5**, 403 (1974).

135. W. T. Chang and L. Weinstein, Antiviral activity of isoprinosine *in vitro* and *in vivo. Am. J. Med. Sci.,* **265**, 143 (1973).

136. R. L. Muldoon, L. Mezny, and G. G. Jackson, Effect of isoprinosine against influenza and some other viruses causing respiratory diseases. *Antimicrob. Agents Chemother.,* **2**, 224 (1972).

137. R. H. Waldman and R. Ganguly, Therapeutic efficacy of isoprinosine in rhinovirus infection. *Ann. N. Y. Acad. Sci.,* **284**, 153 (1977).

138. W. H. Wickett, Jr. and J. L. Bradshaw, Clinical effectiveness of the immunopotentiating agent, inosiplex, in herpes virus infections. *Am. Soc. Microbiol.,* 78 (1976).

139. V. A. Najjar, M. K. Chaudhuri, D. Konopinska, B. D. Plek, P. P. Layne, and L. Linehan, Biology of Tuftsin: A possible role in cancer suppression and therapy. In E. Hersh, M. A. Chirigos, and M. J. Mastrangelo, Eds., *Augmenting Agents in Cancer Therapy,* Vol. 16, Raven, New York, 1981, p. 459.

140. G. M. Edelman, B. A. Cunningham, W. E. Gall, P. D. Gottlieb, V. Rutishauser, and M. J. Waxdal, The covalent structure of an entire gamma G immunoglobulin molecule. *Proc. Natl. Acad. Sci. (USA),* **63**, 78 (1969).

141. V. A. Najjar, Physiological role of gamma globulin. In A. Meister, Ed., *Advances in Enzymology,* Vol. 41, Wiley, New York, 1974, pp. 129–278.

142. A. Constantopoulos and V. H. Najjar, Pepsin, a natural and general phagocytosis stimulating peptide affecting macrophage and polymorphonuclear granulocytes, *Cytobiosynthesis,* **6**, 97 (1972).

143. V. A. Najjar, Molecular basis of familial and acquired phagocytosis deficiency involving the tetrapeptide, Tuftsin. *Exp. Cell. Biol.,* **46**, 114 (1978).

7

Modulation of the Immune Response by Interferons and Their Inducers

HOWARD M. JOHNSON
Department of Microbiology
The University of Texas Medical Branch
Galveston, Texas

1. INTRODUCTION

Interferons are increasingly being recognized as having pleiotropic effects on cell function. These effects may be expressed in the form of antiviral, anticellular, immunoregulatory, and antitumor activities. Interferon was discovered in 1957 by Isaacs and Lindenmann (1,2), and this discovery was based on its antiviral properties with a view toward understanding the nature of host defense against viral infections. It follows, therefore, that most definitions of interferon include the description of its being a glycoprotein that is secreted by virus-infected cells, thus promoting the establishment of an antiviral state in uninfected cells. In this overview of the interferon field, the present-day meaning of interferon will be conveyed in the context of its varied biological activities with emphasis on immunoregulation.

2. THE ANTIVIRAL PROPERTY OF INTERFERON

The production and action of virus-induced interferon at the cellular level is depicted in Figure 1 (3). During the early stages of viral infection of the cell, some event (probably the presence of foreign viral nucleic acid) derepresses cellular genes located on specific human chromosomes that contain the stored genetic information for the interferon protein. Interferon is produced by transcriptional and translational events such as those that occur in normal protein synthesis. The produced interferon does not inactivate the virus by direct interaction; rather, it leaves the cell and then reacts with a specific receptor on the cell membrane of the producing and surrounding cells. This membrane interaction results in the derepression of a gene(s) that codes for the antiviral proteins. The intracellular antiviral proteins are thought to be involved in the actual inactivation with virus. In this chapter we examine the possible identity and mechanism of action of the antiviral proteins.

The interferon system is nonspecific in that it is activated by a variety of viruses and the interferon produced induces cellular resistance against a broad range of viruses. Interferon is the earliest appearing of the known host defenses against viral infections and probably plays an important role in the initial phases of the host protective response. Figure 2 illustrates the early production of interferon in comparison with antibody during experimental infection of humans with influenza virus. This early appearance of interferon has been shown to be important in the ultimate outcome of virus infection (4). Under experimental conditions of viral infections of mice where the produced interferon is neutralized by passively administered anti-interferon antibody, the viral infections are significantly more severe with dramatic increases in animal deaths (5,6). Interferon, then, is probably very important as a natural host defense against viral infections.

3. MOLECULAR ASPECTS OF INTERFERON ACTION

Currently, it is not known precisely how interferon inhibits viral replication. Data have been presented that suggest both a block of transcription of viral RNA and/or inhibition of translation of viral proteins. Inhibition of protein

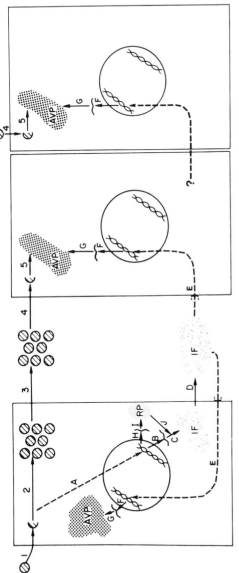

Figure 1. Cellular events of induction and action of interferon (IF). The virus comes into contact with the cell (1) and penetrates the cell membrane. The virus then releases its genetic material, and virus replication occurs (2). The new virus leaves the cell (3) and enters the fluid around the first cell, and some of the replicated virus infects a second cell (4), where the release of the genetic material again takes place (4). During the early stages of infection of the first cell some event (possibly a viral nucleic acid) stimulates a gene in the DNA that contains the stored genetic information for interferon (A). This leads to the production of a messenger RNA for interferon, which leaves (E) the nucleus and is translated by the cell's ribosomes (C) into the interferon protein. Several events now occur more or less simultaneously. Interferon is secreted by the first infected cell (D) and enters the surrounding fluid, where it comes into contact with and stimulates the second cell (E) by interacting with a membrane receptor for interferon. The second cell is thereby induced to produce a new messenger RNA (F) that is translated to a new protein(s) (G), the antiviral protein (AVP). The cell's protein-synthesizing machinery is thereby modified such that cell mRNA is translated into protein but viral RNA is poorly bound or translated, or both. In the first cell processes, E, F, and G may in some instances also operate to form AVP and thereby reduce the virus yield in the first cell. Shortly after interferon is synthesized into the first cell, another mRNA (H) is believed to be synthesized from the cell's DNA that is translated (I) into a regulatory protein (RP) (hypothesized). This regulatory protein combines with the mRNA for interferon, thereby preventing the further synthesis of more interferon (J). There is recent evidence that the antiviral state may be directly transferred between adjacent cells (from second to third cell at right) by the passage of an unknown (?) inducer of the AVP.

243

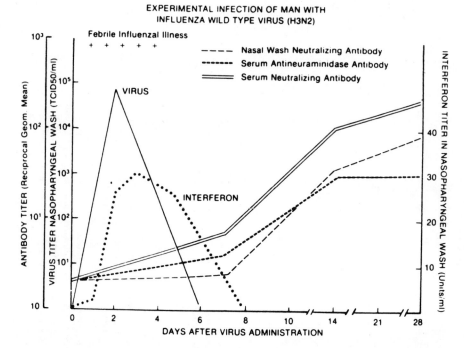

Figure 2. Production of virus, interferon, and antibody during experimental infection of humans with influenza wild-type virus. (From a study by B. Murphy and colleagues at the National Institutes of Health, Bethesda, Maryland.)

synthesis is currently felt to be the primary mode by which interferon exerts its varied biologic effects.

Two mechanisms (Figure 3) by which interferon inhibits protein synthesis have been examined in a number of laboratories. One mechanism involves the induction of a protein kinase, which, in turn, catalyzes the phosphorylation of one of the initiation factors (subunit eIF-2) that is required for protein synthesis (7–12). Subunit eIF-2 is inactive in the phosphorylated state. The second mechanism involves interferon induction of a polymerase, called 2′-5′A synthetase (11–16). This enzyme, in the presence of double stranded RNA, converts ATP to a 2′-5′-linked oligoadenylate(s) (2′-5′A). Then 2′-5′A activates an RNA endonuclease, which catylyzes the degradation of RNA. Destruction of messenger RNA by this enzyme results in inhibition of cellular protein synthesis. Both the protein kinase and endonuclease activities may play a role in a variety of interferon-mediated biological activities. These include inhibition of viral replication, suppression of the immune response, and anticellular effects such as inhibition of tumor growth. Recently, an interferon-induced phosphodiesterase has been described that regulates RNA endonuclease activity by cleavage of 2′-5′A at the 2′ site (12). Additionally, the phosphodiesterase blocks protein synthesis by inhibition of aminoacylation of tRNA (12).

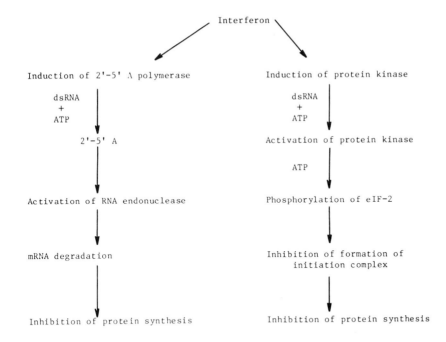

Figure 3. Schematic representation of the effects of interferon on cellular function. Two well-defined pathways have been demonstrated for interferon inhibition of protein synthesis in the cell, involving (1) activation of an endonuclease and (2) induction and activation of a protein kinase. See text for details.

Certainly, the antiviral proteins, described above may be represented by the protein kinase, RNA endonuclease, and phosphodiesterase systems.

4. CLASSIFICATION OF INTERFERONS

Although often presented and spoken of in the singular, there are actually several types of interferon (Table 1). Interferons may be classified into two broad groups, virus type (Type I) (17–19) or immune type (Type II) (20–25), as shown in the following list:

1. Virus type (Type I).
    a. Antigenic types: (i) fibroblast and epithelial cell origin (Beta); (ii) leukocyte cell origin (Alpha).
    b. Inducers: (i) viruses; (ii) polyribonucleotides; (iii) chemicals (Tilorone, etc.); (iv) tumor or heterologous cells (leukocyte interferon).
2. Immune type (Type II).
    a. Antigenic types—only one type known to date (Gamma).
    b. Inducers: (i) antigens; (ii) mitogens (primarily T-cell mitogens).

Virus-type interferons are classically induced by viruses or double-stranded polyribonucleotides. In the human system, and perhaps the mouse system also, there are at least two antigenic types (26). They are called *fibroblast* and *leukocyte interferon,* to indicate their primary or predominant cellular origin. Another interferon, *lymphoblastoid interferon,* which is produced by a transformed human cell line, is thought to be a mixture of leukocyte and fibroblast interferon (19). Recent amino acid (27–29) and DNA (30–32) sequencing data of various virus-type interferons may eventually require further classification of these interferons. Of recent interest is the observation that leukocyte interferon can be induced in some lymphoid cell subpopulations by tumor cells (33,34). This may have some relationship to the antitumor properties of interferon and could possibly represent a host defense response against spontaneous tumors.

Immune interferon (immune type) is either induced in primed T lymphocytes by subsequent exposure to the specific antigen or in unprimed T lymphocytes by T-cell mitogens such as phytohemagglutinin (20,24), concanavalin A (23), and staphylococcal enterotoxin A (25). Immune interferons induced in the mouse systems either by antigen or by several T-lymphocyte mitogens are antigenically the same or very similar to one another (35,36).

5.   MODULATION OF THE IMMUNE RESPONSE BY INTERFERON

The data conclusively indicate that interferon can play a regulatory role in modulation of the immune response at several levels. In fact, interferon is probably the mediator of some forms of suppressor cell activity. Virus-type interferon has been shown to suppress the antibody response in both *in vitro* and *in vivo* systems in the mouse (37–42).

The *in vitro* system for antibody production in the mouse consists of the use of dissociated spleen cells, which are made up of B and T lymphocytes and macrophages, all of which are normally required for an antibody response. Addition of a suitable antigen, such as sheep red blood cells (SRBC), to the spleen cells in culture media under defined conditions stimulates the production of antibody-forming cells. The antibody-forming cells are enumerated by mixing them with a high concentration of SRBC (10%) in a soft agar medium at 37°C for 1 or 2 hours. During this incubation the antibody that is produced by the cells binds to surrounding SRBC. Addition of guinea pig serum, which contains complement, to this complex results in lysis of the SRBC. Thus a plaque or zone of hemolysis surrounds a cell that is producing antibody to SRBC. The antibody-forming cell is frequently referred to as a *plaque-forming cell* (PFC), and the antibody response to SRBC is spoken of as the anti-SRBC PFC response. This system has been of considerable value in looking at a variety of events related to regulation of the antibody response. Advantages over *in vivo* experiments are economy of reagents and better control of the microenvironment of the antibody-forming cell.

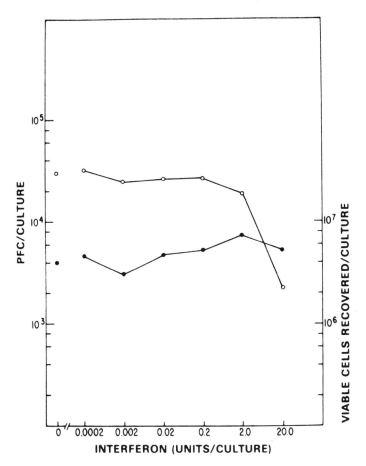

Figure 4.   The effect of highly purified mouse ascites tumor virus-type interferon on the primary *in vitro* PFC response. Direct anti-SRBC PFC/culture (O—O) and viable cells recovered per culture (●—●) were determined on day 5. [Reprinted with permission from H. M. Johnson, B. G. Smith, and S. Baron, *J. Immunol.,* **114**, 403 (1975).]

To determine the effect of interferon on the *in vitro* PFC response, purified interferon is added to the culture at the time of SRBC addition. Five days later the cells are harvested and examined for the PFC response to SRBC. Results of a typical experiment are presented in Figure 4 (41). Virus-type interferon suppressed the *in vitro* PFC response by approximately 99%. Interferon is responsible for the suppression since it is observed with interferon purified to homogeneity (H. M. Johnson, unpublished data) and is specifically blocked by pretreatment of the interferon with specific antibody (41). In general, 20 to 60 units of interferon per milliliter will suppress the *in vitro* PFC response by 90% or more. This represents less than 0.05 ng of interferon per milliliter. This is very potent immunosuppression. Interferon similarly suppresses the antibody response in the mouse, but this requires relatively more interferon ($\geqslant 50,000$ units) (38), and it is impossible to control the concentrations of interferon in the microenvironment of the antibody-producing cell.

We may summarize some of the findings to date on the suppressive effects of interferon on lymphocyte function, both *in vitro* and *in vivo*. Interferon is most effective when added to the system at the time of antigen addition (38,41). Secondary antibody responses are also suppressed (43,44). The suppression of the antibody response could be due to a direct or indirect effect of interferon on the B cell, the cell actually responsible for antibody production. We do have data that show that the B-cell response can be suppressed indirectly by interferon, through interferon induction of a suppressor cell, which releases a soluble factor that actually acts on the B cell (45). The nature of the suppressor factor is not known, but interferon has been shown to induce prostaglandin E in cells, and this molecule can modulate suppressor cell activity (46). This does not preclude a direct effect of interferon on B cells. There are also data that suggest that the mechanism by which interferon suppresses the immune response is through the protein kinase (47) and endonuclease systems (48). Interferon can suppress the cellular immune response in a manner similar to suppression of the antibody response (49–55). It can also enhance the killing of T killer lymphocytes (56). Further, lymphocytes (null cells) that are neither B nor T cells can be stimulated by interferon to have increased killing activity against tumor cells (57–59). Thus interferon may modulate the immune system to have increased antitumor activity. The ability of interferon to activate macrophages may also bear some relationship to its possible antitumor properties in addition to immunoregulatory effects (60). These several findings may be related to the reported activity of interferon as an antitumor agent in certain human neoplasias. The possible sites of interferon action on the immune system are presented as a working model in Figure 5.

Virus-type interferon inducers have been reported to have both enhancing and suppressive effects on the antibody response *in vivo*. Synthetic, double-stranded polyribonucleotides, virus-type interferon inducers, are well known as enhancers or adjuvants of the *in vivo* antibody response (61–63). This enhancement has been ascribed to the effect of these polyribonucleotides on the T lymphocytes (64). Less recognized is the fact that synthetic polyribonucleotides can also inhibit the *in vivo* antibody response under certain conditions (63,64). There is a temporal relationship between enhancement and suppression of the immune response when mice are injected intravenously with poly-riboadenylate:polyribouridylate (poly rA:poly rU) at various times in relation to intravenous injections of bovine gamma globulin (63). Poly rA:poly rU, given 1 day to 12 hours before antigen, profoundly suppressed the antibody response. When given 2 hours before, or at the same time as antigen, a significant enhancement of the antibody response was observed.

The T-lymphocyte mitogens, phytohemagglutinin (PHA), staphylococcal enterotoxin A (SEA), and concanavalin A (Con A), which have been shown to be inducers of immune interferon in lymphoid cell cultures, are also suppres-

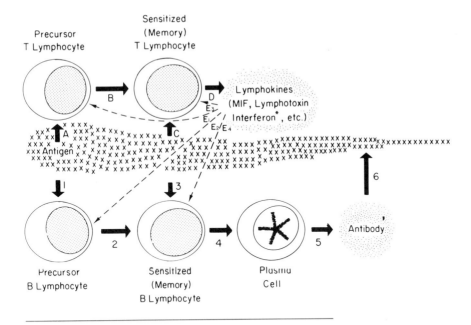

Precursor
T Lymphocyte

Sensitized
(Memory)
T Lymphocyte

Lymphokines
(MIF, Lymphotoxin
Interferon*, etc.)

Antigen

Precursor
B Lymphocyte

Sensitized
(Memory)
B Lymphocyte

Plasma
Cell

Antibody

Time →

Figure 5. Cellular events in the induction and immunosuppressive action of interferons. The antigen comes into contact with a precursor T lymphocyte (A), which undergoes differentiation to a sensitized T lymphocyte (B). This cell, driven by antigen (C), may become a memory cell or may release mediators known as *lymphokines* (D). Among the mediators produced by the T lymphocyte is immune-type interferon. Antigen also reacts with a precursor B lymphocyte (1), which undergoes differentiation to a sensitized B lymphocyte (and memory B cell) (2). The sensitized B cell is further driven by antigen (3) to become a plasma cell (4), which is responsible for most of the antibody (5) produced. This antibody reacts with the specific antigen (6). Both antigen- and virus-induced interferons are capable of suppressing precursor T (E_1) and B (E_2) lymphocytes as well as sensitized T (E_3) and B (E_4) lymphocytes. As differentiation progresses, in part as a result of continued antigen presence, it becomes progressively more difficult to inhibit lymphocyte function by interferons. Plasma cell production of antibody is resistant to inhibition by interferon. The macrophage is not included in the diagram, but interferons may exert their immunosuppressive effects through a required macrophage function in the immune response. Hence the diagrammatic scheme does not necessarily imply a direct effect of the interferons on the lymphocytes.

sors of the antibody response in mice (65,66) and rabbits (67) if the mitogens are injected 1 to 2 days before antigen. It was found in the rabbit that injection of Con A or PHA at the time of antigen had an enhancing effect on the antibody response (67).

In vitro antibody induction studies have shown that poly rA:poly rU can have both a modest enhancing or inhibiting effect on the immune response, depending on the polyribonucleotide concentration and the length of the culture period (68–70). We have obtained consistent suppression of the *in vitro* antibody PFC response with low concentrations (0.1 to 1.0 μg/ml) of polyribonucleotides (71). Functional T lymphocytes are required in the cultures for the polyribonucleotides to be effective as inhibitors, thus demonstrating the thymus dependence of the inhibitions. Suppression of the PFC response by polyribonucleotides is blocked by antibody to mouse virus-type interferon, which suggests that interferon mediates the suppression (43).

T-Cell mitogens are potent inhibitors of the *in vitro* PFC response (72–75). They also induce lymphocytes to produce immune interferon, as indicated previously. In an attempt to obtain some insight into the possible role of immune interferon in the mediation of suppressor T-cell effects, the T-cell mitogens Con A, PHA-P, and SEA were compared for their ability to inhibit the *in vitro* antibody response and to stimulate the production of immune interferon in mouse spleen cell cultures (25). It was found that the ability to inhibit the PFC response to SRBC was proportional to the ability of these mitogens to induce interferon in the cultures. This does not necessarily mean that immune interferon is the mediator of this suppression, since the mitogens do not suppress the PFC response of spleen cells from mice that have T-cell defects, even though immune interferon is induced in the same cultures (76). In our hands immune interferon has not had a clear-cut suppressive effect on the *in vitro* PFC response, even though data by others would suggest that it does (77). Obviously, more work needs to be done, particularly with purified immune interferon, to ensure the removal of possible inhibitors of immune interferon activity from the interferon (78).

6. MODULATION BY CYCLIC AMP

It has been proposed that adenosine 3′:5′-cyclic monophosphate [cyclic AMP (cAMP)] has an inhibitory effect on the immunologic and inflammatory functions of lymphocytes (79). Evidence has been obtained that suggests that cyclic AMP may play a role in regulation of interferon production by lymphocytes and suppression of the *in vitro* PFC response (80). Dibutyryl cAMP, 2×10^{-5} M, inhibited Con A stimulation of immune interferon production by 96%, whereas 1×10^{-4} M inhibited SEA stimulation of interferon production by 85% (80). When the same concentrations of dibutyryl cAMP were added to the supernatant fluids of mouse spleen cell cultures after complete interferon production, no inhibition of antiviral activity of the interferon was observed, so it is concluded that dibutyryl cAMP blocked the production of immune interferon, and not the established activity of produced interferon.

Dibutyryl cAMP also blocks mitogen-induced suppression of the *in vitro* PFC response to SRBC. Staphylococcal enterotoxin inhibits the PFC response by at least 90% when compared to controls (80). Protection of the PFC responses against suppression by SEA is essentially complete when dibutyryl cAMP (1.4×10^{-4} M) is added to cultures along with SEA (Table 1). Dibutyryl

TABLE 1.   Effect of Dibutyryl Cyclic AMP on Mitogen-Induced Suppression of the *in Vitro* **PFC Response to SRBC**

Mitogen	Mitogen Concentration (μ g/ml)	Dibutyryl cAMP (1.4×10^{-4} M)	PFC/10^6 Viable Cells $\pm$ SD
SEA	0.25	−	64 ± 8
SEA	0.50	−	101 ± 11
SEA	0.25	+	5080 ± 820
SEA	0.50	+	5508 ± 1406
—	—	+	4148 ± 296
—	—	−	5206 ± 3626
Con A	1.0	−	7 ± 9
Con A	2.0	−	16 ± 11
Con A	1.0	+	1577 ± 505
Con A	2.0	+	1456 ± 307
—	—	+	3146 ± 537
—	—	−	2571 ± 691

Source: Johnson (80).

cAMP also protects the PFC responses from Con A suppression. Concanavalin A, at 1.0 and 2.0 μg/ml, inhibited the PFC response by $>90\%$ when compared to the controls. Dose-response studies with various concentrations of dibutyryl cAMP showed that the concentrations (1 to 2 $\times$ 10^{-4} M) of the cyclic ribonucleotide that blocked the development of suppressor activity correlated with those concentrations that blocked the production of interferon in spleen cultures stimulated by the T-cell mitogens (81). Dibutyryl guanosine 3′:5′-cyclic monophosphate (cGMP) at the same concentrations has no effect on either mitogen stimulation of interferon production or mitogen-induced suppression of the *in vitro* PFC response.

The effect of dibutyryl cAMP on SEA-induced immunosuppression and interferon production was further explored by adding dibutyryl cAMP (1.4 $\times$ 10^{-4} M) to cultures at various times relative to SEA (0.5 μg/ml) addition and determining the PFC response (Figure 6) (81). In a parallel study SEA induction of interferon under the same conditions was determined (Figure 6). When dibutyryl cAMP was added to the cultures at either -1 or 0 hour, complete blockade of the SEA-induced immunosuppression was observed. An enhancement of the PFC response was obtained when dibutyryl cAMP was added to the cultures at 0 hour; however, subsequent experiments did not always show this enhancement. With increasing time between mitogen addition and dibutyryl cAMP addition to cultures, there was an increasing amount of interferon produced and a corresponding increase in the suppression of the anti-SRBC, PFC response. The data suggest a direct relationship, then, between the effect of dibutyryl cAMP on SEA-induced immunosuppression and on production of interferon by SEA-stimulated cultures. This is further evidence that mitogen-

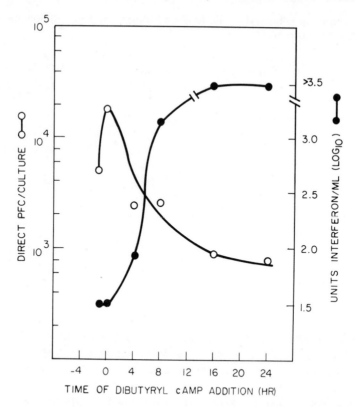

Figure 6. Determination of the PFC response and interferon production after addition of dibutyryl cAMP to spleen cell cultures at various times relative to SEA addition. Staphylococcal enterotoxin A (0.5 μg/ml) and SRBC were added at time 0 to the spleen cells for the PFC response, and dibutyryl cAMP (1.4 × 10⁻⁴ M) was added at the indicated times relative to time 0. Direct anti-SRBC responses were determined on day 5. Mean PFC responses/culture ± SD for the SRBC control and the SEA-suppressed control were 4610 ± 834 and 350 ± 353, respectively. Parallel studies were carried out on interferon production under the same culture conditions, except that SRBC were absent from the cultures and the cultures were incubated 48 hours after SEA addition at time 0. From Ref. 81. [Reprinted with permission from H. M. Johnson, J. E. Blalock, and S. Baron, *Cell. Immunol.,* **33,** 170 (1977).]

induced suppression of the *in vitro* response is related to mitogen induction of immune interferon in the cultures. As mentioned earlier, however, immune interferon has not yet been shown unequivocally to suppress the immune response directly.

Cholera toxin (an enterotoxin produced by *Vibrio cholerae*) raises the endogenous level of cAMP by stimulating adenylate cyclase activity. Adenylate cyclase converts ATP to cAMP. The methyl xanthine 3-isobutyl-1-methylxanthine (IMX) raises the endogenous cAMP level by inhibiting phosphodiesterase activity. Both agents block SEA suppression of the *in vitro* anti-SRBC, PFC response in a manner similar to that observed for dibutyryl cAMP (80). Further, they block SEA stimulation of interferon production in mouse spleen cell cultures at concentrations that block SEA suppressor activity.

Dibutyryl cGMP (10^{-3} to 10^{-7} M) does not affect the ability of dibutyryl cAMP (1.4 × 10^{-4} M) to block the suppression of the PFC response by SEA; nor is the effect of dibutyryl cAMP on mitogen stimulation of interferon affected by dibutyryl cGMP (80). This is further evidence that the phenomena reported here are due to cAMP and are not influenced by cGMP in this system.

The data suggest that immune-induced interferon is associated with mitogen-induced suppressor cell activity and that the interferon induction may possibly be related to such activity, but not necessarily in a direct manner. In related studies, it has been shown that high concentrations (10^{-3} M) of dibutyryl cAMP can inhibit the yield of interferon from PHA-stimulated human peripheral leukocytes (82) and from virus- or polyribonucleotide-stimulated mouse L-cell cultures (83). The data presented here show a logical relationship between cAMP, immune interferon activity, suppressor cell activity, and regulation of the immune response. Preliminary studies on the effect of cAMP on induction of virus-type interferon in mouse spleen cultures suggest that this interferon system is similarly affected by cAMP.

Finally, it is obvious from the preceding discussion that interferons regulate the immune system in a complex fashion involving the interaction of a number of systems. It is not possible at this time to predict in mechanistic terms how these systems function in the antitumor properties of interferon.

7. ANTICELLULAR AND ANTITUMOR EFFECTS

Paucker et al. (84) made the original observation that interferon had an inhibitory effect on cell multiplication. Since then a number of studies *in vitro* and *in vivo* have shown that interferons inhibit the growth of both tumors and normal cells, but not necessarily to the same degree (85–88). Data from clinical trials in progress with human leukocyte interferon and involving osteogenic sarcoma, breast cancer, multiple myeloma, and malignant lymphoma, suggest that interferon may have potential use as an anticancer agent (89–91). As more of the various types of interferon become available for testing, we should have a clearer picture of the nature and mechanism of the antitumor effects of interferon.

8. CONCLUSION

Interferons possess pleiotropic effects on cell function, which are expressed in the form of antiviral, anticellular, immunoregulatory, and antitumor activities. These effects can be exerted through several biochemical mechanisms: (1) increased protein kinase activity, which results in inhibition of initiation of protein synthesis; (2) increased endonuclease activity and thus messenger RNA (mRNA) destruction as the result of stimulation of synthesis of a 2'-5'-linked oligoadenylate; and (3) increased phosphodiesterase activity that blocks aminoacylation of tRNA, which results in inhibition of protein synthesis. The immune system is affected in several ways by interferon: (1) inhibition of antibody synthesis; (2) inhibition of cell-mediated immunity; (3) increased killing by T cells; (4) increased natural killer cell activity; and (5) activation of macrophages. In addition, interferon has anticellular activity, which may be the basis for its observed anticancer properties.

REFERENCES

1. A. Isaacs and J. Lindenmann, *Proc. Roy. Soc. (Lond.), Ser. B,* **147**, 258 (1957).

2. A. Isaacs and J. Lindenmann, *Proc. Roy. Soc. (Lond.), Ser. B,* **147**, 268 (1957).

3. S. Baron and F. Dianzani, *Tex. Rep. Biol. Med.,* **35**, 1–573 (1977).

4. T. Iwasaki and T. Nozima, *J. Immunol.,* **118**, 256 (1977).

5. B. Fauconnier, *Pathol. Biol.,* **19**, 575 (1971).

6. I. Gresser, M. Tovey, M. Bandu, M. Chantal, and D. Brouty-Boye, *J. Exp. Med.* **144**, 1305 (1976).

7. W. K. Roberts, A. Hovanessian, R. E. Brown, M. J. Clemens, and I. M. Kerr, *Nature,* **264**, 477 (1976).

8. A. Zilberstein, P. Federman, L. Shulman, and M. Revel, *FEBS Lett.,* **68**, 119 (1976).

9. B. Lebleu, G. C. Sen, S. Shaila, B. Cabrer, and P. Lengyel, *Proc. Natl. Acad. Sci. (USA),* **73**, 3107 (1976).

10. C. E. Samuel, D. A. Farris, and D. A. Eppstein, *Virology,* **83**, 56 (1977).

11. C. Baglioni, *Cell,* **17**, 255 (1979).

12. M. Revel, Molecular mechanisms involved in the antiviral effects of interferon. In I. Gresser, Ed., *Interferon 1979,* Vol. 1, Academic, New York, 1979, p. 101.

13. W. K. Roberts, M. J. Clements, and I. M. Kerr, *Proc. Natl. Acad. Sci. (USA),* **73**, 3136 (1976).

14. G. E. Brown, B. Lebleu, M. Kawakita, S. Shaila, G. C. Sen, and P. Lengyel, *Biochem. Biophys. Res. Commun.,* **69**, 114 (1976).

15. L. Ratner, G. C. Sen, G. E. Brown, B. Lebleu, M. Kawakita, B. Cabrer, E. Slattery, and P. Lengyel, *Eur. J. Biochem.,* **79**, 565 (1977).

16. I. M. Kerr and R. E. Brown, *Proc. Natl. Acad. Sci. (USA),* **75**, 256 (1978).

17. A. Isaacs, *Adv. Virus Res.,* **10**, (1963).

18. A. K. Field, A. A. Tytell, G. P. Lampson, and M. R. Hilleman, *Proc. Natl. Acad. Sci. (USA),* **58**, 1004 (1967).

19. K. Paucker, *Tex. Rep. Biol. Med.,* **35**, 23 (1977).

20. E. F. Wheelock, *Science,* **149**, 310 (1965).

21. J. A. Green, S. R. Cooperband, and S. Kibrick, *Science,* **164**, 1415 (1969).

22. S. B. Salvin, J. S. Youngner, and W. H. Lederer, *Infect. Immun.,* **7**, 68 (1973).

23. J. Stobo, I. Green, L. Jackson, and S. Baron, *J. Immunol.,* **112**, 1589 (1974).

24. L. B. Epstein, *Tex. Rep. Biol. Med.,* **35**, 42 (1977).

25. H. M. Johnson, G. J. Stanton, and S. Baron, *Proc. Soc. Exp. Biol. Med.,* **154**, 138 (1977).

26. E. A. Havell, B. Berman, C. A. Ogburn, K. Berg, K. Paucker, and J. Vilcek, *Proc. Natl. Acad. Sci. (USA)*, **72**, 2185 (1975).

27. E. Knight, M. W. Hunkapiller, B. D. Korant, R. W. F. Hardy, and L. E. Hood, *Science,* **207**, 525 (1980).

28. K. C. Zoon, M. E. Smith, P. J. Bridgen, C. B. Anfinsen, M. W. Hunkapiller, and L. E. Hood, *Science,* **207**, 527 (1980).

29. H. Taira, R. J. Broeze, B. M. Jayaram, P. Lengyel, M. W. Hunkapiller, and L. E. Hood, *Science,* **207**, 528 (1980).

30. S. Nagata, H. Taira, A. Hall, L. Johnsrud, M. Streuli, J. Ecsodi, W. Boll, K. Cantell, and C. Weissmann, *Nature,* **284**, 316 (1980).

31. N. Mantei, M. Schwarzstein, M. Streuli, S. Panen, S. Nagata, and C. Weissmann, *Gene,* **10**, 1 (1980).

32. T. Taniguchi, N. Mantei, M. Schwarzstein, S. Nagata, M. Muramatsu, and C. Weissmann, *Nature,* **285**, 547 (1980).

33. G. Trincheri, D. Santoli, and B. B. Knowles, *Nature,* **270**, 611 (1977).

34. J. E. Blalock, M. P. Langford, J. Georgiades, and G. J. Stanton, *Cell. Immunol.,* **43**, 197 (1979).

35. L. C. Osborne, J. A. Georgiades, and H. M. Johnson, *IRCS Med. Sci.,* **8**, 212 (1980).

36. L. C. Osborne, J. A. Georgiades, and H. M. Johnson, *Cell. Immunol.,* **53**, 65 (1980).

37. W. Braun and H. B. Levy, *Proc. Soc. Exp. Biol. Med.,* **141**, 769 (1972).

38. T. J. Chester, K. Paucker, and T. C. Merigan, *Nature,* **246**, 92 (1973).

39. R. H. Gisler, P. Lindahl, and I. Gresser, *J. Immunol.,* **113**, 438 (1974).

40. H. M. Johnson, B. G. Smith, and S. Baron, *IRCS Med. Sci.,* **2**, 1616 (1974).

41. H. M. Johnson, B. G. Smith, and S. Baron, *J. Immunol.,* **114**, 403 (1975).

42. H. M. Johnson, Interferon and interferon inducers: Immune Modulation. In D. Stringfellow, Ed., *Interferon and Interferon Inducers,* Dekker, New York, 1980, p. 263.

43. H. M. Johnson and S. Baron, *Cell. Immunol.,* **25**, 106 (1976).

44. B. R. Brodeur and T. C. Merigan, *J. Immunol.,* **113**, 1319 (1975).

45. H. M. Johnson and J. E. Blalock, *Infect. Immun.,* **29**, 301 (1980).

46. D. R. Webb and I. Nowowiejski, *Cell. Immunol.,* **41**, 72 (1978).

47. H. M. Johnson and K. Ohtsuki, *Cell. Immunol.,* **44**, 125 (1979).

48. A. Kimchi, H. Shure, and M. Revel, *Nature,* **282**, 849 (1979).

49. P. Lindahl-Magnusson, P. Leary, and I. Gresser, *Nature,* **237**, 120 (1972).

50. K. R. Rozee, S. H. S. Lee, and J. Ngan, *Nature,* **245**, 16 (1973).

51. L. E. Mobraaten, E. De Maeyer, and J. De Maeyer-Guignard, *Transplantation,* **16**, 415 (1973).

52. J. C. Cerottini, K. T. Brunner, P. Lindahl, and I. Gresser, *Nature,* **242**, 152 (1973).

53. M. S. Hirsch, D. A. Ellis, P. H. Black, A. P. Monaco, and M. L. Wood, *Transplantation,* **17**, 234 (1974).

54. E. De Maeyer, J. De Maeyer-Guignard, and M. Vandeputte, *Proc. Natl. Acad. Sci. (USA),* **72**, 1753 (1975).

55. J. De Maeyer-Guignard, A. Cochard, and E. De Maeyer, *Science,* **190**, 574 (1975).

56. I. Heron, K. Berg, and K. Cantell, *J. Immunol.,* **117**, 1370 (1976).

57. G. Trinchieri and D. Santoli, *J. Exp. Med.,* **147**, 1314 (1978).

58. M. Gidlund, A. Orn, H. Wigzell, A. Senik, and I. Gresser, *Nature,* **273**, 759 (1978).

59. R. B. Herberman, J. R. Ortaldo, and G. D. Bonnard, *Nature,* **277**, 221 (1979).

60. K. Y. Huang, R. M. Donahoe, F. B. Gordon, and H. R. Dressler, *Infect. Immun.,* **4**, 581 (1971).

61. W. Braun, M. Nakano, L. Jaraskova, Y. Yajima, and L. Jimenez, Stimulation of Antibody-Forming cells by oligonucleotides of known composition. In O. J. Plescia and W. Braun, Eds., *Nucleic Acids in Immunology,* Springer-Verlag, New York, 1968, p. 347.

62. A. G. Johnson, J. Schmidtke, K. Merritt, and T. Han, Enhancement of antibody formation by nucleic acids and their derivatives. In O. J. Plescia and W. Braun, Eds., *Nucleic Acids in Immunology,* Springer-Verlag, New York, 1968, p. 379.

63. J. R. Schmidtke and A. G. Johnson, *J. Immunol.,* **106**, 1191 (1971).

64. A. G. Johnson, The adjuvant action of synthetic polynucleotides on the immune response. In E. P. Cohen, Ed., *Immune RNA,* CRC Press, Cleveland, 1976, p. 17.

65. H. Markowitz, D. A. Person, F. L. Gitnick, and R. E. Pitts, *Science,* **163**, 476 (1969).

66. H. S. Egan, W. J. Reeder, and R. D. Ekstedt, *J. Immunol.,* **112**, 63 (1974).

67. C. G. Romball and W. O. Weigle, *J. Immunol.,* **115**, 556 (1975).

68. W. Braun and M. Ishizuka, *Proc. Natl. Acad. Sci. (USA),* **68**, 1114 (1971).

69. M. Ishizuka, W. Braun, and T. Matsumoto, *J. Immunol.,* **107**, 1027 (1971).

70. R. E. Cone and J. J. Marchalonis, *Aust. J. Exp. Biol. Med.,* **50**, 69 (1972).

71. H. M. Johnson, J. A. Bukovic, and B. G. Smith, *Proc. Soc. Exp. Biol. Med.,* **149**, 599 (1975).

72. R. W. Dutton, *J. Exp. Med.,* **136**, 1445 (1972).

73. R. R. Rich and C. W. Pierce, *J. Exp. Med.,* **137**, 205 (1973).

74. J. Watson, R. Epstein, I. Nakoinz, and P. Ralph, *J. Immunol.,* **110**, 43 (1973).

75. B. G. Smith and H. M. Johnson, *J. Immunol.,* **115**, 575 (1975).

76. H. M. Johnson and J. A. Bukovic, *IRCS Med. Sci.,* **3**, 398 (1975).

77. G. Sonnenfeld, A. D. Mandel, and T. C. Merigan, *Cell. Immunol.,* **34**, 193 (1977).

78. W. R. Fleischmann, J. A. Georgiades, L. C. Osborne, F. Dianzani, and H. M. Johnson, *Infect. Immun.,* **26**, 949 (1979).

79. H. R. Bourne, L. M. Lichtenstein, K. L. Melmon, C. A. Henney, Y. Weinstein, and G. M. Shearer, *Science,* **184**, 19 (1974).

80. H. M. Johnson, *Nature,* **265**, 154 (1977).

81. H. M. Johnson, J. E. Blalock, and S. Baron, *Cell. Immunol.,* **33**, 170 (1977).

82. L. B. Epstein and H. R. Bourne, Interferon production by mitogen stimulated lymphocytes: cyclic AMP mediated inhibition by cholera toxin. In J. J. Oppenheim and D. L. Rosenstreich, Eds., *Mitogens in Immunobiology,* Academic, New York, 1976, p. 453.

83. F. Dianzani, P. Neri, and M. Zucca, *Proc. Soc. Exp. Biol. Med.,* **140**, 1375 (1972).

84. K. Paucker, K. Cantell, and W. Henle, *Virology,* **17**, 324 (1962).

85. I. Gresser, D. Brouty-Boye, M. T. Thomas, and A. Macieira-Coelho, *Proc. Natl. Acad. Sci. (USA),* **66**, 1052 (1970).

86. E. Knight, *J. Cell. Biol.,* **56**, 846 (1973).

87. S. B. Salvin, J. S. Youngner, J. Nishio, and R. Neta, *J. Natl. Cancer Inst.,* **55**, 1233 (1975).

88. J. E. Blalock, J. A. Georgiades, M. P. Langford, and H. M. Johnson, *Cell. Immunol.,* **49**, 390 (1980).

89. H. Strander, *Tex. Rep. Biol. Med.,* **35**, 429 (1977).

90. T. C. Merigan, K. Sikora, J. H. Breeden, R. Levy, and S. A. Rosenberg, *New Engl. J. Med.,* **299**, 1449 (1978).

91. J. U. Gutterman, G. R. Blumenschein, R. Alexanian, H.-Y. Yap, A. U. Buzdar, F. Cabanillas, G. N. Hortobagyi, E. M. Hersh, S. L. Rasmussen, M. Harmon, M. Kramer, and S. Pestka, *Ann. Internal Med.,* **93**, 399 (1980).

Immune RNA and Transfer Factor

GLENN STEELE, JR.
BOSCO S. WANG
JOHN A. MANNICK
Department of Surgery, Peter Bent Brigham Hospital
Harvard Medical School
Boston, Massachusetts

1. INTRODUCTION

Despite more than 20 years of investigation, the existence of immune RNA and transfer factor as valid biologic phenomena remains controversial since neither fits into any conventional scheme of immunity or information transfer. Immune RNA and transfer factor differ in their physical characteristics (what is known of them), in their postulated modes of action, in their effects, and even in the justifications for their application to the treatment of humans with various infections, immune deficiencies, allografted organs, or cancer. What is widely accepted, however, is the conceptual appeal of both immune RNA and transfer factor in the therapy of human disease associated with a suboptimal host-immune response. Moreover, at the very least, immune RNA as well as transfer factor (although this is less well studied clinically) have repeatedly been demonstrated not to harm patients.

In this chapter our overall goal will be to evaluate critically the published justifications for presently considering immune RNA and transfer factor in clinical therapy protocols. Important investigations in the definition of immune RNA and transfer factor are reviewed. More recent investigations attempting to identify, characterize, and purify the active elements in immune RNA as well as the development of new *in vitro* and *in vivo* models to test transfer factor are discussed with attention to the presence or absence of appropriate controls and overall experimental design. Finally, preliminary therapeutic applications of both of these biologic phenomena to various animal models and humans with diseases related to inadequate or imbalanced immune response are summarized in an attempt to answer the following questions implicit throughout this chapter:

1. Should either immune RNA or transfer factor be applied clinically now despite an admitted need for more understanding of mechanism of action?
2. Can the optimal conditions for any clinical application be defined at present?
3. If so, who should study these phenomena in humans?
4. How should clinical trials of immune RNA or transfer factor be designed?

2. IMMUNE RNA

The infectivity of ribonucleic acid from numerous viruses for tissue-cultured mammalian cells (including human) has been demonstrated repeatedly and as early as 1956 (1-3). Niu et al. (4) first attempted to show cytoplasmic incorporation of ^{14}C-labeled immune RNA after *in vivo* injection and subsequent autoradiography of single cells obtained from an ascites tumor model. In 1962 investigators postulated that RNA extracted from normal tissues might inhibit tumor isograft growth in rats (5), and RNA extracted from normal human bone marrow cells was used to attempt "redifferentiation" of exposed human leukemic cells (6). However, the first unequivocal demonstration of what seemed to be a legitimate transfer of immunologic information affecting humoral immune response was reported in 1961 by Fishman (7). After incubation of macrophages with bacteriophage T2, a lysate was prepared and filtered and added to a culture of lymph node cells. Antibody directed against T2 was generated by the lysate-exposed lymph node cells. In 1963, Fishman and Adler (8) demonstrated that RNA was most likely the active component in this macrophage extract capable of transferring antibody-forming capacity to the previously unsensitized lymphocytes. Mannick and Egdahl (9,10) in 1962 reported unequivocally that immune responsiveness could be amplified by RNA extracted from lymphoid tissues of specifically immunized animals. They demonstrated in 1964 that on reinfusion, autologous lymphocytes incubated with specific immune RNA *in vitro* could cause second set rejection of skin allografts in rabbits (11). Adoptive transfer of *in vivo* skin allograft immunity by immune RNA was donor specific. Third-party grafts did not undergo second set rejection. In none of the *in vivo* models of Mannick et al. could second-set allograft immunity be adoptively transferred by direct intravenous injection of immune RNA (12). This work was subsequent confirmed by Sabbadini and Sehon (13) and later by Ramming and Pilch (14).

The passive transfer of antibody production *in vitro* by RNA extracted in the manner of Fishman and Adler has been duplicated in many laboratories. All the data indicate a high degree of specificity and justify the conclusion that specific antibody formation can be transferred by immune RNA extracted from the lymphoid tissues of immunized donors. Perhaps the most elegant verifications of this phenomenon have been the experiments of Bell and Dray attempting to show the enhancement of plaque-forming cells after specific immune RNA exposure. By using specific antiallotypic sera, these investigators could demonstrate expression of the immune RNA donor-allotype (presumably not present in the cells of the recipient) on anti-SRBC-directed IgM and IgG after exposure of recipient lymphoid cells to immune RNA from SRBC-immunized rabbits (15–17). Both host and donor immunoglobulin allotypes on the induced anti-SRBC antibody could be shown up to 37 days after immune RNA treatment (17). These investigators speculated that the immune RNA had either an informational role and functioned as a template for protein synthesis through a RNA-dependent DNA polymerase or modified specific regulatory genes in the host lymphoid tissues.

The criticism that allotype transfer by immune RNA has not been a reproducible phenomenon (18) may not be totally accurate since Adler, Fishman, and Dray had shown in 1966 that immune RNA could transfer from one cell to another *in vitro* the ability to produce immunoglobulin molecules possessing both the antibody and allotype specificities of the cells from the RNA donor animal (19). In addition, Fishman, Adler, and numerous co-workers have continued *in vitro* studies focused on the ability of immune RNA to induce specific antibody formation, reproducing their own findings of immune and allotypic specificity and defining the RNAase sensitivity, the pronase and DNAase resistence, the size of the active RNA species (18–30) and the lack of cell proliferation involved in their *in vitro* information transfer models (20–22). A second line of investigation that supports allotypic transfer by immune RNA has provided evidence that RNA fractions from the cytoplasm of myeloma cells could transfer the myeloma idiotype to the cell surface of non-neoplastic lymphocytes (23–25). Subcellular fractions capable of inducing normal mouse lymphocytes to express idiotype specificity of the plasmacytoma have been demonstrated *in vitro* and *in vivo* (23) and have been shown to be RNAase sensitive, $12S$ to $23S$ in size on sucrose density gradients (24), and to contain poly-A sequences (25). Thus, although the phenomenon of transferred idiotype specificity by immune RNA appears reproducible, its explanation is not conventional, and it is perhaps this fact more than any other that inveighs against easy acceptance.

Other lines of evidence have also provided support for the existence of information transfer by immune RNA. For instance, immune RNA extracted from the peritoneal exudate cells of immunized mice has been shown to transfer immunity to *Salmonella enteridites* or *S. tennessee*. *In vivo* humoral antibody transfer was sensitive to RNAase but not DNAase, pronase, or pretreatment of immune RNA with anti-Salmonella flagella antibody, suggesting that there was no antigen contained in the immune RNA fractions (26). Mice treated with immune RNA harvested from peritoneal exudate cells from animals sensitized to *S. enteridites* were resistant to a subsequent lethal challenge of virulent Salmonella (27). The production of cytotoxic antibodies with specificity to a benzpyrene-induced sarcoma by treatment of naive mice with xenogeneic antitumor immune RNA was first reported by Pilch and co-workers in 1976 (28). Antitumor antibody synthesis induced *in vitro* in mouse spleen cells after xenogeneic immune RNA exposure was demonstrated by this same group in 1978 (29), and human lymphoblastoid B-cell lines were shown to be immunizable (to tumor cell-surface specificities) by *in vitro* incubation with the use of immune RNA from specifically immunized sheep. The information transferred to the exposed cell line was shown to be replicated in culture for at least 10 weeks (30).

The initial observation by Mannick and Egdahl that immune RNA could augment specific cell-mediated immune responses has been expanded by numerous investigators in various *in vitro* and *in vivo* systems. Paque, Dray, and associates demonstrated repeatedly their ability to transfer cellular immune response to defined delayed-type hypersensitivity (DTH) antigens (e.g., keyhole limpet hemocyanin, purified protein derivative, or coccidiodin) by *in vitro* incubation of naive lymphocytes with xenogeneic immune RNA obtained from specifically sensitized donors. Recipient lymphocytes included human white cells, and the initial *in vitro* assay was inhibition of macrophage migration. White cells exposed to immune RNA harvested from specifically immunized donors were challenged *in vitro* with KLH, PPD, or COCCI and compared for migration inhibition response with white cells incubated with RNA extracted from the lymphoid tissues of nonsensitized xenogeneic donors (31–33). Using similar *in vitro* assays for migration inhibition factor, Paque et al. (34) demonstrated that specific immune RNA exposure could "restore" DTH responses to the peritoneal exudate cells obtained from strain 13 guinea pigs, and Braun and Dray (35) showed that tumor-specific immune RNA could reestablish the *in vitro* migration inhibition response to peritoneal exudate cells obtained during the "unresponsive" phase 10 to 14 days after plasmacytoma growth in MOPC-315-bearing hosts.

The ability to transfer *in vitro* proliferative responses to xenogeneic lymphocytes challenged with specific antigen has also been shown by immune RNA harvested from lymphoid cells of BCG immunized cattle (36) or tumor-antigen-immunized sheep (37). In both the tumor and the nontumor systems, blastogenesis of antigen-challenged lymphocytes has been monitored by uptake of tritiated thymidine. Specificity controls in the BCG system were provided by comparing nonspecific proliferation after *in vitro* challenge of RNA-treated human lymphocytes with histoplasm with specific proliferation following exposure to PPD.

The most frequently exploited *in vitro* parameter of cell-mediated immune function affected by immune RNA has been the lymphocyte-mediated cytotoxic, cytolytic, or antiadherent effect. Wilson and Wecker first reported the conversion of naive lymphocytes to cytotoxicity after exposure to RNA derived from isologous lymphoid tissues of specifically immunized rats (38). Bondevick and Mannick (39) confirmed this, demonstrating that immune RNA-exposed lymphocytes could be induced to "attack" allogeneic target tissue *in vitro* with a specificity determined by the skin allograft sensitized RNA donor. The initial assay used in their experiments was a 48-hour microcytotoxicity test that included trypan blue staining of residual target cells after effector cell exposure. By using an *in vitro* adherence assay modified from Cohen et al. (40), Pilch and co-workers demonstrated that lymphocytes from nonimmune Fischer rats could be made cytotoxic to methylcholanthrene-induced tumor cells after *in vitro* incubation with the use of immune RNA harvested from spleens of Fischer rats hyperimmunized with methylcholanthrene sarcoma isografts. The concentration of immune RNA effecting this cell-mediated immune transfer was 100 μg/ml. Immune RNA was RNAase sensitive but DNAase and pronase resistant. The level of cytotoxic effect after *in vitro* immune RNA exposure of nonsensitized syngeneic lymphocytes was purported to be similar to lymphocytes harvested from hyperimmunized animals and tested for cytotoxicity directly on the methylcholanthrene sarcoma targets (41). These workers reported similar findings when naive spleen cells obtained from murine donors were exposed to immune RNA harvested from methylcholanthrene sarcoma hyperimmunized rats (42). Almost identical experimental conditions were shown to mediate successfully tumor-specific cytotoxic immune responses after exposure of naive human peripheral blood lymphocytes to xenogeneic immune RNA directed at human tumor targets. Initial xenogeneic donors used for immunization in these experiments were sheep or guinea pigs. Pilch et al. showed not only increased tumor-specific lymphocyte-mediated cytotoxicity (as monitored by the Cohen assay) on human tumor targets, but a lack of effect when these same lymphocytes were incubated with normal human fibroblasts (43–45). In addition, human lymphocytes exposed to tumor-specific allogeneic or xenogeneic RNA demonstrated cell-mediated immunity not only against the specific tumor target used to sensitize the immune RNA donor, but also against other human tumor targets of the same histologic type (46). These findings were confirmed by other groups (47) and extended by Mannick, Wang, and Deckers to models of concommitant tumor immunity. Thus lymphocyte-mediated cytotoxicity against tumor targets could be augmented by *in vitro* immune RNA incubation, even though the exposed lymphocytes were harvested from animals already bearing tumors (48). Augmentation of the cellular immune response after immune RNA exposure of lymph node cells or peripheral blood lymphocytes harvested from animals and humans bearing tumors could be shown *in vitro* by either the ^{125}I IUdR cytotoxicity assay or by proliferation assays monitoring tritiated thymidine uptake after specific antigen exposure of test lymphocytes (49).

Aside from the experiments of Mannick and Egdahl that employed second-set skin allograft models, the earliest *in vivo* demonstrations of immunologic information transfer by immune RNA focused on conventional measurements of the DTH response. Effect of specific immune RNA sensitization on monocytes was hypothesized as at least partially responsible for the *in vivo* protection against experimental Salmonellosis mentioned previously. Immune RNA-treated monocytes did demonstrate marked inhibition of intracytoplasmic bacterial replication (50–53). Additional *in vivo* models of resistance to various parasite infections were postulated to be due to specific immune RNA activation of macrophages in treated recipient mice (54,55). The first direct *in vivo* evidence of adoptive transfer of cell-mediated immunity in humans by immune RNA was claimed in a brief report by Han et al. (56) concerning the transfer of the PPD skin test response from a PPD-positive to a PPD-negative individual by intradermal injection of immune RNA extracted from the peripheral blood lymphocytes of the tuberculin-sensitive human donor. However, nonspecific DTH skin tests were not placed, the PPD skin response remained positive for 4 weeks, and attempts to show an *in vitro* blastogenesis response of the converted individual's lymphocytes after PPD exposure were unsuccessful (56).

The precise definition of immune RNA is much harder to find than the evidence summarized earlier regarding the existence of the various phenomena ascribed to immune RNA. Discussion concerning antigen or antigen fragments in association with RNA in contrast to information transfer by immune RNA without associated antigen continues. The existence of antigen-immune RNA complexes has been reported in cell-free systems (57,58), in numerous *in vitro* cellular systems (59–62), and in various *in vivo* immune RNA transfer models (63–65). Antigen-immune RNA conjugates have been characterized as "super-immunogens," purportedly isolated in the cytoplasm of rat hepatocyte polyribosomes after immunization (65), and postulated to be fundamental as endogenous antibody inducers (63). Although it is harder to prove the absence of something than its presence, an equal number of investigators have maintained that immune RNA functions to provide specific information exchange in the absence of associated antigen (66–69). Despite evidence that endogenous immune RNA in any of its purported "normal" functions as an immune regulator may be heterogeneous (70–72), the likelihood from numerous physical and chemical considerations concerning the hot phenol method of immune RNA preparation used by most investigators (67) and the characteristics of the active immune RNA component after preparation (73,74) is that the probability of antigen-immune RNA conjugates being the active factor in most of the experimental protocols summarized previously is quite small.

Evidence has accumulated that immune RNA has mRNA capability (73–79). Immune RNA fractions have been found to contain the information required to code for the synthesis of IgM in cell-free systems (75). Wang and Mannick (73), Greenup et al. (79), Paque (80), and Kern et al. (81) have determined that immune RNA active in transferring tumor-specific *in vitro* leukocyte-mediated cytotoxicity is an 8 to 16S fraction on 5 to 20% sucrose density gradients, represents 5 to 7% of the total RNA from donor lymphoid tissues, and contains polyadenyllic acid sequences that can be adsorbed to oligo (dT)-cellulose-affinity columns. Investigators using specific antigen such as ARSNAT or KLH (74) have confirmed the work of Wang and Mannick and others, by showing that *in vitro* immune responses can be transferred by oligo (dT) binding fractions obtained from sucrose density gradients (5 to 16S) of whole donor lymphocyte RNA. Purification procedures have been demonstrated to increase the specific activity of immune RNA (76), and this purified fraction remains RNAase sensitive but pronase and DNAase resistant (80).

The kinetics of optimal immunization prior to immune RNA harvest from donor lymphoid tissues has been described by Mannick and his associates and by Pilch and his group. Both groups agree that the most effective immune RNA is harvested from allogeneic or xenogeneic donors 14 to 21 days after immunization (81,82). In these studies immune RNA donors have been immunized with specific antigen in combination with complete Freund's adjuvant. Wang and Mannick have shown that the probable source of donor immune RNA is the macrophage (83) and that there is a requirement for T cells among the cytotoxic effectors in their *in vitro* lymphocyte-mediated cytotoxicity systems (82,84). Even in these *in vitro* systems, however, the effects of immune RNA are undoubtedly multiple and complicated. When more than one response has been looked for, more than one response has been found. Thus immune RNA-exposed lymphocytes have been shown to contain at least two subsets, one stimulated by immune RNA to produce specific tumor target cell killing and a second stimulated by immune RNA to proliferate in mixed lymphocyte-tumor cultures. Wang and Mannick have postulated that proliferation in this system is not necessary for lymphocyte-mediated cytotoxicity after tumor-specific immune RNA incubation (85). Other investigators using completely different methodology have also documented multiple effects on lymphocytes after exposure to xenogeneic immune RNA (86).

Finally, the first prerequisite for all the preceding immune RNA effects—its entrance into recipient lymphoid cells—was claimed as early as 1961 by Niu et al. (4), confirmed in 1964 by Mannick (87), and reproduced in various systems by numerous investigators with the use of a variety of radioisotope and RNA-DNA hybridization techniques (88–94).

In summary, then, despite numerous inconsistencies and disagreements concerning the mechanism of immune RNA action, the preceding investigations focusing specifically on immune RNA as well as more detailed nonimmune RNA studies in molecular biology [e.g., the capacity of single-stranded RNA to act as a messenger for specific cell-free synthesis *in vitro* (95), the characterization of RNA-directed DNA polymerase (96), and the implication that thymocyte cytoplasmic RNA sequences may be homologous to cell-surface immunoglobulin α-chain RNA (97)] all support the conclusion that immune RNA not only exists, but functions as well.

The first application of tumor-specific xenogeneic immune RNA to the *in vivo* therapy of tumors was reported by Deckers and Pilch in 1971 (98). These investigators showed that murine isograft challenge resistance could be altered by five alternate-day footpad injections of tumor-specific xenogeneic immune RNA. Direct injection of immune RNA without an RNAase inhibitor (sodium dextransulfate) did not effect *in vivo* isograft challenge resistence. In 1975 Schlager and Dray (99) reported the successful therapy of an already established strain 2 guinea pig hepatoma by injection of either syngeneic or xenogeneic tumor-specific immune RNA plus naive syngeneic lymphocytes plus tumor-specific antigen vaccine. Regression was obtained not only in the primary injected tumors, but also at secondary noninjected sites. Survival was prolonged in the animals in which tumor regression was obtained. No specificity controls were reported (99).

deKernion et al. published the first anecdotal reports of xenogeneic immunotherapy in humans with a variety of malignant lesions in 1975 (100). This group's progress in treating human cancer with immune RNA was updated in 1976 (101,102) and again in 1977 (103,104). Despite earlier animal experience demonstrating the ineffectiveness of direct immune RNA injection without RNAase inhibitors, their protocol for immunotherapy in humans consisted of direct xenogeneic i.v. immune RNA injection. Immune RNA was harvested from sheep or guinea pigs immunized preferably with the patient's own tumor or if that were impossible, with "tissue-type-specific" human tumor. Treated patients had a variety of cancer diagnoses including melanoma, renal cell carcinoma, sarcoma, and gastric and breast carcinoma, and no uniform conclusions concerning tumor response or effect on survival could be made. Nevertheless, there was no evidence of acute toxicity from the immunotherapy regimen and no evidence that tumor course in any of these patients was exacerbated by immunotherapy. Most of these studies also included *in vitro* tests of lymphocyte-mediated cytotoxicity (as monitored by the Cohen assay with the use of autologous or allogeneic "tissue-type-specific" target cells). In general, host-cell-mediated cytotoxicity seemed to be stimulated immediately after immune RNA treatment, but strict relationships between *in vitro* parameters and *in vivo* response were not obvious, and *in vitro* specificity controls were not always available.

In 1976 Deckers et al. (105) attempted to establish a therapeutic effect on murine sarcoma isograft outgrowth after xenogeneic tumor-specific immune RNA treatment (105). Although they showed a temporary and significant delay in isograft outgrowth among animals treated with tumor-specific xenogeneic immune RNA, isograft growth in treated animals soon caught up with those in non-tumor-specific treated controls. These investigators did, however, show a specific *in vitro* augmentation of splenocyte-mediated antitumor effect in tumor-bearing animals. The major difference in the protocol of Mannick and associates from that of Pilch and colleagues was the *in vitro* incubation of syngeneic splenocytes with xenogeneic tumor-specific immune RNA prior to injection of the treated effector cells into the mice bearing sarcoma isografts. This presumably obviated the need for RNAase inhibitors since Mannick et al. had found direct injection of immune RNA to be ineffective *in vivo* (105).

The minimal effect of immune RNA in preventing isograft outgrowth was disappointing but felt to be a consequence of the particular tumor model chosen and its extremely rapid outgrowth. A more suitable model with at least a superficial analogy to the human "minimal residual disease" situation was first reported by Pilch et al. in 1976 (101). Using a metastasizing rat mammary carcinoma, Pilch claimed that tumor-specific immune RNA in combination with an RNAase inhibitor could prevent development of metastases after primary isograft excision. Animals protected against metastases were long-term survivors. Although this immunotherapy protocol included animals treated with RNAase-neutralized immune RNA and RNA harvested from nonimmunized donors, tumor specificity controls were absent. In 1978 Wang et al. (106) confirmed the efficacy of tumor-specific immune RNA in preventing metastases. Again, as in the Pilch experiments, long-term survival was increased in animals protected from metastases (106). Using B16 melanoma isografts in C57BL/6J mice, these investigators consistently demonstrated prevention of spontaneous metastases after isograft excision and long-term survival in approximately 50% of treated animals when compared to RNAase-neutralized immune RNA, normal RNA, or 3LL (Lewis lung carcinoma)-specific immune RNA-treated animals. Their immune RNA treatment protocol consisted of multiple intraperitoneal injections with the use of xenogeneic (guinea pig) B16 immune RNA incubated syngeneic splenocytes in the C57BL/6J mice after B16 isograft excision. Splenocytes harvested from the B16 immune RNA-treated mice showed progressive augmentation of *in vitro* cytotoxicity directed at B16 target cells after sequential immune RNA treatment. Cell-mediated immunity in these experiments was monitored not only by the standard ^{125}I IUdR (Cohen) assay but also by parallel lymphocyte-mediated cytotoxicity assays using a "long-term" ^{51}Cr release technique and microcytotoxicity tests with visual counting of adherent target cells after 48 hours of exposure to effector cells (107). Splenocytes harvested from control animals treated with RNAase-neutralized immune RNA or 3LL-specific immune RNA showed no significant augmentation of cytotoxic effect when tested on B16 target cells. Animals in groups demonstrating increased *in vitro* B16 target killing were those with a decreased incidence of pulmonary metastases and greater chance of long-term survival. A possible explanation for the effectiveness of B16 immune RNA treatment in this particular adjuvant model has been postulated to be the increased immunogenicity and antigenicity among clones of B16 melanoma predisposed to metastasis (108,109).

The present investigators have also recently completed a Phase I human trial of immune RNA in patients with far-advanced renal cell carcinoma or melanoma. Although their protocol differs from Pilch in the use of autologous tumor-specific immune RNA treatment of the patients' own lymphocytes with reinfusion of stimulated lymphocytes after each treatment, results were similar to the earlier results published by Pilch and his colleagues. No acute toxicity was noted despite multiple injections of xenogeneic tumor-specific immune RNA-treated autologous lymphocytes, and no exacerbation of tumor course was noted in any of the treated patients (110). As in any Phase I trial, effect on tumor (although promising among these patients) could not be positively related to therapy. As opposed to the earlier animal studies, all the patients treated showed long-term serial increase in their lymphocyte-mediated cytotoxicity against "tissue-type-specific" human tumor targets regardless of their ultimate tumor course (111). At present, no prospective, randomized Phase III trial using tumor-specific immune RNA treatment of patients with minimal residual disease has been reported.

3. TRANSFER FACTOR

In 1955 Lawrence (112) extended the work of Dr. Meryl Chase and demonstrated the transfer in humans of delayed skin sensitivity to streptococcal-M substance and to tuberculin by using not only whole leukocytes, but also a suspension of leukocytes disrupted by either distilled water treatment or repeated freeze-thaw cycling. The substance or substances responsible for this transfer of DTH, "transfer factor" (TF), was resistent to RNAase and DNAase. Extracts of leukocytes from patients not sensitive to streptococcal-M substance or to tuberculin had no effect in transferring *in vivo* DTH responses. Sensitized recipients remained capable of wheal-and-flair skin reactions after challenge by specific antigens for more than 7 months. Lawrence and Pappenheimer (113) next showed that human leukocyte extracts from patients sensitized to diphtheria toxin could transfer diphtheria-toxin-specific DTH without increasing antitoxin titers in the TF-treated recipients (113). Lawrence and co-workers extended their observations on cell-mediated transfer by TF when they reported in 1960 the *in vivo* transfer of accelerated skin allograft rejection by treatment of graft recipients with TF from specifically sensitized human donor leukocytes. Again, TF was resistent to RNAase and DNAase. The effectiveness of TF producing second-set rejection was specific to donor sensitization. Third-party allografts were rejected as first-set grafts. The effectiveness of TF increased as donor sensitization increased, and donor serum was shown to be an ineffective source of transfer factor.

Other investigators confirmed the work of Lawrence and associates (114), demonstrated antigenic specificity by using keyhole limpet hemocyanin (KLH) and purified protein derivative of tuberculin (PPD) crisscross *in vivo* controls, and began to establish purification procedures by defining a low-molecular-weight active substance after column chromatography on Sephadex G25 (115). The first indication that an *in vitro* correlate of DTH might be affected by transfer factor was reported by Fireman et al. in 1966 (116), who postulated lymphocyte stimulation after transfer factor exposure by demonstrating an increased number of large lymphocytes with high mitotic indices after *in vitro* antigen recall. A more quantitative *in vitro* correlate of transfer factor effect in triggering the DTH response awaited the report of Asher et al. in 1974 (117), who showed that antigen-triggered lymphocyte blastogenesis as monitored by tritiated thymidine incorporation correlated with the transfer factor-induced DTH response *in vivo*. The possible effect of transfer factor on mixed lymphocyte culture reactivity was reported by Good and his associates (118), who postulated a nonspecific increase in *in vitro* MLC reactivity by nonspecific augmentation of responder cell stimulation or by induction of changes in the expression of histocompatibility determinants after TF exposure. The *in vitro* effects were an offshoot in the investigators' attempts to treat three patients suffering from combined immunodeficiency diseases with pooled normal human transfer factor. No therapeutic effect was observed.

In addition to the problem of very few substantiated *in vitro* assays for TF, until recently there have been no animal models in which transfer factor could be studied. In 1970, however, Baram and Condoulis (119) reported their ability to transfer KLH sensitivity to monkey and human lymphocytes with extracts of peripheral blood lymphocytes harvested from sensitized monkeys. Not only was this the first report of successful transfer factor passage across a species barrier, but the *in vitro* assay for successful transfer was novel and unconfirmed at that time. The authors claimed an increased thymidine uptake 6 to 9 days after transfer factor incubation when recipient lymphocytes were again exposed to KLH (119). The *in vivo* applicability of transfer factor in monkey models was confirmed in 1972 by a report of Madison et al. (120) demonstrating the successful transfer of DTH responses to *Schistosoma mansoni* and tuberculin. Allogeneic and xenogeneic transfer factor have been shown capable of the *in vivo* transfer of DTH responses to PPD in recipient monkeys, but successful *in vitro* correlation with the use of PPD-stimulated lymphocyte blastogenesis has not been consistent (121).

Investigations of the mechanisms of transfer factor activity have, of course, been limited when compared to similar studies with immune RNA since transfer factor affects a lesser number of immune responses than immune RNA (TF function has thus far been shown only in DTH responses *in vivo* and some DTH *in vitro* correlates) and because very few animal models for the study of transfer factor have been available. Preliminary fractionation of leukocyte extracts capable of transferring DTH responses have revealed that transfer factor is probably a low-molecular-weight material with the electrophoretic mobility of slow gamma globulin but with no reactivity to anti-immunoglobulin antisera. Unfortunately, the physicochemical characteristics of distilled water or freeze-thaw leukocyte extracts from normal donors and from TF-sensitized donors are exactly the same (122). Although the immunologic activity of transfer factor is limited, it is secure, but hypotheses concerning the informational character of TF remain almost impossible to test (123), and its possible composition (a short polypeptide chain joined with a three- or four-base segment of RNA) difficult to verify.

Despite the lack of readily reproducible *in vitro* assays for TF effect, the lack of readily available animal models, or even a hint of any successful experimental therapeutic effects, the conceptual appeal of the application of transfer factor to clinical therapy has been great. Treatment of a limited number of patients with a variety of immunodeficiencies has produced mixed results. Griscelli et al. (124) have postulated that TF treatment from pooled normal humans produces a nonspecific stimulation of already acquired but not expressed reactivities in patients with immunodeficiency diseases. Wybran et al. (125) reported an increase in rosette-forming cells (RFCs) among three patients with Wiskott-Aldrich syndrome treated with TF from pooled normal humans. In none of these patients with immunodeficiency diseases was a change in disease course documented (125). Effects of transfer factor from pooled normal donors or from purportedly specifically tumor-immune donors in a variety of patients with various kinds of cancer have been reported in anecdotal fashion (126–129). However, organized Phase I trials have not been reported. Prior to establishing in a formal manner the lack of toxicity or other untoward effects of transfer factor treatment in patients with cancer or immune-deficiency diseases, prospective, randomized, properly controlled Phase III trials would seem premature.

4. CONCLUSION

Both immune RNA and TF seem securely established as real immunologic phenomena. Immune RNA appears to have a much greater range of abilities to transfer immunologic information as well as more numerous *in vitro* and *in vivo* models available for studying its mechanism of action. In addition, preliminary application of immune RNA to animal tumor models (isograft tumor prevention, isograft tumor therapy, and prevention of metastases after isograft excision) all make immune RNA a more easily evaluated immunotherapeutic candidate. Nevertheless, both immune RNA and transfer factor offer the appeal of specific information transfer without possibly harmful additional sensitization of the recipient. Obviously, the judgment as to how much one should know concerning mechanisms of action prior to attempting clinical application is difficult. Nevertheless, this problem might be approached by attempting to answer the following admittedly oversimplified questions:

1. Will the treatment harm the recipient? Agreement is uniform with respect to animal and Phase I human studies with the use of immune RNA. At the very least, immune RNA does not hurt the treated host. As for TF, it is impossible to ascertain from the anecdotal cases thus far reported whether transfer factor benefits or harms the treated patient. In all probability, it does not harm. However, it is possible that the recognition of histocompatibility determinants (as monitored by *in vitro* LMC) is affected by transfer factor (118).

2. What is the probability that any systemic therapy (including immuno-
    therapy) will completely cure the tumor-bearing host? Certainly with
    the increasing awareness of complicated host immune/tumor interac-
    tions, the myriad of feedback controls regulating both humoral and
    cellular immune responses in normals and tumor bearers, the only pos-
    sible conclusion is that the outcome of any particular immunothera-
    peutic protocol depends upon many factors imperfectly understood.
    With the shrinking likelihood of any all-or-none effect, the success of
    immune RNA or TF therapy undoubtedly should depend on tumor
    volume, timing of therapy, and the establishment in preliminary studies
    of optimal conditions for treatment and optimal assays to monitor
    altered host-immune responses during and after therapy. Multiple ani-
    mal models for establishing optimal conditions and for designing *in
    vitro* tests to be followed during and after therapy have been reviewed
    for immune RNA treatment regimens. Preliminary human Phase I
    toxicity studies have been designed for the use of these animal data. The
    establishment of such optimal conditions and the design of *in vitro*
    correlates for any TF immunotherapy trial is at present extraordinarily
    difficult. The end point of any such TF trial, therefore, can be only
    increased survival in treated patients since the best conditions for TF
    treatment or the activity of the TF to be used can probably not be estab-
    lished.

3. Who should apply immune RNA or TF clinically? Any group com-
    mitted to Phase I or ultimately Phase III trials of such new therapeutic
    approaches should be composed of people familiar with the basic re-
    search in their chosen therapeutic modality, as well as medical and sur-
    gical oncologists familiar not only with the overall design of clinical
    trials, but specifically with the natural history of the diseases they wish
    to treat and, finally, statistical consultants who can specifically predict
    if the study design has a reasonable chance of producing an answer,
    even a negative one.

4. How should the clinical trials be designed? Phase I studies of therapeu-
    tic protocols are not compilations of anecdotal case reports. They are
    attempts to define in a formal way the lack of toxicity of a particular
    rigidly applied new regimen. As reviewed previously, such Phase I trials
    have been performed with several modes of immune RNA therapy in
    animals and in patients with far-advanced cancers. Hints concerning
    beneficial effects on tumor course and promising *in vitro* correlates
    should be confirmed not by further Phase I approaches, but by random-
    ized, prospective, controlled therapeutic trials. Clinicians interested in
    applying immunotherapy should learn from previous chemotherapy
    trials in which initially favorable results applying a variety of agents to
    a variety of tumors in nonrandomized fashion were modified dramatic-
    ally by subsequent controlled prospective trials (130).

REFERENCES

1. A. Gierer and G. Schramm, Infectivity of ribonucleic acid from tobacco moser virus. *Nature,* **177,** 702–703 (1956).

2. H. E. Alexander, G. Koch, I. M. Mountain, and O. VanDamme, Infectivity of ribonucleic acid from pilio virus in human cell monolayers. *J. Exp. Med.,* **108,** 493–506 (1958).

3. K. A. O. Ellem and J. S. Colter, The interaction of infectious ribonucleic acid with a mammalian cell line. III. Kinetics of the formation of infectious centers. *Virology,* **12,** 511–520 (1960).

4. M. C. Niu, C. C. Cordova, and L. C. Niu, Ribonucleic acid-induced changes in mammalian cells. *Proc. Natl. Acad. Sci.,* **47,** 1689–1700 (1961).

5. N. N. Aksenova, V. M. Bresler, V. I. Vorobyev, and J. M. Olenov, Influence of ribonucleic acids from the liver on implantation and growth of transplantable tumours. *Nature,* **196,** 443–444 (1962).

6. S. DeCarvalho, Effect of RNA from normal bone marrow on leukemic marrow *in vivo. Nature,* **197,** 1077–1080 (1963).

7. M. Fishman, Antibody formation *in vitro. J. Exp. Med.,* **114,** 837–856 (1961).

8. M. Fishman and F. L. Adler, Antibody formation initiated *in vitro* II. Antibody synthesis in X-irradiated recipients of diffusion chambers containing nucleic acid derived from macrophages incubated with antigen. *J. Exp. Med.,* **117,** 595–602 (1964).

9. J. A. Mannick and R. H. Egdahl, Ribonucleic acid in "transformation" of lymphoid cells. *Science,* **137,** 976–977 (1962).

10. J. A. Mannick and R. H. Egdahl, Transformation of nonimmune lymph node cells to state of transplantation immunity by RNA. *Ann. Surg.,* **156,** 356–366.

11. J. A. Mannick and R. H. Egdahl, Transfer of heightened immunity to skin homografts by lymphoid RNA. *J. Clin. Invest.,* **43,** 2166–2177 (1964).

12. J. A. Mannick, Transfer of "adoptive" immunity to homografts by RNA: A preliminary report. *Surgery,* **56,** 249–255 (1964).

13. E. Sabbadini and A. H. Sehon, Acceleration of allograft rejection induced by RNA from sensitized donors. *Int. Arch. Allergy Appl. Immunol.,* **32,** 55–63 (1967).

14. K. P. Ramming and Y. H. Pilch, Transfer of transplantation immunity by ribonucleic acid. *Transplantation,* **7,** 296–299 (1968).

15. C. Bell and S. Dray, Expression of allelic immunoglobulin in homozygous rabbits injected with RNA extract. *Science,* **171,** 199–201 (1970).

16. C. Bell and S. Dray, Conversion of homozygous lymphoid cells to produce IgM antibodies and IgG immunoglobulins of allelic light-chain allotype by injection of rabbits with RNA extracts. *Cell. Immunol.,* **5,** 52–65 (1972).

17. C. Bell and S. Dray, RNA conversion of lymphoid cells to synthesize allogeneic immunoglobulins *in vivo. Cell. Immunol.,* **6,** 375–393 (1973).

18. S. Sell, Immune RNA—Questions not answered. In M. A. Fink, Ed., *Immune RNA and Neoplasia,* Academic, New York, 1975, pp. 293–301.

19. M. Fishman and F. L. Adler, Correct Status of Immune RNA. In M. A. Fink, Ed., *Immune RNA and Neoplasia,* Academic, New York, 1975, p. 53.

20. H. K. Meiss and M. Fishman, Formation of antibody in rabbit spleen cell cultures stimulated with immunogenic RNA. *J. Immunol.,* **108,** 1172–1178 (1972).

21. A. E. Schaefer, M. Fishman, and F. L. Adler, Studies on antibody induction *in vitro.* III. Cellular requirements for the induction of antibody synthesis by solubilized T_2 phage and immunogenic RNA. *J. Immunol.,* **112,** 1981–1986 (1974).

22. F. L. Adler and M. Fishman, *In vitro* studies on information transfer in cells from allotype-suppressed rabbits. *J. Immunol.,* **115,** 129–134 (1975).

23. N. Bhoopalam, V. Yakulis, N. Costea, and P. Heller, Surface immunoglobulins of circulating lymphocytes in mouse plasmacytoma. II. The influence of plasmacytoma RNA on surface immunoglobulins of lymphocytes. *Blood, 39* (4) (1972), p. 465.

24. D. Giacomoni, V. Yakulis, S. R. Wang, A. Cooke, S. Dray, and P. Heller, *In vitro* conversion of normal mouse lymphocytes by plasmacytoma RNA to express idiotypic specificities on their surface characteristic of the plasmacytoma immunoglobulin. *Cell. Immunol.,* **11,** 389–400 (1979).

25. J. Katzmann, D. Giacomoni, V. Yakulis, and P. Heller, Characterization of two plasmacytoma fractions and their RNA capable of changing lymphocytes surface immunoglobulins (cell conversion). *Cell. Immunol.,* **18,** 98–109 (1975).

26. S. Mitsuhashi, S. Kurashige, M. Kawakami, and T. Nojima, Immune ribonucleic acid which induces antibody formation to Salmonella flagella. *Jap. J. Microbiol.,* **12,** 261–268 (1968).

27. M. R. Venneman, N. J. Bigley, and L. J. Berry, Immunogenicity of ribonucleic acid preparations obtained from *Salmonella typhimurium. Infect. Immun.,* **1,** 574–582 (1970).

28. D. Fritze, D. H. Kern, N. Chon, and Y. H. Pilch, Production of cytotoxic antibody to a benz(a)pyrene-induced sarcoma in mice receiving xenogeneic antitumor immune RNA. *Cancer Immunol. Immunother.,* **1,** 245–250 (1976).

29. D. H. Kern and Y. H. Pilch, Antitumor antibody synthesis *in vitro* induced in mouse spleen cells by xenogeneic immune RNA. *J. Natl. Cancer Inst.,* **60,** 599–603 (1978).

30. D. Viza, C. Boucheix, D. H. Kern, and Y. H. Pilch, Human lymphoblastoid cells in culture replicate immune information carried by xenogeneic RNA. *Differentiation,* **11,** 181–184 (1978).

31. R. E. Paque and S. Dray, Monkey to human transfer of delayed hypersensitivity *in vitro* with RNA extracts. *Cell. Immunol.,* **5,** 30–41 (1972).

32. R. E. Paque, M. S. Meltzer, B. Zhar, H. J. Rapp, and S. Dray, Transfer of tumor-specific relayed hypersensitivity *in vitro* to normal guinea pig peritoneal exudate cells using RNA extracts from sensitized lymphoid tissues. *Cancer Res.,* **33,** 3165–3171 (1973).

33. R. E. Paque and S. Dray, Transfer of delayed hypersensitivity to nonsensitive human leukocytes with rhesus-monkey lymphoid RNA extracts. *Transplant. Proc.,* **6,** 203–207 (1974).

34. R. E. Paque, M. Ali, and S. Dray, RNA extracts of lymphoid cells sensitized to DNP-oligolysines convert nonresponder lymphoid cells to responder cells which release migration inhibition factor. *Cell. Immunol.,* **16,** 261–268 (1975).

35. D. P. Braun and S. Dray, Immune RNA-mediated transfer of tumor antigen responsiveness to unresponsive peritoneal exudate cells from tumor-bearing animals. *Cancer Res.,* **37,** 4138–4144 (1977).

36. B. S. Wang, P. A. Stuart, and J. A. Mannick, Interspecies transfer by "immune" RNA of lymphocyte proliferative response to specific antigen. *Cell. Immunol.,* **12,** 114–118 (1974).

37. M. R. Coates and Y. H. Pilch, Conversion of normal human lymphocytes to tumor-specific immunoreactivity by xenogeneic immune RNA: Blastogenic responses to soluble tumor antigens. *Cancer Immunol. Immunother.,* **3,** 145–152 (1977).

38. D. B. Wilson and E. E. Wecker, Quantitative studies on the behavior of sensitized lymphoid cells *in vitro*. III. Conversion of "normal" lymphoid cells to an immunologically active status with RNA derived from isologous lymphoid tissues of specifically immunized rats. *J. Immunol.,* **97,** 512–516 (1966).

39. H. Bondevik and J. A. Mannick, RNA-mediated transfer of lymphocyte versus target cell activity. *Proc. Soc. Exp. Biol. Med.,* **129,** 264–268 (1968).

40. A. M. Cohen, J. F. Burdick, and A. S. Ketcham, Cell-mediated cytotoxicity: an assay using ^{125}I-iododeoxyuridine-labeled target cells. *J. Immunol.,* **107,** 895–898 (1971).

41. D. H. Kern, C. R. Drogemuller, and Y. H. Pilch, Immune cytolysis of rat tumor cells mediated by syngeneic "immune" RNA. *J. Natl. Cancer Inst.,* **52,** 299–302 (1974).

42. D. H. Kern and Y. H. Pilch, Immune cytolysis of murine tumor cells mediated by xenogeneic "immune" RNA. *Internatl. J. Cancer,* **13,** 679–688 (1974).

43. L. L. Veltman, D. H. Kern, and Y. H. Pilch, Immune cytolysis of human tumor cells mediated by xenogeneic "immune" RNA. *Cell. Immunol.,* **13,** 367–377 (1974).

44. Y. H. Pilch, L. L. Veltman, and D. H. Kern, Immune cytolysis of human tumor cells mediated by xenogeneic "immune" RNA: Implications for immunotherapy. *Surgery,* **76,** 23–34 (1974).

45. D. H. Kern, D. Fritze, C. R. Drogemuller, and Y. H. Pilch, Mediation of cytotoxic immune responses against human tumor-associated antigens by xenogeneic immune RNA. *J. Natl. Cancer Inst.,* **57,** 97–103 (1976).

46. D. H. Kern, D. Fritze, P. M. Schick, N. Chon, and Y. H. Pilch, Mediation of cytotoxic immune responses against human tumor-associated antigens by allogeneic immune RNA. *J. Natl. Cancer Inst.,* **57,** 105–109 (1976).

47. F. Singh, K. Y. Tsang, and W. S. Blakemore, Effects of xenogeneic immune RNA on normal human lymphocytes against human osteosarcoma cells *in vitro. J. Natl. Cancer Inst.,* **58,** 505–510 (1977).

48. P. J. Deckers, B. S. Wang, P. A. Stuart, and J. A. Mannick, Augmentation of tumor-specific immunity with immune RNA. *Transplant. Proc.,* **7,** 259–263, 1975.

49. B. S. Wang and P. J. Deckers, The augmentation of concommitant tumor immunity with RNA. *J. Surg. Res.,* **20,** 183–194 (1976).

50. K. Saito and S. Mitsuhashi, Experimental Salmonellosis. VI. *In vitro* transfer of cellular immunity of mouse mononuclear phagocytes. *J. Bacteriol.,* **90,** 629–634 (1965).

51. J. Tohoku, Cellular immunity with special reference to monocytes of mice immunized with live vaccine of *Salmonella enteritidis. J. Exp. Med.,* **89,** 307–314 (1966).

52. S. Mitsuhashi, K. Saito, N. Osawa, and S. Kurashige, Monocyte immunity and its transfer agent of RNA nature. *Subviral Carcinogen.,* **1,** 265–272 (1967).

53. S. Mitsuhashi, K. Saito, N. Osawa, and S. Kurashige, Experimental Salmonellosis. XI. Induction of cellular immunity and formation of antibody by transfer agent of mouse mononuclear phagocytes. *J. Bacteriol.,* **94,** 907–913 (1967).

54. F. O. Araujo and J. S. Remington, Protection against *toxoplasma gondii* in mice immunized with *toxoplasma* cell fractions, RNA and synthetic polyribonucleotides. *Immunology,* **27,** 711–721 (1974).

55. M. L. Barr, E. J. Cabrer, P. H. Silverman, and J. E. Heidrich, Transfer of immunity to *plasmodium berghei* by spleen and lymph node immune RNA. *Cell. Immunol.,* **33,** 447–451 (1977).

56. T. Han, J. L. Pauly, and A. Mittelman, Adoptive transfer of cell-mediated immunity to tuberculin using RNA from tuberculin-sensitive subjects. *Immunology,* **28,** 127–132 (1975).

57. H. B. Herscowitz and P. Stelos, The induction of bacteriophage-neutralizing antibody by mouse spleen immunogenic RNA. II. Evidence for the presence of *phage antigen* in immunogenic RNA. *J. Immunol.,* **105,** 779–782 (1970).

58. M. Fishman and F. L. Adler, The formation of immunogenic RNA-antigen complexes in a cell-free system. *Cell. Immunol.,* **8,** 221–234 (1973).

59. H. B. Herscowitz and P. Stelos, The induction of bacteriophage-neutralizing antibody by mouse spleen immunogenic RNA. *J. Immunol.,* **105,** 771–778 (1970).

60. C. C. Williams and W. G. Wu, Immunoparalysis induced by pneumococcal polysaccharide. *J. Immunol.,* **107,** 163–171 (1971).

61. J. S. Garvey, H. Rinderknecht, B. G. Weliky, and D. H. Campbell, The use of a nucleo-peptide fraction from injected rabbits to study the nature of antigen fragment RNA. *Immunochemistry,* **9,** 187-206 (1972).

62. K. Nakamura, The proliferation of plasma cells from mouse bone marrow *in vitro*. Stimulation of IgG-producing cells by an RNAase-sensitive thymocyte homogenate. *Cell. Immunol.*, **25**, 163–177 (1976).

63. L. Yuan and D. H. Campbell, The *in vivo* and *in vitro* immunogenicity and antigenic specificity of lymphoid antigen fragment-oligoribonucleopeptide conjugates. *Immunochemistry*, **9**, 1–8 (1972).

64. S. L. White and A. G. Johnson, Studies on the cellular site of action of macrophage RNA-antigen complexes. *Cell. Immunol.*, **21**, 56–69 (1976).

65. E. B. Reilly, and J. S. Garvey, Biological and chemical characterization of an immune antigen-RNA species derived from hepatocyte polysomes. *Cell. Immunol.*, **41**, 20–34 (1978).

66. D. S. Juras and P. Abramoff, *In vitro* induction of sulfanick acid-specific antibodies by RNA extracted from rat spleen. *J. Immunol.*, **105**, 1244–1252 (1970).

67. G. E. Roelants, J. N. Goodman, and H. O. McDevitt, Binding of a polypeptide antigen to ribonucleic acid from macrophage, hela, and escherichia coli cells. *J. Immunol.*, **106**, 1222–1226 (1971).

68. A. A. Gottlich, R. H. Schwartz, and S. R. Waldman, Competition between L- and D-synthetic copolymers at the level of the macrophage. *J. Immunol.*, **108**, 719–725 (1972).

69. S. I. Schlager, S. Dray, and R. E. Paque, Atomic spectroscopic evidence for the absence of a low-molecular-weight (486) antigen in RNA extracts shown to transfer delayed-type hypersensitivity *in vitro*. *Cell. Immunol.*, **14**, 104–122 (1974).

70. S. Arnott, W. Fuller, A. Hodgson, and I. Drutton, Molecular conformations and structure transitions of RNA complementary helices and their possible biological significance. *Nature*, **220**, 561–564 (1968).

71. M. L. Egan, R. P. Smyth, and P. H. Maurer, Association of polypeptides with ribonucleic acid. *J. Immunol.*, **107**, 540–546 (1971).

72. L. J. Duke, and S. Harshman, *In vitro* induction of anti-DNP antibody by immunogenic RNA from rabbit liver. *Immunochemistry*, **8**, 431–445 (1971).

73. B. S. Wang and J. A. Mannick, Fractionation of immune RNA capable of transferring tumor-specific cellular cytotoxicity. *Cell. Immunol.*, **37**, 358–368 (1978).

74. R. E. Paque and T. Nealow, A comparative study of RNA fractions mediating delayed sensitivity to a chemically defined antigen *in vitro*. *Cell. Immunol.*, **43**, 48–61 (1979).

75. P. Bilello, M. Fishman, and G. Koch, Evidence that immune RNA is messenger RNA. *Cell. Immunol.*, **23**, 309–319 (1976).

76. H. Mikami, M. Kanakami, and S. Mitsuhashi, Transfer agent of immunity. VII. Partial purification of immune ribonucleic acid. *Jap. J. Microbiol.*, **15**, 169–174 (1971).

77. T. Honjo, D. Swan, M. Nau, B. Norman, S. Packman, F. Polsky, and P. Leder, Purification and translation of an immunoglobulin α-chain messenger RNA from mouse myeloma. *Biochemistry*, **15**, 2775–2779 (1976).

78. R. E. Paque and T. Nealon, RNA extracts with polyadenylic acid sequences transfer specific sensitivity for a low molecular weight antigen (MW 486). *Cell. Immunol.*, **34**, 279–288 (1977).

79. C. J. Greenup, D. A. Vallera, K. J. Pennline, B. J. Kolodziej, and M. C. Dodd, Antitumor cytotoxicity of poly(A)-containing messenger RNA isolated from tumor-specific immunogenic RNA. *Br. J. Cancer*, **38**, 55–63 (1978).

80. R. E. Paque, Isolation and localization of RNA fractions able to transfer tumor-specific delayed hypersensitivity *in vitro*. *Cancer Res.*, **36**, 4530–4536 (1976).

81. D. H. Kern, N. Chon, and Y. H. Pilch, Kinetics of synthesis and immunologically active fraction of anti-tumor immune RNA. *Cell. Immunol.*, **24**, 58–68 (1976).

82. B. S. Wang, P. J. Deckers, and J. A. Mannick, Kinetics of the transfer of tumor-specific cytotoxicity with immune RNA. *Clin. Immunol. Immunopathol.*, **9**, 218,228 (1978).

83. B. S. Wang, S. R. Onikul, and J. A. Mannick, Identification of the principal cell type yielding immune RNA capable of transferring tumor-specific cellular cytotoxicity. *Cell. Immunol.,* **39**, 27–35 (1978).

84. D. H. Kern, N. Chon, and Y. H. Pilch, Lymphocyte populations participating in cellular antitumor immune responses mediated by immune RNA. *J. Natl. Cancer Inst.,* **60**, 335–344 (1978).

85. B. S. Wang and J. A. Mannick, Relationship between lymphocyte proliferation and tumor-specific cytotoxicity after immune RNA treatment. *J. Immunol.,* **123**, 1057–1061 (1979).

86. P. J. Kmieck, C. B. Bagwell, J. L. Hudson, and G. L. Irvin, Multiparameter kinetic analysis of killer cell initiation by using immune RNA. *J. Histochem. Cytochem.,* **27**, 491–495 (1979).

87. J. A. Mannick, Inhibition by RNA of the transfer reaction following homograft. *J. Clin. Invest.,* **43**, 740–748 (1964).

88. M. C. Niu, L. C. Niu, and A. Guha, The entrance of exogenous RNA into the mouse ascites cell. *Proc. Soc. Exp. Biol. Med.,* **128**, 550–555 (1968).

89. H. A. John, M. C. Birnstiel, and K. W. Jones, RNA-DNA hybrids at the cytological level. *Nature,* **223**, 582–587 (1969).

90. K. Saito and S. Mitsuhashi, Inhibitory effect of rifamycin derivatives of immunogenic RNA. *J. Antibiot.,* **25**, 477,479 (1972).

91. A. R. Wang, D. Giacomoni, and S. Dray, Physical and chemical characterization of RNA incorporated by rabbit spleen cells. *Exp. Cell. Res.,* **78**, 15–24 (1973).

92. G. M. Kolodny, Cell to cell transfer of RNA into transformed cells. *J. Cell. Physiol.,* **79**, 147–150 (1972).

93. D. H. Kern, J. B. deKernion, and Y. H. Pilch, Intracellular localization of anti-tumor immune RNA. *Cell. Immunol.,* **22**, 11–18 (1978).

94. M. K. Legler and E. P. Cohen, Estimation of the number of nucleotide sequences in mouse DNA complementary to messenger RNAs specifying a complete mouse immunoglobulin. *Biochemistry,* **15**, 4390–4399 (1976).

95. D. H. Levin, D. Kyner, G. Acs, and S. Silverstein, Messenger activity in mammalian cell-free extracts of reovirus single-stranded RNA prepared *in vitro. Biochem. Biophys. Res. Commun.,* **42**, 454–461 (1971).

96. S. Spiegelman, A. Burny, M. R. Das, J. Keyder, J. Schlom, M. Travnicek, and K. Watson, Characteriziation of the products of RNA-directed DNA polymerases in oncogenic RNA viruses. *Nature,* **227**, 563 (1970).

97. R. I. Near and V. Storb, RNA sequences homologous to the 3′ portion of immunoglobulin ν-chain mRNA in thymus-derived lymphocytes. *Biochemistry,* **18**, 964–972 (1979).

98. P. J. Deckers and Y. J. Pilch, Transfer of immunity to tumour isografts by the systemic administration of xenogeneic "immune" RNA. *Nature New Biol.,* **231**, 181–182 (1971).

99. S. I. Schlager and S. Dray, Tumor regression at an untreated site during immunotherapy of an identical distant tumor. *Proc. Natl. Acad. Science,* **72**, 3680–3682 (1975).

100. J. B. deKernion, K. P. Ramming, P. Brower, D. G. Skinner, and Y. H. Pilch, Immunotherapy for malignant lesions in man using immunogenic ribonucleic acid. *Am. J. Surg.,* **130**, 575–578 (1975).

101. Y. H. Pilch, D. Fritze, J. B. deKernion, K. P. Ramming, and D. A. Kern, Immunotherapy of cancer with immune RNA in animal models and cancer patients. *Ann. N. Y. Acad. Sci.,* **277**, 592–608 (1976).

102. Y. J. Pilch, J. B. deKernion, D. G. Skinner, K. P. Ramming, P. M. Schick, D. Fritze, P. Brower, and D. H. Kern, Immunotherapy of cancer with "immune" RNA. *Am. J. Surg.,* **132**, 631–637 (1976).

103. K. P. Ramming and J. B. DeKernion, Immune RNA therapy for renal cell carcinoma: Survival and immunologic monitoring. *Ann. Surg.,* **186**, 459–467 (1977).

104. Y. H. Pilch, K. P. Ramming, and J. B. deKernion, Preliminary studies of specific immunotherapy of cancer with immune RNA. *Cancer,* **40**, 2747–2757 (1977).

105. P. J. Deckers, B. S. Wang, and J. A. Mannick, Immunotherapy of murine tumors with immune RNA. *Ann. N. Y. Acad. Sci.,* **277**, 575–591 (1976).

106. B. S. Wang, S. R. Onikul, and J. A. Mannick, Prevention of death from metastases by immune RNA therapy. *Science,* **202**, 59–60 (1978).

107. B. S. Wang, G. Steele, Jr., J. A. Mannick, M. Fallon, and S. R. Onikul, *In vivo* effects and parallel *in vitro* cytotoxicity of splenocytes harvested from treated or control C57BL/6J mice after adjuvant immunotherapy of pulmonary metastases using xenogeneic RNA specific to B16 murine melanoma. *Cancer Res.,* **39**, 1702–1707 (1979).

108. G. Steele, Jr., J. Richie, B. S. Wang, J. A. Mannick, and R. E. Wilson. Increased immunogenicity of B16 melanoma clones selected for their ability to metastasize from a heterogeneous primary tumor. *Surg. Forum,* **30**, 132 (1979).

109. G. Steele, Jr., B. S. Wang, G. Ghavamzadah, M. Fallon, J. Richie, R. E. Wilson, and J. A. Mannick, Antigenic differences among B16 melanoma variants selected for their differing abilities to metastasize: a possible mechanism for effective adjuvant immunotherapy. *J. Surg. Oncol.,* **15**, 71 (1980).

110. G. Steele, Jr., B. S. Wang, J. Richie, T. Ervin, R. Yankee, and J. A. Mannick, Results of xenogeneic I-RNA therapy in patients with metastatic renal cell carcinoma. *Cancer,* **47**, 1286 (1981).

111. G. Steele, Jr., B. S. Wang, J. Richie, R. E. Wilson, T. Ervin, R. Yankee, M. Fallon, and J. A. Mannick, *In vivo* effect and parallel *in vitro* lymphocyte-mediated tumor cytolysis after Phase I xenogeneic I-RNA treatment of patients with widespread melanoma or metastatic renal cell carcinoma. *Cancer Res.,* **40**, 2377 (1980).

112. H. S. Lawrence, The transfer in humans of delayed skin sensitivity to streptococcal M substance and to tuberculin with disrupted leukocytes. *J. Clin. Invest.,* **34**, 219–230 (1955).

113. H. S. Lawrence and A. M. Pappenheimer, Transfer of delayed hypersensitivity to diptheria toxin in man. *J. Exp. Med.,* **104**, 321–336 (1956).

114. P. Baram and M. M. Mosko, A dialysable fraction from tuberculin-sensitive human white blood cells capable of inducing tuberculin-delayed hypersensitivity in negative recipients. *Immunology,* **8**, 461–474 (1965).

115. K. S. Zuckerman, J. A. Neidhart, S. P. Balcerzak, and A. F. LoBugle, Immunologic specificity of transfer factor. *J. Clin. Invest.,* **54**, 997–1000 (1974).

116. P. Fireman, M. Boesman, Z. H. Haddad, and D. Gitlin, Passive transfer of tuberculin reactivity *in vitro. Science,* **155**, 337–338 (1966).

117. M. S. Ascher, W. J. Schneider, F. T. Valentine, and H. S. Lawrence, *In vitro* properties of leukocyte dialysates containing transfer factor. *Proc. Natl. Acad. Science,* **74**, 1178–1182 (1974).

118. B. Dupont, M. Ballon, J. A. Hansen, C. Quick, E. J. Yunis, and R. A. Good, Effects of transfer factor therapy on mixed lymphocyte culture reactivity. *Proc. Natl. Acad. Science,* **71**, 867–871 (1974).

119. P. Baram and W. Condoulis, The *in vitro* transfer of delayed hypersensitivity to rhesus monkey and human lymphocytes with transfer factor obtained from rhesus monkey peripheral white blood cells. *J. Immunol.,* **104**, 769–779 (1970).

120. S. F. Maddison, M. D. Hicklin, B. P. Conway, and I. G. Kagan, Transfer factor: Delayed hypersensitivity to schistosoma mansoni and tuberculin in macaca mulatta. *Science,* **178**, 757–759 (1972).

121. J. M. Anelli and W. H. Adler, Transfer factor—transfer of tuberculin cutaneous sensitivity in an allogeneic and xenogeneic monkey model. *Cell. Immunol.,* **15**, 475–478 (1975).

122. M. P. Arala-Chaves, E. G. Lebalq, and J. F. Heremans, Fractionation of human leukocyte extracts transferring delayed hypersensitivity to tuberculin. *Internatl. Arch. Allergy,* **31**, 353–365 (1967).

123. A. A. Gottlieb, L. G. Foster, and S. R. Waldman, What is transfer factor? *Lancet*, **2**, 822–823 (1973).

124. C. Griscelli, J. P. Revillard, H. Betvel, C. Herzog, and J. L. Touraine, Transfer factor therapy in immunodeficiencies. *Biomedicine*, **18**, 220–227 (1973).

125. J. Wybran, A. S. Levin, L. E. Spitler, and H. H. Fudenberg, Rosette-forming cells, immunologic deficiency diseases and transfer factor. *New Engl. J. Med.*, **288**, 710–713 (1973).

126. H. F. Oettgen, L. J. Old, J. H. Farrow, F. T. Valentine, H. S. Lawrence, and L. Thomas, Effects of dialyzable transfer factor in patients with breast cancer. *Proc. Natl. Acad. Science*, **71**, 2319–2323 (1974).

127. J. A. Neidhart and S. LoBuglio, Transfer factor therapy of malignancy. *Semin. Oncol.*, **1**, 379–385. (1974).

128. A. S. Levin, V. S. Byers, H. H. Fudenberg, J. Wybran, A. J. Hackett, J. O. Johnston, and L. E. Spitler, Immunologic parameters before and during immunotherapy with tumor-specific transfer factor. *J. Clin. Invest.*, **55**, 487–499 (1975).

129. M. S. Ascher, A. A. Gottlieb, and C. H. Kirkpatrick, *Transfer Factor: Basic Properties and Clinical Applications*, Academic, New York, 1976.

130. C. G. Moertel, Chemotherapy of gastrointestinal cancer. *New Engl. J. Med.*, **299**, 1049–1052 (1978).

Monoclonal Antibodies: Prospects for Cancer Treatment

IRWIN D. BERNSTEIN
ROBERT C. NOWINSKI
PETER W. WRIGHT
*Pediatric Oncology, Tumor Virology,
Medical Oncology, and Tumor Immunology
Fred Hutchinson Cancer Research Center
Seattle, Washington
Departments of Pediatrics, Microbiology, and Medicine
University of Washington
Seattle, Washington*

This work was supported in part by Grant CA 26386 from the National Cancer Institute.

1. INTRODUCTION

The use of immune serum for treating neoplastic disease has been considered for many years. Definite therapeutic effects of antisera, particularly for leukemias and lymphomas, have been observed in animals. Objective antitumor effects of tumor-immune sera have also been reported in humans, although these effects have typically been short-lived or of trivial or no clinical importance. The reasons for the limited effectiveness of serum treatment have not been fully explored, however, and the failure to demonstrate clinically important antitumor effects of antibody could presumably be due to the use of antibodies in insufficient quantities or antibodies of an inappropriate specificity, low avidity, or inactive isotype. With the recent development of techniques of somatic cell hybridization, which can be used for the production of hybridomas, virtually unlimited amounts of monoclonal antibody of defined specificity and isotype can now be produced for clinical trials. The use of these antibodies should allow characterization of the mechanism by which antibody can influence tumor growth *in vivo*, as well as permit a critical assessment of their therapeutic potential.

Monoclonal antibodies selected for studies of their therapeutic potential ideally would react with antigens present exclusively on tumor cells, and not on normal cells. Unfortunately, monoclonal antibodies detecting antigens unique to malignant cell surfaces have yet to be convincingly demonstrated. Nonetheless, antibodies reactive with normal differentiation antigens expressed by tumor cells are presently available for clinical investigation. Antibodies that detect differentiation or organ-specific antigens on tumor cells may have potential therapeutic efficacy, provided that the destruction of normal cells that may result from the use of such antibodies can be tolerated by the host with acceptable toxicity.

The purpose of this chapter is to evaluate the prospects of antibody therapy of neoplastic diseases. Several reviews concerning past experience with serotherapy using conventional complex antisera have been published (1–4). Because of this and because of numerous recent developments concerning hybridoma-produced monoclonal antibodies, this chapter is intended to provide only an initial brief review of past studies that have used complex antisera followed by a more detailed consideration of recent studies involving the development and therapeutic use of hybridoma-produced monoclonal antibodies. We restrict this discussion to antibodies that may directly affect tumor and do not consider the more speculative use of antibody to eliminate T-cell subsets that may inhibit host antitumor responses.

2. SEROTHERAPY WITH THE USE OF CONVENTIONAL COMPLEX ANTISERA

2.1. Animal Tumor Model Systems

Serotherapy of allogeneic tumors has been extensively investigated (5,6). In now classical experiments initiated in the 1940s and 1950s, it was demonstrated that passively administered antibodies (depending on their method of preparation) could result either in enhancement or inhibition of tumor growth. Fractionation of hyperimmune mouse sera produced against allogeneic tumor cell antigens demonstrated that immunoglobulin G (IgG) was responsible for enhancement and immunoglobulin M (IgM) for inhibition of tumor growth *in vivo* (7), although more recent exceptions have been reported (8,9). Similar observations were later made in syngeneic tumor systems. For example, 19S fractions (presumably IgM antibodies) of antiserum obtained from mice hyperimmunized with syngeneic methylcholanthrene-induced sarcomas resulted in inhibition of tumor growth, whereas 7S fractions (presumably IgG antibodies) of the same antiserum resulted in acceleration of tumor growth (10).

Growth inhibition after treatment with immune sera has been predictably observed for several tumors of lymphoid origin. For example, Old et al. (11) demonstrated that passive immunization with antisera prepared against syngeneic Gross virus-positive leukemia cells in inbred rats protected mice against the growth of a syngeneic Gross virus-induced leukemia. The protective effects of serum treatment were dose related, and significant inhibitory effects of the antiserum could be seen as late as 3 days after intravenous inoculation of leukemia cells. Under certain circumstances 100% of serum-treated mice could be completely protected by immune serum treatment. Inhibitory effects of serum have been reported for numerous lymphoid and hematopoietic tumors (12–35) and several nonlymphoid tumors, including adenocarcinomas of breast (36–37) and ovary (38), melanomas (39), neuroblastomas (40), hepatomas (41,42), and virus-induced sarcomas (43–51).

The nature of the antigens that serve as the targets for the inhibitory effect of antibody has never been explicitly defined. Studies with virus-induced tumors have indicated that both virus and nonvirus antigens may serve as targets for tumor growth inhibition by antibody. For example, Schafer et al. (30) showed that the viral envelope glycoprotein gp70 was of particular importance for antibody-mediated inhibition of F-MuLV and R-MuLV (Friend and

Rauscher murine leukemia virus) induced tumors in mice. Antibodies to gp70 protected mice against massive infection with either F-MuLV or Rauscher leukemia virus (R-MuLV), provided that the treatment was initiated not later than 6 to 7 days after viral infection. It has also been established that antibodies directed at virus-coded nonvirion antigens can also result in inhibition of tumor growth. For example, sera obtained from chickens immunized with the reticuloendotheliosis (RE) virus contain antiviral antibodies and have the ability to inhibit virus-induced tumor growth when passively administered to normal birds (52). Removal of antiviral antibodies by absorption with whole virus had no effect on the inhibitory activity of the serum. By contrast, absorption with RE virus-induced tumor cells completely removed all *in vivo* antitumor activity.

In the context of this discussion it is important to note that treatment with antibodies against other cell surface components has also been attempted with some success. Treatment with monospecific antibody to alphafetoprotein (AFP) resulted in decreased AFP production and inhibition of an AFP-secreting hepatoma (41). In another instance, the feasibility of treatment with antibodies against organ-specific antigens was demonstrated using an antiserum against organ-specific antigens expressed by normal and malignant ovarian cells (38).

The role of antibody in treating naturally occurring neoplasms deserves special comment. All the evidence cited in the preceding paragraphs has concerned the effects of antibodies on long-transplanted tumors and only on a few primary tumors that were induced in the laboratory. The question of the role of antibody in the prevention and/or therapy of naturally occurring spontaneous neoplasms has not been extensively studied. In this context evidence is now available suggesting that antibodies to the feline oncornavirus-associated cell membrane antigen (FOCMA) are of principal importance in the prevention of FeLV-related malignancies in cats under natural conditions (53–58). Epidemiologic studies have demonstrated that healthy cats from leukemia clusters or cats purposefully placed in a leukemia cluster household have a high incidence of exposure to FeLV (54,55), whereas healthy cats isolated from virus-positive carrier cats have a low risk of virus exposure (56). In these studies a correlation was observed between the presence of antibodies to FOCMA and tumor progression. In a prospective epidemiological study on healthy cats from a single large leukemia cluster household it was noted that cats that subsequently developed leukemia or lymphoma had lower FOCMA antibody titers than did cats that remained healthy in the same household. Cats that remained healthy for a 2.5-year observation period had mean titers of FOCMA antibody that were tenfold higher than those of cats that developed leukemia (57). In more recent studies cats with spontaneous lymphosarcoma have been treated with feline blood products. In one trial eight of nine cats receiving normal cat serum had either complete or partial regression of their disease. There were no responses observed in three cats receiving leukemic cat serum (58).

Evidence suggests that the antitumor effect of cat serum could be attributed to FOCMA antibody. Complete regressions were observed in 8 of 15 cats receiving small amounts (2 to 5 ml administered three times per week for 2 weeks) of a higher-titer FOCMA antiserum. The amount of complement activity present in these small volumes of sera was thought to be insufficient to explain its antitumor effects (unpublished observations).

2.2.   Serotherapy of Human Cancer

Initial reports of attempted serotherapy for the treatment of human cancer appeared in the late nineteenth century. Although most observations reported (often describing dramatic clinical improvement after serotherapy) remain unsubstantiated, several more recent studies have demonstrated unambiguous effects of passively administered antiserum on the growth of human neoplasms. Laszlo et al. (59) treated patients with chronic lymphocytic leukemia by infusion of plasma containing anti-HLA antibodies. Multiple infusions of five different antisera obtained from donors immunized with normal lymphocytes were administered in volumes ranging from 20 to 200 ml in three patients. A prompt reduction in the number of leukemic lymphocytes in the peripheral blood was observed within 24 hours following transfusion. The effects of antiserum treatment were usually short-lived, with leukemic blood cell counts returning to preinfusion levels within a few days. In one patient, however, leukemic cell counts were reduced for several weeks. Similar results with alloantisera were observed by Herberman et al. (60). In a more recent study treatment of a patient with Sezary's syndrome (a diffuse, undifferentiated lymphoma of T-cell origin) with antithymocyte globulin was associated with a 75% reduction in adenopathy and complete resolution of skin erythema (61). These effects were observed despite the patient's previous extensive treatment with electron beam radiation and combination chemotherapy.

Serotherapy has been most extensively evaluated in patients with malignant melanoma. Interest in serotherapy of malignant melanoma was stimulated by an early report of Sumner and Foraker (62) demonstrating complete regression of metastatic melanoma in a patient receiving 250 ml of whole blood from a patient who had previously undergone a spontaneous regression of melanoma. A similar experience was also later reported by Teimourian and McCune (63), who described partial regression of pulmonary metastases in a patient transfused with blood (amount unspecified) from a donor with a melanoma of the back and bilateral axillary metastases in remission 10 years following surgery. However, a more recent and systematic attempt to evaluate serotherapy in patients with malignant melanoma has failed to demonstrate any objective benefit of this approach (64). Nevertheless, the result of serotherapy trials indicate that certain human cancers, particularly leukemias and lymphomas, are at least potentially responsive to treatment with passively administered antiserum.

2.3. Conclusions Concerning Serum Therapy of Malignant Disease with the Use of Complex Antisera

Several generalizations can be drawn from previous studies of serotherapy both in animal models and humans:

1. Passively administered antisera can have inhibitory effects on tumor growth *in vivo*.

2. These inhibitory effects, however, are generally transient, and permanent tumor cure is rarely achieved.

3. The effects are quantitative. Inhibitory effects of antibody are usually seen only when the antiserum is administered coincidently with, or shortly after, a small inoculum of tumor cells. Frequently, no effects may be observed if the antiserum treatment is delayed, or the size of the tumor inoculum is increased.

4. Inhibitory effects are more readily demonstrable with leukemias and/or lymphomas than with solid tumors. Concern exists that antisera may be more likely to enhance rather than inhibit the growth of solid tumors.

5. Inhibitory effects of antisera have typically been demonstrated with virus- or chemically-induced tumors of demonstrable antigenicity that have long been established through many transplant generations. The relevance of studies with such tumors to spontaneously occurring neoplasms has been much debated. In this context, therefore, the results of recent studies showing regression of feline leukemias and lymphomas after treatment with FOCMA antibodies are of particular interest.

3. DEVELOPMENT OF HYBRIDOMA-PRODUCED MONOCLONAL ANTIBODIES

The recent development of techniques for the production of monoclonal antibodies promises to revolutionize future approaches to serotherapy. Kohler and Milstein (65,66) first demonstrated the feasibility of establishing permanent antibody-producing hybrid cell lines. These cell lines have been prepared by fusion of lymphocytes from immune donors with myeloma cells in the presence of Sendai virus or polyethylene glycol (PEG). The fused hybrid cells produce the immunoglobulin chains of both parent cells, and it is possible by appropriate selection to isolate cell lines that produce antibodies of a desired specificity. Subsequently, hybrid cells that synthesize antibody can be cloned and inoculated into syngeneic animals where they produce tumors (hybridomas) that secrete extremely high levels (5 to 40 mg/ml) of monoclonal antibodies into the serum or ascites fluid.

The technical details of the hybridization procedure and various modifications are available from several sources (67,68). In brief, azaguanine-resistant or bromodeoxyuridine-resistant mouse myeloma cells that lack the enzyme hypoxanthine-guanine phosphoribosyl transferase or thymidine kinase, respectively, and are unable to grow in selective medium, containing hypoxanthine, amethopterin, and thymidine (HAT) are fused in the presence (69–71) of PEG with immune lymphoid cells. Myeloma-lymphoid cell hybrids possess the enzyme from the parent lymphocyte and are identified by their ability to grow under the selective conditions utilized. Hybridoma cells are cloned and can be selected for their capacity to produce antibody of a desired specificity. The probability of isolating hybrid clones producing antibody of a given specificity is greatly enhanced by the fact that lymphoid cells obtained from recently immunized donors undergo preferential fusion with mouse myeloma cells at frequencies several orders of magnitude greater than do nonimmune lymphoid cells. This hybridization technique has already been utilized to produce monoclonal antibodies against a variety of tumor cell-surface antigens potentially useful for therapeutic purposes.

3.1. Monoclonal Antibodies Reactive with Human Tumor Cell-Surface Antigens

Hybridoma-produced monoclonal antibodies have been developed against several different human tumors and human tumor cell lines, including malignant melanoma (72–76), neuroblastoma (77,78), colorectal carcinoma (79), and leukemias and lymphomas (80–84). Here we focus on the most extensively studied malignancies, melanomas and leukemias.

Melanoma-Associated Antigens. A variety of antigens have been detected by using monoclonal antibodies produced against human melanomas. Koprowski et al. (72) fused splenic lymphocytes obtained from mice immunized against the human melanoma cell line SW691 with the BALB/C myeloma cell line P3-63AG8. Antibody-producing hybridomas were screened for reactivity with a panel of melanoma and nonmelanoma tumor cell lines and normal cell lines. Nine antibodies with antimelanoma activity were described. Eight of these nine showed cross-reactivity with colorectal carcinoma and normal human cell lines. One of the antibodies, 691-13, however, showed reactivity that was restricted to the immunizing melanoma cell line 691 and two additional melanoma cell lines but had no demonstrable reactivity against the other tumor and normal cell lines included in the test panel. These results indicated that hybridoma-produced monoclonal antibodies may be developed that detect common melanoma-associated antigens. In subsequent studies with these hybridomas, selected monoclonal melanoma antibodies were found to mediate antibody-dependent cell-mediated cytotoxicity (ADCC) reactions against melanoma cell lines *in vitro* and to inhibit the growth of melanoma xenografts in nude mice (86).

Yeh and associates (73) used a similar scheme to produce monoclonal antibodies against the human melanoma cell line M1804. Three hybrid cell lines were developed that produced antibodies that bound to the immunizing M1804 melanoma, but not to autologous skin fibroblasts. Extensive specificity testings of two of these antibodies indicated that they reacted strongly with the M1804 cell line and to a much weaker (although significant degree) with two additional melanoma cell lines, M1801 and SKMEL28, and with one breast carcinoma cell line, CO295. No reactivity with these antibodies was observed, however, against a large panel of additional cell lines. The panel included 9 melanoma cell lines, 11 nonmelanoma tumor cell lines, and 11 fibroblast cell lines. It was concluded from these studies that hybridoma-produced monoclonal antibodies can be developed that identify cell surface antigens expressed by a small proportion of melanoma cell lines.

In a series of recent studies immunochemical methods have been used to explicitly identify antigens detected by hybridoma-produced monoclonal melanoma antibodies. Woodbury et al. (74) have reported that hybridoma 4.1 generated by fusion of spleen cells from mice immunized against the melanoma cell line SKMEL28 with the myeloma cell line NS1 produced a monoclonal IgG_1 immunoglobulin that identified a cell membrane protein of 97,000 molecular weight. This antigen (p97) was found to be present in high concentrations in cell membrane extracts from the immunizing melanoma cell line, but not from autologous fibroblasts. This antigen was also identified in other melanoma and some nonmelanoma tumor cell lines and in biopsy material from patients with melanoma and one patient with breast carcinoma. No p97 was found, however, in surgical samples of eight normal adult human tissues. Brown et al. (75) have utilized similar immunoprecipitation techniques to describe eight distinct antigens present on the human melanoma cell line KZ-2. One of these was identical to the p97 antigen previously described by Woodbury. Another antigen, p80, like p97, was present on the immunizing melanoma cell line but was not detected on autologous fibroblasts. In recent studies Brown et al. (76) have developed two sensitive radioimmunoassays (RIAs) to quantitate the expression of the p97 antigen in cultured cells and in surgical samples of neoplastic and normal adult and fetal tissues. These studies have indicated that although p97 may be detected in small amounts in normal adult tissues, it is present in much larger amounts in most melanomas and often to a significant but lesser degree in nonmelanoma tumors and fetal tissues.

Because of the difference in the quantitative expression of p97 between neoplastic and normal adult cells, p97 may represent a useful marker for tumor diagnosis and therapy with the use of monoclonal antibodies. In preliminary studies, ^{125}I-labeled anti-p97 antibodies have shown significant tumor localization when injected intravenously in athymic nude mice transplanted with human melanoma xenografts expressing p97 (P. W. Wright et al., unpublished observation). These studies suggest the possibility of tumor imaging with radiolabeled anti-p97 monoclonal antibodies in patients with malignant melanoma and possibly other human tumors that express the p97 antigen.

Leukemia-Associated Antigens. Monoclonal antibody techniques are currently being applied in a number of laboratories for the study of human leukemia-associated antigens. In most instances the monoclonal antibodies produced thus far have been shown to be reactive with both the malignant cell lines used for immunization and subpopulations of normal lymphoid cells, indicating that they represent antibodies directed at normally occurring antigens rather than antigens uniquely associated with leukemia (80–84). There is, however, at least one antigen detected on lymphoma cells that remains as a candidate for tumor-specific determinant (85).

A major question with respect to immunodiagnosis of leukemia and lymphoma is to what extent phenotypically distinct subsets defined by these monoclonal antibodies represent clinically distinct groups. This will be of particular importance if the prognosis of the subgroups is sufficiently disparate that they require significantly different therapeutic approaches. Monoclonal antibodies have already been used to define phenotypically distinct subsets within the T-, B-, or non-T- non-B-(null) cell acute lymphocytic leukemias. It is clear that antibodies detecting T-cell differentiation antigens can be used to define subtypes of T-cell leukemias. For example, Rheinherz et al. (82) have used a series of monoclonal antibodies reactive with T-cell differentiation antigens. These antibodies have detected functionally distinct subsets of normal T-cells (helper cell, suppressor cell, etc.) and have shown a variety of antigenic patterns displayed by different T-cell leukemias. There is less evidence as to the extent to which null leukemias can be subdivided. Most null-cell leukemias, including those with the best prognoses, express the common acute lymphocytic leukemia (ALL) antigen (87); monoclonal antibodies against this antigen are now available (83). Recent data have suggested that the use of antibodies to thymocytes (81) as well as to neuroblastoma cells (84) may be useful in defining phenotypically distinct subsets of common ALL.

4. TREATMENT OF TUMORS WITH MONOCLONAL ANTIBODY

Antibodies against tumor-associated antigens are now available for therapeutic trials. A review of experimental and clinical data using these antibodies is presented in the paragraphs that follow. We examine recent laboratory data demonstrating a role for monoclonal antibody treatment directed against normal differentiation antigens and the clinical evidence demonstrating the feasibility of administering these antibodies to patients with cancer. The potential role of monoclonal antibodies in combination with bone marrow transplantation and as carriers of drugs or radioactive isotopes is also briefly discussed.

4.1. Treatment of Experimental Tumors

A series of studies designed to evaluate the use of monoclonal antibodies against a normal differentiation antigen for the treatment of murine leukemias has been initiated by Bernstein et al. (88,89). In these studies monoclonal antibodies of different immunoglobulin isotypes with specificity against a normal T-cell antigen, Thy-1.1, have been used to treat transplantable and spontaneous T-cell leukemias in AKR mice. Results of studies examining the effectiveness of these antibodies and their mechanisms of action, their biodistribution in the host, and factors that may limit antibody effectiveness are summarized in the following paragraphs.

In initial experiments the passive administration of IgG_{2a} monoclonal antibody resulted in prolonged survival and a significant cure rate in mice challenged with a lethal inoculum of leukemia cells (88). For example, AKR/J mice carrying a transplant of 10^5 AKR/J SL2 syngeneic leukemic cells were cured of disease by a combination of ascites fluid containing IgG_{2a} anti-Thy-1.1 antibody and rabbit serum (as a source of complement). In this study treatment consisted of an intravenous infusion of 100 μl of ascites fluid and 100 μl of complement 1 to 2 hours after the tumor challenge and intraperitoneal inoculation of 50 μl of ascites fluid and complement on days 3, 7, 10, and 14. In contrast, mice that were not treated or that received complement alone all expired. Moreover, surviving mice showed no obvious side effects as a result of the presumed interaction of the anti-T-cell antibody and their normal T cells. Hence this particular experiment demonstrated that monoclonal antibody directed against a normal differentiation antigen could influence tumor growth *in vivo* without significant adverse effects.

The availability of monoclonal antibodies also enabled a precise analysis of the antitumor activity and mechanisms of action of antibody of distinct subclasses. Significant differences were observed in the ability of antibodies of different isotypes to mediate antitumor effects *in vitro* and *in vivo*. Monoclonal antibodies of the IgG_{2a} and IgG_3 isotype lysed tumor cell targets *in vitro* either in combination with complement or with nonimmune effector cells. In contrast, IgM antibodies were lytic only in combination with complement. These differences associated with antibody isotype were also observed *in vivo* where the IgG_{2a} antibodies demonstrated significant antitumor effects, whereas equivalent amounts of IgM antibodies failed to exert a discernable influence on tumor growth or recovery from disease; the effects of the IgG_3 antibodies were intermediate. These differences thus suggested that cell-dependent, and not complement-dependent, cytotoxicity may be of primary importance *in vivo*.

Additional studies have also indicated that antibody does not require the participation of complement in inhibiting metastatic disease. In these experiments groups of AKR mice were treated with the IgG_{2a} antibody alone or in combination with complement. The results showed that mice treated with antibody alone experienced the same median survival as did mice treated with the same antibody in combination with complement. Since these mice are known to be deficient in the fifth component of complement, the effectiveness of antibody alone and the lack of an effect with exogenous complement suggests that antibody inhibits the development of systemic disease primarily by combining with nonimmune effector cells rather than complement. This would explain the association of *in vivo* effects only with antibodies that mediated cell-dependent cytotoxicity (IgG_{2a}, IgG_3, and not IgM). There may, however, be some amplification by complement of antibody-mediated effects against solid tumor, rather than metastases, since in some experiments the addition of complement caused a decreased incidence of solid lymphomas at the site of tumor inoculation.

Differences in the effectiveness of antibody of differing isotype may also reflect variation in antibody half-life or distribution in tissues. For example, the failure of IgM to mediate antitumor effects may have resulted from its short half-life, which is significantly less than that of IgG_{2a} molecules *in vivo* (90). To control this variable, IgM antibodies were administered frequently (in some experiments every other day), but antitumor effects were still not observed.

Studies on the biodistribution of antibody in tissues have revealed the existence of sites in which tumor may escape antibody-mediated destruction. A careful assessment of the biodistribution of a homogeneous antibody of IgG_{2a} subclass in AKR mice has demonstrated an initially high uptake of antibody in lymph node, spleen, liver, kidney, and stomach (90). In contrast, relatively small amounts of antibody entered the thymus, brain, skin, and testes. In this particular experiment, where small amounts of radiolabeled antibodies were infused, the existence of potential "sanctuary" sites in which tumor cells may escape antibody-mediated lysis was demonstrated. Whether there are differences in the sites that can serve as sanctuaries in the case of other immunoglobulin isotypes as compared to the IgG_{2a} antibody requires determination. Moreover, differences in distribution between antibody isotypes and the extent to which these differences may contribute to differences in effectiveness between these isotypes remains to be investigated. In this context it should be noted that sanctuary sites may also occur as a result of impaired access of cofactors required for antibody-mediated lysis, such as complement or effector cells. For example, when high doses of anti-Thy-1 antibody were administered to AKR/J mice, a significant depletion of peripheral T-cells, but not thymocytes, was observed. The thymocytes, however, were coated with the infused antibody *in vivo* and when incubated *in vitro* with complement, showed virtually complete lysis.

The limitations on the effectiveness of antibody also require consideration. The existence of "sanctuary" sites in which cells can escape antibody have been discussed previously. In addition, there also appears to exist within a given population of tumor cells antigen-negative variants that are insusceptible to antibody-mediated lysis. For example, a certain proportion of mice inoculated with a relatively high dose of SL2 leukemia cells and treated continuously (twice weekly) with anti-Thy-1 antibody developed systemic leukemia. When the leukemic cells were obtained from these mice and examined for Thy-1 expression, the results showed that the metastatic leukemic cells were variants lacking the Thy-1 antigen. Moreover, on subsequent passage, these leukemic cells remained Thy-1 negative, demonstrating them to be stable genetic variants (unpublished observation). Importantly, these results suggest that antibody therapy should be most effective when antibodies directed against different antigenic determinants are used in combination.

4.2.   Treatment of Human Tumors

There have been attempts to treat leukemias with monoclonal antibody reactive with leukemia-associated antigens. Perhaps the best documented is the experience of Ritz et al. (91), who treated ALL with monoclonal antibodies against the common ALL antigen. This antigen, first described by Greaves et al. (87) using a heteroantiserum, is expressed by leukemic cells from a proportion of patients with ALL that express neither T-cell markers nor surface immunoglobulin; the antigen is also expressed by a small proportion of bone marrow cells in normal individuals. Ritz et al. (83) have produced a cytotoxic IgG_2 monoclonal antibody reactive with the common ALL antigen designated J-5. This antibody has been used to treat a series of patients with common ALL-positive leukemia who had experienced multiple relapses. In these studies side effects were minimal and consisted solely of fevers. In an initial patient a significant reduction in circulating lymphoblasts occurred following infusion of 5 mg/kg of the J-5 antibody given over a 4-hour period. The patient received additional doses of antibody (10 mg/kg) at 24 and 48 hours. By the third day the circulating lymphoblast count began to rise, and lymphoblasts obtained from peripheral blood and bone marrow did not express the common ALL antigen. In fact, loss of reactivity of the patient's leukemic cells with the J-5 antibody was observed at 90 minutes after the start of the initial infusion. Interestingly, 8 days after initiation of therapy and at a time when the patient was no longer in antibody excess, the cells once again expressed the common ALL antigen. The rapidity of the changes which were observed in common ALL antigen expression suggests that its absence on exposure to J-5 antibody may occur as a result of "antigenic modulation," which has been confirmed by subsequent *in vitro* studies.

Nadler et al. (85,92) infused monoclonal antibody against a lymphoma-associated antigen into a patient (N. B.) with a diffuse poorly differentiated B-cell lymphoma resistant to drug therapy. The antibody (Ab89) mediated complement-dependent lysis and was reactive with a subset of B-cell non-Hodgkin's lymphoma, but not with the other normal and malignant target cells that were tested (85). Transient decreases in circulating tumor cells resulted from the antibody infusion in the absence of significant clinical toxicity. However, only small amounts of antibody were detected on the tumor cell surface, and free antibody was not detected in the serum. The observation that the amount of cell-free tumor antigen present in serum decreased following administration of large doses of antibody suggested that the antibody combined with the circulating antigen and was thereby prevented from binding in significant amounts to tumor cells. A transient decrease was noted in the creatinine clearance following each antibody infusion, and this presumably resulted from deposition of antigen-antibody complexes in the kidney.

The experience to date with monoclonal antibody therapy of human tumors has demonstrated the need to select, as targets, antigens that do not modulate on exposure to antibody and, as subjects, patients without large tumor burdens and circulating antigen. Nonetheless, these experiments have also demonstrated the feasibility of administering monoclonal antibody to patients with malignant diseases.

4.3.   Bone Marrow Transplantation

Monoclonal antibodies may be useful in situations where bone marrow transplantation has proved useful, such as acute leukemia, and where a histocompatible donor is not available. Marrow removed from the patient during remission could be treated with antibody and complement to remove contaminating tumor cells (93). After treatment of the patient with total body irradiation and drugs to eliminate residual tumor, the marrow could then be returned. Although it is not known whether reinfusion of contaminating tumor cells with the "autologous" marrow reinfusion would subsequently give rise to tumor recurrence, it will likely prove advantageous to eliminate any tumor cells present in the marrow. Of course, insusceptible antigen-negative tumor cell variants in the marrow may escape lysis, but if combinations of antibody against multiple cell-surface antigens are used to treat marrow cells from patients in remission, the probability that tumor cells will survive antibody-complement treatment and be reinfused with the marrow is highly improbable. Importantly, the antibody treatment used to eliminate tumor must not eliminate stem cells that are required for marrow engraftment.

An additional use of monoclonal antibodies will be to eliminate T cells from allogeneic bone marrow grafts in efforts to prevent the occurrence of graft-versus-host disease. This possibility has been suggested by the results of studies in mice showing that engraftment with marrow pretreated with anti-Thy-1 antibody can be obtained across major histocompatibility barriers without the occurrence of graft-versus-host disease (94,95). There are also preliminary clinical results suggesting that this approach may prevent graft-versus-host response in HLA-identical marrow transplants (96). Thus all individuals with or without histocompatible donors may benefit from marrow transplants.

4.4.   Monoclonal Antibodies as Carriers for Cytotoxic Agents

Antibody has been considered for use as a carrier that can localize conjugated drugs or isotopes at tumor sites, although results with the use of cytotoxic drugs or radioisotopes conjugated with heteroantisera have not been striking (97–99). This has possibly resulted from the fact that only a small percentage of antibodies in antisera raised by conventional techniques specifically combine with the tumor and that the specific antibody-drug or isotope conjugates may, on the other hand, localize in a highly efficient manner to the tumor. Thus the conjugated toxic agent may be delivered almost solely to the cells expressing the target antigen while avoiding nonspecific effects on cells otherwise susceptible to the cytotoxic agent.

Studies with radiolabeled monoclonal antibody have already demonstrated the exquisite ability of monoclonal antibody to localize at cells expressing the target antigen. For example, radiographic imaging methods have demonstrated a monoclonal antibody against teratocarcinoma cells to specifically localize into tumor tissues *in vivo* (100). Houston et al. (90) have examined the ability of homogenous IgG_{2a} monoclonal antibody against Thy-1.1 antigen to selectively bind to cells expressing the target antigen *in vivo*. Localization of this antibody was examined in AKR/J (Thy-1.1 mice) as compared to AKR/Cu (Thy 1.2) mice. Radiolabeled antibody selectively localized to lymphatic tissues; at optimal times (20 hours postinjection) the amount of radiolabel within lymph nodes of AKR/J mice was ninefold greater than in the lymph nodes of AKR/Cu mice. Localization of F(ab')$_2$ fragments of the antibody was even more striking. Although clearance of the F(ab')$_2$ from blood was extremely rapid, by 16 hours after injection there was a 144-fold greater amount of the antibody present in the lymph nodes of AKR/J mice than in those of AKR/Cu mice. When localization of the monoclonal anti-Thy-1.1 antibody versus nonimmune IgG_{2a} was examined, there was 475- and 250-fold greater amount of the specific antibody in spleen and lymph node, respectively, in AKR/J mice. Thus monoclonal antibodies against normal differentiation antigen Thy-1.1 localize in a highly selective manner to the appropriate target tissue *in vivo*, and the degree of selectivity is improved when F(ab')$_2$ fragments are used. These studies not only dramatically demonstrate the potential ability of monoclonal antibodies to deliver toxic agents to tumors but also demonstrate the exquisite *in vivo* specificity of these antibodies.

In the near future numerous studies examining the localization and antitumor effectiveness of monoclonal antibody conjugated with toxic agents will be forthcoming. Future studies using radiolabeled monoclonal antibodies for radioimaging should also provide an additional method of defining antibody specificity *in vivo*. These studies should define whether the injected antibodies localize preferentially to sites of tumor and also the extent to which normal cells share antigenic expression with tumor cells and can compete for the injected antibody.

5. CONCLUSIONS CONCERNING MONOCLONAL ANTIBODY TREATMENT OF MALIGNANT DISEASE

Monoclonal antibodies reactive with tumor-associated antigens are available for therapeutic purposes. Although clinical experiments have demonstrated the safety of administering these antibodies to recipients with cancer, their ultimate usefulness is unknown. Studies with mice have shown the effectiveness of antibody treatment directed at normal differentiation antigens expressed by tumor cells. They have also demonstrated the superiority of particular antibody isotypes and have defined factors that limit the effectiveness of antibody. These factors, which include the existence of "sanctuary" sites and insusceptible tumor cell variants, are also those that limit the effectiveness of chemotherapy. Thus monoclonal antibodies will likely prove useful as antitumor reagents but, as with drugs, will probably need to be used as combinations of antibodies to eliminate insusceptible variants and in conjunction with other therapies to eliminate tumor cells in sanctuary sites.

There is much additional information to be acquired before we can design clinical experiments that are most likely to be successful. In particular, we must elucidate the mechanisms by which antibody can influence tumor *in vivo*. With this information, we will know which cofactors are required for antibody-mediated effects and whether inadequate amounts of cofactors such as complement or effector cells (lymphocytes or macrophages) may limit the effectiveness of antibody. If deficiencies of required cofactors are identified, it may be possible to administer them along with the antibody. Alternatively, it may be possible to circumvent the need for cofactors and render antibody more effective by conjugating the antibodies to radioactive isotopes or cytotoxic drugs.

For the potential of antibody therapy to be fully realized, it will be necessary to produce monoclonal antibodies of human origin since, presumably, these antibodies could be administered for a longer period of time than mouse antibody without significant problems resulting from a host response. Recently, techniques for the production of human antibodies have become available. Human lymphoid cells can be fused with mouse (101) or human myeloma cells (102,103) and stable hybrid clones producing monoclonal antibody of defined specificity obtained.

Additional information regarding potentially limiting toxicities other than allergic responses that may result from antibody therapy is also needed. For example, immune complex formation may be of significance, as exemplified by the occurrence of a transient decrease in renal function observed in a serotherapy trial (92). Toxicity resulting from the effects of antibody on normal cells expressing the target determinant must also be assessed for each antibody that will be used therapeutically.

In addition to studies on the *in vivo* behavior of antibody, we should know more about the *in vivo* specificity of monoclonal antibodies against tumor-associated antigens. This is particularly true of monoclonal antibodies against nonlymphoid tumors where the specificity analyses of monoclonal antibodies have been limited to date primarily to *in vitro* studies with the use of established cell lines. Because of selection and/or adaption that may occur to cells in culture, antigenic expression of cells *in vitro* may not be accurately reflected *in vivo*. Thus specificity analyses of monoclonal antibodies should include studies performed on fresh suspensions or biopsies of normal and malignant cells. Attention should be given to the possibility that monoclonal antibodies that detect antigens on tumor cells may also identify antigens present on a subpopulation of normal cells that, although present in limited numbers, may nevertheless play an important biological role *in vivo*.

Further information about the antigens themselves may also lead to improved therapeutic approaches. As mentioned earlier, we need to specifically select, as targets for monoclonal antibody therapy, antigens that do not "modulate" on exposure to antibody. Further, an understanding of the biochemical pathways associated with antigenic expression may suggest ways to prevent modulation from occurring and render antibodies such as the anti-common ALL antibody effective therapeutic agents.

Perhaps the most critical information must come from studies that use antibody to treat naturally occurring disease. Does antibody induce remission alone or in combination with chemotherapeutic agents? To what extent can antibody eliminate residual leukemia cells following cytoreductive therapy? To what extent are host cofactors depleted by the tumor, antileukemic drugs or radiation? Would antibody conjugated to a drug or radioisotope prove more effective? Can alternate therapies be combined with antibody to eliminate tumor at sites of low or absent antibody concentrations? And, finally, can antibody used alone or in combination with drugs increase survival? Our current efforts in treating spontaneous AKR lymphomas have been directed toward each of these questions in experimental models. Hopefully, conditions for optimal use of antibodies in these experimental therapeutic settings can be defined, and the pitfalls inherent in past empirical approaches to clinical immunotherapy can be avoided in future trials.

REFERENCES

1. A. Fefer, Experimental approaches to immunotherapy of cancer. *Rec. Res. Cancer Res.,* **36,** 182 (1971).

2. P. W. Wright, K. E. Hellström, I. D. Hellström, and I. D. Bernstein, Serotherapy of malignant disease. *Med. Clin. N. Am.,* **60,** 607 (1976).

3. S. A. Rosenberg and W. D. Terry, Passive immunotherapy of cancer in animals and man. *Adv. Cancer Res.,* **25,** 323 (1977).

4. P. W. Wright and I. D. Bernstein, Serotherapy of malignant disease. *Progr. Exp. Tumor Res.,* **25,** 140 (1980).

5. N. Kaliss, The elements of immunological enhancement: A consideration of mechanisms. *Ann. N. Y. Acad. Sci.,* **101,** 64 (1962).

6. K. E. Hellström and G. Möller, Immunological and immunogenetic aspects of tumor transplantation. *Progr. Allergy,* **9,** 158 (1965).

7. M. Takasugi and W. H. Hildemann, Regulation of immunity toward allogeneic tumors in mice. I. Effect of antiserum fractions on tumor growth. *J. Natl. Cancer Inst.,* **43,** 843 (1969).

8. T. Chard, Immunological enhancement by mouse isoantibodies: The importance of complement fixation. *Immunology,* **14,** 583 (1968).

9. P. C. Fuller and H. J. Winn, Immunochemical and biological characterization of alloantibody activity in immunological enhancement. *Transplant. Proc.,* **5,** 585 (1973).

10. J. Bubenik, J. Ivanyi, and P. P. Koldovsky, Participation in 7S and 19S antibodies in enhancement and resistance to methylcholanthrene-induced tumors. *Folia Biol.,* **11,** 426 (1965).

11. L. J. Old, E. Stockert, E. A. Boyse, and G. Geering, A study of passive immunization against a transplanted G+ leukemia with specific antiserum. *Proc. Soc. Exp. Biol. Med.,* **124,** 63 (1967).

12. P. A. Gorer and D. B. Amos, Passive immunity in mice against C57B1 leukosis EL4 by means of iso-immune serum. *Cancer Res.,* **16,** 338 (1956).

13. J. L. McCoy, A. Fefer, and J. P. Glynn, Inhibition and enhancement of syngeneic Friend virus-induced lymphoma cells by passive transferred anti-Friend serum. *Exp. Hematol.,* **16,** 24 (1968).

14. B. Wahren, Immunotherapy in Friend virus leukemia. II. Prevention of Friend leukemia by passive administration of immune serum and cells to young mice. *J. Natl. Cancer Inst.,* **41,** 931 (1968).

15. E. Mihich, Combined effects of chemotherapy and immunity against leukemia L1210 in DBA/2 mice. *Cancer Res.,* **29,** 848 (1969).

16. A. E. Reif and C. H. Kim, Leukemia L1210 therapy trials with antileukemia serum and Bacillus Calmette-Guerin. *Cancer Res.,* **31,** 1606 (1971).

17. H. S. Shin, N. Kaliss, and D. Borenstein, Antibody-mediated suppression of grafted lymphoma cells. I. Participation of a host factor(s) other than complement. *Proc. Soc. Exp. Biol. Med.,* **139,** 684 (1972).

18. W. P. Drake, P. C. Ungaro, and M. R. Mardiney, Jr., Passive administration of antiserum and complement in producing anti-EL4 cytotoxic activity in the serum of C57B1/6 mice. *J. Natl. Cancer Inst.,* **50,** 909 (1973).

19. G. R. Pearson, L. W. Redmon, and L. R. Bass, Protective effect of immune sera against transplantable Moloney virus-induced sarcoma and lymphoma. *Cancer Res.,* **33,** 171 (1973).

20. G. R. Pearson, L. W. Redmon, and J. W. Pearson, Serochemotherapy against a Moloney virus-induced leukemia. *Cancer Res.,* **33,** 1854 (1973).

21. P. J. Smith, C. M. Robinson, and A. E. Reif, Specificity of antileukemia sera prepared by immunization with leukemia cells admixed with normal antigen-blocking sera. *Cancer Res.,* **34,** 169 (1974).

22. M. Yutoku, A. L. Grossberg, and D. Pressman, Suppression of *in vivo* growth of mouse myelomas by purified rabbit antibodies against mouse myeloma cells. *J. Natl. Cancer Inst.,* **53,** 201 (1974).

23. J. Zighelboim, B. Bonavida, and J. L. Fahey, Antibody-mediated *in vivo* suppression of EL4 leukemia in a syngeneic host. *J. Natl. Cancer Inst.,* **52,** 879 (1974).

24. G. Hunsmann, V. Moennig, and W. Schäfer, Properties of mouse leukemia viruses. IX. Active and passive immunization of mice against Friend leukemia with isolated viral GP$_{71}$ glycoprotein and its corresponding antiserum. *Virology,* **66,** 327 (1975).

25. H. S. Shin, M. Hayden, S. Landly, N. Kaliss, and M. R. Smith, Antibody-mediated suppression of grafted lymphoma. III. Evaluation of the role of thymic function, non-thymus-derived lymphocytes, macrophages, platelets, and polymorphonuclear leukocytes in syngeneic and allogeneic hosts. *J. Immunol.,* **114,** 1255 (1975).

26. G. A. Carlson and G. Terres, Antibody-induced killing *in vivo* of L1210/MTX-R cells quantitated in passively immunized mice with ^{131}I-iododeoxyuridine-labelled cells and whole body measurement of retained radioactivity. *J. Immunol.,* **117,** 822 (1976).

27. B. Chesebro and K. Wehrly, Studies on the role of the host immune response in recovery from Friend virus leukemia. I. Antiviral and anti-leukemia cell antibodies. *J. Exp. Med.,* **143,** 73 (1976).

28. G. J. O'Neill, Control of an EL4 lymphoma in nude mice by passively administered antibody. *Eur. J. Cancer,* **12,** 749 (1976).

29. A. E. Reif, C. M. Robinson, and P. J. Smith, Preparation and therapeutic potential of rabbit antisera with "directed" specificities for mouse leukemias. *Ann. N. Y. Acad. Sci.,* **277,** 647 (1976).

30. W. Schafer, H. Schwarz, H. J. Thiel, E. Wecker, and D. P. Bolognesi, Properties of mouse leukemia viruses. XIII. Serum therapy of virus induced mouse leukemias. *Virology,* **75,** 401 (1976).

31. H. S. Shin, J. S. Economou, G. R. Pasternack, R. J. Johnson, and M. L. Hayden, Antibody-mediated suppression of grafted lymphoma. IV. Influence of time of tumor residency *in vivo* and tumor size upon the effectiveness of suppression by syngeneic antibody. *J. Exp. Med.,* **144,** 1274 (1976).

32. H. S. Shin, N. Kaliss, and D. Borenstein, Antibody-mediated suppression of grafted lymphoma cells. I. Participation of a host factor(s) other than complement. *Proc. Soc. Exp. Biol. Med.,* **139,** 684 (1972).

33. T. Ghose, A. Guclu, J. Faulkner, and J. Tai, *In vivo* suppression of EL4 lymphoma by rabbit antitumor sera. *J. Natl. Cancer Inst.,* **58,** 693 (1977).

34. A. E. Reif, R. W. Li, and C. M. Robinson, Passive immunotherapy for mouse leukemia with antisera of "directed" specificity: Synergism with the action of cyclophosphamide. *Cancer Treat. Rep.* **61,** 1499 (1977).

35. J. J. Collins, F. Sanfilippo, L. Tsong-Chou, R. Ishizaki, and R. S. Metzgar, Immunotherapy of murine leukemia. I. Protection against Friend leukemia virus-induced disease by passive serum therapy. *Internatl. J. Cancer,* **21,** 51 (1978).

36. J. Vaage and S. Agarwal, Serum therapy for radiation-induced impairment of immune resistance to metastasis. *Cancer Res.,* **37,** 3556 (1977).

37. D. E. Haagensen, Jr., G. Rolosen, J. J. Collins, S. A. Wells, Jr., D. P. Bolognesi, and H. J. Hansen, Immunologic control of the ascites form of murine adenocarcinoma 755. I. Protection with syngeneic immune serum or lymphoid cells. *J. Natl. Cancer Inst.,* **60,** 131 (1978).

38. S. E. Order, V. Donahue, and R. Knapp, Immunotherapy of ovarian carcinoma—an experimental model. *Cancer,* **32,** 573 (1973).

39. G. J. Hill and K. Littlejohn, B16 melanoma in C57B1/6J mice: kinetics and effects of heterologous serum. *J. Surg. Oncol.,* **3,** 1 (1971).

40. J. E. Byfield, R. Zerubavel, and E. W. Fonkalsrud, Murine neuroblastoma cured *in vivo* by an antibody-dependent cellular cytotoxicity reaction. *Nature,* **264,** 783 (1976).

41. G. J. Mizejewski and R. P. Allen, Immunotherapeutic suppression in transplantable solid tumours. *Nature,* **250,** 50 (1974).

42. H. G. Smith, M. S. Meltzer, and E. J. Leonard, Suppression of tumor growth in strain 2 guinea pigs by xenogeneic antitumor antibody. *J. Natl. Cancer Inst.,* **57,** 809 (1976).

43. L. W. Law, R. C. Ting, and M. E. Stanton, Some biologic, immunogenic, and morphologic effects in mice after infection with a murine sarcoma virus. I. Biologic and immunogenic studies. *J. Natl. Cancer Inst.,* **40,** 1101 (1968).

44. A. Fefer, Immunotherapy and chemotherapy of Moloney sarcoma virus-induced tumors in mice. *Cancer Res.,* **29,** 2177 (1969).

45. I. Hellström, K. E. Hellström, G. E. Pierce, and A. Fefer, Studies on immunity to autochthonous mouse tumor. *Transplant. Proc.,* **1,** 1 (1969).

46. S. C. Bansal and H. O. Sjögren, "Unblocking" serum activity *in vitro* in the polyoma system may correlate with antitumor effects of antiserum *in vivo. Nature New Biol.,* **233,** 76 (1971).

47. H. O. Sjögren and K. Borum, Tumor-specific immunity in the course of primary polyoma and Rous tumor development in intact and immunosuppressed rats. *Cancer Res.,* **31,** 890 (1971).

48. S. C. Bansal and H. O. Sjögren, Counteraction of the blocking of cell-mediated tumor immunity by inoculation of unblocking sera and splenectomy: Immunotherapeutic effects on primary polyoma tumors in rats. *Internatl. J. Cancer,* **9,** 490 (1972).

49. S. C. Bansal and H. O. Sjögren, Correlation between changes in antitumor immune parameters and tumor growth *in vivo* in rats. *Internatl. J. Cancer,* **9,** 165 (1973).

50. S. C. Bansal and H. O. Sjögren, Regression of polyoma tumor metastasis by combined unblocking and BCG treatment: Correlation with induced alterations in tumor immunity status. *Internatl. J. Cancer,* **12,** 179 (1973).

51. G. E. Pierce, Inhibitory effects of xenogeneic antiserum on the growth of Moloney virus-induced sarcomas. *J. Surg. Oncol.,* **9,** 249 (1977).

52. C. Hu and T. J. Linna, Serotherapy of avian reticuloendotheliosis virus-induced tumors. *Ann. N. Y. Acad. Sci.,* **277,** 634 (1976).

53. W. Jarrett, O. Jarrett, L. Mackey, H. Laird, W. Hardy, Jr., and M. Essex, Horizontal transmission of leukemia virus and leukemia in the cat. *J. Natl. Cancer Inst.,* **51,** 833 (1973).

54. M. Essex, A. Sliski, S. M. Cotter, R. M. Jakowski, and W. D. Hardy, Jr., Immunosurveillance of naturally occurring feline leukemia. *Science,* **190,** 790 (1975).

55. W. Hardy, Jr., P. W. Hess, E. G. MacEwen, A. A. Hayes, R. L. Kassel, N. K. Day, and L. J. Old, "Treatment of feline lymphosarcoma with feline blood constituents. In J. Clemmesen and D. S. Yohn, Eds., *Comparative Leukemia Research,* Karger, Basel, 1976, p. 518.

56. W. D. Hardy, Jr., A. J. McClelland, E. E. Zuckerman, P. W. Hess, M. Essex, S. M. Cotter, E. G. MacEwen, and A. A. Hayes, Prevention of the contagious spread of the feline leukemia virus between pet cats. In J. Clemmesen and D. S. Yohn, Eds., *Comparative Leukemia Research,* Karger, Basel, 1976, p. 511.

57. M. Essex, S. M. Cotter, A. H. Sliski, W. D. Hardy, Jr., J. R. Stephenson, S. A. Aaronson, and O. Jarrett, Horizontal transmission of feline leukemia virus under natural conditions in a feline leukemia cluster household. *Internatl. J. Cancer,* **19,** 90 (1977).

58. M. Essex, S. M. Cotter, J. R. Stephenson, S. A. Aaronson, and W. D. Hardy, Jr., Leukemia, lymphoma, and fibrosarcoma of cats as models for similar diseases of man. In H. Hiatt, J. D. Watson, and J. A. Winston, Eds., *Origins of Human Cancer,* Cold Spring Harbor Laboratories, New York, 1978, p. 1197.

59. J. Laszlo, C. E. Buckley, and D. B. Amos, Infusion of isologous immune plasma in chronic lymphocytic leukemia. *Blood,* **31,** 104 (1968).

60. R. B. Herberman, G. N. Rogentine, and M. E. Oren, Bioassay of anti-tumor effects of human alloantisera. *Clin. Res.,* **17,** 328 (1969).

61. R. I. Fisher, T. T. Kubota, G. L. Mandell, S. Broder, and R. C. Young, Regression of a T-cell lymphoma after administration of anti-thymocyte globuline. *Ann. Int. Med.,* **88,** 799 (1978).

62. W. C. Sumner and A. G. Foraker, Spontaneous regression of human melanoma: Clinical and experimental studies. *Cancer,* **13,** 79 (1960).

63. B. Teimourian and W. S. McCune, Surgical management of malignant melanoma. *Am. J. Surg.,* **29,** 515 (1963).

64. P. W. Wright, K. E. Hellström, I. Hellström, G. Warner, R. Prentice, and R. F. Jones, Serotherapy of malignant melanoma. In W. Terry and D. Windhorst, Eds., *Immunotherapy of Cancer: Present Status of Trials in Man,* Raven, New York, 1978, P. 135.

65. G. Köhler and C. Milstein, Continuous cultures of fused cells secreting antibody of predefined specificity. *Nature,* **256,** 495 (1975).

66. G. Köhler and C. Milstein, Derivation of specific antibody-producing tissue culture and tumor lines by cell fusion. *Eur. J. Immunol.,* **6,** 51 (1976).

67. F. Melchers, M. Potter, and N. Warner, Eds., *Current Topics in Microbiology and Immunology,* Vol. 81, *Lymphocyte Hybridomas,* Springer-Verlag, New York, 1978, pp. 246.

68. **R. H. Kennett, T. J. McKearn, and K. B. Bechtol, Eds., *Monoclonal Antibodies, Hybridomas: A New Dimension in Biological Analyses,* Plenum, New York, 1980, pp. 423.**

69. M. T. Hakala, Prevention of toxicity of Amethopterin for Sarcoma-180 cells in tissue culture. *Science*, **126**, 255 (1957).

70. M. T. Hakala and E. Taylor, The ability of purine and thymine derivatives and of glycine to support the growth of mammalian cells in culture. *J. Biol. Chem.*, **234**, 126 (1959).

71. W. Szybalski, E. H. Szybalska, and G. Ragni, Genetic studies with human cell lines. *Nat. Cancer Inst. Monogr.*, **7**, 75–89 (1962).

72. H. Koprowski, Z. Steplewski, D. Herlyn, and M. Herlyn, Studies of antibodies against human melanoma produced by somatic cell hybrids. *Proc. Natl. Acad. Sci. (USA)*, **75**, 3405 (1978).

73. M.-Y. Yeh, I. Hellström, J. P. Brown, G. A. Warner, J. A. Hansen, and K. E. Hellström, Cell surface antigens of human melanoma identified by monoclonal antibody. *Proc. Natl. Acad. Sci. (USA)*, **76**, 2927 (1979).

74. R. G. Woodbury, J. P. Brown, M.-Y. Yeh, I. Hellström, and K. E. Hellström, Identification of a cell surface protein, p97, in human melanomas and certain other neoplasms. *Proc. Natl. Acad. Sci. (USA)*, **77**, 2183 (1980).

75. J. P. Brown, P. W. Wright, C. E. Hart, R. G. Woodbury, K. E. Hellström, and I. Hellström, Proteins antigens of normal and malignant human cells identified by immunoprecipitation with monoclonal antibodies. *J. Biol. Chem.*, **255**, 4980 (1980).

76. J. P. Brown, R. G. Woodbury, C. E. Hart, I. Hellström, and K. E. Hellström, Quantitative analysis of melanoma-associated antigen p97 in normal and neoplastic tissues. *Proc. Natl. Acad. Sci.*, **78**, 539 (1981).

77. R. H. Kennett and F. Gilbert, Hybrid myelomas producing antibodies against a human neuroblastoma antigen present on fetal brain. *Science*, **203**, 1120 (1979).

78. R. C. Seeger, Y. L. Danon, P. M. Zeltzer, J. E. Maidman, and S. A. Rayner, Expression of fetal antigen by human neuroblastoma cells. In A. E. Evans, Ed., *Advances in Neuroblastoma Research,* Raven, New York, 1980, p. 199.

79. M. Herlyn, Z. Steplewski, D. Herlyn, and H. Koprowski, Colorectal carcinoma-specific antigen: Detection by means of monoclonal antibodies. *Proc. Natl. Acad. Sci. (USA)*, **76**, 1438 (1979).

80. R. Levy, J. Dilley, and L. A. Lampson, Human normal and leukemia cell surface antigens. Mouse monoclonal antibodies as probes. In F. Melchers, M. Potter, and N. Warner, Eds., *Current Topics in Microbiology and Immunology,* Vol. 81, *Lymphocyte Hybridomas,* Springer-Verlag, New York, p. 164.

81. R. Levy, J. Dilley, R. I. Fox, and R. Warnke, A human thymus leukemia antigen defined by hybridoma monoclonal antibodies. *Proc. Natl. Acad. Sci. (USA)*, **76**, 6552 (1979).

82. E. L. Rheinherz, P. C. Kung, G. Goldstein, R. H. Levey, and S. F. Schlossman, Discrete stages of human intrathymic differentiation: Analysis of normal thymocytes and leukemic lymphoblasts of T-cell lineage. *Proc. Natl. Acad. Sci. (USA)*, **77**, 1588 (1980).

83. J. Ritz, J. M. Pesando, J. Natis-McConarty, H. Lazarus, and S. F. Schlossman, A monoclonal antibody to human acute lymphoblastic leukemia antigen. *Nature*, **283**, 583 (1980).

84. M. F. Greaves, W. Verbi, J. Kemshead, and R. Kennett, A monoclonal antibody identifying a cell surface antigen shared by common acute lymphoblastic leukemias and B lineage cells. *Blood*, **56**, 1141 (1980).

85. L. M. Nadler, P. Stashenko, R. Hardy, and S. F. Schlossman, A monoclonal antibody defining a lymphoma associated antigen in man. *J. Immunol.* **125**, 570 (1980).

86. D. Herlyn, M. Herlyn, Z. Steplewski, and H. Koprowski, Monoclonal antibodies in cell-mediated cytotoxicity against human melanoma and colorectal carcinoma. *Eur. J. Immunol.*, **9**, 657 (1979).

87. M. F. Greaves, G. Brown, N. T. Rapson, and T. A. Lister, Antisera to acute lymphoblastic leukemia cells. *Clin. Immunol. Immunopathol.*, **4**, 67 (1975).

88. I. D. Bernstein, M. R. Tam, and R. C. Nowinski, Mouse leukemia: Therapy with monoclonal antibodies against a thymus differentiation antigen. *Science,* **207**, 68 (1980).

89. I. D. Bernstein, R. C. Nowinski, M. R. Tam, B. McMaster, L. L. Houston, and E. A. Clark, Monoclonal antibody therapy of mouse leukemia. In R. H. Kennett, T. J. McKearn, and K. B. Bechtol, Eds., *Monoclonal Antibodies,* Plenum, New York, 1980, p. 275.

90. L. L. Houston, R. C. Nowinski, and I. D. Bernstein, Specific *in vivo* localization of monoclonal antibodies directed against the Thy 1.1 antigen. *J. Immunol.* (in press).

91. J. Ritz, J. M. Pesando, S. E. Sallau, L. A. Clavell, J. Notis-McConarty, P. Rosenthal, and S. F. Schlossman, Monoclonal antibodies: Use as diagnostic and therapeutic reagents in acute lymphoblastic leukemia. *Blood,* **58**, 141 (1981).

92. L. M. Nadler, P. Stashenko, R. Hardy, W. D. Kaplan, L. N. Button, D. W. Kufe, K. H. Antman, and S. F. Schlossman, Serotherapy of a patient with a monoclonal antibody directed against a human lymphoma-associated antigen. *Cancer Res.,* **40**, 3147 (1980).

93. B. Netzel, R. J. Haas, H. Rodt, H. J. Kolb, and S. Thierfelder, Immunological conditioning of bone marrow for autotransplantation in childhood acute lymphoblastic leukemia. *Lancet,* **I**, 1330 (1980) (6/21/80).

94. W. Müller-Ruchholtz, H. U. Wottge, and H. K. Müller-Hermelink, Bone marrow transplantation in rats across strong histocompatibility barriers by selective elimination of lymphoid cells in donor marrow. *Transplant. Proc.,* **8**, 537 (1976).

95. K. Onoe, G. Fernandes, and R. A. Good, Humoral and cell-mediated immune responses in fully allogeneic bone marrow chimera in mice. *J. Exp. Med.,* **151**, 115 (1980).

96. H. Rodt, H. J. Kolb, B. Netzel, J. Haas, K. Wilms, Ch. B. Götze, H. Birk, S. Thierfelder, and the Munich Cooperative Group of BMT, Prevention of GvHD by incubation of bone marrow grafts with anti T-lymphocyte globulin. *Transplant. Proc.,* **XII**, 257 (1981).

97. W. F. Bale and I. L. Spar, Studies directed toward the use of antibodies as carriers of radioactivity for therapy. In J. H. Lawrence and C. O. Tobias, Eds., *Advances in Biological and Medical Physics,* Vol. 5, Academic, New York, 1957 p. 285.

98. T. Ghose, S. T. Norvell, A. Guclu, D. Cameron, A. Bodurtha, and A. S. MacDonald, Immunochemotherapy of cancer with chlorambucil-carrying antibody. *Br. Med. J.,* **3**, 495 (1972).

99. C. McGaughey, Feasibility of tumor immunotherapy using radioiodinated antibodies to tumor-specific cell membrane antigens with emphasis on leukemias and early metastases. *Oncology,* **29**, 302 (1974).

100. B. Ballou, G. Levine, T. R. Hakala, and D. Solter, Tumor location detected with radioactively labeled monoclonal antibody and external scintigraphy. *Science*, **206**, 844 (1979).

101. R. Nowinski, C. Berglund, J. Lane, et al., Human monoclonal antibody against Forssman antigen. *Science,* **210**, 537 (1980).

102. L. Olsson and H. Kaplan, Human–human hybridoma secretory monoclonal antibody of predefined antigen specificity. *Proc. Natl. Acad. Sci. (USA),* **78**, 3199 (1981).

103. C. M. Groce, A. Liumenbach, W. Halt, Z. Steplewski, H. Koprowski, Production of human hybridomas secreting antibodies to measles virus. *Nature,* **288**, 488 (1981).

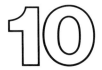

Bone Marrow Transplantation in the Treatment of Neoplastic Diseases

E. DONNALL THOMAS
ALEXANDER FEFER
RAINER STORB
Division of Oncology, Department of Medicine
University of Washington School of Medicine
Fred Hutchinson Cancer Research Center
Seattle, Washington

This investigation was supported by Grant Numbers CA 18029 and CA 15704, awarded by the National Cancer Institute, DHEW. Dr. Thomas is a recipient of a Research Career Award AI 02425 from the National Institute of Allergy and Infectious Diseases, and Dr. Fefer is an American Cancer Society Professor of Clinical Oncology.

1.   INTRODUCTION

Beginning in 1949, the experiments of Jacobson et al. (1) and Lorenz et al. (2) showed that mice could be protected against otherwise lethal total body irradiation (TBI) by shielding the spleen or by an infusion of bone marrow. By 1955 several investigators had shown that the "radiation protection effect" was due to the transplantation of living bone marrow cells of donor origin into the lethally irradiated recipient (reviewed in reference 3). Shortly thereafter efforts to transplant marrow in humans were undertaken. The early attempts were largely unsuccessful. However, two patients with leukemia were given supralethal TBI followed by a marrow transplant from an identical twin (4). Although the leukemia recurred after a few months, the results demonstrated that humans given supralethal irradiation could survive with full hematopoietic restoration when given a transplant of histocompatible marrow.

In 1959 Uphoff and Law (5) demonstrated that the outcome of a marrow graft in mice depended on histocompatibility similarities between donor and recipient. In the 1960s many laboratories continued to study the problems of marrow transplantation biology. Notable was the demonstration in the dog, an outbred model for marrow transplantation in humans, that donor recipient pairs matched for the major histocompatibility complex (DLA) resulted in a high frequency of long-term healthy chimeras (6). These observations, coupled with a rapid advancing knowledge of the major histocompatibility complex in humans (known as HLA) and in supportive care for patients lacking bone marrow function, set the stage for a rational renewal of marrow transplantation efforts in humans. The first successful transplant utilizing an HLA identical sibling donor was described in a patient with severe combined immunologic deficiency disease (7). Within a very short time similarly successful transplants were described in patients with acute leukemia and aplastic anemia. The past decade has witnessed a steadily increasing number of long-term healthy human chimeras, a continuing improvement in overall survival rate, and an application of marrow transplantation to an ever-increasing number of diseases (reviewed in reference 3).

The simplistic view of marrow transplantation is that it represents "supportive care," which permits the destruction of leukemic cells and also the normal marrow cells by chemoradiotherapy with replacement of normal marrow function by the transplanted marrow. This concept may well explain the apparent cure of some patients with end-stage leukemia, but the significance of marrow transplantation, both practical and theoretical, is far broader. Marrow transplantation involves not only the transplantation of donor myeloid cells, but also the replacement of the lymphoid system and the monocyte-macrophage system. Fascinating questions in immunology arise from efforts to understand the nature of the reaction of transplanted lymphoid cells against the tissues of the host (the graft-versus-host reaction) and the nature of the stable chimerism that is observed in the healthy long-term survivors of marrow transplantation. These questions lead to much ongoing research involving the role of humoral factors, the role of B cells, and the role of T cells and subsets of T cells. Interesting questions arise regarding the mechanism of leukemic relapse in some leukemia patients, the mechanism of eradication of leukemia in those patients who appear to be cured, the role of putative leukemia-associated antigens, the role of the graft-versus-leukemia effect, and the nature of the malignant transformation in a few patients whose leukemia has recurred in cells of donor origin. Finally, a number of interesting studies are directed at the nature of the immunologic deficiency following marrow transplantation, the process of immunologic reconstitution, and the origin and management of opportunistic infections, particularly cytomegalovirus infections, in the transplant recipient.

1.1. Histocompatibility

The nature and remarkable heterogeneity of the HLA region is now generally appreciated (reviewed in reference 8). The HLA region, constituting a haplotype located on chromosome 6, contains at least three loci that are thought to be of importance in marrow transplantation. The alleles of HLA-A and HLA-B are detected serologically in a microcytotoxicity assay; HLA-D governs reactivity in the mixed leukocyte culture, and HLA-D typing can be carried out by using homozygous typing cells. More recently D-related antigens can be recognized serologically by typing of B cells. Syngeneic marrow transplants in humans (between identical twins) involve donor-recipient pairs who are perfectly matched not only for the HLA region, but for all other genetic loci that might govern so-called minor transplantation antigen systems. Most allogeneic marrow transplants in humans have involved sibling donor-recipient pairs who are HLA identical by virtue of having inherited the same HLA haplotypes, one from each parent. More recently, a significant number of transplants are being carried out by utilizing donor-recipient pairs in which one haploytpe is genetically identical and the other haplotype similar but not identical. These transplants, of course, involve family members. A few transplants have now been done between unrelated donor-recipient pairs who are apparently identical at the HLA-A, -B, and -D loci. The relative significance or "strength" of these loci and the importance of other closely linked but undetected loci are unknown.

2.   CLINICAL ASPECTS OF MARROW TRANSPLANTATION

Patients with severe combined immunologic deficiency disorders do not require immunosuppressive therapy before transplantation. Patients with nonmalignant hematologic disorders require immunosuppressive therapy before transplantation to condition the host to permit the acceptance of an allogeneic graft. A commonly used regimen involves the administration of cyclophosphamide (CY), 50 mg/kg on each of 4 days followed 36 hours later by the marrow infusion. Patients with leukemia or other hematologic malignancy require immunosuppressive therapy for graft acceptance as well as intensive chemoradiotherapy for destruction of the malignant cells. A commonly used regimen is CY, 60 mg/kg on each of 2 days followed 3 days later by 1000 rad of TBI.

The marrow transplant is technically easy, involving multiple aspirations from the pelvic bones of the donor under anesthesia and sterile conditions (9). Marrow is collected in heparin, screened to break up the particles, and administered to the recipient by simple i.v. infusion.

Following the transplant a period of 2 to 4 weeks is required for the graft to grow and become functional. During this time intensive supportive care is required, involving isolation, platelet and granulocyte transfusions, and antibiotic therapy for bacterial infections. After recovery of the blood counts there is still a long period—from months to years—of subnormal immunologic competence of the recipient with susceptibility to opportunistic infections. About one-half of the recipients of marrow from an HLA identical sibling will develop acute graft-versus-host disease (GVHD) sometime within the first 3 months after grafting, and about one-fourth of the long-term survivors will have some degree of chronic GVHD. Despite these problems, there are now many long-term healthy transplant recipients. The clinical results are summarized below. Subsequent sections will analyze the immunologic aspects and the problems encountered.

2.1.   Nonmalignant Disorders

Infants with *severe combined immunologic deficiency disease* are prepared by the nature of the disease for the acceptance of an allogeneic graft. Although the number of these patients diagnosed each year is very small, they have provided an opportunity for study of the problems of transplantation biology in recipients not exposed to intensive chemoradiotherapy. The first such patient transplanted with marrow from an HLA identical sibling is alive and well now 11 years later. The overall results are good in that approximately 50% of the patients with an HLA identical donor became long-term healthy survivors and many of the deaths that have occurred are related to advanced infections and other problems at the time of transplantation. Results from the use of donors who are not HLA identical with the recipient have been somewhat encouraging in that four of eight patients are living (10). One of these received marrow from an unrelated donor and is living with chronic GVHD.

Acquired *aplastic anemia* is the prototype disease for marrow transplantation in recipients who do not have a malignant disease (11). Several hundred such transplants have now been carried out, and a prospective study has shown marrow transplantation to be superior to conventional treatment if an HLA-identical sibling is available to serve as the marrow donor (12). The initial 73 patients transplanted in Seattle showed a long-term survival rate of 43%, a figure comparable to that reported subsequently by several other marrow transplant groups. The problems encountered were advanced illness and infection at the time of transplantation, graft rejection, acute GVHD, and opportunistic infections. More recently it has been demonstrated that the problem of graft rejection can be avoided if transplantation is carried out before blood transfusions are initiated (13). Recent studies in transfused patients indicate that the administration of additional donor buffy coat cells or the administration of total nodal irradiation will also largely overcome the problem of graft rejection. The long-term survival of these more recent patients appears to be in the range of 75%.

2.2. Acute Leukemia in Relapse

For obvious ethical reasons, most marrow transplant teams began their studies of marrow transplantation in leukemia with patients who were in an apparently refractory end-stage relapse who could not expect to benefit from additional combination chemotherapy. The first 110 such patients transplanted with marrow from HLA-identical siblings in Seattle showed a high mortality rate from advanced disease at the time of transplantation, acute GVHD, opportunistic infections, and recurrent leukemia (14). However, 14 of these patients, who never received maintenance chemotherapy after transplantation, are living in remission and with a marrow graft 4.5 to 9.5 years after transplantation. Similar results were obtained in 16 patients with refractory hematologic neoplasia given a marrow graft from an identical twin, six of whom are alive in remission 6.5 to 9.5 years later (15). The survival curves for these patients are shown in Figure 1. Of course, although the overall results in this series of patients were unsatisfactory, the important point is that there are some long-term survivors

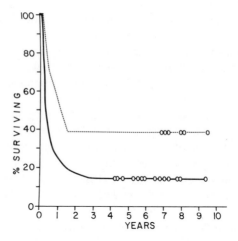

Figure 1.   Kaplan-Meier plot of the probability of survival (as of January 1, 1980) of 110 patients
with acute leukemia who received marrow from an HLA identical sibling (solid line)
and 16 recipients of identical twin marrow (dashed line). The open circles indicate
living patients.

where none would be expected on any chemotherapy regimen. In fact, the surviving patients are now well out on a "plateau," and the length of time since
transplantation indicates a high probability that these patients are cured of the
disease (16). Other marrow transplant teams, as well as our own experience
since 1975, have confirmed these observations, showing that long-term survival of 10 to 15% can be achieved by allogeneic marrow transplantation even
with patients with end-stage refractory leukemia (reviewed in reference 17).

2.3.   Acute Leukemia in Remission

Encouraged by the long-term survivors described in Section 2.2, early in 1976
we began the study of marrow transplantation for patients with acute leukemia
in remission who were considered to have a relatively poor prognosis. The
donors were HLA-identical siblings. The initial series of patients was composed of those with acute lymphoblastic leukemia (ALL) in second or subsequent remission and those with acute nonlymphoblastic leukemia (ANL) in
first remission. Transplantation in remission should offer the advantage of
transplantation when the body burden of leukemic cells is minimal, when these
cells have not become refractory to therapeutic agents, and when the patient is
in excellent condition and thus better able to undergo the preparative regimens
and marrow grafting.

We have reported an initial series of 22 patients with ALL transplanted in
second or subsequent remission (18). The median survival of these patients
was 13 months. Most importantly, however, eight are still in remission 26 to 42
months after transplantation. Figure 2 shows the survival curve for these patients.

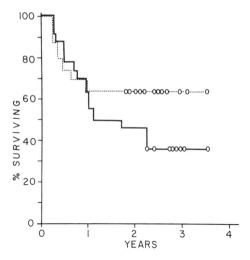

Figure 2. Kaplan Meier plot of the probability of survival (as of January 1, 1980) of 22 patients with ALL transplanted in second or subsequent remission (solid line) and 19 patients with ANL transplanted in first remission (dashed line). The open circles indicate living patients.

We have also reported an initial series of 19 patients with ANL transplanted in first remission (19). Twelve of these 19 patients are in remission 22 to 43 months following transplantation. Figure 2 also shows the survival curve for these patients. The median remission duration for this group of 19 patients will not be less than 2 years.

2.4. "Mismatched" Donors for Patients with Acute Leukemia

In an effort to make marrow transplantation available to the many patients without identical twins or genotypically HLA-identical siblings, we have initiated a cautious exploration of the use of other donors. Twenty-eight transplants were performed in patients with acute leukemia by the end of 1979 in which the donor-recipient pairs were genotypically HLA identical for one haplotype and had a varying degree of similarity for the other (20). In one case the donor was an uncle of the recipient, 13 donors were siblings, and 14 were parents of the recipients. Five recipients were phenotypically identical with their parent donors and all other combinations were mismatched for one or more HLA loci. None of the five patients with phenotypically HLA-matched donors developed GVHD. The frequency and severity of GVHD in the mismatched patients was not noticeably different from that seen in transplants between genotypically HLA-identical siblings. The outcome of these transplants was disease related in the same way as for recipients of HLA-identical sibling marrow. Thus of 17 recipients whose leukemia was in relapse at the time of transplantation, 4 are long-term survivors, whereas of 11 patients transplanted in remission 7 are long-term survivors. None of the patients transplanted in remission died of leukemia. Ten patients were mismatched with their donors at the D locus. Of these, six were in relapse at the time of transplantation and all of these died, whereas three of four transplanted in remission are long-term survivors. Thirteen patients were matched at the D locus with their donors but mismatched at other loci. Seven of these patients were transplanted in relapse, with two long-term survivors and 6 were transplanted in remission with three long-term survivors. The identification of suitable "mismatched" donor-recipient pairs requires a careful evaluation of family HLA typing.

One patient with ALL in second remission received a marrow transplant from a donor who was completely unrelated but phenotypically HLA identical at the HLA-A, -B, -D, and -DR loci. She did not develop GVHD and is in remission 5 months after transplantation. This patient illustrates the feasibility of use of unrelated donors, and this approach could be used more generally given a large pool of donors of known HLA type.

2.5. Chronic Myelogenous Leukemia (CML)

Patients with CML have a rather benign course until the onset of the accelerated or "blast crisis" phase of the disease. The median survival for patients with CML is approximately 30 months. Most patients in blast crisis do not respond to chemotherapy, and survival for the few who do respond is only a few months. Chemoradiotherapy and marrow transplantation for patients in blast crisis has also proved to be very difficult, with major support problems and many deaths from infection (reference 21 and unpublished data). In our first 18 such patients treated with marrow transplantation from an HLA-identical sibling, only two are in remission beyond 2 years. One of six recipients of syngeneic marrow is in remission at 4 years. Despite these discouraging overall results, the three long-term survivors are unique and indicate the feasibility of cure of the disease by intensive chemoradiotherapy and marrow transplantation.

In view of the bleak outlook for patients with CML in the accelerated phase, we began a cautious study of transplantation earlier in the course of the disease. Initially we studied four patients with Philadelphia chromosome positive CML in the chronic phase of the disease (22). They were prepared with dimethyl busulfan, CY, and TBI followed by a marrow transplant from identical twins who were hematologically and cytogenetically normal. A complete hematologic and cytogenetic remission was induced in all four patients, but one patient relapsed back into the chronic phase of the disease 30 months after transplantation. The other three remain hematologically and cytogenetically well at 35, 38, and 43 months after marrow transplantation. These results suggest that it is possible to eradicate the Philadelphia chromosome positive abnormal clone in some patients. With these encouraging results, a study of marrow transplantation for patients with CML in chronic phase utilizing HLA-identical sibling donors is now under way.

2.6. Autologous Marrow Transplantation

Autologous marrow transplantation consists of removing and setting aside a portion of an individual's bone marrow, administering intensive chemotherapy and/or radiotherapy, and returning the marrow to the individual to avoid lethal marrow aplasia. The feasibility of this approach to protection against lethal irradiation was first demonstrated in mice (see Section 1), and clinical application was attempted in the late 1950s. In the late 1950s and early 1960s it was demonstrated that marrow could be preserved for long periods of time at low temperatures in either glycerol or dimethyl sulfoxide. Both *in vitro* and *in vivo* studies have now demonstrated that human marrow can be cryopreserved with retention of effective viability. Thus, although cryopreservation techniques have been available for 20 years, it is disappointing that there has been no clear demonstration as yet of the value of autologous marrow transplantation to clinical problems (reviewed in reference 23).

In considering autologous marrow transplantation, the following major points must be kept in mind:

1. Autologous marrow can be of value only in protecting the patient against lethal toxicity to the hematopoietic system. Chemotherapy limited by lethal toxicity to other organ systems (liver, heart, etc.) cannot be improved by the use of autologous marrow.

2. The tumor being treated must show a dose response curve such that unusually intensive treatment can result in a significantly enhanced tumor response. Unfortunately, with currently available agents, only a few tumors appear to fall into this category.

3. The clinical experiment must be designed in such a way that the role of autologous marrow can be convincingly demonstrated. For example, in animal systems it is easy to demonstrate that the administration of 800 to 1000 rad of TBI will result in death whereas the administration of autologous or syngeneic marrow following the TBI will protect against lethality.

For obvious ethical reasons, this kind of controlled experiment cannot be undertaken in humans. For most cancer chemotherapeutic agents, it has been difficult to demonstrate, even in animal systems, that autologous marrow can protect against lethal hematopoietic toxicity because the marrow sometimes shows a surprising ability to recover from large doses of drug and because such large doses may uncover unexpected toxicity to other organ systems. Failure to recognize these three principles accounts for much of the current uncertainty about the value of autologous marrow transplantation in the treatment of patients with cancer.

Nevertheless, the potential use of autologous marrow is undergoing a new wave of interest, and some results are encouraging. We reported a study in seven patients with CML whose marrow was stored during the chronic phase of the disease and, following the onset of blast crisis, returned to the patient after the administration of high-dose CY and 1000 rad TBI (24). As with other patients in blast crisis described previously, major problems were encountered, but recovery of marrow function was demonstrated, and one patient exhibited a return to the chronic phase for 4 months before relapse into the blastic phase. The study demonstrated that stored autologous marrow could effect hematopoietic reconstitution following lethal irradiation and demonstrated the general feasibility of the approach. Goldman has reported a similar study with a few encouraging remissions utilizing cryopreserved peripheral blood buffy coat cells as a source of stem cells for marrow repopulation (25). Dicke et al. (26) have described a series of patients with acute nonlymphoblastic leukemia whose marrow was stored in remission and, on relapse, returned to the patient after intensive chemoradiotherapy. Because of the advanced illness of the patients, there were many early deaths, but there were a few remissions of significant duration. The high relapse rate in the patients who did achieve remission is not surprising in view of the similar high relapse rate for such patients given syngeneic or allogeneic marrow as described previously. Several preliminary reports have described successful hematopoietic reconstitution following intensive chemoradiotherapy for selected solid tumors (27). The tumors that might be expected to show a significant improvement in response to high-dose chemoradiotherapy include the leukemias, lymphoma, small-cell cancer of the lung, testicular tumors, and ovarian tumors. Results of ongoing studies at several centers utilizing autologous marrow transplantation to treat human tumors should provide data for a better evaluation of this approach.

3. IMMUNOLOGIC ASPECTS OF MARROW TRANSPLANTATION

3.1. Marrow Graft Rejection

"Marrow graft rejection" describes a phenomenon in which the marrow graft functions briefly but, after a few days or few weeks, fails to produce new cells. The peripheral blood counts suddenly drop, and marrow aspiration and/or biopsy shows the marrow to be devoid of myeloid elements. In some instances the graft may be rejected so quickly that graft function is never established. Marrow graft rejection has accounted for 25 to 60% of the deaths of patients given marrow grafts for severe aplastic anemia. For reasons to be described later, graft rejection is generally thought to be due to sensitization of the recipient by minor histocompatibility antigens contained in blood products given to these patients before transplantation. However, since histologic proof of marrow graft rejection (in contrast to other organ grafts) cannot be obtained, it must be kept in mind that other mechanisms may be responsible for failure of a marrow graft. Possible mechanisms include (1) inadequate immunosuppressive therapy before grafting, (2) defective or inadequate numbers of "stem cells" in the donor marrow, (3) allogeneic resistance not associated with HLA, (4) sensitization to non-HLA antigens through immunization with cross-reacting environmental antigens, and (5) susceptibility of the donor marrow to the same etiologic mechanism responsible for the original disease process.

In the canine model for marrow grafting with the use of DLA-identical littermates and preparation with TBI, the following observations were made: (1) marrow graft rejection almost never occurred when the recipient was a normal dog; (2) a single small blood transfusion from the intended marrow donor given to the recipient 10 days before grafting resulted in a 75% incidence of graft rejection; (3) blood transfusions from nine unrelated donors given 1 to 2 weeks before marrow transplantation resulted in rejection of the DLA-identical marrow in approximately one-third of the recipients (reviewed in reference 28).

In the initial studies of marrow transplantation for aplastic anemia, marrow grafting was carried out only after the failure of conventional treatment. Thus the vast majority of patients had had multiple blood transfusions before coming to marrow transplantation (29). In the initial 73 patients with severe aplastic anemia treated in Seattle by marrow grafts from HLA identical siblings, 21 rejected the graft. Since all but 3 of the 73 patients had had multiple blood transfusions, the role of such transfusions in graft rejection could not be evaluated. A logistic regression analysis identified two factors that correlated strongly with graft rejection: a positive relative response index in mixed leukocyte culture, indicating sensitization of the patient's lymphocytes against cells of the donor and a low number of marrow cells used for transplantation. Subsequently, a positive reaction of patient lymphocytes against donor cells in a chromium release assay was also found to be predictive of subsequent graft rejection.

In view of these observations, two possible approaches to the resolution of the graft rejection problem were apparent: (1) to carry out marrow transplantation before transfusions are given and (2) for patients already transfused, to explore methods of overcoming the immunologic reaction of the host's lymphoid system against cells of the donor. With regard to the first approach, 30 "untransfused" patients with severe aplastic anemia have now been reported (13). All 30 had prompt initial marrow engraftment that was sustained in 27. Twenty-five patients are alive from 1 to 7 years after transplantation. For patients who have already received transfusions before coming to marrow transplantation, three approaches have been utilized in an effort to overcome sensitization and prevent rejection.

The first approach involves more intensive immunosuppressive therapy before grafting. The Seattle group attempted to do this by administering CY and TBI; however, although graft rejection appeared to be reduced, overall survival was not improved because of the toxicity of the regimen (29). Studies in dogs had shown that the administration of procarbazine and antithymocyte globulin (ATG) before TBI was effective in preventing graft rejection. However, the use of procarbazine and ATG before the standard CY regimen did not alter the incidence of graft rejection for patients with aplastic anemia in a controlled study.

The second approach, which is currently being explored by the Minneapolis group, involves the administration of total nodal irradiation (750 rad) on the day following the CY administration and preceding marrow transplantation. Nine previously transfused patients were transplanted (30). No patient suffered graft rejection, and seven of the nine became long-term survivors.

The third approach, carried out by the Seattle group, is to give additional living cells of donor origin following the marrow transplant (29). The need for more donor-type cells was suggested by the observation, cited previously, that the larger the dose of marrow cells, the less the likelihood of graft rejection. As we were unable to obtain more marrow cells despite a maximal effort through multiple aspirations of the anterior and posterior iliac crests and the sternum, we turned to the donor's peripheral blood as an added source of cells. These cells are of interest since they might contribute additional hematopoietic and/or lymphoid cells that could enhance engraftment. Previous work in mice, guinea pigs, dogs, and baboons has shown that pluripotent hematopoietic stem cells circulate in the blood, and, although evidence for pluripotent stem cells in humans is still missing, studies have shown the presence of circulating committed hematopoietic stem cells in humans. Peripheral blood (and thoracic duct) lymphoid cells have been shown experimentally to enhance marrow engraftment *in vivo* and to increase erythropoiesis *in vitro*. For these reasons, we decided to give peripheral blood leukocytes from the donor in addition to the marrow inoculum for patients who, on the basis of *in vitro* test results of sensitization, were thought to be at high risk for graft rejection (29). Thirteen of 16 such sensitized patients given only marrow rejected the graft, whereas 3 of 23 given marrow plus peripheral blood leukocytes rejected. Survival in the two groups was 25 and 71%, respectively. The addition of peripheral blood leukocytes did not appear to change the incidence or severity of GVHD.

3.2. Acute Graft-Versus-Host Disease

A "wasting disease" or "runt disease" was described many years ago in newborn mice or rodents exposed to lethal TBI and given infusions of allogeneic hematopoietic cells. Soon these observations were confirmed for other species and were recognized to be the consequence of an immunologic reaction of engrafted lymphoid cells against the tissue of the host (31). This disease is now referred to as "GVHD" and is one of the major complications besetting the field of marrow transplantation in humans. Despite the initial restriction of the human donor-recipient pairs to HLA-identical siblings and the "prophylactic" use of methotrexate (MTX), GVHD is a serious problem in humans. In a series of 262 patients, 116 (44%) developed moderate to severe GVHD.

The principal target organs of GVHD in both animals and humans are skin, gastrointestinal tract, and liver (3). The host's marrow, if present, may also be a target organ. A skin rash is usually the first sign of GVHD. Intestinal involvement presents mainly in the form of diarrhea but may progress to abdominal pain and ileus. Liver disease is manifested by rises in bilirubin, serum glutamic oxaloacetic transaminase, and alkaline phosphatase. Severe immunologic deficiency accompanies GVHD, and death from infection is frequently the terminal event. The distinction between illness due to an active immunologic assault against host tissues and the consequences of this assault—deranged organ function and infection—is subtle, and for the purpose of this discussion, both are considered part of GVHD.

The graft-versus-host reaction is thought to be primarily T-cell mediated. Immunologically competent donor lymphocytes recognize host alloantigens, undergo proliferation, and generate cytotoxic lymphocytes. The nature of the graft-versus-host reaction in mice has been reviewed extensively (31). Recent studies were carried out in dogs by using DLA-mismatched donor-recipient pairs shown to be reactive in mixed leukocyte culture (32). Dogs with acute GVHD showed the continued presence of lymphocytes (of donor origin) in the circulating blood that reacted to cryopreserved host cells in mixed leukocyte culture. Lymphocytes from dogs that became stable long-term survivors did not react in mixed leukocyte culture with cryopreserved host cells. Whether antibody plays a role in acute GVHD is unclear.

Because of the presumed immunologic etiology of GVHD, efforts to prevent the development of GVHD with immunosuppressive therapy have been carried out in animals. The literature on this topic has been reviewed recently (28). To be effective, treatment with immunosuppressive agents must be started before GVHD becomes apparent. Of the many agents studied MTX and CY have been found useful. Methotrexate was found to ameliorate GVHD in mice, dogs, and monkeys when given immediately after grafting. Studies in dogs have shown that MTX was most effective when continued for a long time (3 months), and stable long-term chimerism was achieved in some DLA-incompatible recipients. Cyclophosphamide has had some effect in mice, rats, and monkeys but was ineffective in dogs. Studies with the use of cytosine arabinoside, procarbazine, and antilymphocyte serum in the immediate postgrafting period have been disappointing, whereas 6-mercaptopurine has shown some beneficial effect. Prevention of GVHD has been attempted with the use of antilymphocyte serum just before grafting in rodents, dogs, and monkeys with only slight prolongation of survival.

The most frequent postgrafting regimen used for human transplantation is based on canine studies and consists of MTX, 15 mg/m^2 on the first day after grafting and 10 mg/m^2 on the third, sixth, and eleventh days and weekly thereafter for the first 100 days. Others have used CY 7.5 mg/kg for 5 doses on alternate days, beginning on the first day after marrow grafting followed by additional doses at irregular intervals. Controlled clinical trials of these regimens have not been carried out in humans.

Only a few studies in rodent systems have been reported in which established GVHD was treated either with chemicals or with antilymphocyte or antithymocyte serum. For the most part, the agents used failed to influence the course of events or the investigators failed to document sustained chimerism. A review of these studies has been presented recently (33). An exception was the study by Owens and Santos (34), who inoculated (C57BL/6 × DBA/2)F₁ hybrid mice with Balb/c spleen cells and were able to suppress clinically established GVHD with CY.

We attempted to influence established GVHD by treating canine recipients of marrow grafts with rabbit antidog thymocyte serum (33). Unrelated histoincompatible donor-recipient pairs were used, which constitute a severe test model for any immunosuppressive regimen. Survival was prolonged significantly with the median survival at 46 days compared with 19 days in dogs not given antithymocyte serum. Prednisone at high doses was ineffective.

Subsequently, we treated GVHD in human recipients of HLA-identical marrow with rabbit or goat antithymocyte globulin (35), and improvement was observed in some patients. In a clinical trial without untreated controls because of ethical considerations, and in contrast to the results in DLA-mismatched dogs, prednisone and horse ATG gave results equivalent to those of treatment of established human GVHD in recipients of HLA-matched marrow (36). An attempt to prevent GVHD from occurring by the "prophylactic" use of antithymocyte globulin in humans was unsuccessful (37). It is clear from these studies that the treatment of acute GVHD is unsatisfactory and that new approaches in preventing or treating GVHD must be sought.

More recently an immunosuppressive agent with unique properties, cyclosporin A, has been described. It was reported to suppress plaque formation in gel, hemagglutinin titers, lymphocyte-mediated cytolysis, and skin reactivity to oxazolone and to prevent lymphocyte blastogenesis to concanavalin A (Con A) and phytohemagglutinin (PHA) in various species, including humans (reviewed in reference 38). The survival of allografts of hearts in rats and pigs and of kidneys in rabbits, dogs, and humans was prolonged with cyclosporin A. In histoincompatible mice and rats, amelioration or prevention of GVHD was observed. The data in rats suggested the emergence of suppressor cells maintaining a stable chimeric state. We found cyclosporin A to be a very powerful immunosuppressant in the dog, prolonging skin graft survival *in vivo* and suppressing various *in vitro* functions, including mixed leukocyte culture reactivity and cell-mediated lympholysis. However, it failed to induce persistent immunologic unresponsiveness in that immunosuppression depended on the continued presence of the drug. Only preliminary data for the use of cyclosporin A in clinical marrow grafting are available. More studies are needed to determine its ultimate place in the prevention and treatment of human GVHD.

Recently interest has been focused on treating the marrow inoculum *in vitro* in an attempt to eliminate immune-competent cells but retain hematopoietic stem cells. One approach has involved albumin gradient separation (39), but in human transplants the results were either failure of engraftment or death from GVHD when histoincompatible marrow was used. Other attempts have involved treatment of the marrow inoculum *in vitro* by specifically absorbed antithymocyte globulin. Richie et al. treated marrow from A strain mice with Fab fragments of antilymphocyte globulin before injection into lethally irradiated C57 × (A)F$_1$ mice and observed an improvement in the mortality rate from GVHD during the first 15 days postgrafting (40). Müller-Ruchholtz et al. (41) treated marrow of CAP rat donors with xenogeneic antilymphocyte globulin absorbed on rat lymphocytes, cultured peritoneal cells, and fetal liver cells before infusion into lethally irradiated LEW rats (RtH-1 incompatible). They observed 75% 50-day survival, compared to 0% survival for rats given untreated marrow. Similarly, Rodt et al. (42) treated H-2 incompatible parental spleen cells with xenogeneic antimouse T-cell globulin before infusion into irradiated F$_1$ hybrids and saw complete suppression of GVHD while hematopoiesis was restored by donor cells. These same authors have absorbed rabbit antihuman antithymocyte globulin with liver-kidney homogenate as well as cells from lymphoblastoid cell lines and from patients with chronic lymphocytic leukemia (CLL). They found that activity against bone marrow cells was removed while anti-T-cell activity was preserved. Korngold and Sprent prevented GVHD in mice differing for minor histocompatibility antigens by removal of T cells from the marrow with an anti-Thy 1.2 serum (43). Kolb et al. (44) used absorbed rabbit ATG and reported prevention of GVHD in a number of dogs given DLA nonidentical grafts. The recent development of monoclonal antibodies that react with human T cells or subsets of T cells points toward greatly improved methods of *in vitro* treatment of marrow. These attractive approaches for the prevention of GVHD require intensive study for application in human marrow transplantation.

Finally, interesting results have been reported in mice and rats with the use of total lymphoid irradiation, in a manner analogous to that used for the treatment of Hodgkin's disease, as a conditioning regimen for marrow transplantation (45). Approximately 30% of the mice have become long-term chimeras that tolerate skin grafts from the marrow donors. The remainder either have not become chimeras or have died from complications associated with the treatment. The results in large animals, particularly dogs, are as yet not convincing in respect to the establishment of permanent chimerism and tolerance of organ grafts across a major histocompatibility barrier. This approach is already being applied to patients with aplastic anemia (see Section 2).

3.3. Chronic Graft-Versus-Host Disease

Chronic GVHD, a recently recognized syndrome, occurs in approximately one-fourth of the long-term recipients of marrow from an HLA-identical sibling. The syndrome may range from mild to severe and may develop as an extension of acute GVHD or *de novo* after a period of well-being (46). The protean manifestations may include skin disease, keratoconjunctivitis, buccal mucositis, esophageal strictures, small and large intestinal involvement, pulmonary insufficiency, chronic liver disease, and generalized wasting. Histologically, the disease resembles the systemic collagen vascular diseases, especially morphea and lupus erythematosus profundus. The analogy between chronic GVHD and collagen vascular diseases is further underlined by the finding of circulating autoantibodies and of immunoglobulin and complement deposition at the dermoepidermal junction. Chronic GVHD is also characterized clinically by recurrent (and occasionally fatal) bacterial infections.

The success of treatment has been limited. Short courses of ATG or prolonged treatment with prednisone were found to be ineffective. More recently, in a series of 21 patients, we attempted to use combinations of prednisone and either procarbazine, CY, or azathioprine, all at 1.5 mg/kg/day for a median of 10 months (47). Combination therapy was generally well tolerated with only modest and reversible myelotoxicity. Four of the 21 patients died with chronic GVHD and 17 are alive, most with Karnofsky scores above 90%. In six patients treatment has been discontinued for up to 3 years without recurrence of chronic GVHD. Thus combination therapy can modify the course of chronic GVHD in a beneficial way and, in some cases, permanently arrest the disease. In other patients, however, immunosuppressive therapy has introduced additional infectious complications. New approaches must be sought to treat or to prevent chronic GVHD.

We propose the hypothesis that chronic GVHD is the result of an immunoregulatory imbalance that, in turn, is caused by the absence of the thymus. This hypothesis is based, in part, on the observation of a striking and highly significant correlation between chronic GVHD and increasing patient age. Bach et al. (48) have described the involution of thymic function with increasing age. Thymic function decreases above age 30, is very low at age 40, and ceases above age 50 years.

Further support for the hypothesis comes from a number of observations from this and other laboratories. Patients with chronic GVHD exhibit significantly decreased cell-mediated and humoral immune reactivity when compared to long-term survivors without GVHD. They show a striking inability to form antibodies to new antigens such as bacteriophage ϕX174 and keyhole limpet hemocyanin. On repeated antigenic challenge, they seem unable to convert from IgM to IgG antibody production, although quite frequently they have significantly higher than normal serum levels of polyclonal IgG. *In vitro* studies show deficient IgM responses after *Staphylococcus aureus* stimulation (49), and yet examination of biopsies of skin shows impressive IgM and complement deposits at the dermoepidermal junction. In contrast to patients without GVHD, patients with chronic GVHD show circulating nonspecific suppressor cells in a high percentage of cases, which, along with polyclonal elevation of IgG and circulating autoantibody, appear to be another inappropriate immunologic expression of this disease (50). Specific suppressor cells, present in long-term survivors without GVHD, presumably mediating transplantation tolerance, are conspicuously absent in patients with chronic GVHD. Histologic examination of lymph nodes from seven patients with severe chronic GVHD showed lymphocytopenia in T-dependent areas, whereas germinal centers were present in six of the seven, and, indeed, plasma cell infiltration was prominent in the medullary cords. Another group of investigators studied six patients with chronic GVHD and found lack of Th2-positive cells (i.e., suppressor cells) in two patients and an increase in four (51). Two of these four patients had Th-positive, Ia-positive T cells, suggesting *in vivo* activation of suppressor cells. They also noted active suppression by these cells of *in vitro* immune responses, which is in line with the hypothesis that immunoregulatory cells may profoundly affect the overall immune response.

In summary, the immunologic mechanisms involved in chronic GVHD are as yet poorly understood but point toward a complex immunodysregulation. New approaches to prevent or remove the immunoregulatory imbalance, perhaps by transplants of thymic epithelial monolayers or thymic fragments or by the use of thymic factors, must be explored.

3.4. Recovery of Immunologic Function

Approximately one-third of patients who achieve a functional allogeneic marrow graft develop fatal interstitial pneumonitis, and one-half of these have evidence of cytomegalovirus infection (52). Candida septicemia, *Pneumocystis carinii* pneumonia, and a variety of other infections have been observed in these patients. The high incidence of infection is presumably the result of poor immunologic reactivity, the sum of a variety of conditions: (1) the patient's own immune system is destroyed by either the disease or the conditioning regimen; (2) the postgrafting phase, even of recipients of syngeneic grafts, is characterized by a slow return of immunologic reactivity that is probably simply a function of a slow repopulation of the lymphoid system by donor cells; (3) the postgrafting treatment with immunosuppressive agents used to prevent GVHD also suppresses the immune response to other antigens; (4) the graft-versus-host reaction may lead to destruction of donor lymphoid cells (allergic death) by an excess of host antigens; or (5) ATG and steroid therapies used to treat established GVHD also result in nonspecific immunosuppression. An understanding of the immunologically deficient state and the development of possible means of its prevention are of great importance.

The immunologic system in recipients of marrow grafts is derived from cells of donor origin. The pattern of immunologic recovery has already been defined to some extent in several animal models. In inbred rodent radiation chimeras, immunologic reactivity was found to be very low in the immediate postgrafting period, regardless of whether they were recipients of syngeneic or allogeneic marrow (reviewed in reference 49). Some months after transplantation, syngeneic chimeras were found to have complete recovery of immunologic reactivity. Allogeneic and xenogeneic rodent chimeras were in general less immunologically reactive than their syngeneic counterparts, even when studied as late as 300 days postgrafting.

We surveyed the immune status of 50 allogeneic and five autologous canine chimeras for periods of up to 8 years after grafting (53). They showed a severe combined immune deficiency during the first 200 days of postgrafting, with quantitatively and qualitatively impaired humoral antibody responses to sheep red blood cells and the neoantigen bacteriophage ϕX174. Similarly, first- and second-set allogeneic skin graft survivals were prolonged. Long-term canine chimeras showed a return of immune function to the normal range. They were able to live in an unprotected environment with no increase in the incidence of infection as compared to normal dogs.

We have reported a study of immune function in 56 long-term survivors after marrow grafting from HLA-identical siblings and have reviewed the earlier reports (49). All patients had survived for 1 to 5 years postgrafting. Immunologic studies on the marrow donor served to establish the normal range for the tests used. All patients had pronounced impairment of all immunologic parameters studied during the first 4 months postgrafting. Differences existed in regard to the tempo and the pattern of immunologic reconstitution between patients who never had GVHD and those who developed chronic GVHD. Antibody responses, both quantitatively and qualitatively, to neoantigens such as bacteriophage ϕX174 or keyhold limpet hemocyanin returned to the normal range within the first year in GVHD-free patients, whereas patients with chronic GVHD continued to show profoundly deficient antibody responses. Similarly, GVHD-free patients showed return of positive skin test responsiveness to dinitrochlorobenzene and keyhole limpet hemocyanin, whereas patients with chronic GVHD showed little or no return. Polyclonal IgG levels in the serum were significantly higher in patients with chronic GVHD than in those without GVHD.

One striking finding was that despite the poor *in vivo* immune reactivity during the first months following transplantation, many *in vitro* parameters of immunity rapidly returned to the normal range. For instance, total-lymphocyte counts and the numbers of T and B cells in the peripheral blood were normal by 3 months, and cells involved in natural killing, antibody-dependent killing, or lectin-dependent killing were generally normal by 1 month. Many patients showed good responsiveness in mixed leukocyte culture and to various mitogens by 1 to 2 months postgrafting. These findings suggest that the currently used *in vitro* tests and lymphocyte markers are not good indicators of the real immunologic status after marrow grafting and demonstrate the necessity of developing new *in vitro* methodology to study these patients.

Studies of B-cell function *in vitro* assessed by direct and indirect hemolysis in gel assays were carried out (54,55). No plaque-forming cells could be induced after *Staphylococcus aureus* stimulation during the first 3 or 4 months after marrow transplantation, which correlates well with a lack of *in vivo* antibody responses. Similar findings were made with the indirect plaque-forming assay, which allowed determination not only of cells secreting IgM antibodies, but also those of other immunoglobulin classes. *In vitro* B-cell function returned to normal within 1 year in patients without chronic GVHD but remained abnormal in those with chronic GVHD. These results suggest that the plaque-forming assays might be useful for studying the mechanisms involved in deficient B-cell function *in vivo* seen early after marrow transplantation. For instance, coculture studies with various lymphocyte subpopulations from the marrow donor might clarify whether the B-cell deficiency is due to an intrinsic defect of B cells, a lack of helper cells, or an excess of suppressor cells.

3.5. Tolerance

In a healthy long-term chimera, the immunologically competent foreign graft does not mount a harmful reaction against the host. At least three possible mechanisms for the maintenance of stable graft-host tolerance are discussed in the following subsections.

Blocking Factors. In dogs, stable chimeras had lymphocytes exclusively of donor origin that were capable of reaction against host fibroblasts, and this lymphocyte response was inhibited by serum from the chimera. These data were obtained by using the colony inhibition assay (56). Subsequently, similar data were reported for tetraparental mice, mice made neonatally tolerant, and rodent radiation chimeras (reviewed in reference 57). These observations gave rise to the concept of tolerance mediated by a serum blocking factor. One study reported the presence of blocking factors after marrow transplantation in humans.

We reexamined the question of serum blocking factors in DLA-matched donor-recipient dogs (57). By sensitization to skin grafts, it was easily demonstrated that the cell inhibition assay was able to detect immunity against minor histocompatibility systems. Both long- and short-term chimeras occasionally demonstrated cell inhibition of chimeric fibroblasts, but serum blocking factors were usually not present. In an effort to demonstrate blocking factors *in vivo,* we infused large volumes of chimeric plasma into dogs given skin grafts, but survival of the skin grafts was not altered. More recent data in DLA nonidentical dogs with the use of mixed leukocyte culture assay also failed to show evidence for serum blocking factors (32).

We then studied the phenomena of cellular inhibition and serum blocking factors in human patients given marrow grafts from HLA-identical siblings (58). Of 14 long-term chimeras studied, lymphocytes from 11 did not show cell inhibition, and only three showed cell inhibition that was blocked in the presence of chimera serum. Short-term survivors with and without GVHD showed a spectrum of *in vitro* reactivity, with only about one-half of the patients showing evidence of serum blocking factors. There was no correlation with presence or absence of GVHD. From these studies in humans and in dogs, it was concluded that maintenance of stable graft-host tolerance after marrow grafting did not depend on the presence of serum blocking factors.

Central Tolerance. A number of investigators using rodents rendered neonatally tolerant suggested that tolerance was due to a central failure of immune responsiveness (reviewed in reference 32): (1) spleen cells from tolerant animals failed to produce GVHD when injected into animals of the tolerated strain; (2) GVHD activity of normal spleen cells was not abolished by serum from tolerant animals; (3) attempts to prolong skin graft survival by passive transfer of serum from tolerant animals failed; (4) it was possible to abrogate tolerance by adoptive transfer of normal spleen cells; (5) the mixed leukocyte culture response of tolerant lymphocytes to cells of the tolerated strain was negative whereas the response to third party lymphocytes was positive; (6) lymphocytes from mouse radiation chimeras were unable to kill tumor cells of host anti-genicity *in vitro*; and (7) serum from these animals did not prevent immune cells of donor type from being cytotoxic to cells of the host type. Von Boehmer and Sprent (59) could find no evidence for suppressor cells in the maintenance of tolerance to histocompatibility antigens in murine parent to F_1 hybrid radiation chimeras with either the mixed leukocyte culture or cell-mediated lympho-lysis assays and concluded that clonal deletion was the responsible mechanism.

We studied canine chimeras without GVHD that had received marrow from DLA identical littermates. The donors were given 1200 R and marrow from the chimera (of donor origin) followed by a skin graft from the chimera. The skin grafts were rejected, suggesting that the clone(s) capable of reacting against the chimera- (host-) histocompatible antigens were still present in the donor marrow in the chimera.

Suppressor Cells. Evidence for the presence of suppressor cells was re-ported from studies in tetraparental mice (reviewed in reference 50). It was found that spleen cells from these mice could block mixed leukocyte culture reactivity between the two parental cell types, but not between those of un-related strains. Others presented evidence of suppressor T cells in mice tolerant to skin allografts and to fowl immunoglobulin. Splenic and thymic suppressor cells have been reported to inhibit GVHD activity in mice. A study by Tutschka et al. (60) in rats involving transplantation of chimeric cells supported the sup-pressor cell concept. In contrast, Wilson and Nowell (61) reported that toler-ant cells did not interfere with nontolerant cells in mixed leukocyte culture. Similar negative findings have been reported by Elkins (62).

We investigated the effect of infusion of large numbers of lymphocytes from the marrow donor into stable chimeras. None of the 14 chimeras given lym-phocytes from normal donors developed GVHD (63). In contrast, 8 of 12 chimeras given lymphocytes from donors specifically sensitized against the chimera by grafts of the chimera skin developed GVHD. Results with lympho-cytes from nonsensitized donors are not consistent with clonal deletion, but rather suggest the presence of an active mechanism suppressing recognition of host antigen by donor lymphocytes. This mechanism apparently can be over-come by infusion of donor lymphocytes that have already recognized host antigens and become sensitized.

We also studied healthy chimeras that had received marrow from DLA non-identical (mixed leukocyte culture reactive) donors (32). Circulating lympho-cytes from these chimeras (of donor origin) failed to react in mixed leukocyte culture against cryopreserved host lymphocytes while retaining good reactivity to third-party cells. Mixing experiments did not show evidence of suppressor cells, and serum blocking factors could not be demonstrated. These data are thus in keeping with clonal deletion as the mechanism for tolerance in canine radiation chimeras and are in apparent contrast to our previous findings that favored a cellular suppressor mechanism. To reconcile these seemingly opposing findings, it may be that clonal "abortion" is operative, that is, with inactivation or destruction of newly generated lymphoid cells capable of reacting with host antigen by a cellular suppressor mechanism residing in central lymphoid tissues and requiring the continuous presence of host antigen.

It is clear that we do not as yet have a good understanding of the immunologic mechanism(s) of the tolerance observed in stable, long-term marrow graft recipients. It is difficult to reconcile the differing results of observation made *in vitro* or *in vivo* in different species and in differing degrees of donor-host histocompatibility. It seems likely that more than one mechanism is involved.

3.6. Role of Interferon in Marrow Transplantation

Recent data suggest that interferons may have great potential in clinical marrow transplantation (reviewed in reference 64). The interferons are inducible glycoproteins produced by cells in response to viruses and other stimuli (see Chapter 7). Their potential role in marrow transplantation derives from their effects on resistance to certain viruses, their manifold effects on various components of the immune response, and their increasingly documented antitumor activities. The three effects may ultimately be translated into clinical benefits by helping to alleviate the three major clinical problems posed by allogeneic marrow transplantation, namely, cytomegalovirus (CMV) infections, GVHD, and recurrence of leukemia (3).

The antiviral activities of the interferons have been documented *in vitro* in experimental animals and, increasingly, in humans. In three patients with chronic active hepatitis administration of human leukocyte interferon (HuLeIF) was associated with a rapid and reproducible fall in all Dane particle markers. Moreover, controlled studies showed that HuLeIF decreases the progression and dissemination of herpes zoster in cancer patients, promotes the healing of herpes simplex virus interstitial keratitis, and reduces the incidence of herpes labialis reactivation after trigeminal ganglion decompression (65). Finally, a study in immunosuppressed renal transplant recipients showed that prophylactic HuLeIF delayed the shedding of CMV and decreased the incidence of viremia after transplantation (66). The delay in onset of active infection and the decrease in viremia observed could be very beneficial in marrow transplant recipients because the period of greatest risk for CMV pneumonia is the first 3 months after the transplant, and HuLeIF administered during that time could conceivably decrease the incidence of fatal CMV pneumonia.

Interferons have been demonstrated to have many effects on the immune response by mechanisms not yet established. B-cell, T-cell, natural killer cell, and macrophage functions have been affected, with enhancement or suppression partly depending on the timing of interferon administration, the antigens involved, and the particular response studied. Thus, although the proliferative response of lymphocytes is depressed by interferon, the cytotoxic responses by T cells and natural killer cells are enhanced (64). In animal models interferons have been reported to increase or decrease the graft-versus-host reaction. It is difficult to predict the potential effect of interferon therapy on GVHD in marrow transplant recipients.

Finally, interferons have been shown to have an effect against various viral and nonviral primary and transplanted tumors in animals and, more recently, in humans. Encouraging preliminary results have been obtained with HuLeIF in patients with osteogenic sarcoma, nodular poorly differentiated lymphocytic lymphoma (NPDLL), multiple myeloma, breast cancer, and acute leukemia. Patients with osteogenic sarcoma treated prophylactically with HuLeIF after surgical resection of the primary tumor were reported to have a lower incidence of metastases than did noninterferon treated historical or contemporary controls (67). At Stanford University Medical Center, three of three patients with NPDLL showed a dramatic response to HuLeIF as the sole form of therapy (68), and so did three of six patients with NPDLL treated by Gutterman et al. (69). Multiple myeloma has been reported to be unusually responsive to HuLeIF. Two complete and two partial responses were reported in four patients in Sweden (70) and objective responses were also observed in 6 of 10 myeloma patients by Gutterman et al. (69). Patients with breast cancer treated with HuLeIF also showed objective responses in 7 of 17 cases (69). Finally, HuLeIF has been reported (71) to have shown some antitumor effect in four children with acute leukemia as reflected by transient reduction in the peripheral blood blast count and, to a lesser extent, in the marrow.

The preliminary data available show that HuLeIF can exert objectively measurable antitumor effects in some patients with some malignancies. However, the overall efficacy of such therapy and its potential as an adjunct to other modes of therapy such as chemoradiotherapy and marrow transplantation remains unknown. In rodent models, interferon when combined with cytotoxic chemotherapy, has yielded synergistic antitumor effects (64). However, such use has not yet been reported in humans.

It must be emphasized that the antitumor therapeutic results reported in humans have been obtained with empirically derived, variable, and probably suboptimal regimens of HuLeIF and have used material that is only approximately 0.1% pure. It is, therefore, likely that the therapeutic results will be more impressive when more purified interferon preparations became available and are administered in optimal doses and schedules. Finally, since all the clinical results cited were obtained with HuLeIF, no predictions can yet be made about the potential utility of fibroblast interferon or of immune interferon produced by T cells in response to antigens. Nevertheless, the results to date suggest that interferon may have an important role in marrow transplantation for its antitumor and antiviral effects and possibly for its effects on immunologic reactivity.

4. STUDIES OF RECURRENT LEUKEMIA AFTER GRAFTING

4.1. Recurrence of Leukemia After Grafting

In 1978 we reported an analysis of 139 patients with acute leukemia in relapse who were given intensive chemoradiotherapy followed by a marrow transplant that indicated that the long-term survivors were probably cured (14,15). Now, after an additional 3 years of follow-up, these patients continue in remission, lending support to our previous hypothesis that these patients are cured (Figure 1). A Kaplan-Meier plot of the probability that a patient will be in remission at any given time after grafting disclosed a rather constant rate of recurrence of leukemia in the first year, a decreasing rate in the second year and no recurrences thereafter. This analysis, which compensates for the death of patients due to causes other than leukemia, showed that only approximately 35% of the patients would be cured whereas 65% would be destined to relapse. A review of reports by other marrow transplant groups showed, in general, a similar experience with recurrence of leukemia (17). Our experience during the past 4 years with patients transplanted in remission (Figure 2 and patients transplanted more recently) was analyzed by a Kaplan-Meier plot to project the expected percent of patients who would relapse by the end of 2 years. Thirty-nine patients with ALL transplanted in second or subsequent remission showed an expected relapse fraction of 55%, which may not be significantly different from the expected relapses for patients transplanted in relapse. Most impressive, and rather unexpected, was the finding that only 2% (1 of 45) of patients with ANL transplanted in first remission relapsed subsequently. The 19 patients with ANL transplanted in second remission showed a relapse fraction of 35%.

The results show quite clearly that patients transplanted in first remission have a very low rate of subsequent recurrence of leukemia, whereas patients transplanted in second or subsequent remission are destined to have a much higher rate of recurrence. Our results suggest that patients in first remission may, indeed, have a relatively small number of leukemic cells whereas those in second or subsequent remission may have a relatively large number of leukemic cells, perhaps just below the level of clinical detection. Another possible contributing factor may be that the leukemic cells of patients in first remission may not yet have acquired resistance to therapeutic agents.

4.2. Nature of Recurrent Leukemia

By utilizing blood genetic markers and cytogenetic techniques, it is possible to identify the origin of both the normal and abnormal cells following marrow grafting. All patients given 1000 rad TBI, with or without additional chemotherapy, have invariably showed normal marrow cells only of donor type. In our initial series of patients prepared with 1000 rad TBI without additional chemotherapy, five of six patients with ALL suffered a recurrence of leukemia. Two of these patients were girls, and the marrow donor was a brother. Cytogenetic studies showed the recurrent leukemia to be in donor type cells (72,73). Two patients with AML in relapse given allogeneic marrow grafts have also relapsed in donor-type cells (74,75).

The theoretical implications and possible mechanisms for the recurrence in donor cells have been discussed previously. A possible explanation might be the existence of a leukemogenic virus in the host, perhaps induced by the TBI (76). However, there is at present no evidence for the existence of leukemogenic viruses in humans. Further, recent observations indicate that both viral and nonviral transforming genes can be transferred to and expressed in certain types of recipient cells (e.g., NIH/3T3) following transfection with free DNA and/or chromatin (77–80). Thus an alternative possibility is that cellular genes responsible for malignant transformation may have been transferred to donor cells. It is important to note that donor cells were infused into the recipient within a few hours after the administration of TBI at a time when the large mass of leukemic cells was undergoing rapid disintegration. Thus exposure of marrow stem cells to DNA or chromatin fragments from host leukemic tissue may have occurred.

Since that early experience we have always administered the two large doses of CY 5 and 4 days before TBI. Thus, at the time of TBI and marrow administration, extensive destruction of leukemic cells has already occurred. With the use of this regimen, the recurrent leukemia observed in more than 50 patients with a donor of opposite sex has always been in host-type cells. In many instances the recurrent leukemic cell population has displayed a marker chromosome characteristic of the disease before transplantation.

4.3. Efforts to Prevent Recurrence of Leukemia After Grafting

The reappearance of the original leukemic cell clone after the administration of CY and 1000 rad TBI indicates a remarkably resistant population of cells. Regardless of whether this resistance was acquired during previous therapy, it seemed logical to attempt more vigorous antileukemic chemotherapy prior to the TBI. Our group and several other marrow transplant teams have attempted to do this with combinations of drugs such as daunomycin, cytosine arabinoside, 6-thioguanine, and BCNU. The results, reviewed elsewhere (81), have been discouraging in that recurrence of leukemia has continued to be a major problem and a reduction in the recurrence rate of leukemia, if any, has been offset by increased toxicity, thus preventing improvement of overall survival rate. A major problem may be that most of the patients had already been exposed to the most effective agents, and the likelihood of leukemic cell resistance to these agents would be expected to be high. Protection by marrow transplantation makes it possible to explore some agents that otherwise could not be used because of marrow toxicity. Busulfan and dimethyl busulfan are two such agents currently being explored (17). Most attractive are agents whose mechanism of action is entirely different from that of chemoradiotherapy. Examples of such new agents include the use of interferon and the use of monoclonal antibodies reacting specifically with leukemic cells. The utility of such agents might be best demonstrated when applied following marrow graft, when the number of leukemic cells is minimal.

4.4. Graft-Versus-Leukemia

In the first studies of marrow transplantation in a murine leukemia model, Barnes et al. (82) pointed out that a small residual population of leukemic cells might be killed off by a reaction of the engrafted marrow against the leukemic cells. Subsequently Mathe et al. (83) enlarged upon this concept and coined the term "adoptive immunotherapy." More recently Bortin (84) and Fefer et al. (85) have presented evidence in support of a graft-versus-leukemia effect in murine systems.

Evidence supporting the existence of a graft-versus-leukemia effect in human recipients of allogeneic bone marrow grafts has been difficult to obtain because of the large number of deaths from other causes among patients with severe GVHD. Some recipients of allogeneic marrow have had no GVHD but have remained free of leukemia for 2 to 9 years. Other patients have developed severe acute GVHD but have suffered a recurrence of leukemia within a few months after grafting. Recently, utilizing sophisticated statistical methodologies, we have been able to account for differing intervals and competing causes of risk to study the rate of leukemic relapse in 46 recipients of syngeneic marrow, 117 recipients of allogeneic marrow with no or minimal GVHD, and 79 recipients of allogeneic marrow with moderate to severe or chronic disease (86). The relative relapse rate was 2.5 times less in allogeneic marrow recipients with GVHD than in recipients without it. This apparent antileukemic effect was more marked in patients with lymphoblastic than nonlymphoblastic leukemia and in those who received transplants during relapse rather than during remission and was most evident during the first 130 days after transplantation. Survival of all patients was comparable since the lesser probability of recurrent leukemia in patients with GVHD was offset by a greater probability of other causes of death. More recent studies (unpublished) support these initial observations, except that overall survival now seems to be better in patients with moderate to severe GVHD.

Thus, from studies in murine systems and in humans, it appears that the graft-versus-host reaction does have a significant antileukemic effect, suggesting that a therapeutic advantage might be achieved utilizing this effect. In 1968 Boranic described a treatment plan of this type (87). Leukemic mice were given transplants of allogeneic immunocompetent cells to initiate a potentially lethal graft-versus-host reaction. The mice were rescued from the graft-versus-host reaction by repeated injections of CY and a transplant of syngeneic marrow cells.

A general problem with this kind of therapeutic approach, particularly so in outbred species such as dogs and humans, is the fact that the graft-versus-host reaction, once initiated, is extremely difficult to control. In fact, with DLA- or HLA-matched donor-recipient pairs, the graft-versus-host reaction, which must be ascribed to antigenic incompatibilities outside the major histocompatibility complex, is nevertheless quite often lethal. As advances are made in the management of acute and chronic GVHD, it may be appropriate to explore the therapeutic potential of the graft-versus-host reaction. Perhaps the current studies of monoclonal antibodies against human T-cell subsets will lead to an ability to terminate or modulate an ongoing graft-versus-host reaction.

4.5. Role of Nature Killer Cells in Relation to Recurrence of Leukemia

Natural killing is a newly discovered mechanism thought to be involved in surveillance against cancer, especially leukemia. We have recently carried out a study involving 88 patients with acute leukemia given marrow grafts from HLA-identical siblings (88). Patients were studied at 30-day intervals after transplantation for the presence of natural killer activity. With some variability, natural killer activity returned to normal by 30 days after grafting. Twenty-four of the 88 leukemic patients studied developed recurrent leukemia after transplantation. We have analyzed our data on the degree of natural killer activity in these patients with respect to recurrence of leukemia and failed to show a significant association. This lack of association held even when other factors known to affect the risk of leukemic recurrence (type of leukemia, remission or relapse status at transplant, residual leukemia at day 7 post-transplantation and GVHD) were taken into account.

There are a number of possible explanations for this lack of association. First, the target cell used, K562, may not be an appropriate indicator for all natural killer activity. Second, it is possible that the tumor load was never sufficiently reduced to a level low enough to be handled successfully by a natural killer mechanism *in vivo*. Third, it could be argued that the leukemias were resistant to natural killer cells. In this vein, all tumors should have already escaped a natural killer surveillance mechanism. Finally, of course, natural killer activity *in vitro* may not represent a surveillance mechanism against leukemia *in vivo*.

4.6. Role of Leukemia-Associated Antigens (LAA) in Marrow Transplantation

It is generally assumed that the end results of marrow transplantation for leukemia reflect solely the antitumor effects of the chemotherapy and TBI and that the only function of the infused donor marrow is hematopoietic restoration and prevention of iatrogenic death. Moreover, although the marrow restores some of the measurable immunologic functions suppressed by chemoradiotherapy, such restored function may perhaps help prevent infections but does not demonstrably contribute to the antitumor effects. Indeed, no relationship between recovery of measurable immunologic function and recurrence of leukemia in marrow transplant recipients has been demonstrated. If the preceding assumptions are valid, then the characteristics that distinguish those marrow transplant recipients who relapse and those who do not must be the tumor load at the time of the chemoradiotherapy and the tumor sensitivity to the chemoradiotherapy. Consequently, the major effort for the future must be directed at approaches to reduce further the tumor load, such as by transplanting while in complete remission as discussed previously, or by developing chemoradiotherapy regimens that will be more effective against the tumor.

It is possible, however, that the infused marrow does exert some specific effect against the tumor. This possibility is raised because eradication of leukemia in animals by radiation alone requires far larger doses than the TBI used in humans (89) and because it is deemed unlikely that the dose of TBI employed can exert such a great cytoreductive and, occasionally, curative antileukemic effect in patients who have large tumor burdens.

The only indirect evidence for the view that allogeneic marrow may contribute to the ultimate antitumor effects observed in our patients is the statistical demonstration mentioned previously to the effect that the leukemic relapse was significantly lower in recipients of *allogeneic* marrow than in recipients of *syngeneic* marrow. (This does not, of course, rule out the possibility that syngeneic marrow also contributes to an antileukemic effect, but to a lesser extent than that exerted by allogeneic marrow.) The graft-versus-host leukemia effect probably reflects a reaction directed against alloantigens present on leukemic cells as well as on normal host cells—a reaction that might be facilitated by an intrinsic increased sensitivity of leukemic cells to immunologic attack. It is also possible, however, that cells from the allogeneic marrow react not only to the normal alloantigens on the leukemic cells, but also against LAA to which the marrow is already sensitized or has become sensitized in the host. Such a reaction to LAA could conceivably be exerted by both allogeneic and syngeneic marrow.

The existence of human LAA has been suggested by many serologic and cellular studies (90-92). Moreover, peripheral blood lymphocytes from some prospective syngeneic or allogeneic HLA-identical sibling marrow donors have been reported to respond in mixed leukocyte culture to leukemic cells from future marrow recipients (93,94). However, there is no evidence that such LAA are recognized *in vivo* by infused marrow or that they are the target of an attack by the infused marrow against host leukemic cells.

Rodent models utilizing supralethal TBI directly analogous to marrow transplantation in humans have not received the requisite investigative attention in recent years. However, models have been developed in which mice bearing disseminated syngeneic tumors have been saved by a combination of noncurative sublethal chemotherapy plus donor lymphocytes specifically sensitized to TAA (95). Although the models are not strictly analogous to the marrow transplant model in humans nor can yet be directly extrapolated to humans, studies in the models have identified problems that, if resolved, may eventually suggest how to take advantage of the existence of putative LAA in humans and alter the role of human marrow transplantation for the treatment of malignant disease. In syngeneic adoptive chemoimmunotherapy (ACIT) models, the demonstration that the most effective cells are T cells immune to TAA has stimulated attempts to sensitize cells to TAA *in vitro* and render them more effective *in vivo* (96,97). A variety of subpopulations of lymphoid cells have been generated—including cytotoxic effector cells as well as suppressor cells that prevent the therapeutic efficacy of immune cells (98). The results have raised the issue of how to generate preferentially the requisite effector cells and/or to eliminate suppressor cells.

Studies in allogeneic ACIT models involving varying degrees of donor-host histoincompatibility have emphasized the role of the major histocompatibility complex in determining both the immunogenicity and the immunosensitivity of tumor cells (99), the need for viable donor lymphocytes to persist in the host for some time, and the problems and challenges posed by GVHD (95).

Finally, the problem of obtaining adequate numbers of lymphocytes for possible therapy is being explored by using factors to grow long-term cultures of cytotoxic lymphocytes *in vitro* (100). The characterization of such cells and their function *in vitro* and, especially, their possible therapeutic efficacy in appropriate animal models *in vivo* is under active investigation.

If the above-mentioned problems identified in animal models are postulated to be relevant to the future development in humans of an approach similar to ACIT and analogous to the present marrow transplantation in humans, there are several potential implications (99). If cells sensitized to TAA are essential for efficacy, then in autologous marrow transplantation autologous cells may be considered as already primed to TAA, and secondary sensitization *in vitro* to TAA would represent a potential way of increasing the quantity of effector cells and bypassing the mechanisms that presumably limit effective sensitization *in vivo*. The principal problem is likely to be contamination of the infused marrow by tumor. For syngeneic marrow transplantation, it may be necessary to attempt to sensitize normal twin lymphocytes to patient tumor *in vitro*. For allogeneic marrow transplantation, *in vitro* sensitization to patient tumor may, of course, also result in sensitization to patient alloantigens and potentially increase the risk of GVHD. Accordingly, methods must be developed to either control GVHD *in vivo* or somehow specifically deplete GVHD-inducing cells *in vitro* while retaining those cells that have an antileukemic effect.

The principal point, however, is that if methods can be developed to generate donor cells that will have an effector function against the tumor to be treated, it is conceivable that we might either add such cells to the present regimen of high-dose chemoradiotherapy and marrow transplantation or may eventually be able to rely more on the specific antitumor effect of infused effector cells and less on the antitumor effect of the chemoradiotherapy. Moreover, since the reason for extraordinarily high doses of chemoradiotherapy now employed is for both maximal antileukemic effect and for immunosuppression so as to allow hematopoietic engraftment, if potent antileukemic cells do require only a relatively short time in the host to exert their antitumor effect, long-term or life-long chimerism may not be necessary. The requisite transient engraftment might then be achieved with far lower and less toxic doses of chemoradiotherapy than are now being employed.

In short, although it is assumed that the antitumor effect observed with marrow transplantation reflects the antitumor effect of chemoradiotherapy and no antitumor effect of the infused marrow, studies in rodent models suggest the possibility that either an additional antitumor effect may be obtained by the infusion of specific antitumor effector cells and/or that marrow transplantation in the future may rely more on the antitumor effect of infused cells and may, therefore, require less chemoradiotherapy.

REFERENCES

1. L. O. Jacobson, E. K. Marks, M. J. Robson, E. O. Gaston, and R. E. Zirkle, Effect of spleen protection on mortality following x-irradiation. *J. Lab. Clin. Med.,* **34**, 1538 (1949).

2. E. Lorenz, C. Congdon, and D. Uphoff, Modification of acute irradiation injury in mice and guinea-pigs by bone marrow injections. *Radiology,* **58**, 863 (1951).

3. E. D. Thomas, R. Storb, R. A. Clift, A. Fefer, F. L. Johnson, P. E. Neiman, K. G. Lerner, H. Glucksberg, and C. D. Buckner, Bone-marrow transplantation. *New Engl. J. Med.,* **292**, 832, 895 (1975).

4. E. D. Thomas, H. L. Lochte, Jr., J. H. Cannon, O. D. Sahler, and J. W. Ferrebee, Supralethal whole body irradiation and isologous marrow transplantation in man. *J. Clin. Invest.,* **38**, 1709 (1959).

5. D. E. Uphoff and L. W. Law, An evaluation of some genetic factors influencing irradiation protection by bone marrow. *J. Natl. Cancer Inst.,* **22**, 229 (1959).

6. R. B. Epstein, R. Storb, H. Ragde, and E. D. Thomas, Cytotoxic typing antisera for marrow grafting in littermate dogs. *Transplantation,* **6**, 45 (1968).

7. R. A. Gatti, H. J. Meuwissen, H. D. Allen, R. Hong, and R. A. Good, Immunological reconstitution of sex-linked lymphopenic immunological deficiency. *Lancet,* **2**, 1366 (1968).

8. W. F. Bodmer, The HLA system. *Br. Med. Bull.,* **34**, 213–316 (1978).

9. E. D. Thomas and R. Storb, Technique for human marrow grafting. *Blood,* **36**, 507 (1970).

10. B. Dupont, R. J. O'Reilly, M. S. Pollack, and R. A. Good, Use of HLA genotypically different donors in bone marrow transplantation. *Transplant. Proc.,* **11**, 219 (1979).

11. E. D. Thomas, C. D. Buckner, R. Storb, P. E. Neiman, A. Fefer, R. A. Clift, S. J. Slichter, D. D. Funk, J. I. Bryant, and K. G. Lerner, Aplastic anaemia treated by marrow transplantation. *Lancet,* **1**, 284 (1972).

12. B. M. Camitta, E. D. Thomas, D. G. Nathan, R. P. Gale, K. J. Kopecky, J. M. Rappeport, G. Santos, E. C. Gordon-Smith, and R. Storb, A prospective study of androgens and bone marrow transplantation for treatment of severe aplastic anemia. *Blood,* **53**, 504 (1979).

13. R. Storb, E. D. Thomas, C. D. Buckner, R. A. Clift, H. J. Deeg, A. Fefer, B. W. Goodell, G. E. Sale, J. E. Sanders, J. Singer, P. Stewart, and P. L. Weiden, Marrow transplantation in thirty "untransfused" patients with severe aplastic anemia. *Ann Intern. Med.,* **92**, 30 (1980).

14. E. D. Thomas, C. D. Buckner, M. Banaji, R. A. Clift, A. Fefer, N. Flournoy, B. W. Goodell, R. O. Hickman, K. G. Lerner, P. E. Neiman, G. E. Sale, J. E. Sanders, J. Singer, M. Stevens, R. Storb, and P. L. Weiden, One hundred patients with acute leukemia treated by chemotherapy, total body irradiation, and allogeneic marrow transplantation. *Blood,* **49**, 511 (1977).

15. A. Fefer, C. D. Buckner, E. D. Thomas, M. A. Cheever, R. A. Clift, H. Glucksberg, P. E. Neiman, and R. Storb, Cure of hematologic neoplasia with transplantation of marrow from identical twins, *New Engl. J. Med.,* **297**, 146 (1977).

16. E. D. Thomas, N. Flournoy, C. D. Buckner, R. A. Clift, A. Fefer, P. E. Neiman, and R. Storb, Cure of leukemia by marrow transplantation. *Leukemia Res.,* **1**, 67 (1977).

17. G. W. Santos, G. J. Elfenbein, and P. J. Tutschka, Bone marrow transplantation—present status. *Transplant. Proc.,* **11**, 182 (1979).

18. E. D. Thomas, J. E. Sanders, N. Flournoy, F. L. Johnson, C. D. Buckner, R. A. Clift, A. Fefer, B. W. Goodell, R. Storb, and P. L. Weiden, Marrow transplantation for patients with acute lymphoblastic leukemia in remission. *Blood,* **54**, 468 (1979).

19. E. D. Thomas, C. D. Buckner, R. A. Clift, A. Fefer, F. L. Johnson, P. E. Neiman, G. E. Sale, J. E. Sanders, J. W. Singer, H. Shulman, R. Storb, and P. L. Weiden, Marrow transplantation for acute nonlymphoblastic leukemia in first remission. *New Engl. J. Med.,* **301**, 597 (1979).

20. R. A. Clift, J. A. Hansen, E. D. Thomas, C. D. Buckner, J. E. Sanders, E. M. Mickelson, R. Storb, F. L. Johnson, J. W. Singer, and B. W. Goodell, Marrow transplantation from donors other than HLA-identical siblings. *Transplantation,* **28**, 235 (1979).

21. K. Doney, C. D. Buckener, G. E. Sale, R. Ramberg, C. Boyd, and E. D. Thomas, Treatment of chronic granulocytic leukemia by chemotherapy, total body irradiation and allogeneic bone marrow transplantation. *Exp. Hematol.,* **6**, 738 (1978).

22. A. Fefer, M. A. Cheever, E. D. Thomas, C. Boyd, R. Ramberg, H. Glucksberg, C. D. Buckner, and R. Storb, Disappearance of Ph¹-positive cells in four patients with chronic granulocytic leukemia after chemotherapy, irradiation and marrow transplantation from an identical twin. *New Engl. J. Med.,* **300**, 333 (1979).

23. C. D. Buckner, F. R. Appelbaum, and E. D. Thomas, Bone marrow and fetal liver. In A. M. Karow and D. E. Pegg, Eds., *Organ Preservation for Transplantation,* Dekker, Chapter 16, pp. 355–375, 1981.

24. C. D. Buckner, R. A. Clift, A. Fefer, P. E. Neiman, R. Storb, and E. D. Thomas, Treatment of blastic transformation of chronic granulocytic leukemia by high dose cyclophosphamide, total body irradiation and infusion of cryopreserved autologous marrow. *Exp. Hematol.,* **2**, 138 (1974).

25. J. M. Goldman, Autografting cryopreserved buffy coat cells for chronic granulocytic leukaemia in transformation. *Exp. Hematol.,* **7**, (Suppl. 5), 389 (1979).

26. K. A. Dicke, A. Zander, G. Spitzer, D. S. Verma, L. Peters, L. Vellekoop, K. B. McCredie, and J. Hester, Autologous bone-marrow transplantation in relapsed adult acute leukaemia. *Lancet,* **1**, 514 (1979).

27. R. P. Gale, Autologous bone marrow transplantation in patients with cancer. *JAMA,* **243**, 540 (1980).

28. R. Storb, P. L. Weiden, H. J. Deeg, B. Torok-Storb, K. Atkinson, T. C. Graham, and E. D. Thomas, Marrow graft studies in dogs. In S. Thierfelder, H. Rodt, and H. J. Kolb, Eds., *Immunobiology of Bone Marrow Transplantation,* Springer-Verlag, Heidelberg, (1980), p. 43.

29. R. Storb and E. D. Thomas (for the Seattle Marrow Transplant Team), Marrow transplantation for treatment of aplastic anaemia. In E. D. Thomas, Ed., *Clinics in Haematology,* Vol. 7, Saunders, London, 1978, p. 597.

30. N. K. C. Ramsay, T. Kim, M. E. Nesbit, W. Krivit, P. F. Coccia, S. H. Levitt, W. G. Woods, and J. H. Kersey, Total lymphoid irradiation and cyclophosphamide as preparation for bone marrow transplantation in severe aplastic anemia, *Blood,* **55**, 344 (1980).

31. W. L. Elkins, Cellular immunology and the pathogenesis of graft versus host reactions. *Progr. Allergy,* **15**, 78 (1971).

32. K. Atkinson, R. Storb, P. L. Weiden, H. J. Deeg, L. Gerhard-Miller, and E. D. Thomas, *In vitro* tests correlating with presence or absence of graft-*vs*-host disease in DLA nonidentical canine radiation chimeras: Evidence that clonal abortion maintains stable graft-host tolerance. *J. Immunol.* **124**, 1808 (1980).

33. R. Storb, H. J. Kolb, T. C. Graham, H. Kolb, P. L. Weiden, and E. D. Thomas, Treatment of established graft-versus-host disease in dogs by antithymocyte serum or prednisone. *Blood,* **42**, 601 (1973).

34. A. H. Owens, Jr. and G. W. Santos, The effect of cytotoxic drugs on graft-versus-host disease in mice. *Transplantation,* **11**, 378 (1971).

35. R. Storb, E. Gluckman, E. D. Thomas, C. D. Buckner, R. A. Clift, A Fefer, H. Glucksberg, T. C. Graham, F. L. Johnson, K. G. Lerner, P. E. Neiman, and H. Ochs, Treatment of established human graft-versus-host disease by antithymocyte globulin. *Blood,* **44**, 57 (1974).

36. P. L. Weiden, K. Doney, R. Storb, and E. D. Thomas, Anti-human thymocyte globulin (ATG) for prophylaxis and treatment of graft-versus-host disease in recipients of allogeneic marrow grafts. *Transplant. Proc.,* **10**, 213 (1978).

37. P. L. Weiden, K. Doney, R. Storb, and E. D. Thomas, Antihuman thymocyte globulin for prophylaxis of graft-versus-host disease. A randomized trial in patients with leukemia treated with HLA-identical sibling marrow grafts. *Transplantation,* **27**, 227 (1979).

38. H. J. Deeg, R. Storb, L. Gerhard-Miller, H. M. Shulman, P. L. Weiden, and E. D. Thomas, Cyclosporin A, a powerful immunosuppressant *in vivo* and *in vitro* in the dog, fails to induce tolerance. *Transplantation,* **29**, 230 (1980).

39. K. A. Dicke and D. W. Van Bekkum, Allogeneic bone marrow transplantation after elimination of immunocompetent cells by means of density gradient centrifugation. *Transplant. Proc.,* **3**, 666 (1971).

40. E. R. Richie, M. T. Gallagher, and J. J. Trentin, Inhibition of the graft-versus-host reaction. II. Prevention of acute graft-versus-host mortality by Fab fragments of antilymphocyte globulin. *Transplantation,* **15**, 486 (1973).

41. W. Müller-Ruchholtz, H.-U. Wottge, and H. K. Müller-Hermelink, Bone marrow transplantation in rats across strong histocompatibility barriers by selective elimination of lymphoid cells in donor marrow. *Transplnt. Proc.,* **8**, 537 (1976).

42. H. Rodt, S. Thierfelder and M. Eulitz, Anti-lymphocytic antibodies and marrow transplantation. III. Effect of heterologous anti-brain antibodies on acute secondary disease in mice. *Eur. J. Immunol.,* **4**, 25 (1974).

43. R. Korngold and J. Sprent, Lethal graft-versus-host disease after bone marrow transplantation across minor histocompatibility barriers in mice. Prevention by removing mature T cells from marrow. *J. Exp. Med.,* **148**, 1687 (1978).

44. H. J. Kolb, I. Rieder, H. Rodt, B. Netzel, H. Grosse-Wilde, S. Scholz, E. Schäffer, H. Kolb, and S. Thierfelder, Antilymphocytic antibodies and marrow transplantation. VI. Graft-versus-host tolerance in DLA-incompatible dogs after *in vitro* treatment of bone marrow with absorbed antithymocyte globulin. *Transplantation,* **27**, 242 (1979).

45. S. Slavin, Z. Fuks, H. S. Kaplan, and S. Strober, Transplantation of allogeneic bone marrow without graft-versus-host disease using total lymphoid irradiation. *J. Exp. Med.,* **147**, 963 (1978).

46. H. M. Shulman, K. M. Sullivan, P. L. Weiden, G. B. McDonald, G. E. Striker, G. E. Sale, R. Hackman, M. S. Tsoi, R. Storb, and E. D. Thomas, Chronic graft-versus-host syndrome in man: A clinicopathologic study of 20 Seattle patients, *Am. J. Med.,* **69,** 204 (1980).

47. K. M. Sullivan, H. M. Shulman, R. Storb, P. L. Weiden, R. P. Witherspoon, and E. D. Thomas, Human chronic graft-vs-host disease (C-GVHD): Course and treatment. *Blood,* **54,** (Suppl. 1) (624), 231a (1979).

48. J. F. Bach, M. Dardenne, J. M. Pleau, and M. A. Bach, Isolation, biochemical characteristics and biological activity of a circulating thymic hormone in the mouse and in the human. In H. Friedman, Ed., *Thymus Factors in Immunity,* New York, 1975, p. 186, **249.**

49. D. R. Noel, R. P. Witherspoon, R. Storb, K. Atkinson, K. Doney, E. M. Mickelson, H. D. Ochs, R. P. Warren, P. L. Weiden, and E. D. Thomas, Does graft-versus-host disease influence the tempo of immunologic recovery after allogeneic human marrow transplantation? An observation on 56 long-term survivors. *Blood,* **51,** 1087 (1978).

50. M. S. Tsoi, R. Storb, S. Dobbs, K. J. Kopecky, E. Santos, P. L. Weiden, and E. D. Thomas, Nonspecific suppressor cells in patients with chronic graft-*vs*-host disease after marrow grafting, *J. Immunol.,* **123,** 1970 (1979).

51. E. L. Reinherz, R. Parkman, J. Rappeport, F. S. Rosen, and S. F. Schlossman, Aberrations of suppressor T cells in human graft-versus-host disease, *New Engl. J. Med.,* **300,** 1061 (1979).

52. J. D. Meyers and E. D. Thomas, Infection complicating bone marrow transplantation. In L. S. Young and R. H. Rubin, Eds., *Clinical Approach to Infection in the Immunocompromised Host,* Plenum, New York (in press), Chapter 15.

53. H. D. Ochs, R. Storb, E. D. Thomas, H. J. Kolb, T. C. Graham, E. Mickelson, M. Parr, and R. H. Rudolph, Immunologic reactivity in canine marrow graft recipients, *J. Immunol.,* **113,** 1039 (1974).

54. O. Ringden, R. P. Witherspoon, R. Storb, E. Ekelund, and E. D. Thomas, Increased *in vitro* B-cell IgG secretion during acute graft-versus-host disease and infection. Observations in 50 human marrow transplant recipients. *Blood,* **55,** 179 (1980).

55. O. Ringden, R. Witherspoon, R. Storb, E. Ekelund, and E. D. Thomas, B cell function in human marrow transplant recipients assessed by direct and indirect hemolysis-in-gel assays. *J. Immunol.,* **123,** 2729 (1979).

56. I. Hellström, K. E. Hellström, R. Storb, and E. D. Thomas, Colony inhibition of fibroblasts from chimeric dogs mediated by the dogs' own lymphocytes and specifically abrogated by their serum. *Proc. Natl. Acad. Sci.,* **66,** 65 (1970).

57. M. S. Tsoi, R. Storb, P. L. Weiden, M. L. Schroeder, and E. D. Thomas, Canine marrow transplantation: Do serum blocking factors maintain stable graft-vs.-host tolerance? *Transplant. Proc.,* **7,** 841 (1975).

58. M. S. Tsoi, R. Storb, P. L. Weiden, and E. D. Thomas, Studies on cellular inhibition and serum-blocking factors in 28 human patients given marrow grafts from HLA identical siblings. *J. Immunol.,* **118,** 1799 (1977).

59. H. von Boehmer and J. Sprent, T cell function in bone marrow chimeras: Absence of host-reactive T cells and cooperation of helper T cells across allogeneic barriers. *Transplant. Rev.,* **29,** 3 (1976).

60. P. J. Tutschka, L. Smith, and G. W. Santos, Is the immunodeficiency seen after marrow transplantation maintained by suppressor cells? *Exp. Hematol.,* **6,** (Suppl. 3), 67 (1978).

61. D. B. Wilson and P. C. Nowell, Quantitative studies on the mixed lymphocyte interaction in rats. IV. Immunologic potentiality of the responding cells, *J. Exp. Med.,* **131,** 391 (1970).

62. W. L. Elkins, Correlation of graft-versus-host mortality and positive CML assay in the mouse. *Transplant. Proc.,* **8,** 343 (1976).

63. P. L. Weiden, R. Storb, M. S. Tsoi, T. C. Graham, K. G. Lerner and E. D. Thomas: Infusion of donor lymphocytes into stable canine radiation chimeras: Implications for mechanism of transplantation tolerance, *J. Immunol.*, **116**, 1212 (1976).

64. E. C. Borden: Interferons—Rationale for clinical trials in neoplastic disease. *Ann. Int. Med.*, **91**, 472 (1979).

65. G. J. Pazin, J. A. Armstrong, M. T. Lam, G. C. Tarr, P. J. Jannetta, and M. Ho, Prevention of reactivated herpes simplex infection by human leukocyte interferon after operation on the trigeminal root. *New Engl. J. Med.*, **301**, 225 (1979).

66. S. H. Cheeseman, R. H. Rubin, J. A. Stewart, N. E. Tolkoff-Rubin, A. B. Cosimi, K. Cantell, J. Gilbert, S. Winkle, J. T. Herrin, P. H. Black, P. S. Russell, and M. S. Hirsch, Controlled clinical trial of prophylactic human-leukocyte interferon in renal transplantation. Effects on cytomegalovirus and herpes simplex virus infections. *New Engl. J. Med.*, **300**, 1345 (1979).

67. U. Adamson, T. Aparisi, L. A. Brostrom, et al., Adjuvant interferon treatment of human osteosarcoma. *Cancer Immunol. Immunother.* (in press).

68. T. C. Merigan, K. Sikora, J. H. Breeden, R. Levy, and S. A. Rosenberg, Preliminary observations on the effect of human leukocyte interferon in non-Hodgkin's lymphoma, *New Engl. J. Med.*, **299**, 1449 (1978).

69. J. Gutterman, Y. Yap, A. Buzdar, R. Alexanian, E. Hersh, F. Cabanillas, and S. Greenberg, Leukocyte interferon (IF) induced tumor regression in patients (pts) with breast cancer and B cell neoplasms. *Proc. Am. Assoc. Cancer Res.*, **20**, (674), 167 (1979).

70. H. Mellstedt, A. Ahre, M. Björkholm, G. Holm, B. Johansson, and H. Strander, Interferon therapy in myelomatosis. *Lancet*, **1**, 245 (1979).

71. N. O. Hill, E. Loeb, A. S. Pardue, G. L. Dorn, A. Khan, and J. M. Hill, Response of acute leukemia to leukocyte interferon. *J. Clin. Hematol. Oncology*, **9**, 137 (1979).

72. P. J. Fialkow, E. D. Thomas, J. I. Bryant, and P. E. Neiman, Leukaemic transformation of engrafted human marrow cells *in vivo*. *Lancet*, **1**, 251 (1971).

73. E. D. Thomas, J. I. Bryant, C. D. Buckner, R. A. Clift, A. Fefer, F. L. Johnson, P. Neiman, R. E. Ramberg, and R. Storb, Leukaemic transformation of engrafted human marrow cells *in vivo*. *Lancet*, **1**, 1310 (1972).

74. K. Goh and M. R. Klemperer, *In vivo* leukemic transformation: Cytogenetic evidence of *in vivo* leukemic transformation of engrafted marrow cells. *Am. J. Hematol.*, **2**, 283 (1977).

75. G. J. Elfenbein, D. S. Brogaonkar, W. B. Bias, W. H. Burns, R. Saral, L. L. Sensenbrenner, P. J. Tutschka, B. S. Zaczek, A. R. Zander, R. B. Epstein, J. D. Rowley, and G. W. Santos, Cytogenetic evidence for recurrence of acute myelogenous leukemia after allogeneic bone marrow transplantation in donor hematopoietic cells. *Blood*, **52**, 627 (1978).

76. H. S. Kaplan, On the natural history of the murine leukemias: Presidential Address. *Cancer Res.*, **27**, (Part 1), 1325 (1967).

77. A. Karpas and C. Milstein, Recovery of the genome of murine sarcoma virus (MSV) after infection of cells with nuclear DNA from MSV transformed non-virus producing cells. *Eur. J. Cancer*, **9**, 295 (1973).

78. P. Andersson, M. P. Goldfarb, and R. A. Weinberg, A defined subgenomic fragment of *in vitro* synthesized Moloney sarcoma virus DNA can induce cell transformation upon transfection. *Cell*, **16**, 63 (1979).

79. C. Shih, B.-Z. Shilo, M. P. Goldfarb, A. Dannenberg, and R. A. Weinberg, Passage of phenotypes of chemically transformed cells via transfection of DNA and chromatin. *Proc. Natl. Acad. Sci. (USA)*, **76**, 5714 (1979).

80. N. G. Copeland, A. D. Zelenetz, and G. M. Cooper, Transformation of NIH/3T3 mouse cells by DNA of Rous sarcoma virus. *Cell*, **17**, 993 (1979).

81. E. D. Thomas, C. D. Buckner, A. Fefer, J. E. Sanders, and R. Storb, Efforts to prevent recurrence of leukemia in marrow graft recipients. *Transplant. Proc.,* **10**, 163 (1978).

82. D. W. H. Barnes, M. J. Corp, J. F. Loutit, and F. E. Neal, Treatment of murine leukaemia with x rays and homologous bone marrow. Preliminary communication, *Br. Med. J.,* **2**, 626 (1956).

83. G. Mathe, J. L. Amiel, L. Schwarzenberg, A. Cattan, and M. Schneider, Adoptive immuntherapy of acute leukemia: Experimental and clinical results. *Cancer Res.,* **25**, 1525 (1965).

84. M. M. Bortin, Graft versus leukemia. In F. H. Bach and R. A. Good, Eds., *Clinical Immunobiology,* Vol. 2, Academic, New York, 1974, p. 287.

85. A. Fefer, Adoptive tumor immunotherapy in mice as an adjunct to whole-body X-irradiation and chemotherapy. A review, *Isr. J. Med. Sci.,* **9**, 350 (1973).

86. P. L. Weiden, N. Flournoy, E. D. Thomas, R. Prentice, A. Fefer, C. D. Buckner, and R. Storb, Antileukemic effect of graft-versus-host disease in human recipients of allogeneicmarrow grafts. *New Engl. J. Med.,* **300**, 1068 (1979).

87. M. Boranic, Transient graft-versus-host reaction in the treatment of leukemia in mice. *J. Natl. Cancer Inst.,* **41**, 421 (1968).

88. S. Livnat, M. Seigneuret, R. Storb, and R. L. Prentice, Analysis of cytotoxic effector cell function in patients with leukemia or aplastic anemia before and after marrow transplantation. *J. Immunol.,* **124**, 481 (1980).

89. J. H. Burchenal, H. F. Oettgen, E. A. D. Holmberg, S. C. Hemphill, and J. A. Reppert, Effect of total-body irradiation on the transplantability of mouse leukemias. *Cancer Res.,* **20**, 425 (1960).

90. M. A. Baker, J. A. Falk, W. H. Carter, R. N. Taub, and the Toronto Leukemia Study Group, Early diagnosis of relapse in acute myeloblastic leukemia: Serologic detection of leukemia-associated antigens in human marrow. *New. Engl. J. Med.,* **301**, 1353 (1979).

91. B. G. Leventhal, J. Mirro, Jr., and G. S. Yarbro, Immune reactivity to tumor antigens in leukemia and lymphoma. *Semin. Hematol.,* **15**, 157 (1978).

92. R. S. Metzgar and T. Mohanakumar, Tumor-associated antigens of human leukemia cells. *Semin. Hematol.,* **15**, 139 (1978).

93. A. Fefer, E. Mickelson, and E. D. Thomas, Leukaemia antigens: Mixed leucocyte culture tests on twelve leukaemic patients with identical twins. *Clin. Exp. Immunol.,* **18**, 237 (1974).

94. A. Fefer, E. Mickelson, and E. D. Thomas, Leukaemia antigens: Stimulation of lymphocytes in mixed culture by cells from HL-A identical siblings. *Clin. Exp. Immunol.,* **23**, 214 (1976).

95. A. Fefer, A. B. Einstein, Jr., and M. A. Cheever, Adoptive chemoimmunotherapy of cancer in animals: A review of results, principles and problems. *Ann. N. Y. Acad. Sci.,* **277**, 492 (1976).

96. M. A. Cheever, P. D. Greenberg, and A. Fefer, Tumor neutralization, immunotherapy, and chemoimmunotherapy of a Friend leukemia with cells secondarily sensitized *in vitro:* II. Comparison of cells cultured with and without tumor to noncultured immune cells. *J. Immunol.,* **121**, 2220 (1978).

97. E. Kedar, Z. Raanan, and M. Schwartzbach, *In vitro* induction of cell-mediated immunity to murine leukemia cells. *Cancer Immunol. Immunother.,* **4**, 161 (1978).

98. P. D. Greenberg, M. Cheever, and A. Fefer, Suppression of the *in vitro* secondary response to syngeneic tumor and of *in vivo* tumor therapy with immune cells by culture-induced suppressor cells. *J. Immunol.,* **123**, 515 (1979).

99. J. F. A. P. Miller, Influence of the major histocompatibility complex on T-cell activation. *Adv. Cancer Res.,* **29**, 1 (1979).

100. F. W. Ruscetti, D. A. Morgan, and R. C. Gallo, Functional and morphologic characterization of human T cells continuously grown *in vitro. J. Immunol.,* **119**, 131 (1977).

Lymphocyte Transfer as Potential Cancer Immunotherapy

ALEXANDER FEFER
MARTIN A. CHEEVER
PHILIP D. GREENBERG
Division of Oncology, Department of Medicine
University of Washington School of Medicine
Fred Hutchinson Cancer Research Center
Seattle, Washington

This investigation was supported by Grant CA 10777 and Contract CB 84247-31 awarded by the National Cancer Institute, DHEW. Dr. Greenberg is an American Cancer Society Junior Faculty Fellow, and Dr. Fefer is an American Cancer Society Professor of Clinical Oncology. The authors wish to thank M. Bolton, S. Emery, R. Hung, and B. Keniston for their expert technical assistance and J. Hoak, J. Ryan, and L. Sutch for their assistance in manuscript preparation.

1. INTRODUCTION

The use of lymphocytes as adoptive tumor immunotherapy is predicated on the following assumptions: (1) the tumor possesses antigens (TAA) that can serve as a target for an immune response; (2) the antitumor reaction is facilitated or mediated largely by the type of cell to be infused; (3) an antigenic tumor normally grows progressively either because no antitumor response is evoked or because such a response is quantitatively or qualitatively inadequate, defective or inappropriate; and (4) infusion of large numbers of the requisite cells can overcome that problem and directly or indirectly cure the tumor-bearing host. The validity of these assumptions has not been established, but support for some of them is presented in the other chapters of this book.

An evaluation of the potential for this approach to therapy in humans requires that its effectiveness be demonstrated in animal models and that the models be used to identify problems to be resolved before adoptive immunotherapy can be applied to humans. About a decade ago some adoptive therapy models began to be developed in animals. Concurrently a series of empiric attempts to use lymphocytes to treat advanced cancer in humans were reported, with largely inconclusive results.

There has recently been a resurgence of interest in lymphocyte transfer as therapy due to several developments that favor the likelihood of its eventual clinical application. These include the following: (1) additional animal models have been developed in which syngeneic or allogeneic cells, alone or as an adjunct to other modalities of therapy, can eradicate advanced tumor; (2) methods have been developed for sensitizing lymphocytes to tumor *in vitro* and for using them for therapy in animals; (3) methods have been developed for maintaining lymphocytes in long-term culture with growth factors, thereby increasing the potential for cloning cells for therapeutic purposes; (4) more knowledge has been generated about lymphocyte subpopulations and their interactions with the help of antibodies to lymphocyte membrane antigens; (5) very encouraging results have been obtained in treating leukemic patients with supralethal chemoradiotherapy and syngeneic or allogeneic bone marrow transplantation—an approach that may reflect or involve adoptive immunotherapy; (6) evidence has increased for the existence of a graft-versus-tumor reaction by allogeneic cells in animal models; and (7) evidence has been reported for a graft-versus-leukemia reaction by allogeneic marrow grafts in humans.

In this chapter we review the use of syngeneic or allogeneic lymphocytes for the treatment of tumors in animal models, identify some of the prerequisites for efficacy, explore some of the problems posed by those prerequisites for potential application of immunotherapy to humans, summarize the past attempts at empiric adoptive immunotherapy in humans, and suggest directions for future studies. Some of the information has been previously reviewed (1–4). We are especially indebted to the reviews by Rosenberg and Terry (5) and Kedar and Weiss (6).

2. ANIMAL STUDIES

2.1. Immunotherapy with the Use of Syngeneic Lymphocytes

Models in which the lymphocyte donor, the tumor-bearing host, and the tumor are all syngeneic enable one to study immunotherapy and its mechanisms without the complications of transplantation immunology and with the assurance that the therapy is not directed against normal histocompatibility antigens. Moreover, the results obtained can be potentially extrapolated directly to clinical studies in which the lymphocytes are to be derived from a genetically identical twin (syngeneic) or directly from the patient (autologous).

Adoptive Immunotherapy (AIT) with Syngeneic Lymphocytes. Cells from syngeneic animals immunized to tumor are often effective when administered shortly before or after tumor challenge (2). However, even under optimal conditions—when the tumor is immunogenic and sensitive to an induced response and when large numbers of lymphocytes demonstrably immune to tumor can be administered—it is rarely possible to affect a tumor by AIT alone once the tumor has become established in the host (1,7). Nevertheless, impressive complete regressions of advanced tumors have been reported after treatment with lymphocytes from syngeneic donors immunized to tumor *in vivo*. This approach has been curative against an established murine methylcholanthrene sarcoma (8), palpable murine sarcoma virus (MSV)-induced tumors growing progressively in newborn or immunologically suppressed adult mice (9–11), an established hepatoma with lymph node metastases in guinea pigs (12), and a large methylcholanthrene tumor in T-cell-deficient mice (13). In all the preceding models only cells from immune donors were effective, whereas normal lymphocytes were not.

Similar studies have recently been performed by using lymphocytes sensitized *in vitro*. The most widely used method for sensitizing lymphocytes to tumor *in vitro* is to cultivate lymphocytes and tumor cells in suspension cultures for several days (6). This usually induces proliferation of the stimulated cell and the generation of cytotoxic lymphocytes. A less frequently used approach to *in vitro* sensitization has been to culture lymphocytes on antigen-fed macrophage or tumor monolayers (6). Primary sensitization of normal lymphocytes to tumor *in vitro* may be the best way to potentially generate specific anti-tumor effector cells without exposing a normal donor to tumor material. However, although normal cells primarily sensitized to tumor antigens *in vitro* can kill tumor cells *in vitro* and can occasionally protect against tumor in a neutralization assay (6, 14–16), they have not yet been reported to be significantly and reproducibly effective therapeutically when used as the sole form of therapy (14–16). For example, in two plasmacytoma models lymphocytes sensitized *in vitro* were effective in a tumor neutralization assay but failed to prevent tumor growth when administered at a site away from the tumor (16).

Cells primed to tumor antigen *in vivo*—that is, cells from animals immunized once—can be secondarily sensitized to tumor *in vitro* for potential antitumor therapy *in vivo*. Such syngeneic cells secondarily sensitized to tumor *in vitro* have been therapeutically effective against several rodent tumors. For example, a transplantable progressively growing MSV tumor—already established and clinically detectable in preirradiated rats—totally regressed after treatment with syngeneic cells secondarily sensitized to the tumor *in vitro,* but not after treatment with cells secondarily sensitized to an antigenically unrelated tumor or with primed cells not secondarily sensitized at all (17,18). Lymphocytes secondarily sensitized to tumor *in vitro* were also effective against a Friend leukemia (FBL-3) in normal mice, whereas cells cultured without any antigen or with unrelated alloantigens were not effective (19). Finally, Mills et al. (20) reported that spleen cells from mice bearing a syngeneic progressively growing mastocytoma (P815) secondarily sensitized for 5 days with P815 *in vitro* in the presence of a T-cell growth factor, Interleukin 2 (IL-2) (discussed below), were therapeutically effective when transferred to other syngeneic hosts 2 hours or 2 days after they had been inoculated with P815. The lymphocyte activity in this model was not, however, specific in that both L1210 leukemia and P815 were killed regardless of which of the two tumors was used as the immunogen *in vivo* or *in vitro*. The role or function of IL-2 in this short-term culture system is not clear.

Several factors determine the success of AIT in the models studied. Among the most important are the tumor load and the positive or negative influences of the host on the antitumor effect of the infused donor cells.

Adoptive immunotherapy is less effective when used against a large tumor burden or when used at a later time after tumor inoculation. For example (12), immune lymphocytes administered 7 days after inoculation of guinea pig hepatoma cells were less effective therapeutically for a larger initial tumor inoculum than for a smaller one. Moreover, for a given tumor inoculum, treatment on day 14 was less effective than on day 7 (12). Time was also critical in the AIT of a murine Friend leukemia (FBL-3) (3). Although mice inoculated with 10^4 FBL-3 cells on day 0 were saved by 5×10^6 immune cells infused on day 1, when treatment was delayed to day 3, even 10^8 immune cells exerted no effect. Although these results may reflect simply a higher ratio of tumor cells to effector cells at a later time after tumor inoculation, factors other than this ratio must be involved since in the FBL-3 model that ratio is calculated to be approximately 1 to 250 on day 1 and 1 to 1000 on day 3.

An alternative or additional explanation for the decreased effectiveness of immune cells administered against a large tumor or late after tumor inoculation is that under those conditions there may be generation of host factors that interfere with the therapeutic efficacy of infused donor cells. The factors may include suppression by the tumor itself, by circulating tumor antigen, by blocking antibodies, or by suppressor cells (21–24). The principal circumstantial evidence for a host suppressor cell as a limiting factor in the effectiveness of AIT is provided by the finding that in some models (17,18,20) AIT is decidedly more effective in a preirradiated host than in a normal host, suggesting that the elimination of radiation-sensitive host suppressor cells can increase the efficacy of AIT. More definitively, in the model reported by Berendt and North (13) AIT against a large methylcholanthrene sarcoma was far more effective in a thymectomized T-cell deficient mouse than in a normal recipient. Although immune cells were effective in normal recipients if infused no later than 3 to 4 days after tumor implantation (25), immune cells administered 7 days after tumor inoculation were still effective in T-cell-deficient recipients, but not in normal recipients (13). The efficacy of AIT in T-cell-deficient recipients was abrogated by an infusion of T cells from T-cell-intact tumor-bearing donors who had lost their concomitant immunity (13). The results strongly suggest that a normal host with a progressively growing tumor generates suppressor T cells that interfere with the therapeutic effectiveness of AIT. Their results may explain why it is so difficult to use syngeneic AIT alone to treat a clinically detectable tumor in normal animals.

AIT with Syngeneic Lymphocytes as an Adjunct to Other Therapies.

Since AIT potentially provides unique antitumor specificity but is limited, at least in part, by the tumor load and/or by suppressive factors associated with a large tumor load, it has long been considered that AIT might be best used to specifically destroy tumor cells remaining after surgery, radiation, or chemotherapy. Effective syngeneic AIT after surgery has been reported by Treves et al. (26). Spleen cells from normal mice sensitized in vitro to syngeneic Lewis lung carcinoma (3 LL) prevented microscopic pulmonary metastases when administered to mice whose primary 3 LL tumor had been surgically removed. The results were better than those achieved with surgery alone, or with surgery plus unsensitized cells or cells sensitized against normal syngeneic fibroblasts. Cells from 3 LL-bearing mice, when sensitized secondarily to 3 LL in vitro, were also therapeutically effective, but not as effective as were sensitized lymphocytes from normal mice (26,27).

The use of AIT as an adjunct to radiation therapy has received too little investigative attention. The principal studies that may or may not have involved or reflected such an approach have consisted of treating tumor-bearing mice with supralethal doses of total body irradiation (TBI) to destroy tumor cells and infusing syngeneic marrow to repopulate the hemopoietic system of the host, and, possibly, to "destroy by the reaction of immunity these residual leukemic cells" (28). This approach was occasionally effective against murine lymphoid tumors (29), especially if instituted shortly after inoculation of a small number of tumor cells and especially if lymph node cells were also added (30). Subsequent reports, reviewed elsewhere (31), were disappointingly negative. Variations in the results probably reflected variable radiosensitivity and antigenicity of the various tumors studied by different groups at different times. Moreover, no attempts were made to increase the potential immunotherapeutic effectiveness of the syngeneic cells by using donors immune to tumor. Thus most of the syngeneic marrow transplant results in the animal models were negative and involved too many variables to establish whether the end results reflected any effect against tumor on the part of the infused donor cells.

Syngeneic marrow and spleen cells have also been used as an adjunct to lethal chemotherapy in mice. Normal cells infused after lethal dimethylmyleran were quite effective against a Moloney leukemia (32), but not against a Friend or Rauscher leukemia (33). The results may reflect differences in the sensitivity of the tumors to the drug and/or differences in host responses to them.

During the past decade animal models have been developed that have involved lower nonlethal doses of chemotherapy and greater reliance on the immunotherapeutic effect of syngeneic cells immune to tumor. The results in such adoptive chemoimmunotherapy (ACIT) models have clearly demonstrated that antigenic syngeneic advanced tumors can be eradicated by a combination of nonlethal, noncurative chemotherapy plus lymphoid cells immune to tumor antigen. The approach has been effective in several strains of mice against several advanced syngeneic tumors (3), especially Moloney leukemias (6,34), L1210 leukemia (35,36), Friend leukemia (FBL-3) (37,38), EL-4 leukemia (6,39,40), and a Rauscher leukemia (RBL-5) (33), as well as against L_2C leukemia in guinea pigs (41). Although all the prerequisites for efficacy have not yet been identified, studies in those models have suggested that for maximal immunotherapeutic efficacy, the syngeneic cells should be immune T-cells capable of proliferating in the host and persisting in the host for several days.

The efficacy and problems of ACIT can be illustrated by studies with a syngeneic antigenic transplantable Friend virus-induced leukemia (FBL-3) in C57BL/6 mice. This tumor (FBL-3) is fatal, even at a dose of 100 cells. It possesses antigens which cross-react with those on other tumors induced by Friend, Moloney, or Rauscher (FMR) viruses (42). Spleen cells from mice immunized to FBL-3 are active by the Winn assay for tumor neutralization (37) and can save mice when administered 1 day after FBL-3 inoculation (3).

A model for treating advanced FBL-3 with ACIT using cyclophosphamide (CY) and syngeneic spleen cells was developed with the following experimental design: adult C57BL/6 mice were inoculated i.p. with $1 \times 10^7 - 5 \times 10^7$ FBL-3 cells on day 0. Five days later, when tumor cells are known to be present in blood and spleen (43), the mice were treated with a nonlethal dose of CY (180 mg/kg) and 6 hours later—after the CY had disappeared from the blood (44)—with C57BL/6 spleen cells.

A summary of early experiments (37) with lymphocytes sensitized *in vivo* is shown in Figure 1. All 97 tumor-bearing mice, untreated or treated with immune cells but without CY, died rapidly. Treatment with CY alone or CY plus syngeneic cells that were nonimmune or immune to unrelated antigens doubled the median survival time (MST) but was not curative. By contrast, treatment with CY plus cells specifically immune to FBL-3 cured most of the 88 mice treated. Concurrent studies with EL-4, a C57BL/6 chemically induced leukemia antigenically distinct from FBL-3, showed that ACIT was immunospecific. Cells from mice immunized against FBL-3 or other FMR tumors sharing anti-

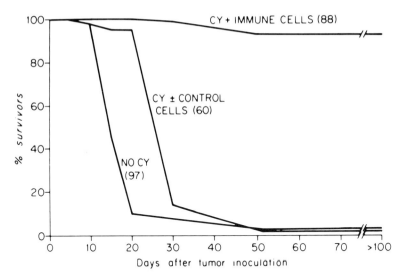

Figure 1. Syngeneic adoptive chemoimmunotherapy of Friend leukemia (FBL-3). The C57BL/6 mice given 1×10^7 to 5×10^7 FBL-3 cells on day 0 were treated on day 5 with cyclophosphamide (CY), 180 mg/kg, with or without C57BL/6 spleen cells. "Control cells" = from donors that were normal or immune to unrelated antigens; "immune cells" = from donors immunized with FBL-3. Numbers in parentheses represent the number of tumor-bearing mice treated.

gens with FBL-3 were effective against FBL-3, but not against EL-4, whereas cells from mice immunized against EL-4 were quite effective against EL-4, but not against FBL-30 (40).

Similar studies have been performed by using normal cells sensitized primarily *in vitro* or cells from animals primed *in vivo*, that is, immunized once to tumor, and secondarily sensitized to tumor *in vitro*. Cells primarily sensitized to tumor *in vitro* and used as an adjunct to chemotherapy against tumors already growing in the host have been reported (39) to be effective against EL-4 and against a Moloney leukemia when ACIT was administered 1 to 3 days after tumor inoculation, that is, when the tumors were small and curable by chemotherapy alone in 20 to 60% of the mice. More recently, an advanced Balb/c Moloney leukemia (LSTRA) of Balb/c origin and EL-4 of C57BL/6 origin were eradicated by treatment with CY plus syngeneic lymphocytes cultured with irradiated tumors (45). The *in vitro* sensitization employed and the *in vivo* therapeutic effect induced were immunospecific. This was shown by studies in (Balb/c $\times$ C57BL/6)F$_1$ (CBF$_1$) mice by using the two tumors that were syngeneic to CBF$_1$ but possessed no cross-reacting tumor antigens. Normal CBF$_1$ lymphocytes cultured with LSTRA exhibited a substantially enhanced ability to eradicate established LSTRA, but not EL-4, in CBF$_1$ mice, whereas CBF$_1$ lymphocytes cultured with EL-4 eradicated established EL-4, but not LSTRA. Thus normal lymphocytes can be sensitized specifically *in vitro* to become therapeutically effective in ACIT against advanced leukemia (45).

Cells from mice primed to tumor antigens *in vivo* and then secondarily sensitized to tumor *in vitro* have been most extensively studied for therapy in the FBL-3 model. Such cells were concurrently tested for cytotoxicity *in vitro* for tumor neutralization, for AIT of early FBL-3, and for ACIT of advanced FBL-3 (19,40,46,47). Cells primed *in vivo* and secondarily sensitized by co-culture with FBL-3 *in vitro* became more cytotoxic *in vitro* and more effective in tumor neutralization and in AIT than were freshly primed cells that were not cultured (19,46). Secondarily sensitized cells were also significantly more effective in ACIT of advanced FBL-3 (19,46). However, they were not *always* more effective than nonsensitized cells—their greater efficacy depended on the particular *in vivo* priming regimen used prior to culture and could not be predicted by results of any of the other *in vivo* or *in vitro* assays (46,47).

The results reviewed thus far show that a number of models have been developed in which syngeneic lymphocytes, alone or as an adjunct to other modalities of therapy, can eradicate established progressively growing antigenic tumors. The precise prerequisites for success have not yet been identified. However, several relevant observations have been made regarding the donor effector cells, the possible influence of the host on the end results of therapy, and the potential functions of chemotherapy.

Although a variety of non-T effector cells may be involved in the cytolytic process, especially *in vitro* [including natural killer (NK) cells, macrophages, or non-T cells acting through the antibody-dependent cell-mediated cytotoxicity. mechanism] (6), the critical effector cell *in vivo* in all the AIT and ACIT models tested has been a T cell whose therapeutic efficacy was decreased or abolished by treatment with antibody directed against T-cell antigens (6,11,13,18,45,48). In one rat AIT model the donor cell responsible for the elimination of the large established tumor *in vivo* was found to be an antigenically identifiable subset of rat T cells that was poorly cytotoxic *in vitro* (18). However, the specific subset of T cells required in any murine therapy model has not yet been identified in terms of its Lyt phenotype and represents an important question. T-cell subsets cytotoxic *in vitro* may differ from those active *in vivo* (6). Indeed, different Lyt subsets have even been reported (50) to protect against different tumors *in vivo*.

The effector cell for effective AIT or ACIT must be not only a T cell, but also one that is immune to tumor (3,6, 11–13, 17–20, 27,40, 45–48). The major exception to this generalization is a report that, in an unusually sensitive model, an advanced Moloney leukemia was eradicated by CY plus normal nonimmune syngeneic spleen cells (49). Although immune cells were far more therapeutically effective in concurrent studies, the nonimmune cells did have significant efficacy. Unlike the effective *immune* cells—which were T cells— the effective *nonimmune* cells were nonadherent lymphocytes not sensitive to anti-Thy plus complement and present in the spleens of T-deficient nude mice as well as in the spleens of normal mice (49). They were, therefore, thought to be NK cells. However, unlike classical NK cells, they were not cytotoxic *in vitro* and were not effective in tumor neutralization (49). It must be emphasized that even in this study in which non-T cells obtained from nonimmune donors were effective therapeutically, T cells obtained from immune donors were significantly more effective.

The mechanism by which immune donor T cells exert their antitumor effects has not yet been established. It is clear that the cells may be quite therapeutic *in vivo* even if not demonstrably cytotoxic *in vitro* (6,18,19,46). To be therapeutic, the cells must be able to proliferate in the host—lethal irradiation of the cells abolishes their efficacy (3). It is thought that those cells that are already cytotoxic *in vitro* may or may not act by immediate direct cytotoxicity *in vivo* whereas those that are not demonstrably cytotoxic *in vitro* may become cytotoxic after exposure to the relevant antigens in the host. It is likely, however, that the donor T cells do not exert all their anti-tumor effect by direct cytotoxicity but may also help, amplify, or recruit other donor or host cells to destroy the tumor (3,6,27,51,52). This is suggested by the finding in two AIT models that after the infusion of donor cells, the tumor continued to grow for some time before beginning to regress (13,18), possibly reflecting the eventual effect of recruitment of host cells for maximal efficacy of AIT.

A host contribution to the end results of ACIT has been further suggested by the observation that just before ACIT of FBL-3 is instituted, the peripheral blood of tumor-bearing hosts contains both FBL-3 cells—which kill secondary hosts—and lymphocytes that are effective in ACIT against FBL-3 in a secondary host (53). Thus the blood of mice destined to die with FBL-3 contained FBL-3 cells that coexisted with lymphocytes that could not prevent progressive growth of FBL-3 in the primary host but could be curative when used as an adjunct to CY in a secondary host.

On the other hand, a negative host influence on donor T-cell efficacy is implied by the observation that in the successful AIT models, infused donor cells are more effective in tumor-bearing hosts that have been preirradiated, rendered T-cell deficient (13,18,20), or pretreated with cyclophosphamide (6,54). This suggests that a radiosensitive or CY-sensitive host suppressor T cell may interfere with the effectiveness of donor cells. Thus the role of the tumor-bearing host in AIT and ACIT can be both positive and negative. The positive contribution may be represented by potentially reactive antitumor cells in the host that may be recruited by donor cells, whereas the negative influence is best represented by the potential generation of suppressor cells capable of interfering with the efficacy of infused donor cells.

Finally, the chemotherapy in syngeneic ACIT may have several functions. The chemotherapy may decrease the tumor load to be handled by the lymphocytes. This is probably not its sole function because syngeneic immune lymphocytes can be curative even when used as an adjunct to a chemotherapeutic agent that inherently has only a very modest antitumor effect (33). Moreover, some antitumor drugs, especially CY, are known to enhance T-cell-mediated immunity (55,56) and to have a preferential effect against suppressor cells in the host (57). Such activity may be very helpful if not crucial to the efficacy of ACIT. Finally, CY used *in vivo* has been reported to alter tumor antigenicity (58) and to enhance the susceptibility of tumor cells to immune-mediated lysis (59). Given the various effects of chemotherapy, it is likely that different chemotherapeutic agents may be more or less effective in various ACIT models, depending on which of its particular activities is most critical for efficacy in the given model. Undoubtedly, however, the two major functions of chemotherapy in ACIT with syngeneic lymphocytes are to reduce the tumor load and to preferentially destroy those host cells that might interfere with the therapeutic efficacy of infused donor cells or with recruitment.

A major requirement for effective AIT and ACIT is for large numbers of the requisite effector cells—cells that may exist *de novo* in the suspension in low frequency. This highlights the need for sensitizing lymphocytes *in vitro* so as to generate the cells required. *In vitro* sensitization of normal lymphocytes represents a way for preferentially generating a therapeutically effective cell from a normal suspension of cells whereas secondary sensitization *in vitro* of cells primed *in vivo* represents a way to generate a larger number of effector cells or effector cells with an enhanced antitumor reactivity. In addition, secondary sensitization *in vitro* may bypass those mechanisms that limit effective sensitization *in vivo*—for example, immunosuppression by suppressor cells (23), by tumor (21), by blocking factors (22), or by tumor antigens and other mechanisms that limit the generation and/or expression of the requisite antitumor effector cells in the tumor-bearing host (27).

Techniques for sensitization to tumor *in vitro* are critical for any eventual clinical application of ACIT because (1) the patient is likely to require large quantities of cells immune to tumor, (2) cells from a *normal* donor might be rendered immune by exposing them to a tumor *in vitro* without exposing the donor to tumor *in vivo,* and (3) if the lymphocytes of the tumor-bearing patient have already become reactive to tumor, but the expression of effective reactivity is suppressed in the host, the reactivity of those cells might be enhanced by secondary sensitization to tumor *in vitro* and cells might then be reinfused for potential therapy.

The results reported to date with lymphocytes primarily sensitized *in vitro* for specific killing of tumor *in vitro* and for specific tumor therapy *in vivo* are still quite sparse. However, the results have been obtained largely with empirically derived sensitization regimens. Better results will hopefully be obtained when optimal methods are developed for generating requisite effector cells *in vitro*. The development of such methods for use in therapy models against established tumors represents a major area for investigation.

The studies reviewed using lymphocytes primed *in vivo* and secondarily sensitized to tumor *in vitro* have been more extensive and have shown significant and immunospecific therapeutic efficacy against established tumors by such cells when used alone or as an adjunct to other therapies. Several major problems, however, have been noted. First, there is too little correlation between different assays for anti-tumor activity (6,16,17,19,46,47). For example, cells that lack detectable cytotoxic reactivity *in vitro* may be quite effective therapeutically *in vivo,* whereas cells that are cytotoxic *in vitro* may or may not be therapeutically effective. Thus extensive studies in the FBL-3 model emphasize that although cells secondarily sensitized *in vitro* can become more effective in ACIT, their enhanced efficacy varies with the priming regimen and cannot be predicted from the usual enhanced reactivity of such cells demonstrable by other assays (46). The results suggest that the effector mechanism in ACIT may be different from or subject to immunoregulatory mechanisms different from those operative in the AIT of early tumor, in tumor neutralization, or in *in vitro* cytotoxicity.

The second problem is the possibility of generating the wrong cell. For example, in the FBL-3 studies, cells primed *in vivo* were modestly effective in ACIT of FBL-3 and were rendered significantly more effective by secondary sensitization to tumor *in vitro* (19). However, primed cells cultured *without* tumor (i.e., without secondary sensitization to tumor,) became *less* effective in ACIT than were primed cells that were *never* cultured (46). This loss of therapeutic effectiveness by cells cultured without tumor was postulated to be due to the generation of suppressor cells in culture. The hypothesis was tested in the FBL-3 model (60).

During culture of normal spleen cells, radiosensitive T suppressor cells are generated that can nonspecifically inhibit an *in vitro* allogeneic response (61). In the FBL-3 model, cells with the same suppressor activity were generated not only by culturing normal cells, but also by culturing tumor-immune cells for 5 days with or without tumor (60). Moreover, normal spleen cells cultured without tumor were shown to suppress the generation of *in vitro* cytotoxic reactivity to FBL-3 by secondary *in vitro* sensitization (60). Most importantly, the normal cells cultured without tumor dramatically inhibited the therapeutic effectiveness of immune cells in ACIT when injected concurrently into a tumor-bearing CY-treated host (60). Thus secondarily sensitized cells were rendered therapeutically less effective by the *in vivo* administration of culture-induced suppressor cells (60). The results show that the suppressor cells or their precursors are generated during some *in vivo* priming regimens and are enhanced during *in vitro* sensitization and that culturing cells can promote the expression of a nonspecific suppressor cell that can significantly inhibit the therapeutic efficacy of immune cells in ACIT of advanced FBL-3. The results emphasize the need to study ways to preferentially generate *in vitro* the particular cells desired for therapy and prevent or decrease the generation of those cells that might be deleterious to the host.

A third and very important problem that limits the effectiveness of this type of culture system for the generation of secondarily sensitized effector cells for therapy is the quantity of effector cells generated. After 5 days in culture for secondary sensitization, only a small fraction of cells remain viable. To overcome the problem of inefficient and insufficient expansion of effector cells during secondary sensitization *in vitro,* numerical expansion *in vitro* by culture with T-cell growth factor, now designated Interleukin 2 (IL-2) (62), is being explored.

Interleukin 2, a protein produced by stimulated amplifier T-cells (63,64), induces activated T-cells to proliferate *in vitro* and makes it possible to continuously maintain the cells in culture even without the continued presence of antigen (65,66). Thus, by continually supplementing cultures with IL-2, large numbers of specific subclasses of activated T-lymphocytes have been generated and maintained in culture (65,67).

Long-term cultured T lymphocytes (LTCL), maintained in the presence of IL-2, have been reported to be cytotoxic to tumor *in vitro* and to inhibit the growth of syngeneic tumors in a neutralization assay (65,66,68). Moreover, such cells have recently been shown to retain the subpopulation of cells necessary for adoptive therapy (69,70). Cells primed to tumor *in vivo* and secondarily sensitized by 7-day culture with FBL-3 *in vivo* were maintained in culture through day 19 with IL-2. The cells increased in number by over 700%, exhibited specific reactivity *in vitro,* and were effective in ACIT of FBL-3 (69,70). Concurrent studies in the EL-4 ACIT model confirmed the fact that the *in vivo* therapeutic efficacy of LTCL was immunologically specific.

The approach provides a potential way to generate and maintain large quantities of cells with specific antitumor reactivity *in vitro* and with therapeutic potential *in vivo.* However, therapy studies with LTCL are still relatively rare and preliminary, and the principal problems have not yet been identified. The results *in vivo* may be strongly influenced by at least two factors: (1) the possibility that the LTCL may become dependent on the IL-2 and may, therefore, require the continual presence of IL-2 in the host to retain efficacy and (2) the possibility that the efficacy of LTCL may be affected positively or negatively by changes in the homing characteristics of cells maintained in culture for long periods of time (16,39). Both areas require future investigation in appropriate syngeneic adoptive immunotherapy models.

3.   IMMUNOTHERAPY WITH THE USE OF ALLOGENEIC LYMPHOCYTES

The use of *non*syngeneic lymphocytes for therapy, alone or with other modes of therapy, is far more complex and presents additional issues and problems not posed by syngeneic cells. These include the rejection of donor lymphocytes by the host, induction of graft-versus-host reaction or disease by donor cells, the influence of chemotherapy or radiation on those reactions, and the effect of GVH disease on the tumor.

3.1.   AIT with Allogeneic Lymphocytes

Although normal or immune allogeneic lymphocytes can protect an animal against subsequent tumor challenge, such cells have, with very rare exceptions

(1,2,5), been impressively ineffective when administered after tumor cell inoculation (1,2,5,12,71). The most recent and unique report of successful tumor therapy by allogeneic cells alone involved the treatment of PVG T-cell leukemia in PVG rats by lymphocytes from AUG rats (72). The two strains of rats share the major histocompatibility complex (MHC) antigens but differ at minor loci, including the loci that code for differentiation antigens expressed on normal peripheral T lymphocytes. The infused AUG lymphocytes were therapeutically effective if their donors were preimmunized against either the PVG T cell leukemia or normal PVG T lymphocytes. Thus AIT was effective with allogeneic lymphocytes immune to antigens shared by the host leukemia target and by the peripheral T cells of the host. In this AIT model, donor cell immunity need not be directed to antigens specific for or restricted to the tumor, but can be directed against differentiation antigens shared by tumor and some nontumor tissue.

We suspect that one reason for the usual *failure* of allogeneic lymphocytes alone to affect an established tumor may be that the infused donor cells may have to persist in the host for some time to be effective (4) and that an untreated tumor-bearing host is likely to be sufficiently immunologically competent to reject the donor cells before they can affect the tumor. This view is supported by results in the model of Westcott et al. (72) in which immune MHC-compatible AUG cells were effective against PVG leukemia in *normal* PVG rats, but not in PVG rats who had been *preimmunized* against donor (AUG) histocompatibility antigens and who would, therefore, be expected to reject donor lymphocytes more rapidly. Interestingly, in that same model, MHC-compatible immune lymphocytes were effective, but immune lymphocytes from donors MHC-*incompatible* with PVG were not effective (72). Among the possible explanations is the anticipated more rapid rejection of MHC-incompatible than of MHC-compatible lymphocytes by a normal host.

Thus the few reported successes and the many failures of immunotherapeutic treatments with allogeneic lymphocytes against a growing tumor when used alone suggest that the prime impediment to therapeutic efficacy of immune allogeneic lymphocytes is their failure to persist in the host for some unknown, though probably brief, period of time and the large tumor burden that such cells encounter when used alone.

3.2. AIT with Allogeneic Lymphocytes as an Adjunct to Other Therapies

One way to meet the requirements for a reduced tumor load and delayed rejection of donor lymphocytes by the host is to use allogeneic lymphocytes as an adjunct to chemotherapy and/or radiation that would be both cytotoxic and immunosuppressive and would, therefore, decrease the tumor load and suppress graft rejection. The principal examples of these approaches are represented by bone marrow transplantation after supralethal chemoradiotherapy and the use of lymphocyte infusions after sublethal chemotherapy or chemoradiotherapy.

Barnes et al. (73) first suggested that allogeneic marrow given to a lethally irradiated tumor-bearing host would not only restore normal hematopoiesis, but would also "destroy by the action of the immunity these residual leukemic cells, and perhaps the host." Subsequent studies demonstrated that this approach with MHC-incompatible marrow with or without lymphocytes would cause GVHD that could exert an antitumor effect but would, with rare exceptions, kill the host (30, 74–77). Mathe et al. (78) first suggested the use of graft-versus-host reaction as an antitumor weapon—that is, inducing a graft-versus-host reaction and then arresting the GVHD so as to save the cured host. However, despite rare encouraging reports (79,80), the problem remains formidable because GVHD once established, is extraordinarily difficult to control even in a nontumor-bearing host, whereas early treatment of GVHD may interfere with its antitumor effect (81,82). The various problems encountered with marrow transplantation in animal models have now also been observed in humans. The results are summarized and discussed in Chapter 10.

In ACIT with chemotherapy and/or radiation that is not lethal but is sufficiently immunosuppressive to prevent rapid rejection of donor cells, GVH disease remains a problem. However, although any promotion of rejection of donor cells might prevent fatal GVHD, it might also prevent the therapeutic antitumor effect of the infused cells—if, indeed, donor cells must persist to be effective against tumor. The need for donor cell persistence for antitumor efficacy has been strongly suggested by studies in which F_1 hybrid donor lymphocytes sensitized to parental tumor were used to treat tumor in parental hosts— a setting in which the infused cells cannot react against the normal host antigens, but the host can potentially react against the F_1 alloantigens and reject the F_1 cells. It was observed that (Balb/c × DBA/2)F_1 lymphocytes immune to a Balb/c Moloney leukemia (LSTRA) had no effect when administered to an immunologically competent LSTRA-bearing Balb/c host but were effective against advanced LSTRA when used as an adjunct to CY in doses known to be sufficiently immunosuppressive to prevent rapid donor-cell rejection by the host (83). More cogent evidence was provided (82) in a model in which Balb/c mice bearing advanced LSTRA were reproducibly cured by CY plus immune spleen cells from (Balb/c × C57BL/6)F_1 donors. Antiserum cytotoxic to C57BL/6 alloantigens (present on donor cells) administered within 2 days after infusion of the F_1 cells abolished their immunotherapeutic efficacy, whereas antiserum infused 3 days or later did not interfere with therapy (82). The results suggested that immune F_1 donor cells had to persist in the host for 2 days to be therapeutic. Studies in a MSV model (10), using H2-compatible allogeneic cells under conditions that would promote or would not promote their rapid rejection by the host, yielded results consistent with the above-mentioned need for donor cell persistence.

The need for allogeneic lymphocytes to persist to be immunotherapeutically effective against established tumor and the consequent need to prevent such rejection of donor cells by an immunosuppressive agent has reemphasized the centrality of the GVH disease problem in animal models. Nevertheless, allogeneic lymphocytes have been employed with some success as an adjunct to noncurative, nonlethal chemotherapy to treat a Moloney leukemia (6,34,39, 84,85), L1210 leukemia (36), a Moloney sarcoma (10), a Gross virus leukemia (86,87), and a rat sarcoma (88).

Two experimental settings for allogeneic ACIT that would be unlikely to be associated with frequent fatal GVH disease include the use of donor cells that are MHC compatible with the host or donor cells that are MHC incompatible but are administered in such a low dose as to make GVHD induction unlikely.

Adoptive chemoimmunotherapy with MHC-compatible allogeneic cells has been reported to be immunotherapeutically effective without GVHD, but only with cells immune to tumor (34,36,84,86). For example, Balb/c mice bearing an advanced disseminated Balb/c Moloney leukemia (LSTRA) were treated with sublethal CY plus spleen cells from H-2-compatible DBA/2 donors that were either nonimmune, immune to normal host alloantigens, or immune to TAA. Only cells from mice specifically immunized to TAA had a significant antitumor effect (34,84). The role of the GVH reaction, if any, could not be assessed since no detectable GVH disease occurred. Similar results were reported against a Gross leukemia (86). As an adjunct to CY, normal CBA lymphocytes had no significant therapeutic effect against the leukemia in H-2-compatible AKR hosts, whereas such cells immunized against TAA were quite effective (86).

The use of H-2-incompatible lymphocytes—especially in large numbers—in ACIT, as an adjunct to any chemotherapeutic agent that is sufficiently immunosuppressive to prevent rapid rejection of donor cells is likely to cause GVHD. The GVHD may or may not be fatal to the host and may or may not exert an antitumor effect. The likelihood that GVHD will occur and that it will exert a graft-versus-tumor effect is not predictable (87–90). Even an intense GVHD need not necessarily exert a significant GVT effect. Moreover, the GVT effect may vary with the tumor type. For example, severe GVHD induced by cells from normal donors exerted no significant effect against sarcomas (10) or against an adenocarcinoma (90).

Severe GVH disease in ACIT may be avoided by infusing a relatively small number of H-2-incompatible lymphocytes (91). To determine whether a significant anti-tumor effect might still be achieved under such conditions and whether preimmunization of the lymphocyte donor might still impart some specific or preferential anti-tumor activity, Balb/c mice (H-2^d) bearing disseminated LSTRA (H-2^d) were treated with CY plus spleen cells from C57BL/6 mice (H-2^b). The donors were either normal or had been immunized with normal Balb/c spleen cells, with LSTRA or with antigenically related MSV. Cumulative results (4,85), shown in Figure 2, demonstrate that as an adjunct to CY, normal cells did exert a significant antitumor effect and that cells immunized with LSTRA or MSV were significantly more effective in prolonging survival and increasing the number of long-term tumor-free survivors. It is not known whether the results reflect donor cell reactivity to alloantigens on the tumor, specific reactivity to tumor antigens, or both. Although no obvious

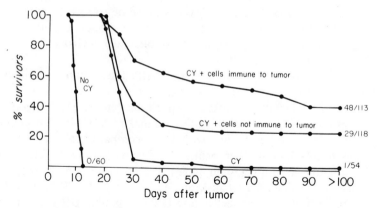

Figure 2.   Allogeneic adoptive chemoimmunotherapy of a Balb/c Moloney lymphoma (LSTRA). Balb/c mice bearing LSTRA were treated on day 4 with CY, 180 mg/kg with or without C57BL/6 spleen cells. "Cells not immune to tumor" = from donors that were normal or immunized with normal Balb/c spleen cells; "cells immune to tumor" = from donors immunized with LSTRA or with antigenically related MSV (Moloney). Numbers at end of curves represent number of tumor-free survivors of the total number treated.

GVH disease was observed, it is possible that a subclinical GVH reaction occurred and was effective against tumor, even when induced by normal cells, but that the GVH reaction was rendered immunotherapeutically more effective when induced by cells immune to tumor. A similar therapeutically effective GVT reaction was induced by normal nonimmune MHC-incompatible cells in ACIT against L1210 leukemia (36) and a rat sarcoma (88). A methylcholanthrene sarcoma in rats was successfully treated 3 days after tumor inoculation by ACIT in the form of ftorafur plus lymphoid cells from grossly histoincompatible normal rats (88).

The results of immunotherapy with the use of allogeneic lymphocytes in animal models highlight the problems posed by the need for immune cells and the variable likelihood of inducing GVHD. Lymphocytes from MHC-compatible donors have no therapeutic effect against established tumors unless preimmunized to tumor and can occasionally, though not predictably, cause significant GVHD (87,92,93). A novel approach to this problem was recently reported on the basis of the observation that tumor cells can express genetically inappropriate or "alien" histocompatibility antigens (94) and that cells primed with pooled alloantigens can become cytotoxic to tumor or virus-infected targets (95). Bortin et al. (96) reported that cells from CBA ($H-2^k$) mice alloimmunized *in vivo* against a variety of tumor or nontumor tissue of different H-2 composition exerted a significant GVT effect when transplanted into lethally preirradiated AKR ($H-2^k$) mice bearing an AKR leukemia. The GVT effect was documented by bioassay in a secondary host, was mediated by T cells, and was not associated with increased GVH disease (96). One possible explanation for this effect is that the cytotoxic T cells were generated by sensitization to allo-antigens cross-reactive with antigens present on the leukemia target cells.

In contrast to MHC-compatible lymphocytes, *MHC-incompatible* lympho-cytes have a significant therapeutic effect in the animal models studied, even if nonimmune (4,6,10, 85–88) and may become more effective if preimmu-nized (4,6,10,85). Thus, for maximal antitumor efficacy, MHC-incompatible lymphocytes should be preimmunized with host tumor or with material con-taining antigens cross-reacting with those on the tumor to be treated. Unfor-tunately, the GVHD that can so often be induced by normal MHC-incompa-tible lymphocytes is significantly increased when the lymphocytes are preim-munized to host alloantigens (6,97).

The use of a third-party tumor as an immunogen—to avoid sensitization to host alloantigens—is potentially complicated by the problem of H-2 restric-tion. Specific T-cell responses are stimulated by relevant antigens, such as viral or tumor antigens, in association with products of the H-2 complex, and cells thus stimulated react to the relevant antigens in association with the H-2 product recognized during sensitization (98). Thus there is H-2 restriction of cytotoxic T cell responses; sensitization to TAA will evoke a response by effec-tor cells that will recognize the TAA only in the context of the H-2 antigens on the tumor cells used for immunization. Therefore, donor T cells will be cyto-toxic *in vitro* to only those tumor targets that express both TAA and donor-type MHC.

If H-2 restriction were to be operative *in vivo,* tumor used as an immunogen should possess not only TAA cross-reactive with the tumor to be treated, but also the same MHC as that of the lymphocyte donors. However, it has been shown that cells from mice immunized with MHC incompatible tumor were therapeutically effective in ACIT against an MHC-compatible tumor (38). For example, lymphocytes from C57BL/6 (H-2^b) donors immunized *in vivo* with a Balb/c (H-2^d) Moloney leukemia became therapeutically effective in ACIT of a C57BL/6 Friend virus-induced leukemia in C57BL/6 hosts (38). Thus thera-peutically effective cells were generated *in vivo* with an immunogen that had cross-reacting antigens with TAA on the tumor to be treated despite the fact that the MHC of the immunogen and the tumor to be treated were different. Although the results might suggest that H-2 nonrestricted effector cells are generated, they can also be interpreted as showing that the lymphocytes gener-ated were still H-2 restricted but that antigen processing of the cross-reactive tumor antigens *in vivo* permitted the presentation of the tumor antigens on a syngeneic cell (99). Thus it may be possible to use alloantigenic tumors to gen-erate syngeneic restricted effector cells for ACIT.

Various ways to control or prevent GVHD have been studied with only limited success in non-tumor-bearing animals and only rare success in tumor-bearing hosts (4). For example, some tumor-bearing mice undergoing poten-tially fatal GVHD have been saved by being kept in germ-free environments (87,100) or by receiving drugs and/or infusion of syngeneic or histocompatible lymphocytes (79,80,101). However, the problem remains formidable in that it is still extremely difficult to reproducibly prevent GVH disease or—more importantly—to control its severity or duration. The main approaches in non-tumor-bearing animals have included provision of germ-free environments (87,100), infusion of lymphocytes identical to or histocompatible with the host (77,79,80,101), immunosuppressive drugs (102–107), antisera directed against donor isoantigens (82), adsorption of donor lymphocytes on mono-layers possessing host antigens (108), and "suicide" techniques involving the exposure of donor cells to host antigens *in vitro* and addition of lethal doses of radioactive material to kill the responding proliferating donor lymphocytes (109,110). Most recently attention has focused on a new immunosuppressive agent named *cyclosporin A* (111), on total lymphoid irradiation of the host (112), and on depletion of T cells from the suspension of donor cells infused (92,113). The former two are already being actively tested in allogeneic bone marrow transplantation in humans (114,115), and the latter is anticipated to be testable with an appropriate monoclonal antibody to human T cells.

4. SUMMARY OF AND CONCLUSIONS FROM ANIMAL STUDIES

A number of effective models for adoptive immunotherapy and chemoimmunotherapy of advanced progressively growing antigenic tumors have been developed. Some of the prerequisites for efficacy have been determined, and some of the problems to be resolved before clinical application have been identified.

The most extensive studies have been performed in totally syngeneic systems so as to avoid the problems of transplantation immunology. Syngeneic lymphocytes sensitized *in vivo* to TAA can occasionally eradicate even large tumors. This approach is limited largely by the tumor load and by suppressive factors—especially suppressor cells—in the tumor-bearing host. Sensitized lymphocytes are more effective, therefore, when used as an adjunct to radiation therapy and, especially, chemotherapy that can potentially decrease both the tumor load and the suppressor cells in the host. The critical donor effector cell for therapy is a T cell that acts with or without recruitment of host cells. The requisite effector cells can now increasingly be generated and/or their reactivity enhanced by sensitization to TAA *in vitro*. However, this is complicated by the potential generation of suppressor cells capable of interfering with the therapeutic efficacy of the antitumor effector cells. Finally, the requisite lymphocyte can now increasingly be maintained in long-term culture with retention of some specific cytotoxic and therapeutic antitumor activity.

Studies with allogeneic donor lymphocytes are far more complex and difficult. Allogeneic lymphocytes when used alone are rarely therapeutically effective but have exerted a significant therapeutic effect against established tumors when used with radiation and, especially, chemotherapy. For maximal antitumor therapeutic efficacy, the allogeneic lymphocytes should be immune to tumor and should be able to persist and proliferate in the host for some period of time. These requirements raise the difficult problem of the appropriate immunogens, the conditions for sensitization, the need for immunosuppressive therapy to prevent rapid rejection of donor lymphocytes by the host, and the resultant problem of potentially fatal GVH disease. However, GVH disease represents a double-edged sword. Although its harmful effects on normal host tissue represent a major impediment to allogeneic adoptive chemoimmunotherapy, GVH disease also exerts demonstrable significant effects against some tumors.

The results of the animal studies reviewed thus far emphasize the need to continue studies in several relevant areas:

1. The critical effector cell operative in eradicating tumor must be more precisely identified and the interactions of that cell with other donor or host cells must be explored so as to better appreciate the positive and negative influences on its effectiveness.

2. Methods for sensitizing lymphocytes *in vitro* must be studied so as to develop regimens that might decrease the generation of cells or responses that might be deleterious to the host, while enhancing the generation of those effector mechanisms that exert antitumor effects.

3. Approaches to long-term maintenance in culture and to cloning the requisite effector cell(s) must continue to be developed.

4. Prerequisites and limitations of material that can be used as an immunogen *in vivo* and *in vitro* must be determined, including the problems of MHC restriction and the opportunities presented by the existence of "alien" antigens and differentiation antigens on tumor cells.

5. Approaches should continue to be studied to prevent or control GVHD and use it for its antitumor activity, with special emphasis on ways to impart preferential and/or specific antitumor activity to the graft-versus-host reaction.

6. Finally, the role or contribution of a tumor-bearing host to the end results of immunotherapy as well as the influence of the usually cytotoxic antitumor drugs or radiation on the host or donor cell reactivity to tumor must be investigated so as to develop optimal combinations and conditions for effective immunotherapy.

5. HUMAN STUDIES

Many empiric attempts have been made to treat cancer patients by infusion of lymphoid cells (2,5), with largely negative or inconclusive results. However, the conditions of the clinical studies have not been consistent with the apparent prerequisites for effective adoptive therapy as derived from animal models, namely, tumor-immune lymphocytes capable of persisting and proliferating in a host bearing a small tumor load.

In one report (116) of syngeneic AIT in humans, a patient with advanced malignant melanoma received lymphocytes from an identical twin whose melanoma had been cured and whose lymphocytes were reactive to the melanoma cells in mixed culture. No therapeutic benefit was detected.

Normal allogeneic lymphocytes, whether fresh or cultured, have often been used to treat cancer patients—all without convincing therapeutic effect (2,5). However, the lymphocytes were *not* immune to tumor and were administered to patients who had a *large* tumor load and who were *not* immunosuppressed and would, therefore, be expected to *reject* the donor lymphocytes.

Lymphocytes considered "immune" because they were obtained from patients cured of their own tumors have been reported to benefit two patients. Moreover, such cells infused by the intralymphatic route into one melanoma patient were associated with long-term tumor-free survival (117).

To further satisfy the need for immune cells, cancer patients have been treated with cells from allogeneic donors immunized with the patient's tumor cells or tumor homogenates. The most extensive studies (118–120) involved cross-immunization with killed tumor cells from patients with the same type of tumor followed by cross-transfusions of lymphocytes. Objective responses of variable degree and variable documentation were reported in about 20% of the patients. Under the conditions of the study, the donor lymphocytes infused would be expected to be rapidly rejected by the host because the host, having been exposed to donor tumor cells, would have been immunized to the normal histocompatibility antigens of the donor cells.

On the reasonable assumption that rejection of allogeneic cells would be less rapid if donor and host were identical at the major histocompatibility complex, patients with disseminated cancer of different types were treated with lymphocytes from normal donors who were HLA identical with the recipients (121,122). Objective responses were reported in two of six patients, but in one of the two the response could be attributed to concurrently administered chemotherapy.

To comply with the need for a reduced tumor load, Neff and Enneking (123) used immunotherapy against patients with minimal residual tumor. They treated 32 patients after radical surgery for osteogenic sarcoma with lymphocytes from allogeneic donors immunized with patient tumor cells. No significant difference was observed between the results in this group and a comparable historical control group treated by surgery alone.

Infusion of allogeneic cells sensitized to normal host alloantigens is not innocuous but can, in fact, induce GVHD even in a patient who is not on chemotherapy. The risk was raised by a report (124) of a patient with melanoma who received thoracic duct lymphocytes from the mother who had been immunized with patient melanoma cells. The patient died 9 days later. Some donor lymphocytes were demonstrated to persist in the host and a clinical syndrome compatible with GVHD was noted. There was no antitumor therapeutic effect.

The possibility has been entertained that cancer patients may generate an antitumor response whose full expression is suppressed *in vivo* and could be unmasked or enhanced by *in vitro* manipulation with exposure to either tumor cells or other materials such as PHA or BCG. Several studies (5, 125–128) with the use of such autologous lymphocytes for reinfusion into the patient or into tumor nodules have involved too many variables and/or inadequate followups and have not yielded reproducibly positive responses.

The use of lymphocytes in combination with other modes of tumor therapy in humans is best represented by studies in which leukemia patients were treated with supralethal doses of chemotherapy, TBI, and bone marrow infusion from a normal syngeneic (identical twin) or allogeneic donor, or directly from the patient. The present status of clinical bone marrow transplantation has been reviewed (Chapter 10). Although the principal function of the infused marrow is hemopoietic restoration, it is considered likely that cells from the donor marrow may also exert an immunotherapeutic antileukemic effect.

Patients with hematologic malignancies treated with identical twin marrow transplantation have experienced significant long-term complete remissions and, in many instances, cures (129). The principal problem has been a significant incidence of leukemic relapse. Infusion of normal twin peripheral blood lymphocytes had no detectable influence on the incidence of leukemic relapse in a small number of patients (129).

Allogeneic marrow transplantation for acute leukemia has involved largely marrow from MHC-identical normal siblings. The results show that leukemic relapse remains a significant problem (Chapter 10). However, relapses can be markedly reduced if the transplantation is performed when the patient is in chemotherapy-induced complete remission. The principal problem is a high incidence of acute and/or chronic GVHD, which occurs despite the MHC identity between donor and host and despite methotrexate prophylaxis for GVHD.

However, in humans, as in animal models, GVHD is a double-edged sword —it may be either fatal or beneficial (130–133). A recent statistical analysis revealed (131,132) that in patients transplanted for acute leukemia the incidence of leukemia recurrence after marrow transplantation was lowest (131) and survival longest (132) in those patients who exhibited significant GVHD as compared to allogeneic or syngeneic marrow recipients who exhibited no GVHD. The results suggest that GVHD induced by normal marrow has an antileukemic effect. The target antigens for the effect have not been defined. A variety of approaches, similar to those studied in animal models (discussed previously), have been and are being explored for the control of GVHD in humans.

Autologous marrow transplantation is being used in humans in conjunction with supralethal chemoradiotherapy to treat hematologic and some nonhematologic malignancies (134–136). The main problems anticipated are the resistance of the malignancy to chemoradiotherapy and the likelihood of tumor cell contamination of the infused marrow. As discussed in Chapter 9, attempts are in progress to selectively eliminate contaminating tumor cells from infused marrow by using specific monoclonal antibodies.

6. CONCLUSIONS REGARDING LYMPHOCYTE TRANSFER AS POTENTIAL CANCER THERAPY IN HUMANS

The application of adoptive immunotherapy to the clinical situation should ideally be based on the apparent prerequisites for efficacy derived from animal models, namely, a minimal tumor load and a large number of viable effector lymphocytes immune to TAA and capable of persisting in the host for some period of time. Accordingly, the cancer patient to be treated should have no evidence of disease after surgery, chemotherapy, or radiation, but should have a high probability of tumor recurrence. For ACIT, the chemotherapy should be administered in doses that would have an antitumor effect and would also be sufficiently immunosuppressive to delay rejection of infused lymphocytes if they are allogeneic to the host. If the dose of chemotherapy and/or radiotherapy is potentially lethal due to myelosuppression, then bone marrow stem cells—in addition to lymphocytes—may have to be infused so as to ensure complete hemopoietic restoration. Until effective approaches to controlling GVH disease are developed, the lymphocytes should be obtained from donors who are either genetically identical twins or MHC-identical siblings rather than MHC-mismatched individuals.

To avoid exposing normal lymphocyte donors to tumor material, the lymphocytes should be sensitized by cocultivation with material containing TAA. Evidence for the existence of unique as well as shared antigens on some human tumors is being accumulated with the aid of potent monoclonal antibodies as reviewed in Chapters 1 and 9. Future studies will determine whether the optimal immunogen for *in vitro* sensitization will be the tumor to be treated, another tumor with cross-reactive TAA, or differentiation antigens shared by the tumor. Indeed, recent studies suggest that even pooled normal alloantigens may act as effective immunogens for the generation of antitumor effector cells in animals (98) and humans (137). For example, cocultivation of human lymphocytes with irradiated normal lymphocytes pooled from unrelated individuals led to the generation of T cells that were cytotoxic to autologous lymphoblastoid cell lines, but not to normal autologous lymphocytes (137).

The conditions used for *in vitro* sensitization will have to be those that are likely—on the basis of studies in animal models—to generate the lymphocyte effector cell subpopulations required for an antitumor effect *in vivo* but that are not likely to concurrently generate suppressor cells. In rodents specific lymphocyte subpopulations have been antigenically and functionally identified, and their role in therapy is being studied. In humans such subpopulations are also being similarly identified (138). Once the desired cells with specific antitumor activity are identified and generated, they may be either expanded *in vitro* with the help of T-cell growth factors and/or they may be cloned for their specific cytotoxic reactivity (139,140).

Tumor-immune lymphocytes may also be available from related or unrelated donors whose own tumors have regressed and who might have demonstrable reactivity against tumor to be treated. Such cells might be secondarily sensitized to TAA *in vitro* prior to being used.

Autologous lymphocytes, that is, cells obtained directly from the patient, may also be therapeutically effective in ACIT. However, since it is assumed that whatever immunologic antitumor reactivity those cells possess failed to prevent the progressive growth of the tumor, those lymphocytes should be secondarily sensitized with killed autologous tumor cells *in vitro* in an effort to circumvent or bypass whatever mechanisms existed *in vivo* that had interfered with the full expression of antitumor reactivity. Since patients in complete remission are more likely to have lymphocytes reactive to tumor, autologous lymphocytes might be best obtained from patients in complete remission and might be cryopreserved. The patients might then receive vigorous chemoradiotherapy and infusion of their own lymphocytes while still in complete remission with minimal residual disease. Additional manipulations such as plasmaphoresis may be required to remove humoral factors that might interfere with cellular reactivity.

In conclusion, during the past decade the rationale for the use of adoptively transferred lymphocytes for tumor therapy has been solidified, animal models for adoptive therapy have been developed, and some of the prerequisites for immunotherapeutic efficacy in those models have been determined, and the major problems posed by those prerequisites for possible clinical application have been identified. Concurrent progress in cellular immunology in the generation and maintenance of cytotoxic lymphocytes *in vitro* and in human marrow transplantation has identified additional areas deserving increased investigative attention and has greatly increased the likelihood that adoptive immunotherapy will eventually have an important role in the treatment of malignant disease in humans.

REFERENCES

1. P. Alexander, Immunotherapy of cancer. Experiments with primary tumors and syngeneic tumor grafts. *Progr. Exp. Tumor Res.,* **10**, 22 (1968).

2. A. Fefer, Tumor immunotherapy. In A. C. Sartorelli and D. G. Johns, Eds., *Handbook of Experimental Pharmacology.* Springer Verlag, New York, Vol. 38, 1974, p. 528.

3. A. Fefer, A. B. Einstein, M. A. Cheever, and J. R. Berenson, Models for syngeneic adoptive chemoimmunotherapy of murine leukemias. *Ann. N. Y. Acad. Sci.,* **276**, 573 (1976).

4. A. Fefer, A. B. Einstein, and M. A. Cheever, Adoptive chemoimmunotherapy of cancer in animals: A review of results, principles and problems. *Ann. N. Y. Acad. Sci.,* **277**, 492 (1976).

5. S. A. Rosenberg and W. D. Terry, Passive immunotherapy of cancer in animals and man. *Adv. Cancer Res.,* **25**, 323-88; 347-65; 366-69 (1977).

6. E. Kedar and D. W. Weiss, Cell-mediated tumor immunity induced *in vitro.* In R. Borek, Ed., *Immunogenicity,* 2nd ed., Springer Verlag, Heidilley (in press).

7. P. Alexander and J. G. Hall, The role of immunoblasts in host resistance and immunotherapy of primary sarcomata. *Adv. Cancer Res.,* **13**, 37 (1970).

8. H. Borberg, H. F. Oettgen, K. Choudry, and E. J. Beathie, Inhibition of established transplants of chemically induced sarcomas in syngeneic mice by lymphocytes from immunized donors. *Internatl. J. Cancer,* **10**, 539 (1972).

9. A. Fefer, Immunotherapy and chemotherapy of Moloney sarcoma virus-induced tumors in mice. *Cancer Res.,* **29**, 2177 (1969).

10. A. Fefer, Immunotherapy of primary Moloney sarcoma virus-induced tumors. *Internatl. J. Cancer,* **5**, 327 (1970).

11. D. Colavo, P. Zanovello, E. Leuchars, A. J. S. Davies, L. Chieco-Bianchi, and G. Biasi, Moloney murine sarcoma virus oncogenesis in T-lymphocyte-deprived mice: Biologic and immunologic studies. *J. Natl. Cancer Inst.,* **64**, 97 (1980).

12. H. G. Smith, R. P. Harmel, M. G. Hanna, B. S. Zwilling, B. S. Zbar, and H. J. Rapp, Regression of established intradermal tumors and lymph node metastases in guinea pigs after systemic transfer of immune lymphoid cells. *J. Natl. Cancer Inst.,* **58**, 1315 (1977).

13. M. J. Berendt and R. J. North, T-cell-mediated suppression of antitumor immunity. An explanation for progressive growth of an immunogenic tumor. *J. Exp. Med.,* **151**, 59 (1980).

14. M. Rollinghoff and H. Wagner, *In vivo* protection against murine plasma cell tumor growth by *in vitro* activated syngeneic lymphocytes. *J. Natl. Cancer Inst.,* **51**, 1317 (1973).

15. M. Small and N. Trainin, Inhibition of syngeneic fibrosarcoma growth by lymphocytes sensitized on tumor-cell monolayers in the presence of the thymic humoral factor. *Internatl. J. Cancer,* **15**, 962 (1975).

16. R. C. Burton and N. L. Warner, *In vitro* induction of tumor specific immunity. IV. Specific adoptive immunotherapy with cytotoxic T cells induced *in vitro* to plasmocytoma antigens. *Cancer Immunol. Immunother.,* **2**, 91 (1977).

17. E. Fernandez-Cruz, B. Halliburton, and J. D. Feldman, *In vivo* elimination by specific effector cells of an established syngeneic rat Moloney virus-induced sarcoma. *J. Immunol.,* **123**, 1772 (1979).

18. E. Fernandez-Cruz, B. A. Woda, and J. D. Feldman, Elimination of syngeneic sarcomas in rats by a subset of T lymphocytes. *J. Exp. Med.,* **152**, 823 (1980).

19. M. A. Cheever, R. A. Kempf, and A. Fefer, Tumor neutralization, immunotherapy, and chemoimmunotherapy of a Friend leukemia with cells secondarily sensitized *in vitro. J. Immunol.,* **119**, 714 (1977).

20. G. B. Mills, G. Carlson, and V. Paetkau, Generation of cytotoxic lymphocytes to syngeneic tumors by using co-stimulator (Interleukin 2): *In vivo* activity. *J. Immunol.,* **125**, 1904 (1980).

21. H. Friedman, S. Specter, I. Kamo, and J. Kateley, Tumor-associated immunosuppressive factors. *Ann. N. Y. Acad. Sci.,* **276**, 417 (1976).

22. K. E. Hellström and I. Hellström, Lymphocyte-mediated cytotoxicity and blocking serum activity to tumor antigens. *Adv. Immunol.,* **18**, 209, (1974).

23. S. Fujimoto, M. I. Greene, and A. H. Sehon, Regulation of the immune response to tumor antigens. I. Immunosuppressor cells in tumor-bearing hosts. *J. Immunol.,* **116**, 800 (1976).

24. R. B. Mokyr, D. B. Braun, and S. Dray, Augmentation of antitumor cytotoxicity in MOPC-315 tumor bearer spleen cells by depletion of glass-adherent cells prior to *in vitro* activation. *Cancer Res.,* **39**, 785 (1979).

25. M. J. Berendt, R. J. North, and D. P. Kirstein, The immunological basis of endotoxic-induced tumor regression. Requirement for T cell mediated immunity. *J. Exp. Med.,* **148**, 1550 (1978).

26. A. J. Treves, I. R. Cohen, and M. Feldman, Immunotherapy of lethal metastases by lymphocytes sensitized against tumor cells *in vitro. J. Natl. Cancer Inst.,* **54**, 777 (1975).

27. A. J. Treves, I. R. Cohen, B. Schechter, and M. Feldman, *In vivo* effects of lymphocytes sensitized *in vitro* against tumor cells. *Ann. N. Y. Acad. Sci.,* **276**, 165 (1976).

28. D. W. H. Barnes, J. R. Loutit, and F. E. Neal, Treatment of murine leukemia with x-rays and homologous bone marrow. *Br. Med. J.*, **2**, 626 (1956).

29. J. J. Trentin, Whole body x-ray and bone marrow therapy of leukemia in mice. *Proc. Am. Assoc. Cancer Res.*, **2**, 54 (1957).

30. M. J. DeVries and P. Vos, Treatment of mouse lymphosarcoma by total body x-irradiation and by injection of bone marrow and lymph node cells. *J. Ntl. Cancer Inst.*, **21**, 1117 (1958).

31. A. Fefer, Adoptive tumor immunotherapy in mice as an adjunct to whole-body X-irradiation and chemotherapy. A review. *Isr. J. Med. Sci.*, **9**, 350 (1973).

32. G. L. Floersheim, Treatment of Moloney lymphoma with lethal doses of dimethyl myleran combined with injection of hemopoietic cells. *Lancet*, **1**, 228 (1969).

33. A. B. Einstein, M. A. Cheever, and A. Fefer, The use of dimethyl myleran in adoptive chemoimmunotherapy of two murine leukemias. *J. Natl. Cancer Inst.*, **56**, 609 (1976).

34. A. Fefer, Adoptive chemoimmunotherapy of a Moloney lymphoma. *Internatl. J. Cancer*, **8**, 364 (1971).

35. E. Mihich, Combined effects of chemotherapy and immunity against leukemia L1210 in DBA/2 mice. *Cancer Res.*, **29**, 848 (1969).

36. S. Vadlamudi, M. Padarathsingh, E. Bonmassar, and A Goldin, Effect of combination treatment with cyclophosphamide and syngeneic or allogeneic spleen and bone marrow cells in leukemic (L1210) mice. *Internatl. J. Cancer*, **7**, 160 (1971).

37. L. Fass and A. Fefer, Studies of adoptive chemoimmunotherapy of a Friend virus-induced lymphoma. *Cancer Res.*, **32**, 997 (1972).

38. L. Fass and A. Fefer, Factors related to therapeutic efficacy in adoptive chemoimmunotherapy of a Friend virus-induced lymphoma. *Cancer Res.*, **32**, 2427 (1972).

39. E. Kedar, Z. Raanan, and M. Schwartzbach, *In vitro* induction of cell-mediated immunity to murine leukemia cells. VI. Adaptive immunotherapy in combination with chemotherapy of leukemia in mice, using lymphocytes sensitized *in vitro* to leukemia cells. *Cancer Immunol. Immunother.*, **4**, 161 (1978).

40. M. A. Cheever, P. D. Greenberg, and A. Fefer, Specificity of adoptive chemoimmunotherapy of established syngeneic tumors. *J. Immunol.*, **125**, 711 (1980).

41. D. L. Klein, W. Brown, P. Cote, W. Garner, and J. W. Pearson, Chemoadoptive immunotherapy against a guinea-pig leukemia. *Cancer Immunol. Immunother.*, **6**, 17 (1979).

42. J. L. McCoy, A. Fefer, and J. P. Glynn, Comparative studies on the induction of transplantation resistance in BALB/c and C57BL/6 mice in three murine leukemia systems. *Cancer Res.*, **27**, 1743 (1967).

43. P. D. Greenberg, M. A. Cheever, and A. Fefer, Detection of early and delayed anti-tumor effects following curative adoptive chemoimmunotherapy of established leukemias. *Cancer Res.*, **40**, 4428 (1980).

44. I. Kline, M. Gang, D. D. Tyrer, N. Mantel, J. M . Venditti, and A. Goldin, Duration of drug levels in mice as indicated by residual anti-leukemic efficacy. *Chemotherapy (Tokyo)*, **13**, 28 (1968).

45. M. A. Cheever, P. D. Greenberg, and A. Fefer, Adoptive therapy of established syngeneic leukemia by cells primarily sensitized *in vitro*. *Cancer Res.*, **41**, 2658 (1981).

46. M. A. Cheever, P. D. Greenberg, and A. Fefer, Tumor neutralization, immunotherapy, and chemoimmunotherapy of a Friend leukemia with cells secondarily sensitized *in vitro*: II. Comparison of cells cultured with and without tumor to noncultured immune cells. *J. Immunol.*, **121**, 2220 (1978).

47. M. A. Cheever, P. D. Greenberg, and A. Fefer, Chemoimmunotherapy of a Friend leukemia with cells secondarily sensitized *in vitro*: Effect of culture duration on therapeutic efficacy. *J. Natl. Cancer Inst.*, **67**, 169 (1981).

48. J. R. Berenson, A. B. Einstein, and A. Fefer, Syngeneic adoptive immunotherapy and chemoimmunotherapy of a Friend leukemia: Requirement for T cells. *J. Immunol.*, **115**, 234 (1975).

49. M. A. Cheever, P. D. Greenberg, and A. Fefer, Therapy of leukemia by non-immune syngeneic spleen cells. *J. Immunol.*, **124**, 2137 (1980).

50. J. C. LeClerc and H. Cantor, T-cell mediated immunity to oncornavirus-induced tumors. I. Ly phenotype of precursor and effector cytolytic T lymphocytes. II. Ability of different T-cell sets to prevent tumor growth *in vivo. J. Immunol.*, **124**, 846 (1980).

51. O. Alaba and I. Bernstein, Tumor-growth suppression *in vivo*: cooperation between immune lymphoid cells sensitized *in vitro* and nonimmune bone marrow cells. *J. Immunol.*, **120**, 1961 (1978).

52. G. C. Ting, D. Rodrigues, and T. Igarashi, Studies of the mechanisms for the induction of *in vivo* tumor immunity. III. Recruitment of host helper cells by donor T cells in adoptive transfer of cell-mediated immunity. *J. Immunol.*, **122**, 1510 (1979).

53. A. Fefer and L. Fass, Immunotherapeutic efficacy of lymphocytes from mice bearing lethal Friend leukemia (FBL-3). *Proc. Am. Assoc. Cancer Res.*, **17**, 208 (1976).

54. A. Fefer, M. A. Cheever, and P. D. Greenberg, Unpublished observations.

55. L. Fass and A. Fefer, The application of an *in vitro* cytotoxicity test to studies of the effects of drugs on the cellular immune response in mice. I. Primary response. *J. Immunol.*, **109**, 749 (1972).

56. J. L. Turk, D. Parker, and L. W. Poulter, Functional aspects of the selective depletion of lymphoid tissue by cyclophosphamide. *Immunology*, **23**, 493 (1972).

57. M. Glaser, Regulation of specific cell-mediated cytotoxic response against SV40-induced tumor associated antigens by depletion of suppressor T cells with cyclophosphamide in mice. *J. Exp. Med.*, **149**, 774 (1979).

58. A. Nicolin, S. Vadlamudi, and A. Goldin, Antigenicity of L1210 leukemia sublines induced by drugs. *Cancer Res.*, **32**, 653 (1972).

59. T. Borsos, R. C. Bast, S. H. Ohanian, M. Segerline, B. Zbar, and H. Rapp, Induction of tumor immunity by intratumoral chemotherapy. *Ann. N. Y. Acad. Sci.*, **276**, 565 (1976).

60. P. D. Greenberg, M. Cheever, and A. Fefer, Suppression of the *in vitro* secondary response to syngeneic tumor and of *in vivo* tumor therapy with immune cells by culture-induced suppressor cells. *J. Immunol.*, **123**, 515 (1979).

61. R. J. Hodes, L. M. Nadler, and K. S. Hathcock, Regulatory mechanisms in cell-mediated immune responses. III. Antigen-specific and nonspecific suppressor activities generated during MLC. *J. Immunol.*, **119**, 961 (1977).

62. S. B. Mizel and J. J. Farrar, Revised nomenclature for antigen-nonspecific T-cell proliferation and helper factors. *Cell Immunol.*, **48**, 433 (1979).

63. H. Wagner and M. Rollinghoff, T-T-cell interaction during *in vitro* cytotoxic allograft responses. I. Soluble products from activated Ly 1[+] T cells trigger autonomously antigen-primed Ly 23[+] T cells to cell proliferation and cytolytic activity. *J. Exp. Med.*, **148**, 1523 (1978).

64. J. Shaw, B. Caplan, V. Paetkau, L. M. Pilarski, T. L. Delovitch, and I. F. C. McKenzie, Cellular origins of co-stimulator (IL 2) and its activity in cytotoxic T lymphocyte responses. *J. Immunol.*, **124**, 2231 (1980).

65. S. Gillis and K. S. Smith, Long-term culture of tumor-specific cytotoxic T-cells. *Nature*, **268**, 154 (1977).

66. K. A. Smith, S. Gillis, P. E. Baker, D. McKenzie, and F. W. Ruscetti, T-cell growth factor mediated T-cell proliferation. *Ann. N. Y. Acad. Sci.*, **332**, 423 (1979).

67. S. A. Rosenberg, S. Schwarz, and P. J. Spiess, *In vitro* growth of murine T cells. II. Growth of *in vitro* sensitized cells cytotoxic for alloantigen. *J. Immunol.*, **121**, 1951 (1978).

68. K. A. Smith, S. Gillis, and P. Baker, The inhibition of *in vivo* tumor growth by cytotoxic T-cell lines. *Proc. Am. Assoc. Cancer Res.*, **20**, 93 (1979) (abstract).

69. M. A. Cheever, P. D. Greenberg, and A. Fefer, Specific adoptive therapy of established leukemia with syngeneic lymphocytes sequentially immunized *in vivo* and *in vitro* and non-specifically expanded by culture with Interleukin 2. *J. Immunol.*, **126**, 1318 (1981).

70. M. A. Cheever, P. D. Greenberg, and A. Fefer, Adoptive chemoimmunotherapy in murine leukemia with cells secondarily sensitized *in vitro* and cells numerically expanded by culture with Interleukin 2. In J. P. Saunders, Ed., *Fundamental Mechanisms in Human Cancer Immunology*, International Cancer Symposium Committee, Elsevier/North Holland, New York, 1981.

71. D. P. Osborne and D. H. Katz, The allogeneic effect on tumor growth. II. Suppression of both ascitic and solid MOPC 315 plasmacytoma by the graft-vs-host reaction, with pathologic correlation. *J. Immunol.*, **118**, 1449 (1977).

72. O. Wescott, S. Dorsch, and B. Roser, Adoptive immunotherapy of leukemia in the rat, without graft-vs-host complications. *J. Immunol.*, **123**, 1478 (1979).

73. D. W. H. Barnes and J. F. Loutit, Treatment of murine leukemia with x-rays and homologous bone marrow. *Br. J. Hematol.*, **3**, 241 (1957).

74. G. Mathe and J. Bernard, Essai de traitement, par l'irradiation X suivie de l'administration de cellules myeloides homologues, de souris AK atteintes de leucemie spontanee tres avancee. *Bull. Cancer*, **45**, 289 (1958).

75. G. Mathe and J. Bevnase, Essai de traitement de la leucemie greffe L1210 par l'irradiation X suivie de transfusions de cellules hematopoietique normales. *Rev. Franc. Etud. Clin. Biol.*, **4**, 442 (1959).

76. G. Mathe, J. L. Amiel, and J. Bernard, Traitement de souris AKR a l'age de six mois par irradiation totale suivie de transfusion de cellules hematopoietiques allogeniques incidences respectives de la leucemie et du syndrome secondaire. *Bull. Cancer*, **57**, 331 (1960).

77. M. Boranic and I. Tonkovic, Time pattern of the antileukemic effect of the graft-versus-host reaction in mice. *Cancer Res.*, **31**, 1140 (1970).

78. G. Mathe, J. L. Amiel and J. Niemetz, Greffe de moelle osseuse apres irradiation totale chez des souris leucemiques suivie de l'administration d'un antimitotique pour reduire la frequence du syndrome secondaire et ajouter a l'effet antileucemique. *C. R. Acad. Sci.* (*Paris*), **254**, 3603 (1962).

79. M. Boranic, Transient graft-versus-host reaction in the treatment of leukemia in mice. *J. Natl. Cancer Inst.*, **41**, 421 (1968).

80. M. M. Bortin, W. C. Rose, R. L. Truitt, A. A. Rimm, E. C. Saltzstein and G. E. Rodey, Graft versus leukemia. VI. Adoptive immunotherapy in combination with chemoradiotherapy for spontaneous leukemia-lymphoma in AKR mice. *J. Natl. Cancer Inst.*, **55**, 1227 (1975).

81. M. Boranic and I. Tonkovic, The effect of cyclophosphamide on the ability of graft-versus-host reaction to suppress leukemia in mice. *Eur. J. Clin. Biol. Res.*, **7**, 314 (1972).

82. M. Kende, L. D. Keys, M. Gaston, and A. Goldin, Immunochemotherapy of transplantable Moloney leukemia with cyclophosphamide and allogeneic spleen lymphocytes and reversal of graft-versus-host disease with alloantiserum. *Cancer Res.*, **35**, 346 (1975).

83. J. P. Glynn, B. L. Halpern, and A. Fefer, An immunochemotherapeutic model for the treatment of a transplanted Moloney virus-induced lymphoma in mice. *Cancer Res.*, **29**, 515 (1969).

84. J. P. Glynn and M. Kende, Treatment of Moloney virus-induced leukemia with cyclophosphamide and specifically sensitized allogeneic cells. *Cancer Res.*, **31**, 1383 (1971).

85. A. Fefer, Treatment of a Moloney lymphoma with cyclophosphamide and H-2-incompatible spleen cells. *Cancer Res.*, **33**, 641 (1973).

86. D. L. Putman, P. D. Kind, A. Goldin, and M. Kende, Adoptive immunochemotherapy of a transplantable AKR leukemia (K36). *Internatl. J. Cancer,* **21**, 230 (1978).

87. R. L. Truitt and M. M. Bortin, Adoptive immunotherapy of malignant disease: Model systems and their relevance to human disease. In S. Slavin, Ed., *Organ Transplantation: Present Status, Future Goals,* Elsevier/North Holland, Amsterdam (in press).

88. Y. Yamada, T. Kawamura, E. Gotohda, J. Akiyama, M. Hosokawa, T. Kodama, and H. Kobayashi, Effect of normal allogeneic lymphoid cell transfer in combination with chemotherapy on a transplantable tumor in rats. *Cancer Res.,* **40**, 954 (1980).

89. G. W. Santos, Effect of graft-versus-host disease on a spontaneous adenocarcinoma. *Exp. Hematol.,* **20**, 46 (1970).

90. M. M. Bortin, A. A. Rimm, E. C. Saltzstein, and G. E. Rodey, Graft versus leukemia. III. Apparent independent antihost and antileukemic activity of transplanted immunocompetent cells. *Transplantation,* **16**, 182 (1973).

91. H. Glucksberg and A. Fefer, Chemotherapy of established graft-versus-host disease in mice. *Transplantation,* **13**, 300 (1972).

92. R. Korngold and J. Sprent, Lethal graft-versus-host disease after bone marrow transplantation across minor histocompatibility barriers in mice. *J. Exp. Med.,* **148**, 1687 (1978).

93. M. M. Bortin, A. A. Rimm, W. C. Rose, and E. C. Saltzstein, Graft versus leukemia. V. Absence of antileukemic effect using allogeneic H-2 identical immunocompetent cells. *Transplantation,* **18**, 280 (1974).

94. W. J. Martin, T. G. Gipson, and J. M. Rice, H-2^a-associated alloantigen expressed by several transplacentally-induced lung tumors of C3HF mice. *Nature,* **265**, 738 (1977).

95. M. L. Bach, F. H. Bach, and J. M. Zarling, Pool-priming: A means of generating T lymphocytes cytotoxic to tumor or virus-infected cells. *Lancet,* **1**, 20 (1978).

96. M. M. Bortin and R. L. Truitt, Graft-versus-leukaemia reactivity induced by alloimmunisation without augmentation of graft-versus-host reactivity. *Nature,* **281**, 490 (1979).

97. A. B. Einstein, M. A. Cheever, and A. Fefer, Induction of increased graft-versus-host disease by mouse spleen cells sensitized *in vitro* to allogeneic tumor. *Transplantation,* **22**, 589 (1976).

98. R. M. Zinkernagel and P. C. Doherty, MCH-restricted cytotoxic T cells: Studies on the biological role of polymorphic major transplantation antigens determining T-cell restriction-specificity, function and responsiveness. *Adv. Immunol.,* **27**, 51 (1979).

99. M. J. Bevan, Cytotoxic T-cell response to histocompatibility: The role of H-2. *Cold Spring Harbor Symp. Quant. Biol.,* **41**, 519 (1976).

100. R. L. Truitt, Application of germfree techniques to the treatment of leukemia in AKR mice by allogeneic bone marrow transplantation. In H. Waters, Ed., *The Handbook of Cancer Immunology,* Vol. 5, *Immunotherapy,* Garland STPM Press, New York, 431, 1978.

101. S. J. Chester, A. R. Esparza, L. J. Flinton, J. D. Simon, R. J. Kelley, and M. M. Albala, Further development of a successful protocol of graft versus leukemia without fatal graft-versus-host disease in AKR mice. *Cancer Res.,* **37**, 3494 (1977).

102. A. H. Owens and G. W. Santos, The effect of cytotoxic drugs on graft-versus-host disease in mice. *Transplantation,* **11**, 378 (1971).

103. H. Glucksberg and A. Fefer, Combination chemotherapy for clinically established graft-versus-host disease in mice. *Cancer Res.,* **33**, 859 (1973).

104. R. Storb, J. H. Kolb, T. C. Graham, H. Kolb, P. L. Weiden, and E. D. Thomas, Treatment of established graft-versus-host disease in dogs by antithymocyte serum or prednisone. *Blood,* **42**, 601 (1973).

105. E. R. Richie, M. T. Gallagher, and J. J. Trentin, Inhibition of the graft-versus-host reaction. II. Prevention of acute graft-versus-host mortality by Fab fragments of anti-lymphocyte globulin. *Transplantation,* **15**, 486 (1973).

106. H. L. Lochte, A. S. Levy, D. M. Guenther, E. D. Thomas, and J. W. Ferrebee, Prevention of delayed foreign marrow reaction in lethally irradiated mice by early administration of methotrexate. *Nature (Lond.)* **196**, 1110 (1962).

107. R. Storb, R. B. Epstein, T. C. Graham, and E. D. Thomas, Methotrexate regimens for control of graft-versus-host disease in dogs with allogeneic marrow grafts. *Transplantation,* **9**, 240 (1970).

108. B. Bonavida and E. Kedar, Transplantation of allogeneic lymphoid cells specifically depleted of graft-versus-host reactive cells. *Nature,* **249**, 658 (1974).

109. D. C. Zoschke and F. H. Bach, Specificity of allogeneic cell recognition by human lymphocytes *in vitro. Science,* **172**, 1350 (1971).

110. S. E. Salmon, R. S. Drakauer, and W. F. Whitmore, Lymphocyte stimulation. Selective destruction of cells during blastogenic response to transplantation antigens. *Science,* **172**, 490 (1971).

111. H. J. Deeg, R. Storb, P. L. Weiden, R. Graham, K. Atkinson, and E. D. Thomas, Cyclosporin A—effect on marrow engraftment and graft-versus-host disease in dogs. *Transplant Proc.,* **13** (1), 402 (1981).

112. S. Slavin, Z. Fuks, H. S. Kaplan, and S. Strober, Transplantation of allogeneic bone marrow without graft-versus-host disease using total lymphoid irradiation. *J. Exp. Med.,* **147**, 963 (1978).

113. H. Rodt, S. Thierfelder, and M. Eulitz, Anti-lymphocytic antibodies and marrow transplantation. III. Effect of heterologous anti-brain antibodies on acute secondary disease in mice. *Eur. J. Immunol.,* **4**, 25 (1974).

114. R. L. Powles, H. M. Cliur, D. Spence, G. Morgenstering, J. G. Watson, P. J. Selley, M. Woods, A. Barrett, B. Jamison, J. Sloane, S. D. Lawler, H. E. M. Kay, D. Lawson, T. S. McElwain, and P. Alexander, Cyclosporin A to prevent graft-versus-host disease in man after allogeneic bone-marrow transplantation. *Lancet,* **1**, 327 (1980).

115. N. K. C. Ramsay, T. Kim, M. E. Nesbit, W. Krivit, P. F. Coccia, S. H. Levitt, W. G. Woods, and J. H. Kersey, Total lymphoid irradiation and cyclophosphamide as preparation for bone marrow transplantation in severe aplastic anemia. *Blood,* **55**, 344 (1980).

116. G. A. Nagel, G. S. Arneault, J. F. Holland, D. Kirkpatrick, and R. Kirkpatrick, Cell-mediated immunity against malignant melanoma in monozygous twins. *Cancer Res.,* **30**, 1828 (1970).

117. C. J. McPeak, Intralymphatic therapy with immune lymphocytes. *Cancer,* **28**, 1126 (1971).

118. S. H. Nadler and G. E. Moore, Immunotherapy of malignant disease. *Arch. Surg.,* **99**, 376 (1969).

119. L. J. Humphrey, W. R. Jewell, D. R. Murray, and W. O. Griffen, Immunotherapy for the patient with cancer. *Ann. Surg.,* **173**, 47 (1971).

120. E. T. Krementz, M. S. Samuels, J. H. Wallace, and E. N. Benes, Clinical experiences in immunotherapy of cancer. *Surg. Gynecol. Obstet.,* **133**, 209 (1971).

121. R. H. Yonemoto and P. I. Terasaki, Cancer immunotherapy with HLA-compatible thoracic duct lymphocyte transplantation. A preliminary report. *Cancer,* **30**, 1438 (1972).

122. R. G. Yonemoto, Adoptive immunotherapy utilizing thoracic duct lymphocytes. *Ann. N. Y. Acad. Sci.,* **277**, 7 (1976).

123. J. R. Neff and W. F. Enneking, Adoptive immunotherapy in primary osteosarcoma. *J. Bone Joint Surg.,* **57**, 145 (1975).

124. G. A. Andrews, C. C. Congdon, C. L. Edwards, N. Gengozian, B. Nelson, and H. Vodopick, Preliminary trials of clinical immunotherapy. *Cancer Res.,* **27**, 2535 (1967).

125. J. H. Frenster and W. M. Rogoway, *In vitro* activation and reinfusion of autologous human lymphocytes. *Lancet,* **2**, 979 (1968).

126. H. F. Seigler, W. W. Shingleton, R. S. Metzgar, E. C. Buckley, P. M. Bergoc, D. S. Miller, B. F. Fetter, and M. P. Phaup, Non-specific and specific immunotherapy in patients with melanoma. *Surgery,* 72, 162 (1972).

127. A. R. Cheema and E. R. Hersh, Local tumor immunotherapy with *in vitro* activated autochthonous lymphocytes. *Cancer,* 29, 982 (1972).

128. J. V. Schlosser and E. H. Benes, Immunotherapy of human cancer with PHA stimulated lymphocytes. *Proc. Am. Assoc. Cancer Res.,* 12, 82 (1971) (abstract).

129. A. Fefer, M. A. Cheever, E. D. Thomas, F. R. Appelbaum, C. D. Buckner, R. A. Clift, H. Glucksberg, P. D. Greenberg, F. L. Johnson, H. G. Kaplan, J. E. Sanders, R. Storb, and P. L. Weiden, Bone marrow transplantation for refractory acute leukemia in 34 patients with identical twins. *Blood,* 57, 421 (1981).

130. L. F. Odom, C. S. August, J. H. Githens, J. R. Humbert, H. Morse, D. Peakman, B. Sharma, S. L. Rusnak, and F. B. Johnson, Remission of relapsed leukaemia during a graft-versus-host reaction: a "graft-versus-leukaemia reaction" in man? *Lancet,* 2, 537 (1978).

131. P. L. Weiden, N. Flournoy, E. D. Thomas, R. Prentice, A. Fefer, C. D. Buckner, and R. Storb, Antileukemic effect of graft-versus-host disease in human recipients of allogeneic-marrow grafts. *New Engl. J. Med.,* 300, 1068 (1979).

132. P. L. Weiden, N. Flournoy, E. D. Thomas, A. Fefer, and R. Storb, Antitumor effect of marrow transplantation in human recipients of syngeneic or allogeneic grafts. In J. Okunewich, R. Meredity, Eds., *Graft-Versus-Leukemia in Man and Animal Models,* CRC Press, West Palm Beach, Florida, 22 (1981).

133. R. McIntyre and R. P. Gale, Relationship between graft-versus-leukemia and graft-versus-host in man—UCLA experience. In J. Okunewich and R. Meredity, Eds., *Graft-Versus-Leukemia in Man and Animal Models,* CRC Press, West Palm Beach, Florida (in press).

134. K. A. Dicke, A. Zander, G. Spitzer, D. S. Verma, L. Peters, L. Vellekoop, K. B. McCredie, and J. Hester, Autologous bone-marrow transplantation in relapsed adult acute leukaemia. *Lancet,* 1, 514 (1979).

135. R. P. Gale, Autologous bone marrow transplantation in patients with cancer. *JAMA,* 243, 540 (1980).

136. F. R. Appelbaum, G. P. Herzig, J. L. Ziegler, A. S. Levine, and A. B. Deisseroth, Successful engraftment of cryopreserved autologous bone marrow in patients with malignant lymphoma. *Blood,* 52, 85 (1978).

137. J. M. Zarling, F. H. Bach, and P. C. Kung, Sensitization of lymphocytes against pooled allogeneic cells. II. Characterization of effector cells cytotoxic for autologous lymphoblastoid cell lines. *J. Immunol.,* 126, 375 (1981).

138. E. L. Reinherz and S. F. Schlossman, The differentiation and function of human T lymphocytes. *Cell,* 19, 821 (1980).

139. S. Gillis, P. E. Baker, F. W. Ruscetti, and K. A. Suitte, Long-term culture of human antigen-specific cytotoxic T cell lines. *J. Exp. Med.,* 148, 1093 (1978).

140. H. von Boehmer, W. Haas, H. Pohlit, H. Hengartner, and M. Nabholz, T cell clones: Their use for the study of specificity, induction, and effector-function of T cells. *Springer Semin. Immunopathol.,* 3, 23 (1980).

Specific Active Immunotherapy in Cancer Treatment

P. O. LIVINGSTON
H. F. OETTGEN
L. J. OLD
Memorial Sloan-Kettering Cancer Center
New York, New York

1. INTRODUCTION

The treatment or prevention of cancer with specific vaccines has been a dream of physicians ever since the first vaccines against infectious diseases were developed. Although substantial numbers of cancer patients have been injected with tumor cell preparations, the design and complexity of these studies makes an assessment of the value of this approach impossible. Even with a most carefully designed study, the testing of human cancer vaccines is fraught with difficulties and uncertainties ranging from appropriate type, dose, route, and frequency of vaccine, to suitable patient selection and evaluation of clinical response. What is required for the development of immunogenic cancer vaccines are rapid and objective methods to assess effectiveness that can guide the process of vaccine construction and testing. With regard to vaccines against infectious disease, serologic responses to bacterial or viral antigens have been essential in monitoring development. The lack of comparable serologic tests to monitor the effectiveness of cancer vaccines in human patients has been a major impediment to applying this approach to cancer therapy. With the development of serologic typing systems for defining cell surface antigens of some human cancers, we now have serologic tests of requisite sensitivity and specificity to gauge the immunogenicity of cancer vaccines. It seems timely, therefore, to consider anew what approaches to specific active immunization can be taken in the light of current knowledge of tumor antigens and of the immune responses they elicit.

2. TUMOR-SPECIFIC ANTIGENS IN EXPERIMENTAL ANIMALS

Of the several ways in which tumor-specific antigens of experimental animals can be classified, two are most relevant to the subject of this chapter. First, tumor antigens may be localized on the cell surface or within the cell. We consider only cell-surface antigens because it is their location on the cell surface which makes the cells vulnerable to immunologic attack. Second, tumor antigens may be specific for one individual tumor or shared by many tumors of a particular class. This distinction is of obvious importance in selecting sources of tumor cell vaccines.

2.1. Individually Specific Transplantation Antigens of Chemically Induced Tumors

Sarcomas induced by subcutaneous injection of polycyclic hydrocarbons have been shown to possess characteristic antigenicity in syngeneic hosts. The removal of a growing transplant of a tumor of this type is followed by resistance to subsequent challenge with the same tumor (1,2). The confirmation of these early experiments included a series of important controls that demonstrated as conclusively as possible with transplanted tumors that the immunity observed was specific for the tumor and was not attributable to residual genetic disparity among the inbred animals used (3). Moreover, the primary host itself was shown to be resistant to challenge with its own tumor excised and maintained in passage (4-6).

A consistent and remarkable feature of chemically induced tumors is that each tumor elicits immunity to itself but not to any other tumor. Thus tumors induced by the same carcinogen in the same inbred strain exhibit unique antigens. Even when two tumors are induced in the same animal, each can be shown to have distinct antigens. Although the subject of much speculation, the genetic origin of these new antigens is not known. Determination of the extent as well as the basis of the remarkable antigenic diversity has been hampered by the fact that the antigens have been demonstrable unequivocally only by *in vivo* transplantation studies. Although serologic approaches to these questions would appear to be more promising, it has been exceedingly difficult to raise antibodies to the individually distinct antigens of chemically induced sarcomas. Only recently two such antigens have been defined on methylcholanthrene-induced sarcomas with antibody derived from hyperimmunized mice (7,8). The detection of these antigens provides the first serologic probes in investigation of the nature of these highly restricted cellular antigens.

2.2. Shared Transplantation Antigens of Virus-Induced Tumors

Among the naturally occurring tumors that develop in mice, some are caused by viral agents. Two such agents are the RNA murine leukemia virus (MuLV) and the RNA mammary tumor virus. A number of other viruses have also been shown to cause tumors in laboratory mice, although they seldom do so under normal circumstances. Nevertheless, they have been invaluable tools for uncovering the immunological factors that influence tumor development and growth. Examples of such viruses are the polyoma virus, the SV40, and the adenoviruses.

In studies of tumors induced by the polyoma virus, the surprising observation was made that such transplanted tumors would not grow if the recipient mouse had been previously injected with polyoma virus as an adult (only newborn or immunologically crippled mice develop tumors when injected with polyoma virus) (9,10). This finding can be best understood by assuming that tumor cells do arise in adult mice but are recognized immunologically and rejected, leaving the mouse tumor free and also resistant against subsequent transplants of polyoma tumors. In contrast to the antigenic uniqueness of each chemically induced tumor, transplantation studies have shown that all tumors induced by polyoma virus have the same virus-specified cell surface antigen, so that immunization with any one polyoma tumor confers resistance to any other. The study of tumors induced by other oncogenic viruses has led to the same conclusion. Identical antigens appear in different tumors induced by the same virus. Although it appeared at first that a sharp distinction could be made between chemically induced tumors and virus-induced tumors, it now seems that the distinction is relative rather than absolute. The finding that mammary tumors of the mouse have individually distinct transplantation antigens in addition to shared transplantation antigens (11) indicates that individually distinct transplantation antigens may be characteristic of tumors generally, although this feature will often be overshadowed by the presence of cross-reacting antigens in virus-induced tumors.

2.3. Methods of Measuring Tumor Immunity: The Leading Role of Serology

With the recognition of tumor-specific antigens, many attempts have been made to develop analytical methods that would be faster and less cumbersome than transplantation techniques. An array of techniques has been devised to demonstrate immune reactions to tumor antigens *in vitro*. In recent years much effort has gone into developing methods that measure the reactivity of cellular components of the immune system, particularly the T lymphocyte. Perhaps the most important advance in this area has been the discovery of the T-cell growth factor that permits the continuous culture of sensitized T cells (12). Although considerable progress has been made, further understanding of the conditions required for the function, growth, and analysis of specificity of T cells *in vitro* is needed before these methods can provide the desired precision and flexibility. By far the most advanced and versatile methods are serologic methods that use antibody as the analytical probe. The awesome potential of the hybridoma methodology proposed by Kohler and Milstein (13) applied to production of monoclonal antibodies against tumor antigens promises to further increase the sensitivity and specificity of serologic methods. As these efforts are still at an early stage, we concentrate here on traditional serologic approaches. The analysis of the cell surface antigens of mouse leukemias provides an excellent example of the resolving power of one such approach.

2.4. Serologic Definition of Cell-Surface Antigens of Mouse Leukemia

The great majority of mouse leukemias arise in the thymus, and this has allowed the serologist to study the leukemia cell side by side with its normal counterpart, the thymocyte. As a consequence of these advantages, more is known about the surface antigens of normal and malignant T cells than about any other cell population in the mouse (14–16).

Four general classes of cell surface antigen have been distinguished on mouse leukemias: (1) conventional H-2 alloantigens (major histocompatibility antigens), present on all cells; (2) differentiation alloantigens, such as Thy-1 and the Lyt series and several products of the H-2-Ir and *Q* complex characteristic for cells undergoing T-cell differentiation; (3) MuLV-related antigens specified by endogenous murine leukemia viruses; and (4) TL (thymus-leukemia) antigens that occur as differentiation alloantigens on normal thymocytes of TL-positive strains of mice and as leukemia-specific antigens in TL-negative mouse strains not normally expressing TL antigens. Of these, the latter two classes are of particular interest to the tumor immunologist because in certain circumstances they are tumor-specific antigens.

Before discussing them in more detail, consideration should be given to the methods that were devised to produce antibody to these cell-surface antigens. The challenge was to develop methods of immunization or testing that would eliminate the contribution of H-2 antibodies. This has been accomplished in three principal ways: (1) immunization with H-2 incompatible leukemia cells and testing the resulting antiserum on syngeneic leukemia cells; (2) H-2-compatible immunization; and (3) syngeneic immunization. In addition to antisera prepared by deliberate immunization, naturally occurring antibodies in normal mouse serum have become valuable reagents for defining the spectrum of cell-surface antigens specified by murine leukemia viruses.

The list of MuLV-related antigens recognized by mouse antibody is rapidly growing; it parallels the diversity of MuLV recognizable by virologic and biochemical methods. They can be distinguished on the basis of their strain distribution, tissue distribution, and appearance in leukemias and other tumors of strains that normally do not express these antigens. Their specification by MuLV is shown in two general ways: (1) demonstration of structural relationship to MuLV components (absorption of antibody with purified MuLV proteins or immunochemical characterization of the cell surface molecule) or (2) antigen induction following MuLV infection of permissive cells.

Murine leukemia virus-related antigens may be found on the surface of both normal and malignant cells of normal mice and on cells deliberately infected with MuLV. The two major antigens, GCSA and G_{IX} (the letter "G" is intended to honor Ludwik Gross, the discoverer of this class of viruses), are both structural components of the MuLV particle. When they are glycosylated and inserted into the cell membrane, they become cell-surface antigens. The GCSA antigen appears only when virus is produced, but G_{IX} may also appear on the normal thymocytes of certain strains in the absence of virus production.

The TL system of antigens shows certain similarities to G9 and other MuLV antigens (17), although there is no evidence linking it to MuLV. The antigen is called TL because the only types of cell on which it is found are mouse thymocytes and leukemia cells. Mouse strains can be classified as TL positive or TL negative depending on whether their thymocytes express TL. The characteristic feature of TL (which it shares with G_{IX}) is that when leukemias arise in mice of TL-negative strains, the leukemia cells may express TL. As with G_{IX}, this has been explained on the grounds that all mice have the genetic information for TL but that other genes determine whether it will be expressed. Leukemia affects a change in the genetic control, resulting in the anomalous appearance of TL on the surface of the leukemia cell.

These findings raise interesting questions about antigens that are classified as tumor specific. Antigens GCSA, G_{IX} and TL can be considered tumor specific under conditions where they appear in mice that normally never express them. Yet they are not truly specific in the sense that they only occur on cancer cells. With the range of surface markers that have been identified on T cells of the mouse, the surface phenotype of mouse leukemias is becoming well characterized. To illustrate this point, a comparison of surface antigens of three leukemias with the corresponding normal thymocyte population is shown in Table 1 (18). With regard to TL and MuLV-related antigens, the surface phenotype of the AKR leukemia AKSL2 does not differ from normal thymocytes. On the other hand, the cells of A-strain leukemia RADA1 express $G_{(RADA1)}$, not detected on normal A-strain thymocytes and the cells of leukemia ERLD, originating in a TL⁻ C57BL/6 mouse, express TL.

TABLE 1.   Cell-Surface Phenotype of Normal Murine Thymocytes and Leukemia Cells

	H-2		Lyt	TL^a				MuLV		
	D K	Thy-1	1 2 3	1 2 3 4	GCSA	G_{IX}	$G_{(RADA1)}$	$G_{(ERLD)}$	$G_{(AKSL}$
AKR thymocytes	+ +	+	+ + +	− − − −	+	+	+	+	+
AKR spontaneous leukemia AKSL2	+ +	+	− − −	− − − −	+	+	+	+	+
A-strain thymocytes	+ +	+	+ + +	+ + + −	−	+	−	+	−
A-strain x-ray-induced leukemia RADA1	+ +	+	− − −	+ + + −	−	+	⊞	+	−
C57BL/6 thymocytes	+ +	+	+ + +	− − − −	−	−	−	+	−
C57BL/6 x-ray-induced leukemia ERLD	+ +	+	+ + +	⊞⊞ − ⊞	−	−	−	+	−

Source: Old and Stockert (18).

^{a}Squares ☐ represent leukemia-specific antigens in the strain of origin.

Table 2 summarizes current knowledge about the categories of surface antigens of mouse leukemia cells (15). The term "derepression antigens" has been used to distinguish antigens appearing on the surface of tumor cells that are coded for by normally silent genetic information. The TL- and MuLV-related antigens appearing on leukemias of TL$^-$ and MuLV$^-$ strains are prime examples of derepression antigens. Tumor antigens shared with histocompatibility antigens or coded for by genes active only in embryonic fetal life and completely undetectable in adult cells would also belong to this category. The well-defined F9 antigen that is present on undifferentiated murine teratocarcinoma, embryonal tissues, and sperm cells comes closest to meeting these criteria (19). Despite considerable interest in such tumor antigens, the TL and MuLV antigens present in leukemias of mice not normally expressing these antigens remain the best-defined examples.

TABLE 2. Categories of Serologically Demonstrable Surface Antigens on Mouse Leukemias of Thymic Origin (15)

Conventional alloantigens	H-2D, H-2K
Differentiation alloantigens	Lyt-1,2,3,4, Thy-1, TL.1,2,3
MuLV-related antigens	GCSA, G_{IX}, $G_{(RADA1)}$, $G_{ERLD)}$, $G_{(AKSL2)}$, X.1, FMR
Derepression antigens	TL.1,2,4 in TL$^-$ strains and MuLV-related antigens in strains not normally expressing these antigens
MTV-related antigens	ML
Species antigens	MSLA
Transformation-specific MuLV antigens	None defined
Embryonic and fetal antigens	None defined
Individually distinct (unique) antigens	None defined
Idiotype receptors	None defined

Source: Old and Stockert (15).

Even though important advances have been made, our understanding of the enormous variety of surface antigens on normal and malignant cells of the mouse is still quite limited. The ultimate aim is not, of course, to compile an inventory, but to understand how the cell surface is constructed, how malignant transformation changes that structure, and how the immune system responds to these changes. Another important question is how oncornaviruses such as MuLV are transmitted in nature, not only for the light the answer may shed on the relation between virus and host, but also because the facts are needed for an understanding of how infection may be controlled. The probable ubiquity of the viral genome in mammalian cells accords with the view that it is, in fact, integrated and transmitted as part of the cellular genome.

This mode of infection, which has been termed *vertical transmission* or *transmission by gametes* (20), does not of course exclude horizontal transmission, that is, passage of infection from one individual to another. In chickens there is much evidence of horizontal transmission of leukemia virus, carrying with it a heightened risk of leukemia (21). In the mouse horizontal transmission does not appear to play a role in the natural incidence of leukemia, and so one might assume that horizontal transmission is a negligible factor in mammals generally. But work in the cat indicates the opposite. Again, it was the development of serologic tests for the cat leukemia virus (22–24) that made it possible to study the epidemiology of the virus and its relationship to leukemia in the cat.

2.5. Epidemiology of the Feline Leukemia Virus (FeLV) and Its Relationship to Leukemia; Implications for Prophylactic and Therapeutic Vaccination

Study of the spread of FeLV became possible with the development of an immunofluorescence test on peripheral white cells that identified infected cats (25). A survey of more than 2000 cats showed that all virus-positive cats originated from households in which another cat had previously been diagnosed as suffering from leukemia or another disease caused by FeLV.

In most instances the diseased cats were not immediately related to the infected normal animals identified serologically (26). This clearly points to spread of infection from cat to cat. The crucial point is that the probability of these serologically positive cats becoming leukemic is greatly increased. Subsequently, infected normal cats were removed from households where permission to do so was given, and the tests were repeated at a later date. A dramatic decrease was seen in the incidence of subsequent FeLV infection as compared with households from which FeLV-positive healthy cats had not been removed (27). Three classes of antigen have been found associated with FeLV and FeLV-induced tumor cells. Two are components of the viral envelope (23) or internal structure (22), and the third is the so-called feline oncornavirus-associated cell membrane antigen (FOCMA), specified by this virus but not a structural component (28). Healthy cats can now be classified by three serologic tests. One is the test described previously that detects the internal structural viral antigen in blood leukocytes; it indicates FeLV infection (25). The second test measures antibodies against the viral envelope antigens; they neutralize the virus and protect against FeLV infections (29). The third test measures antibodies against the FOCMA (30,31); they appear to confer resistance against FeLV leukemia (but not FeLV infection) and can be found in cats with or without neutralizing antibodies and even in some cats that show no evidence of FeLV infection. The knowledge of the horizontal spread of FeLV, its relation to leukemia, the antigens found in FeLV and FeLV leukemia cells, the serologic response of cats to these antigens, and the beneficial effect of removing FeLV carriers now serves as a valuable basis for developing protective FeLV vaccines. Similarly, the knowledge that FOCMA antigen is present on FeLV-induced lymphosarcomas and that anti-FOCMA antibodies protect against these malignancies suggests the development of vaccines containing FOCMA for therapeutic trials.

2.6. Apparent Lack of Tumor-Specific Antigens in Certain Tumors

Tumors caused by any agent vary greatly in their immunizing capacity. Tumor-specific antigens are described as "weak" or "strong" depending on how effectively they immunize against subsequent challenge with the same tumor. Naturally occurring tumors of mice have generally been found to be only weakly antigenic, and sometimes not antigenic at all (32). It is possible that the techniques used for detecting them have not been sufficiently sensitive. Whether tumor-specific antigens are characteristic of all cancers or whether cells can become cancerous without gaining these markers cannot be decided on the basis of current evidence.

3. CELL-SURFACE ANTIGENS OF HUMAN CANCERS

Despite the enormous literature that has addressed the question of tumor-specific surface antigens of human cancers, the existence of such antigens must still be considered in the realm of speculation. The general impression that tumor-specific antigens have been demonstrated in many types of human cancer is simply not justified. The critical issue is, of course, the issue of specificity, and defining the specificity of a serologic or cell-mediated immune reaction is much easier in mice than in humans. In laboratory animals the availability of inbred strains permitted the transplantation studies that established the existence of distinctive cell-surface antigens in tumors. The serologic definition of these antigens in the mouse and the rat has also depended on inbred populations to provide the necessary reagents. In the absence of these advantages, the human cancer serologist is still attempting to evolve approaches that can cope with the issue of specificity. Antisera prepared against human cancer cells in foreign species, though at first appearing tumor specific, have in every instance turned out to be directed against normal cellular products, either present in higher concentration in tumor cells or found in restricted normal cell populations. Surveys of human sera for reactivity with cell-surface antigens of allogeneic tumor cells, usually cell lines considered representative of one or another type of cancer, form the basis for a large number of reports in the literature. They are rarely, if ever, interpretable as tumor-specific reactions, however, because the participation of alloantibodies in the reactions observed is extremely difficult to exclude.

   To develop as unambiguous a serologic typing system as possible, several years ago we turned to analyzing autologous serum reactivity to cell-surface antigens of human cancer. As we considered continued availability of target cells for repeated testing essential, our studies have been restricted to tumor types that can be grown in tissue culture with some degree of regularity, malignant melanoma, renal cancer, and astrocytoma. Other essential features included extensive absorption tests to establish specificity by determining the occurrence of antigen on a wide range of normal and malignant tissues and the use of several serologic techniques (mixed hemadsorption, immunoadherence, C3-mixed hemadsorption, protein-A assay) to reduce the possibility that antibody of a particular immunoglobulin class might be missed. Although the same procedure has been applied to the study of malignant melanoma (33–36), renal cancer (37), and astrocytoma (38), the work with melanoma is most advanced and may serve as an example.

Results obtained by testing autologous combinations of serum and melanoma target cells with the four serologic assays are shown in Table 3. Antibody was detected in the serum of 11/39 (i.e., 11 of 39) patients by MHA (titers 1/4 to 1/512), 21/40 patients by IA (titers 1/4 to 1/320), 8/28 patients by PA (titers 1/64 to 1/640), and 25/26 patients by C-3-MHA (titers 1/4 to 1/192). In general, antibodies detected by MHA or PA were reactive at 24°C, whereas antibodies detected by IA or C3-MHA were most reactive at 4°C. As the different assays detect antibodies that belong to different classes of immunoglobulin, the lack of complete concordance between the results of the various assays comes as no surprise. Indeed, the expectation that this would be so was the reason for choosing a battery of serologic assays. Antibodies to surface antigens of cultured autologous fibroblasts were not detected by MHA or IA even though the same sera contained antibodies to surface antigens of cultured autologous melanoma cells. Protein-A and C3-MHA assays have not as yet been applied to the testing of fibroblasts from patients with melanoma.

Positive sera were absorbed with a wide range of cells from autologous, allogeneic, and xenogeneic sources to determine the specificity of the reaction with autologous melanoma cells. The following three categories of melanoma surface antigen have been distinguished on the basis of these absorption tests:

Class 1.   Individually distinct or unique melanoma antigens. These antigens show an absolute restriction to autologous melanoma cells.

Class 2.   Shared melanoma antigens. These antigens are also expressed by some allogeneic melanoma cells and other cells of similar embryologic origin.

Class 3.   Widely crossreacting antigens. These antigens are expressed on an extensive range of normal and malignant cells of human and animal origin.

As shown in Table 2, sera from 3 of 22 patients recognized Class I antigens (AU, BD, BI), sera from 2 patients recognized Class II antigens (AH, BD), and sera from 17 patients recognized Class III antigens. It should be noted that even in the same patient, the specificity of the detected reactions may be different when the same serum sample is tested by different serologic assays or when sera obtained at different times are tested by the same assay. Typical examples of absorption analyses by which antigens of each of the three classes were defined are shown in Tables 4 through 6. Table 4 shows an example of a Class I antigen, detected by patient BD's serum in IA assays. The antibody in BD's serum was absorbed by autologous melanoma cells (SK-MEL-37) but not by a variety of other autologous, allogeneic, or xenogeneic cells, including 12 allogeneic cultured melanoma cell lines. Table 5 shows an example of a Class II antigen, found on 5 of 12 melanoma cell lines but not any other types of cultured or noncultured cells. An example of a Class III antigen, found on autologous, allogeneic and xenogeneic cells, is shown in Table 6. This example underscores the importance of absorption analysis: whereas AV fibroblasts removed reactivity for autologous melanoma cells in absorption tests, they did not react with autologous serum in direct tests. These three classes of antigen have also been found on the cells of renal cancers and astrocytomas by autologous typing (37,38).

Thus it appears that individually specific tumor antigens and shared tumor antigens exist in humans as well as in mice. Moreover, normal humans, as normal mice, have "natural" antibodies to some of these antigens in their serum. An initial survey of over 100 normal nontransfused males showed that IgG antibody to melanoma surface antigens was rare but IgM antibody was more common. In five of these normal individuals, IgM antibody identified an antigen related to the AH melanoma antigen (see Table 5) (39).

The serologic dissection of sera from melanoma patients and healthy individuals tells us which melanoma surface molecules can be recognized as immunogenic by humans. The recently developed hybridoma technology permits us to take a new look at what heterologous species recognize as immunogeneic on human melanoma cells. Several groups have described murine monoclonal antibodies against melanoma cell-surface antigens (40–42). In our laboratory 18 monoclonal antibodies analyzed so far have identified six distinguishable systems of melanoma cell-surface antigens. Two are glycoproteins, as judged by lectin binding and radiolabeling with amino acid and carbohydrate precursors. Other systems have properties of glycolipids, as indicated by heat stability and antibody inhibition tests with glycolipid fractions of reactive cells. One antigen in this system has the most restricted distribution we have seen so far; it is found on melanomas and astrocytomas but may also be present in normal brain and on melanocytes (43). These studies have taught us that what has been shown using conventional immune sera or natural antibodies also applies to monoclonal antibodies: direct serologic tests may be less sensitive than absorption tests for determining the presence of antigen. Several examples of the direct test-negative/absorption test-positive phenotype have been found in our analysis of monoclonal antibodies to melanoma cells. Continued application of hybridoma methodology in its present form should tell us whether the mouse recognizes antigens that are melanoma specific. When techniques for the production of human monoclonal antibodies are perfected, we may be able to determine the full range of melanoma antigens that are recognized by humans.

TABLE 3. Survey of Sera from Patients with Malignant Melanoma for Autologous Antibody to Surface Antigens of Cultured Malignant Melanoma Cells: Summary of Serologic Tests

Target Cell Line	Patient	Range of Antibody Titers				Classification of Antigen by Absorption Analysis
		MHA	PA	IA	C3-MHA	
SK-MEL- 5	AA	1/16 to 1/32		—		
SK-MEL- 6	AB	—				
SK-MEL- 7	AC	—				
SK-MEL- 8	AD	—	—	1/8	1/32	III (C3-MHA)
SK-MEL- 9	AE	—				
SK-MEL-11	AF	—				
SK-MEL-12	AG			—		
SK-MEL-13	AH	1/4	—	1/20 to 1/160		II (C3-MHA), II (IA)
SK-MEL-14	AI	—		—		
SK-MEL-15	BO					
SK-MEL-17	AJ	—				
SK-MEL-18	AK	—				
SK-MEL-19	AL	—		1/4	1/8	
SK-MEL-20	AM					
SK-MEL-21	AN	1/4 to 1/16		1/40 to 1/320	1/16	III (C3-MHA), III (IA)
SK-MEL-22	AO	1/4		1/4		
SK-MEL-23	AP	—	—	1/8	1/32	III (C3-MHA)
SK-MEL-24	AQ	—	—	—	—	
SK-MEL-25	AR	—	—	1/4		
SK-MEL-26	AS	—	>1/64	—	1/32	III (C3-MHA)
SK-MEL-27	AT	1/4 to 1/16	—	1/4 to 1/32	1/128	III (MHA)
SK-MEL-28	AU	1/16 to 1/512	1/64	1/4 to 1/32	1/10	I (MHA), I (PA)
SK-MEL-29	AV	—	1/640	1/4 to 1/16		III (PA), III (PA)
SK-MEL-30	AW	—		—		

Cell line	Code					Reactivity
SK-MEL-31	AX	1/4	—	>1/64	>1/192	III (IA), III (C3-MHA)
SK-MEL-32	AY	—	—	1/4 to 1/32	1/32	III (C3-MHA), III (IA)
SK-MEL-33	AZ	1/4 to 1/16	—	—		
SK-MEL-34	BA					
SK-MEL-35	BB	—				
SK-MEL-36	BC	1/16 to 1/64	—	1/4	1/32	III (C3-MHA)
SK-MEL-37	BD	1/16 to 1/64		1/4 to 1/96	1/8	II (C3-MHA)
SK-MEL-38	BE	—				
SK-MEL-39	BF	—			1/4	
SK-MEL-40	BG	—	1/256	1/4 to 1/128	1/128	III (C3-MHA), III (IA), III (PA)
SK-MEL-41	BH	—	>1/64	—	1/4	III (PA), I (MHA)
MeWo	BI	1/64 to 1/128	>1/64	—		
SK-MEL-42	BR			—	1/16 to 1/64	III (C3-MHA)
SK-MEL-43	BS		—	1/4	1/16	III (C3-MHA), III (PA)
SK-MEL-44	BT		1/256	1/8	1/4	
SK-MEL-45	BU					
SK-MEL-46	BV			—		
SK-MEL-47	BW	—		1/10 to 1/64	1/64	III (C3-MHA)
SK-MEL-49	BZ	—		1/64	1/8	
SK-MEL-51	CB	—		—	1/8	III (C3-MHA)
SK-MEL-52	CC		>1/64	—	1/8	
SK-MEL-55	CF			—		
SK-MEL-56	CG			—		
SK-MEL-57	CH	—		1/8	1/32	III (C3-MHA)
SK-MEL-59	CJ		1/64	1/4	1/8	III (C3-MHA)
SK-MEL-61	CL			—		
SK-MEL-62	CM			—	1/8	
SK-MEL-63	CN			—	1/16	III (C3-MHA)

TABLE 4. Absorption of IA Reactivity from Serum[a] of Patient BD Tested Against Autologous Melanoma Cells (SK-MEL-37)

Positive Absorption	Negative Absorption	
Autologous cultured melanoma cells SK-MEL-37 (BD)	Autologous normal cells	Allogeneic cultured melanoma cells
	Lymphoid cells	SK-MEL-8 (AD)
	Platelets	SK-MEL-13 (AH)
	Granulocytes	SK-MEL-15 (BO)
	Red blood cells	SK-MEL-19 (AL)
		SK-MEL-22 (AO)
	Autologous cultured	SK-MEL-23 (AP)
	normal cells	SK-MEL-27 (AT)
	BD fibroblasts	SK-MEL-28 (AU)
		SK-MEL-29 (AV)
	Allogeneic normal cells	SK-MEL-30 (AW)
	Pooled buffy coat	SK-MEL-36 (BC)
	leukocytes	MeWo (BI)
	A red blood cells	
	B red blood cells	Allogeneic cultured
	AB red blood cells	nonmelanoma cells
	O red blood cells	SK-RC-2 (renal cell cancer)
	Xenoageneic cells and	SK-RC-4 (renal cell cancer)
	serum	T-24 (bladder cancer)
	Sheep red blood cells	J-82 (bladder cancer)
	Guinea pig kidney	ME-180 (cervical cancer)
	Fetal bovine serum	SK-LC-LL (lung cancer)
		SK-L7 (leukemia)
	Oncornaviruses	Sal III (breast cancer)
	SSV-1	
	RD-114	Alloageneic cultured
	MuLV (AKR)	normal cells
		AT fibroblasts
	Microorganisms	
	BCG	Allogeneic cultured fetal cells
		WI-38 (fetal lung fibroblasts)
		PHEL-6 (fetal lung fibroblasts)

Source: Shiku et al. (34).

[a] Serum drawn November 1975.

4. SPECIFIC ACTIVE IMMUNIZATION WITH TUMOR ANTIGENS IN EXPERIMENTAL ANIMALS

The knowledge that tumor antigens exist and that the tumor-bearing host responds to them has provided the rational basis for immunologic approaches to therapy. The first obvious principle to emerge from work in animals is that it is much easier to prevent the establishment of a tumor than to alter the course of an already established tumor. Induction of specific resistance subsequent to tumor transplants has, of course, been accomplished many times by injecting animals with irradiated cells of the same tumor or the temporary growth (followed by removal) of nonirradiated cells or similar maneuvers. As discussed previously, experiments of this sort first established the existence of tumor-specific antigens. There are only a few reports, however, that describe retardation of tumor growth by specific active immunization when treatment was begun after the tumor transplant had been passed, and these are summarized in the paragraphs that follow. In these experiments treatment was generally successful only when given early after inoculation of the tumor cells, that is, at a time when tumors were not yet detectable.

In a study of chemically induced tumors in rats, immunization with a vaccine of viable or irradiated tumor cells mixed with BCG inhibited only tumors of substantial immunogenicity. With the most responsive tumor, the maximum challenge inoculum controlled was 10^6 cells, and treatment had to be given within 1 to 2 days to be predictably successful (44). In another series of experiments with chemically induced sarcomas in mice, treatment with a mixture of C. parvum and irradiated or living tumor cells specifically suppressed tumor growth when given at 6, but not 10, days after tumor challenge (45). In mice inoculated with the Moloney virus-induced leukemia LSTRA, intravenous or intraperitoneal injections of irradiated LSTRA cells beginning 2 days later caused prolongation of survival. The vaccine was not effective when started later (46). Inhibition of tumor growth was also noted when mice bearing transplants of chemically induced sarcomas were injected with neuraminidase-treated tumor cells (47).

The tumor system that has been investigated most in this context is the L10 hepatocarcinoma of strain 2 guinea pigs. Intratumoral injection of BCG caused regression not only of the injected established tumor in the skin, but also of reginal lymph node metastases (48). Moreover, vaccines of BCG mixed with viable irradiated L10 cells were effective in eliminating established visceral micrometastases (49) when given 4 to 10 days after intravenous injection of L10 cells. Similarly, regression after initial growth of cutaneous L10 tumor transplants was seen when the vaccine was injected contralaterally on the day of the tumor transplant (50). A feature common to the injected local tumor and the sites of vaccine injections was the development of a chronic inflammatory reaction. In the vaccine experiments the most important variables on which regression of metastases depended were an adequate dose of BCG and the viability of the tumor cells used to prepare the vaccine. Most of the studies

TABLE 5. Absorption of IA Reactivity from Serum of Patient AH Tested Against Autologous Melanoma Cells (SK-MEL-13)

Positive Absorption	Negative Absorption	

Autologous cultured melanoma cells
  SK-MEL-13 (AH)
 	
Allogeneic cultured melanoma cells
  SK-MEL-23 (AP)
  SK-MEL-27 (AT)
  SK-MEL-29 (AV)
  MeWo   (BI)
	Autologous normal cells
	  Lymphoid cells
	  Platelets
	  Granulocytes
	  Red blood cells
	
	Autologous cultured normal cells
	  AH fibroblasts
	
	Allogeneic normal cells (from patients
	whose cultured melanoma cells absorb
	reactivity from AH serum)
	  AT and AV
	    Lymphoid cells
	    Platelets
	    Granulocytes
	    Red blood cells
	  AP
	    Lymphoid Cells
		Xenogeneic cells or serum
		  Sheep red blood cells
		  Guinea pig kidney
		  Fetal calf serum
		
		Virus
		  SSV-1
		  RD-114
		  MuLV (AKR)
		
		Microorganisms
		  BCG
		  C. parvum
		
		Allogeneic cultured melanoma
		  cells
		  SK-MEL-8 (AD)
		  SK-MEL-15 (BO)
		  SK-MEL-19 (AL)
		
		Allogeneic cultured normal cells
		  AU fibroblasts
		  FB fibroblasts
		  FB normal kidney cells
		
		Allogeneic cultured fetal cells
		  WI-38 (fetal lung fibroblasts)
		  PHEL-6 (fetal lung fibroblasts)

Allogeneic cultured normal cells (from
patients whose cultured melanoma cells
absorb reactivity from AH serum)

AT fibroblasts
AV fibroblasts
BI fibroblasts

Allogeneic normal cells
Pooled buffy coat leukocytes
A red blood cells
B red blood cells
AB red blood cells
O red blood cells

SK-MEL-22 (AO)
SK-MEL-28 (AU)
SK-MEL-30 (AW)
SK-MEL-37 (BD)

Allogeneic cultured
nonmelanoma tumor cells

SK-RC-2   (renal cell cancer)
SK-RC-2   (renal cell cancer)
T-24   (bladder cancer)
J-82   (bladder cancer)
SK-LU1   (lung cancer)
SAL III   (breast cancer)
A1Ab   (breast cancer)
ME 180   (cervical cancer)
HeLa   (cervical cancer)
HT-3   (cervical cancer)
SK-OV-3   (ovarian cancer)
HT-29   (colon cancer)

Source: Shiku et al. (34).

TABLE 6.   Absorption of IA Reactivity from Serum of Patient AV Tested Against Autologous Melanoma Cells (SK-MEL-29)[a]

Positive Absorption	Negative Absorption
Autologous	Autologous
Cultured melanoma cells	Normal cells
SK-MEL-29	Lymphoid cells
Cultured normal cells	Granulocytes
AV fibroblasts	Platelets
	Erythrocytes
Allogeneic	Allogeneic
Cultured melanoma cells	Normal cells and serum
SK-MEL-27	Lymphoid cells
SK-MEL-28	Granulocytes
SK-MEL-30	Platelets
MeWo	Erythrocytes
Cultured normal cells	Sera
AT fibroblasts	
AU fibroblasts	
Allogeneic	Allogeneic
Cultured nonmelanoma cells	Cultured melanoma cells
SK-LMS-1 (leiomyosarcoma)	SK-MEL-13
SK-RC-4 (renal cell cancer)	SK-MEL-37
T-24 (bladder cancer)	Cultured normal cells
ME 180 (cervical cancer)	AH fibroblasts
SK-LC-LL (lung cancer)	BD fibroblasts
Xenogeneic	Xenogeneic cells and serum
Cultured monkey kidney cells	Sheep erythrocytes
Cultured chicken fibroblasts	Fetal bovine serum
Cultured mouse fibroblasts	Mouse erythrocytes
Mouse spleen cells	

[a] *Source:* Shiku et al. (35).

with transplanted tumors included controls that showed that vaccines prepared from the cells of unrelated tumors were ineffective.

Although the applicability of principles derived from experiments with transplanted tumors in animals to the treatment of human cancers may be questioned, there are also some reports of successful treatment of spontaneous primary cancers in domestic animals. Intratumoral injection of a BCG cell-wall vaccine into squamous carcinomas of the eyelid in Hereford cows has frequently resulted in control of the injected tumor and of regional lymph node metastases (51), and treatment of mammary carcinomas in mongrel dogs with vaccines prepared from neuraminidase-treated autologous tumor cells caused tumor regression and prolonged survival (52).

On the whole, specific active immunization of animals inoculated with tumor cells, or bearing small tumors, has been effective only in exceptional circumstances. In general, the successful induction of resistance to subsequent tumor grafts by irradiated tumor cells has been in stark contrast to the failure of the same procedure to control the growth of tumor cells inoculated at the time of, or after, immunization (53). Only little effort has gone into attempts at increasing the immunogenicity of the tumor antigens used in these experiments, and the selection of antigenic tumors as well as the assessment of the effects of immunization has been made solely on the basis of rejection reactions. Serologically defined antigens have not been used in therapy experiments, nor has the immunogenicity of administered vaccines been evaluated in terms of the serologic response. But it is precisely this approach that is feasible in humans, and not procedures involving transplantation. Thus we cannot derive a detailed blueprint for developing immunogenic human cancer vaccines from experiments in animals. Recognizing this state of affairs, we have used our knowledge of human cancer antigens and of mechanisms by which immunogenicity of cell-surface antigens can be increased as a basis for proceeding with the development of immunogenic human cancer vaccines.

5. SPECIFIC ACTIVE IMMUNIZATION WITH TUMOR ANTIGENS IN HUMANS

5.1. Past Experience

Attempts at inducing tumor regression in humans by specific active immunization can be grouped into two categories. The first represents topical application or intratumoral injection of agents that cause a delayed hypersensitivity reaction at the site of treatment. Agents that have been used with success in this context are DNCB, applied in an ointment to basal cell and squamous cell carcinomas of the skin (54,55) and BCG (56–58), MER (59), and DNCB (60) injected into cutaneous metastases of malignant melanomas and some other tumors. It is not entirely clear whether the tumor regression observed in these trials simply reflects the susceptibility of the tumor cells to damage inflicted by products of the delayed hypersensitivity reaction to unrelated antigens or whether it results from specific immunization that is augmented as a consequence of the reaction in the tumor. The fact that simultaneous regression of noninjected lesions is occasionally seen points to that possibility.

Although it is clear that patients with malignant melanoma whose metastases regress after intralesional injection of BCG fare better than do patients who do not show tumor regression, it is not yet known whether this treatment is more effective than other treatments or no treatment in retarding the subsequent progression of malignant melanoma. An answer to this question may soon be forthcoming, albeit in another setting. Results of a pilot study suggested that recurrence of superficial bladder cancer after surgery is delayed by repeated intravesical application of BCG (61). It seems that this suggestion is now confirmed, at least on a short-term basis, by two prospective randomized trials (62,63).

The second category of attempts at specific active immunization makes use of tumor vaccines with the objective of inducing or augmenting systemic tumor immunity. Attempts of this sort have been made for decades. Some 2000 patients have been injected with various preparations of autologous or allogeneic tumor tissue, fresh or cultured, from whole cells, cell homogenates, or fractions, with or without adjuvants. A summary of clinical trials in this category is given in Table 7. They have two features in common: (1) a therapeutic effect was not seen or, if suspected, has not been confirmed; and (2) no acceptable information has been provided regarding the presence of tumor antigens in the vaccines and the immune response of the patients to these antigens. Thus the principle of specific active immunization as a means of cancer therapy has not really been tested in humans, and there is no point in reviewing these trials in detail (for references, see Table 7).

In attempting to develop vaccines against cancer, we should perhaps take a lesson from the successful development of vaccines against infectious diseases. The sequence of events leading to the vaccine that all but eradicated poliomyelitis is particularly instructive. In the early 1930s vaccine trials with the use of crude spinal cord preparations from virus-infected monkeys were started (125,126). These trials were discontinued because the vaccine was quite toxic. This was perhaps a blessing in disguise because nothing was known at the time about different serotypes of the poliomyelitis virus. If the vaccine had been acceptably safe, it might have been insufficiently protective, and the whole approach might have been in disrepute. It was only much later that methods were developed that permitted propagation of poliomyelitis virus *in vitro* on monolayers of nonneural cells (127,128). At the same time epidemiologic surveys showed that poliomyelitis virus occurred in three distinct serotypes and that individuals with antibodies in their serum were protected against the serotype that fitted the antibody (129). These developments made possible the preparation of a vaccine and its initial testing in monkeys and small groups of human subjects to determine the conditions of preparation and administration that provided optimal safety and immunogenicity (130). The success of subsequent large-scale immunization proved the soundness of this stepwise approach (131). The subsequent development of live virus vaccines against poliomyelitis, rubella, and measles has followed the same general principles. There is no reason why they should not also guide our attempts at constructing vaccines against cancer.

5.2.   Current Attempts to Construct Immunogenic Melonoma Vaccines

Relating the currently known well-defined melanoma cell-surface antigens to biological and clinical aspects of melanoma is an important task now under way. Perhaps the most critical challenge involves determining the range of melanoma surface molecules that are or can be made immunogenic in humans.

TABLE 7. Clinical Trials of Tumor Vaccines in Humans[a]

Tumor	Type of Vaccine[b]	Description of Trial[b]	Number Patients Vaccinated	Disease Stages Treated[c]	Clinical Response[d]	Ref.
Melanoma	Aut, WC, Surg	NC, serology	13	All stages	None	64
Melanoma	Aut, Neur, Surg, BCG	NC, serology, CMC	149	All stages	6%	65,66
Melanoma	Aut, Neur, Surg, BCG	NC	120	All stages	5%	66
Melanoma	Aut + Allo, Neur, TC, BCG	NC	719	Stage 1,2	—	67
Melanoma	Aut, WC, Surg, BCG	NC	18	All stages	4 (med. 3 mo)	68
Melanoma	Aut, WC, Surg, BCG	R	8	Stage 2	Early deaths	69
Melanoma	Aut, Neur, Surg, BCG	NC	8	All stages	No effect	70
Melanoma	Aut, WC, Surg	NC, CMC	12	All stages	None	71,72
Melanoma	Aut, Neur, nonviable, Surg	R + CC	44	All stages	No effect	73
Melanoma	Aut, WC, Surg	NC, CMI	8	Stage 3	None	74
Melanoma	Aut, WC, TC	NC, serology	19	All stages	1	75
Melanoma	Aut, Goat, Surg	NC	50	Stage 3	2	76
Melanoma	Aut and/or Allo, VOL	NC, CMC	13	Stage 3	6, ↑ survival	77,78
Melanoma	Aut, WC, Surg	NC, serology CMC	10	All stages	None	79
Melanoma	Aut, WC, Surg, BCG and/or PPD	IL, NC	4	All stages	None	75
Melanoma	Allo, WC, TC, BCG and/or PPD	IL, NC	16	All stages	1	75
Melanoma	Allo, WC, Surg, BCG	Chemo, R	27	All stages	No effect	80
Melanoma	Allo, WC, TC, ± BCG	R, serology	29	Stage 2	No effect	81,82
Melanoma	Allo, WC, Surg, BCG	Chemo, R	31	All stages	No effect	83
Melanoma	Allo, WC, Surg, BCG	Chemo, NC	59	All stages	↑ response rate	84
Melanoma	Allo, WC, Surg, BCG	Chemo, CC	16	Stage 2	Early relapse	85
Melanoma	Allo, HOM, Surg	WBC, NC, serology	105	Stage 3	24%	86,87
Melanoma	Allo, HOM, Surg	WBC, NC	42	Stage 2	↑ DFI	86
Melanoma	Allo, VOL, TC	Chemo, NC	23	All stages	No effect	88,89
Melanoma	Allo, HOM	NC	15	All stages	33%	90

TABLE 7. (Continued)

Tumor	Type of Vaccine[b]	Description of Trial[b]	Number Patients Vaccinated	Disease Stages Treated[c]	Clinical Response[d]	Ref.
Melanoma	Allo or Aut, WC, Surg or TC, BCG or PPD	NC	37	All stages	No effect	91
Sarcoma	Aut, WC, Surg, BCG	NC, serology	9	Advanced	—	92
Osteosarcoma	Allo, WC, TC, BCG	CC	17	All stages	No effect	92,93
Osteosarcoma	Aut, VOL, TC	NC, serology, CMI	3	—	—	94
Osteosarcoma	Allo, VOL, TC	± chemo, NC, serology, CMI	9	—	—	94
Sarcoma	Allo, VOL, TC	CC	14		No effect	95
Sarcoma	Allo, WC, TC	CC	44	All stages	± ↑ DFI	96
Sarcoma	Allo, WC, Surg	HC, WBC	32	All stages	No effect	97
Sarcoma	Aut, HOM, Surg	HC	15	All stages	↑ DFI	98
Osteosarcoma	Allo, WC, TC, BCG	NC	6	All stages	—	99
Lung cancer	Allo, HOM, Surg, CFA	CC + R	29	I, II, NED	↑ DFI, ↑ survival	100
Lung cancer	Allo, HOM, Surg	R	8	All stages	—	101
Lung cancer	Aut, Neur, Surg, CFA	R	15	Stage III	↑ survival	102
Epidermoid cancer	Allo, VOL, TC	NC	35	Advanced	None	103
Breast cancer	Allo, WC, TC	Chemo, NC	10	Stage I	—	104
Breast cancer	Allo, WC, TC	Chemo, R	25	Stage II	—	105
Breast cancer	Aut, WC, Surg	NC, LMI	16	Stages II, III	↑ survival	106,107
Breast cancer	Aut, WC, Surg	NC, CMC	16	Stage I, II, III	—	108
Head and neck epidermoid carcinoma	Aut, Neur, Surg, BCG	Chemo, R	14	Stage III	No effect	109

	Aut, Neur, Surg, BCG	Chemo, CC	11	Stage III	—	110
Head and neck epidermoid carcinoma	Aut, Neur, Surg, BCG	Chemo, CC	11	Stage III	—	110
Colon cancer	Allo, HOM, Surg, BCG	NC, WBC	20	All stages	5	111
Ovarian	Allo, WC, Surg, BCG	CC, chemo	10	All stages	↑ survival	112
Glioblastoma	Aut, WC, Surg	R	27	S/P radical surg.	± ↑ survival	113
Various tumors	Aut, Polym, Surg, PPD	NC	200	All stages	—	114
Various tumors	Aut, VOL, Surg	NC, DH	29	Stages II, III	2	115
Various tumors	Aut, WC or HOM, Surg, CFA	CC	233	Stages II, III	No effect	116
Various tumors	Aut, HOM, Surg, CFA	NC, pathology	12	Stages II, III	7	117
Various tumors	Aut, Neur, Surg	NC, adjuvant	21	NED	—	118
Various tumors	Aut, HOM, Surg, CFA, T.B.A.	NC	20	NED	1	119
Various tumors	Aut, Neur, TJC, BCG	NC, CMC	7	NED	None	120
Various tumors	Aut, HOM, Surg, CFA	NC, serology	21	Advanced	None	121
Various tumors	Aut, WC, Surg Rab.	NC, serology	14	Advanced	14%	122
Various tumors	Allo, WC, Surg	NC, ILY	14	Stages II, III	25%	123
Various tumors	Aut, WC, Surg	NC, ILY	7	Stages II, III	2	123
Various tumors	Allo, WC, Surg, ± CFA	NC, WBC	118	Advanced	19%	124
Various tumors	Aut, WC, Surg, PPD and/or BCG	NC	7	Advanced	None	75

[a] Only trials with more than five solid tumor patients included.

[b] *Abbreviations:*. Allo, allogeneic tumor cells; Aut, autologous tumor cells; CA, Candida albicans antigens; CC, concurrent controls; CFA, complete Freund's adjuvant; DFI, disease-free interval; Goat, goat gamma globulin coupled to tumor cells; HC, historical controls; HOM, acellular omogenate; IL, Freund's adjuvant; DFI, disease-free interval; Goat, goat gamma globulin coupled to tumor cells; HC, historical controls; HOM, acellular omogenate; IL, vaccine administered intralesionally as well as intradermally; ILY, vaccine administered intralymphatically; LMI, leukocyte migration inhibition; NC, no vaccine administered intradermally as well as intradermally; ILY, vaccine administered intralymphatically; LMI, leukocyte migration inhibition; NC, no controls; Neur, neuraminidase-treated whole cells; PPD, purified protein derivative; Polym, polymerized insoluble antigen; R, randomized; Rab., rabbit gamma globulin coupled to tumor cells; Surg, cells obtained from surgical specimen; TBA, typhoid vaccine; TC, cells obtained from tissue; VOL, viral oncolysate; WBC, white blood cell exchanges; WC, whole cells.

[c] Staging: I, minimal residual disease; II, localized or regional disease; III, systemic disease.

[d] Number or percent of patients with greater than 50% reduction in tumor burden.

385

We know from autologous typing that antigens with a high degree of specificity for melanoma cells can be recognized by melanoma patients. We do not know why antibodies to these antigens are so rare in melanoma patients, despite the presence of the antigens on many melanomas. In view of the demonstrable autoimmunogenicity of certain melanoma surface components and the development of serologic methods with the requisite resolving power to monitor the specificity of humoral immune responses to melanoma surface antigens, it seemed both justified and timely to reexplore the effects of active specific immunization in melanoma patients. The two key features of these new trials are (1) the use of vaccines of defined antigenicity and (2) the monitoring of the effects of vaccine administration on the patients' serologic reactivity for their own melanoma cells. The objectives have been first to construct vaccines that are demonstrably and consistently immunogenic and then to test their therapeutic effects. At this point the first objective has been accomplished only in rare cases, so the second objective remains to be addressed.

Vaccines Prepared from Irradiated Cultured Autologous Melanoma Cells. The first type of vaccine we investigated was prepared from irradiated cultured autologous melanoma cells. The reason for emphasizing autologous vaccine in the initial study came from the restriction of Class I antigens to autologous melanoma; if such antigens are important in the immunologic control of human cancer, then autologous vaccines are a logical way to proceed. The disadvantage of this approach is that vaccinations cannot begin until sufficient numbers of autologous melanoma cells can be cultured, and this usually requires 3 to 6 months.

The initial trial involved patients with melanoma whose metastases had been removed as far as possible. The patients were given intradermal injections of autologous irradiated melanoma cells, 2 to 20 $\times$ 10^7 per injection, mixed with BCG, into sites that had been injected with BCG 1 week before. Vaccine injections were given at 3- to 4-week intervals. Of 13 patients who received five or more vaccine injections, 8 developed increased serologic reactivity against cultured autologous melanoma cells. Absorption analysis showed, however, that the antibodies were directed against Class III antigens related to the fetal calf serum in the culture medium in seven cases. In one case the titer of antibodies against a Class I antigen of autologous melanoma cells had initially declined after resection of most of the lymph node metastases in both groins and one axilla. After vaccination, reactivity increased again temporarily (Figure 1). Absorption analysis showed it to be directed against a Class II antigen shared by some other melanoma cells, but not expressed on nonmelanoma cells (Table 8). The patient is still free of recurrence, 5 years after vaccine treatment was started (34,132).

Irradiated Cultured Allogeneic Melanoma Cells. The definition of shared (Class II) melanoma antigens provides the rationale for the use of allogeneic melanoma vaccines. This approach has the advantage of being applicable to

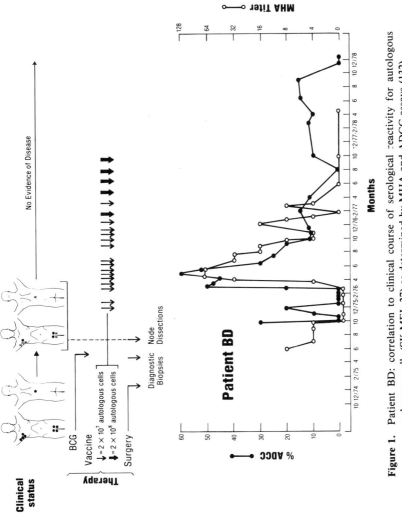

Figure 1. Patient BD: correlation to clinical course of serological reactivity for autologous melanoma cells (SK-MEL-37) as determined by MHA and ADCC assays (132).

387

TABLE 8.   Absorption of MHA Reactivity from Serum of Patient BD (7531) Tested Against Autologous Melanoma Cells (SK-MEL-37)[a]

Positive Absorption	Negative Absorption
Autologous cultured melanoma cells SK-MEL-37	Autologous cultured normal cells BD skin fibroblasts
Allogeneic cultured melanoma cells SK-MEL-13 SK-MEL-41 SK-MEL-42	Allogeneic cultured normal cells AH skin fibroblasts
	Allogeneic cultured melanoma cells SK-MEL-26 SK-MEL-27 SK-MEL-28 SK-MEL-29 SK-MEL-31 SK-MEL-40 MeWo
	Allogeneic cultured nonmelanoma cells T-24 (bladder cancer) ME-180 (cervical cancer) RAOC (ovarian cancer) Raji (Burkitt's lymphoma) MOLT-4F (lymphatic leukemia)
	Allogeneic normal cells Pooled buffy coat lymphocytes Type O, AB erythrocytes
	Xenogeneic cells Sheep erythrocytes

Source: Shiku et al. (36).

[a] Serum drawn May 1976.

patients whose autologous melanoma cells have not yet been established in culture. Another advantage to the use of allogeneic vaccines comes from the theoretical possibility (which has adequate precedent in defined immunologic systems) that foreign determinants present on the allogeneic cell surface may "help" immune recognition of tumor-specific antigens (133). In an initial trial we treated 19 patients with vaccine prepared from a cell line that had been shown to express a Class II antigenic system shared by many melanomas. Serologic analysis showed that 18 of 19 patients developed high titers of antibodies against HLA antigens of the cells in the vaccine. Only one patient developed antibodies that reacted with his own cultured melanoma cells, and these antibodies were shown to be directed against the Class II antigen expressed by the vaccine cells. Thus these early trials have demonstrated both the feasibility and the importance of determining the immunogenicity of melanoma vaccines.

As autologous or allogeneic melanoma vaccines of serologically demonstrated antigenicity induced corresponding serologic reactivity with vaccine recipients only in exceptional circumstances, consideration must be given to possible mechanisms of unresponsiveness and to ways of overcoming them.

6. POSSIBLE MECHANISMS OF IMMUNOLOGIC UNRESPONSIVENESS TO CANCER ANTIGENS

Several mechanisms are known that permit tumors to grow despite clear evidence that the host responds immunologically. They include (1) antigenic modulation, that is, temporary loss of tumor antigens in the presence of antibodies directed against them (17), (2) immunoselection, that is, a shift to cells of decreased antigenicity after elimination of the more antigenic cells by an immune reaction (134,135), and (3) blocking of antibodies or effector cells by shed antigen (136,137). While these maneuvers on the part of the tumor may play a role in the progression of human cancer, we are concerned here only with changes in host reactivity that permit the progressive growth of immunogenic tumors and with manipulations aimed at reversing these changes.

General deficiency of the immune system associated with cancer or its treatment can, of course, include a deficient immune response to cancer antigens. By all standard criteria, however, the general immunologic reactivity of our vaccine recipients was normal. There are other factors that may affect the immune response to cancer antigens in individuals with otherwise normal immunity.

Since it is now clear that immunologic reactions are under genetic control, one possibility for the lack of an immune response to tumor antigens would be the lack of immune response (Ir) genes that are required for certain kinds of tumor-specific antigen. In the mouse the influence of H-2 on susceptibility to leukemia was first suspected from the observation that the strains of mice best known for a high incidence of leukemia were $H-2^k$ and that other $H-2^k$ mice were highly susceptible to inoculation of leukemia virus (138). This association between H-2 types and susceptibility to leukemogenesis was confirmed in formal genetic studies (138). As Ir genes map in the H-2 complex (139), it possibly controls susceptibility to leukemia by affecting immune responsiveness to the antigens of the leukemia virus. Genetically determined unresponsiveness to tumor antigens need not exclude immunologic approaches to tumor control because it may overcome by appropriate modification or presentation of the relevant antigen. Although some experiments in that direction have shown promise, much work remains to be done to define the value of these approaches.

Another mechanism for the specific inhibition of a normal immune system's response to tumor antigens (tolerance) is evident from work on mammary tumors of the mouse. The great majority of these tumors are known to be caused by the mammary tumor virus, which is commonly passed from generation to generation through the milk. If the infant mice are nursed by foster mothers that are not infected with the virus, the infants do not become infected and do not develop mammary tumors. Transplantation experiments have shown that mammary tumors are far more antigenic in mice that lack the virus than in those that acquired it at birth (140). The latter apparently become immunologically tolerant to certain antigens related to the virus and the tumors it induces.

Studies of immunologic tolerance and of ways to overcome it have shown that in a variety of experimental systems T-cell unresponsiveness is more rapidly induced and more easily maintained than B-cell unresponsiveness (141,142). Levels of circulating antigen suitable for maintaining T-cell tolerance frequently fail to maintain B-cell tolerance. Consequently, antibodies can be produced to tolerated T-cell-dependent antigens. Autoimmune thyroiditis may serve as an example. It is caused by antibodies reacting with the autologous thyroglobulin (to which the animal is immunologically tolerant). These autoantibodies can be induced by injecting either chemically altered autologous thyroglobulin, or autologous thyroglobulin complexed with heterologous antibody, autologous thyroglobulin in Freund's adjuvant, or heterologous thyroglobulin. The various induction mechanisms make use of the fact that T cells, but not B cells, are tolerant of the autologous thyroglobulin. T Cells sensitized against related, but not identical, thyroglobulin serve as helper cells for B cells programmed to produce antibody against the autologous thyroglobulin (141). Autoantibodies reacting with autologous thyroglobulin are produced and thyroiditis results. Two features of the resulting disease are pertinent to our subject: (1) the autoimmunity that results is short-lived, repeated injections are required to maintain thyroiditis; and (2) injections of unaltered homologous thyroglobulins simultaneously with the altered thyroglobulin results in persistence of the tolerant state.

In recent years immunologic unresponsiveness mediated by suppressor cells has received much attention. Whereas one subset of T cells, helper T cells, plays a crucial role in activating B cells to become immunoglobulin-secreting plasma cells, another subset, suppressor T cells, has been shown to have the opposite effect. Physiologically, suppressor cells appear to terminate excessive immune reactions and to provide a safeguard against autoimmune reactions. Indeed, there is evidence that immunologic tolerance is brought about through the action of suppressor cells (143) and that impaired suppressor T-cell function can lead to autoimmune disease (144). Certain classes of B cells and macrophages may also exert a suppressor effect. In the mouse, T-cell helper and suppressor activity have been shown to be associated with the I region of the H-2 complex. The I-J subregion contains the genetic information for surface markers found on suppressor T-cells and also for determinants found on soluble suppressor factors derived from such cells (145). Accordingly, intravenous injection of alloantisera directed against I-J determinants has been found to potentiate immune responses by inhibiting suppressor cell function and even to reverse genetic nonresponsiveness to certain polymers (145,146).

Suppressor cells have also been reported to inhibit the immune response of mice to tumor antigens (147–149) causing accelerated tumor growth. Conversely, treatment with anti-I-J serum was found to retard tumor growth (150). More detailed characterization of phenotype and function of regulatory T-cell subsets is now proceeding in the mouse (151), and more recently also in humans (152). These studies are likely to provide new clues to means by which the balance of inducer and suppressor circuits can be reset favorably prior to immunization with tumor vaccines and to the most effective ways in which tumor antigens can be presented to induce a strong cytotoxic and inflammatory response. In this respect several modified melanoma cell vaccines can be envisaged on the basis of existing information.

7. MODIFIED CANCER CELL VACCINES

Modifications that may offer promise of increasing the immunogenicity of cancer cell vaccines include (1) infection with certain viruses, (2) chemical attachment of foreign determinants, (3) introduction of foreign determinants by somatic cell hybridization, and (4) isolation and purification of Class I/II antigens. The approaches to increasing immunogenicity emphasized here do not include immunologic adjuvants such as bacterial products or synthetic adjuvants; however, we do not mean to imply that these will not be useful in further augmenting the immunogenicity of tumor antigens. On the contrary, as the use of these adjuvants is covered at length in other sections of this book (Chapters 3 and 4), it need not be discussed further here.

7.1 Irradiated Cultured Autologous Melanoma Cells Infected with Vesicular Stomatitis Virus

The basis for this approach comes from the finding that the immunogenicity of tumor antigens appears to be augmented following infection of tumor cells by certain viruses, particularly myxoviruses. With the use of mice that were genetically resistant to virus lethality, total tumor destruction could be achieved by infecting tumor-bearing mice with West Nile Virus (153) or influence A (154). Survivors were then found resistant to subsequent challenge with the corresponding tumor. Subsequent work revealed that homogenates prepared from virus-infected tumors (viral oncolysates) were more effective immunogens than comparable preparations of non-infected tumor cells in terms of inducing transplantation immunity (155–157). Application of this approach to the treatment of clinical cancer is now an active area of interest.

The virus we have chosen for the preparation of viral oncolysates of melanoma cells is vesicular stomatitis virus (VSV). This choice is based primarily on the work of Boone et al. (158), who demonstrated that membrane extracts of VSV-infected melanoma cells elicited delayed hypersensitivity reactions in patients with melanoma but rarely in normal volunteers or patients with other types of cancer. Membranes from non-VSV-infected melanoma cells were virtually inactive, as were membranes from fibroblast, regardless of whether they were VSV infected. Before initiating the vaccine program with VSV oncolysates, we determined the influence of VSV infection on the expression of Class I and Class II antigens by melanoma cells, as determined by quantitative absorption analysis at various time intervals after virus infection. The details of viral infection and antigen quantitation have now been worked out, and the testing of VSV-infected melanoma vaccines in patients with melanoma has begun.

7.2   Irradiated Chemically Modified Cultured Autologous Melanoma Cells

A number of different methods have been proposed to augment the immunogenicity of tumor cells by chemical or enzymatic modification of the cell surface (159). A procedure that seems attractive for clinical testing is based on the experiments of Lachmann and Sikora with transplantable methylcholanthrene-induced tumors in syngeneic mice (160). The idea behind their approach was discussed earlier—namely, that effective recognition of tumor-specific antigens requires "helper" determinants on the cell and that these can be provided by foreign histocompatibility antigens, viral antigens, or other classes of antigens physically or chemically coupled to the cell surface. Lachmann and Sikora (160) reasoned that PPD bound to the cell surface might provide effective "help" provided that the host had a preexisting delayed hypersensitivity to BCG. Because BCG is so widely used in clinical immunotherapy testing, they felt that this approach to augmenting the immunogenicity of tumor cells might have particular clinical applicability. Although PPD could be directly coupled to the cell surface, they found it easier to do so by first attaching PPD to Con A and then allowing the Con A-PPD complex to bind to cell surface by the virtually universal Con A receptors on mammalian cells. The tumor-specific immunogenicity of sarcoma cells modified in this fashion was strikingly increased in BCG-primed mice, but not in normal controls.

Two additional forms of vaccines can be envisioned that require more developmental work before they can be applied in the clinic.

7.3   Irradiated Intraspecies or Interspecies Hybrids Expressing Class I/II Antigens Formed by Fusing Autologous Melanoma Cells with (a) Allogeneic Melanoma Cells, (b) Allogeneic B-Cell Lines, or (c) Xenogeneic Cells

Cell hybridization provides another way to introduce foreign "helper" determinants on the surface of melanoma cells (161). The development of this approach will rely on the successful adaptation of the techniques of somatic cell genetics. Our initial analysis of hybrids formed by fusing Chinese hamster ovarian cells and human melanoma cells expressing a Class I antigen has shown that this antigen is expressed constitutively in these interspecies hybrids and that the trait segregates independently of HLA and β_2 microglobulin. (L. Resnick and D. Pravtcheva, unpublished observation).

7.4 Immunogenic Forms of Isolated Class I/II Melanoma Antigens

Earlier in this chapter we referred to the development of viral vaccines as an example that should be followed in attempts at constructing cancer cell vaccines. Although potent viral vaccines have been developed that use whole attenuated viruses, vaccines containing more complex microorganisms such as pneumococci, mennigococci, or influenza bacilli have been considerably less effective than vaccines prepared from isolated capsular polysaccharides of these bacteria. It seems logical, therefore, to explore this approach also in the context of developing cancer vaccines, now that serologic reagents are at hand that permit the testing of the products of purification procedures for the presence of antigen.

One example of solubilized melanoma antigens is a Class I antigen isolated by limited papain digestion from cultured melanoma cells. Maximal yield of this antigen was obtained after very short (5- to 15-minute) digestion in contrast to the more prolonged proteolysis required for maximal release of HLA and β_2 microglobulin. The solubilized antigen showed the same highly restricted Class I specificity as did the antigen on the cell surface in inhibition tests. At least a proportion of the molecules with determinants of this antigen appear to be glycoproteins, as indicated by specific affinity for *Lens culinaris* hemagglutination (LcH). After affinity chromatography on LcH-agarose, the specific activity of the antigen was increased fiftyfold. As determined by gel filtration chromatography, the antigen has a molecular weight in the range of 20,000 to 50,000 (162). More recently, an acidic glycolipid has been isolated from another line of cultured melanoma cells (SK-MEL-13 derived from the melanoma of patient AH) that shows shared melanoma-restricted (Class II) specificity in inhibition tests with autologous serum, similar to the specificity shown by the cells themselves. The reaction patterns seen in inhibition tests with glycolipid preparations from other melanoma cells have also been similar to the patterns seen in absorption tests with the same cells (K. Lloyd and C. Pukel, unpublished observations). Our interest in glycolipid components of melanoma cells as a possible source of melanoma-restricted antigens for vaccine preparation has been further strengthened by the results of an investigation of monoclonal antibodies (43). Of the 18 mouse monoclonal antibodies described in Section 3 of this chapter, six distinct antigenic systems were defined by direct serologic assays and absorption tests by using a large panel of cell lines derived from normal and malignant tissues. Biochemical analysis indicated that two of the antigens were glycoproteins with a molecular weight of 95,000 and 150,000 (gp95 and gp150, respectively). Two other antigenic systems (O_5 and the R_{24} group) are associated with heat-stabile molecules that have the characteristics of glycolipids. The remaining two antigens (M and R) are heat labile, but further molecular characterization has not been possible.

Each antigenic system has a distinctive pattern of distribution on various cell types, varying from a broad representation to more restricted occurrence. The antigen defined by the R_{24} group of antibodies has the most restricted distribution of all. Highest reactivity is found with melanoma and astrocytoma, whereas epithelial cell types, fibroblasts and cells of hematopoietic origin, are, with rare exception, negative for antigen. Interestingly, R_{24} antigen has also been shown to be an acidic glycolipid. Occurrence of gp95, gp150, M, and R distinguished a small subset of melanomas lacking these antigens, whereas R_{24} is expressed on all melanoma cells. The antigen detected by R_{24} may well be another candidate for a glycolipid vaccine.

8. CONCLUDING REMARKS

At the present time serologic methods offer the most advanced and versatile tools to test the immunogenicity of melanoma vaccines in patients with malignant melanoma. Although there is a general impression that increased cellular rather than humoral immunity is the desired end point of immunologic manipulation in patients with cancer, we know too little at present to form a judgment about this matter. Although considerable progress has been made in the area of cellular immunity, further understanding of the conditions required for analyzing cellular immune reactions *in vitro* is needed before these methods can be applied productively to the analysis of immunity induced by melanoma vaccines. We have completed the first substantial study of lymphocyte cytotoxicity restricted to autologous lymphocyte-target cell combinations (163). Apart from eliminating reactions due to alloantigens, the testing of autologous effector cell-target combinations is clearly required for the detection of individually distinct antigens and may be required for the detection of all pertinent antigens if HLA restriction applies to cell-mediated cytotoxicity of human cancers (164,165). Our results indicate that the specificity of observed reactions cannot be determined by direct tests alone. Indirect methods such as cold target cell inhibition and immunoadsorption require further technical improvement. The severe constraints imposed by the limited number of effector cells that are available for such tests may be overcome by expanding them in cultures supplemented with T-cell growth factor, but here again further methodologic refinement is required. At present, serologic techniques are clearly most precise and thus most incisive.

There has been considerable discussion about the possibility that raising the level of humoral immunity to melanoma cells may result in augmented rather than restricted tumor growth; the precedent for this is the well-known phenomenon of immunologic enhancement seen with some experimental allogeneic tumors (166,167). However, antibody-mediated immunologic enhancement has never been convincingly demonstrated with strictly syngeneic or autologous tumors in animal systems, and these are the systems most applicable to the clinical setting.

It has been repeatedly shown in experimental animals and in human patients (168,169) with growing transplanted allogeneic tumors that the immune system is capable of destroying large tumor masses. As it appears that tumor-specific antigens in animals and humans are poorly immunogenic, emphasis must be placed on augmenting their immunogenicity. The ability of experimental animals to mount strong reactions against poor immunogens or normal auto-antigens following vaccination with relevant antigens in association with appropriate adjuvants or modified by "helper" determinants, argues strongly that this approach is feasible.

REFERENCES

1. L. Gross, Intradermal immunization of C3H mice against a sarcoma that originated in an animal of the same line. *Cancer Res., 3*, 326 (1943).

2. E. J. Foley, Antigenic properties of methylcholanthrene-induced tumors in mice of the strain of origin. *Cancer Res., 13*, 835 (1953).

3. R. T. Prehn and J. M. Main, Immunity to methylcholanthrene-induced sarcomas. *J. Natl. Cancer Inst., 18*, 759 (1957).

4. G. Klein, H. O. Sjögren, E. Klein, and K. E. Hellström, Demonstration of resistance against methylcholanthrene-induced sarcomas in the primary autochthonous host. *Cancer Res., 20*, 1561 (1960).

5. E. A. Boyse, Immune responses to experimental tumours. *Guy Hosp. Rep., 112*, 433 (1963).

6. Z. B. Mikulska, C. Smith, and P. Alexander, Evidence for an immunological reaction of the host directed against its own actively growing primary tumor. *J. Natl. Cancer Inst., 36*, 29 (1966).

7. A. B. DeLeo, H. Shiku, T. Takahashi, M. John, and L. J. Old, Cell surface antigens of chemically induced sarcomas of the mouse. *J. Exp. Med., 146*, 720 (1977).

8. A. B. DeLeo, H. Shiku, T. Takahashi, and L. J. Old, Serological definition of cell surface antigens of chemically induced sarcomas of inbred mice. In R. W. Ruddon, Ed., *Biological Markers of Neoplasia: Basic and Applied Aspects,* Elsevier/North-Holland, New York, 1978, p. 25.

9. K. Habel, Resistance of polyoma virus immune animals to transplanted polyoma tumors. *Proc. Soc. Exp. Biol. Med., 106*, 722 (1961).

10. H. O. Sjögren, I. Hellström, and G. Klein, Resistance of polyoma virus immunized mice to transplantation of established polyoma tumors. *Exp. Cell Res., 23*, 204 (1961).

11. D. L. Morton, G. F. Miller, and D. A. Wood, Demonstration of tumor-specific immunity against antigens unrelated to the mammary tumor virus in spontaneous mammary adeno-carcinomas. *J. Natl. Cancer Inst., 42*, 289 (1969).

12. S. Gillis and K. A. Smith, Long term culture of tumour-specific cytotoxic T cells. *Nature, 268*, 154 (1976).

13. G. Kohler and C. Milstein, Continuous cultures of fused cells secreting antibody of pre-defined specificity. *Nature, 256*, 495 (1975).

14. L. J. Old and E. A. Boyse, Current enigmas in cancer research. *Harvey Lect., 67*, 273 (1973).

15. L. J. Old and E. Stockert, Immunogenetics of cell surface antigens of mouse leukemia. *Ann. Rev. Genet., 11*, 127 (1977).

16. E. A. Boyse and L. J. Old, Immunogenetics of differentiation in the mouse. *Harvey Lect., 71*, 23 (1978).

17. L. J. Old, E. A. Boyse, and E. Stockert, Antigenic properties of experimental leukemias. I. Serological studies *in vitro* with spontaneous and radiation-induced leukemias. *J. Natl. Cancer Inst.,* **31,** 977 (1963).

18. L. J. Old and E. Stockert, Serological definition of cell surface antigens of mouse leukemias. In H. C. Morse, III, Ed., *Origins of Inbred Mice,* Academic, New York, 1978, p. 391.

19. F. Jacob, Mouse teratocarcinoma and embryonic antigens. *Immunol. Rev.,* **33,** 3 (1977).

20. L. Gross, "Spontaneous" leukemia developing in C3H mice following inoculation in infancy with AK leukemic extracts or AK embryos. *Proc. Soc. Exp. Biol. Med.,* **76,** 27 (1951).

21. H. Rubin, L. Fanshier, A. Cornelius, and W. F. Hughes, Tolerance and immunity in chickens after congenital and contact infection with an avian leukosis virus. *Virology,* **17,** 143 (1962).

22. W. D. Hardy, Jr., G. Geering, L. J. Old, and E. de Harven, Feline leukemia virus: Occurrence of viral antigen in the tissues of cats with lymphosarcoma and other diseases. *Science,* **166,** 1019 (1969).

23. P. S. Sarma, J. D. Baskar, R. J. Huebner, L. J. Old, and W. D. Hardy, Jr., Detection of group specific viral antigens and infectious virus by complement fixation test. In R. M. Dutcher, Ed., *Comparative Leukemia Research 1969,* Karger, Basel, 1970, p. 368.

24. M. A. Fink, L. E. Sibal, and E. J. Plata, Serologic detection of feline leukemia virus antigens or antibodies. *J. Am. Vet. Med. Assoc.,* **158,** 1070 (1971).

25. W. D. Hardy, Jr., Y. Hirshaut, and P. W. Hess, Detection of the feline leukemia virus and other mammalian oncornaviruses by immunofluorescence. In R. M. Dutcher and L. Chieco-Bianchi, Eds., *Unifying Concepts of Leukemia,* Karger, Basel, 1973, p. 778.

26. W. D. Hardy, Jr., L. J. Old, P. W. Hess, M. Essex, and S. Cotter, Horizontal transmission of feline leukaemia virus. *Nature,* **244,** 266 (1973).

27. W. D. Hardy, Jr., A. J. McClelland, E. E. Zuckerman, P. W. Hess, M. Essex, S. Cotter, E. G. MacEwen, and A. A. Hayes, Prevention of the contagious spread of feline leukaemia virus and the development of leukaemia in pet cats. *Nature,* **263,** 326 (1976).

28. M. Essex, G. Klein, S. P. Snyder, and J. B. Harrold, Feline sarcoma virus (FSV)-induced tumors: Correlation between humoral antibody and tumor regression. *Nature,* **233,** 195 (1971).

29. W. D. Hardy, Jr., P. W. Hess, E. G. MacEwen, A. J. McClelland, E. E. Zuckerman, M. Essex, S. M. Cotter, and O. Jarrett, The biology of feline leukemia virus in the natural environment. *Cancer Res.,* **36,** 582 (1976).

30. M. Essex, R. M. Jakowski, W. D. Hardy, Jr., S. M. Cotter, P. W. Hess, and A. Sliski, Feline oncornavirus-associated cell membrane antigen. III. Antibody titers in cats from leukemia cluster households. *J. Natl. Cancer Inst.,* **54,** 637 (1975).

31. W. D. Hardy, Jr., E. E. Zuckerman, E. G. MacEwen, A. A. Hayes, and M. Essex, A feline leukaemia virus and sarcoma virus-induced tumour-specific antigen. *Nature,* **270,** 249 (1977).

32. H. B. Hewitt, E. R. Blake, and A. S. Walder, A critique of the evidence for active host defense against cancer, based on personal studies of 27 murine tumours of spontaneous origin. *Br. J. Cancer,* **33,** 241 (1976).

33. T. E. Carey, T. Takahashi, L. A. Resnick, H. F. Oettgen, and L. J. Old, Cell surface antigens of human malignant melanoma. I. Mixed hemadsorption assays for humoral immunity to cultured autologous melanoma cells. *Proc. Natl. Acad. Sci. (USA),* **73,** 3278 (1976).

34. H. Shiku, T. Takahashi, H. F. Oettgen, and L. J. Old, Cell surface antigens of human malignant melanoma. II. Serological typing with immune adherence assays and definition of two new surface antigens. *J. Exp. Med.,* **144,** 873 (1976).

35. H. Shiku, T. Takahashi, L. A. Resnick, H. F. Oettgen, and L. J. Old, Cell surface antigens of human malignant melanoma. III. Recognition of autoantibodies with unusual characteristics. *J. Exp. Med.,* **145**, 784 (1977).

36. H. Shiku, T. Takahashi, T. E. Carey, L. A. Resnick, H. F. Oettgen, and L. J. Old, Cell surface antigens of human cancer. In R. W. Ruddon, Ed., *Biological Markers of Neoplasia: Basic and Applied Aspects,* Elsevier/North-Holland, New York, 1978, p. 73.

37. R. Ueda, H. Shiku, M. Pfreundschuh, T. Takahashi, L. T. C. Li, W. F. Whitmore, H. F. Oettgen, and L. J. Old, Cell surface antigens of human renal cancer defined by autologous typing. *J. Exp. Med.,* **150**, 564 (1979).

38. M. Pfreundschuh, H. Shiku, T. Takahashi, R. Ueda, J. Ransohoff, H. F. Oettgen, and L. J. Old, Serological analysis of cell surface antigens of malignant human brain tumors. *Proc. Natl. Acad. Sci. (USA),* **75**, 5122 (1978).

39. A. N. Houghton, M. C. Taormina, H. Ikeda, T. Watanabe, H. F. Oettgen, and L. J. Old, Serological survey of normal humans for natural antibody to cell surface antigens of melanoma. *Proc. Natl. Acad. Sci. (USA),* **77**, 4260 (1980).

40. H. Koprowski, Z. Steplewski, D. Herlyn, and M. Herlyn, Study of antibodies against human melanoma produced by somatic cell hybrids. *Proc. Natl. Acad. Sci. (USA),* **75**, 3405 (1978).

41. M.-Y. Yeh, I. Hellström, J. P. Brown, G. A. Warner, J. A. Hansen, and K. E. Hellström, Cell surface antigens of human melanoma identified by monoclonal antibody. *Proc. Natl. Acad. Sci. (USA),* **76**, 2927 (1979).

42. R. C. Woodbury, J. P. Brown, M.-Y. Yeh, I. Hellström, and K. E. Hellström, Identification of cell surface protein, p97, in human melanomas and certain other neoplasms. *Proc. Natl. Acad. Sci. (USA),* **77**, 2183 (1980).

43. W. G. Dippold, K. O., Lloyd, L. T. C. Li, H. Ikeda, H. F. Oettgen, and L. J. Old, Cell surface antigens of human malignant melanoma: Definition of six new antigenic systems with mouse monoclonal antibodies. *Proc. Natl. Acad. Sci. (USA),* **77**, 6114 (1980).

44. R. W. Baldwin, M. V. Pimm, and R. A. Robins, Active specific immunotherapy: Experimental Studies. In *Proceedings of the Twelfth International Cancer Congress,* Vol. 6, UICC, Talleres Graficos, Buenos Aires, 1978, p. 67.

45. R. Bomford, Active specific immunotherapy of mouse methylcholanthrene-induced tumours with *Corynebacterium parvum* and irradiated tumour cells. *Br. J. Cancer,* **32**, 551 (1975).

46. G. L. Bartlett, J. W. Kreider, and D. M. Purnell, Active specific immunotherapy of murine leukemia. I. Irradiated tumor cell vaccine. *Internatl. J. Cancer,* **24**, 629 (1979).

47. A. Rios and R. L. Simmons, Experimental cancer immunotherapy using a neuraminidase-treated non-viable frozen tumor vaccine. *Surgery,* **75**, 503 (1974).

48. B. Zbar, I. Bernstein, G. L. Bartlett, and H. J. Rapp, Immunotherapy of cancer regression of intradermal tumors and prevention of growth of lymph node metastases after intralesional injection of living *Mycobacterium bovis* (BCG). *J. Natl. Cancer Inst.,* **49**, 119 (1972).

49. B. Zbar, G. Canti, M. P. Ashley, H. J. Rapp, J. T. Hunter, and E. Ribi, Eradication by immunization with mycobacterial vaccines and tumor cells of microscopic metastases remaining after surgery. *Cancer Res.,* **39**, 1597 (1979).

50. L. C. Peters, J. S. Brandhorst, and M. G. Hanna, Jr., Preparation of immunotherapeutic autologous tumor cell vaccines from solid tumors. *Cancer Res.,* **39**, 1353 (1979).

51. S. J. Kleinschuster, H. J. Rapp, D. C. Lueker, and R. A. Kainer, Regression of bovine ocular carcinoma by treatment with mycobacterial vaccine. *J. Natl. Cancer Inst.,* **58**, 1807 (1977).

52. H. H. Sedlacek, M. Weise, A. Lemmer, and F. R. Seiler, Immunotherapy of spontaneous mammary tumors in mongrel dogs with autologous tumor cells and neuraminidase. *Cancer Immunol. Immunother.,* **6,** 47 (1979).

53. H. Boreberg, H. F. Oettgen, K. Choudry, and E. J. Beattie, Jr., Inhibition of established transplants of chemically induced sarcomas in syngeneic mice by lymphocytes from immunized donors. *Internatl. J. Cancer,* **10,** 539 (1972).

54. E. Klein, Tumours of the skin. X. Immunotherapy of cutaneous and mucosal neoplasms. *N. Y. State J. Med.,* **68,** 900 (1968).

55. D. L. Morton, F. R. Eilber, E. C. Holmes, J. S. Hunt, A. S. Ketcham, J. J. Silverstein, and F. C. Sparks, BCG immunotherapy of malignant melanoma; Summary of a seven-year experience. *Ann. Surg.,* **130,** 635 (1974).

56. C. M. Pinsky, Y. Hirshaut, and H. F. Oettgen, Treatment of malignant melanoma by intratumoral injection of BCG. *Natl. Cancer Inst. Monogr.,* **39,** 225 (1973).

57. M. J. Mastrangelo, D. Berd, and R. E. Bellet, Critical review of previously reported clinical trials of cancer immunotherapy with nonspecific immunostimulants. *Ann. N. Y. Acad. Sci.,* **277,** 94 (1976).

58. S. E. Krown, E. Y. Hilal, C. M. Pinsky, Y. Hirshaut, H. J. Wanebo, J. A. Hansen, A. G. Huvos, and H. F. Oettgen, Intralesional injection of the methanol extraction residue of *Bacillus Calmette-Guerin* (MER) into cutaneous metastases of malignant melanoma. *Cancer,* **42,** 2648 (1978).

59. M. H. Cohen, J. Jessup, F. Milburn, J. E. Felix, J. L. Weese, and R. B. Herberman, Intralesional treatment of recurrent metastatic cutaneous malignant melanoma: A randomized prospective study of intralesional *Bacillus Calmette-Guerin vs.* intralesional dinitrochlorobenzene. *Cancer,* **41,** 2456 (1978).

60. M. H. Cohen, E. Felix, J. Jessup, and S. Rosenberg, Treatment of metastatic melanoma by intralesional injection of BCG, organic chemicals and *C. parvum.* In R. G. Crispen, Ed., *Neoplasm Immunity: Mechanisms* (Proceedings of a Chicago Symposium), ITR Press, Chicago, 1975, p. 121.

61. A. Morales and A. Ersil, Prophylaxis of recurrent bladder cancer with *Bacillus Calmette-Guerin.* In D. E. Johnson and M. L. Samuels, Eds., *Cancer of the Genito-Urinary Tract,* Raven, New York, 1979, p. 121.

62. C. M. Pinsky, F. J. Camacho, D. Kerr, D. Braun, Jr., W. F. Whitmore, Jr., and H. F. Oettgen, Treatment of superficial bladder cancer with intravesical *Bacillus Calmette-Guerin* (BCG). In W. D. Terry and S. A. Rosenberg, Eds., *Immunotherapy of Cancer: Present Status of Trials in Man* (in press).

63. D. L. Lamm, V. D. Stogdill, and D. E. Thor, BCG immunotherapy in superficial transitional cell carcinoma of the urinary bladder. *Proc. Am. Soc. Clin. Oncol.,* **21,** 372 (1980).

64. R. L. Ikonopisov, M. G. Lewis, I. D. Hunter-Craig, D. C. Bodenham, T. M. Phillips, C. I. Cooling, J. Proctor, and G. Hamilton-Fairley, Autoimmunization with irradiated tumor cells in human malignant melanoma. *Br. Med. J.,* **2,** 752 (1972).

65. H. F. Seigler, W. W. Shingleton, R. S. Metzgar, C. E. Buckley, and P. M. Bergoc, Immunotherapy in patients with melanoma. *Ann. Surg.,* **178,** 352 (1973).

66. H. F. Seigler, C. E. Buckley, L. B. Sheppard, B. J. Horne, and W. W. Shingleton, Adoptive transfer and specific active immunization of patients with malignant melanoma. *Ann. N. Y. Acad. Sci.,* **277,** 522 (1976).

67. H. F. Seigler, E. Cox, F. Mutzner, L. Shepherd, E. Nicholson, and W. W. Shingleton, Specific active immunotherapy for melanoma. *Ann. Surg.,* **190,** 366 (1979).

68. J. F. Laucius, A. J. Bodurtha, M. J. Mastrangelo, and R. E. Bellet, A Phase II study of autologous irradiated tumor cells plus BCG in patients with metastatic malignant melanoma. *Cancer,* **40,** 2091 (1977).

69. M. B. McIllmurray, M. J. Embleton, W. G. Reeves, M. J. S. Langman, and M. Deane, Controlled trial of active immunotherapy in management of Stage IIB malignant melanoma. *Br. Med. J.,* **1**, 540 (1977).

70. P. B. McCulloch, P. B. Dent, M. Blajchman, W. M. Muirhead, and R. A. Price, Recurrent malignant melanoma: Effect of adjuvant immunotherapy on survival. *Can. Med. Assoc. J.,* **117**, 33 (1977).

71. G. A. Currie, F. Lejeune, and G. Hamilton-Fairley, Immunization with irradiated tumour cells and specific lymphocyte cytotoxicity in malignant melanoma. *Br. Med. J.,* **2**, 305 (1971).

72. G. A. Currie, Effect of autoimmunization with irradiated tumour cells on specific cell-mediated immunity in patients with malignant melanoma. *Proc. Roy. Soc.,* **65**, 144 (1972).

73. G. V. Aranha, C. F. McKhann, T. B. Grage, A. Gunnarsson, and R. L. Simmons, Adjuvant immunotherapy of malignant melanoma. *Cancer,* **43**, 1297 (1979).

74. F. G. Gercovich, J. U. Gutterman, G. M. Mavligit, and E. M. Hersh, Active specific immunization in malignant melanoma. *Med. Pediatr. Oncol.,* **1**, 277 (1975).

75. E. T. Krementz, M. S. Samuels, and J. H. Wallace, Clinical experience in the immunotherapy of cancer. *Surg. Gynecol. Obstet.,* **133**, 209 (1971).

76. W. H. McCarthy, G. Cotton, A. Carlon, G. W. Milton, and S. Kossard, Immunotherapy of malignant melanoma—A clinical trial. *Cancer,* **32**, 97 (1973).

77. D. Murray, W. Cassel, A. Torbin, Z. Olkowski, and M. Moon, Viral oncolysate in the management of malignant melanoma. *Cancer,* **40**, 680 (1977).

78. W. A. Cassel, D. R. Murray, A. H. Torbin, Z. L. Olkowski, and M. E. Moore, Viral oncolysate in the management of malignant melanoma—Preparation of the oncolysate and measurement of immunologic responses. *Cancer,* **40**, 672 (1977).

79. H. R. Shibata, L. M. Jerry, M. G. Lewis, P. W. Mansell, A. Capek, and G. Marquis, Immunotherapy of human malignant melanoma with irradiated tumor cells. Oral *Bacillus Calmette-Guerin* and levamisole. *Ann. N. Y. Acad. Sci.,* **277**, 335 (1976).

80. E. S. Newlands, C. J. Oon, J. T. Roberts, P. Elliott, R. F. Mould, C. Topham, F. J. Madden, K. A. Newton, and G. Westbury, Clinical trial of combination chemotherapy and specific active immunotherapy in disseminated melanoma. *Br. J. Cancer,* **34**, 174 (1976).

81. D. L. Morton, F. R. Eilber, E. C. Holmes, C. M. Townsend, Jr., J. Mirra, and T. H. Weisenburger, Adjuvant therapy in melanoma and sarcomas. In S. E. Salmon and S. E. Jones, Eds., *Adjuvant Therapy of Cancer,* Elsevier/North-Holland, Amsterdam, 1977, p. 391.

82. R. F. Irie, A. E. Glullano, and D. L. Morton, Oncofetal antigen: A tumor-associated fetal antigen immunogenic in man. *J. Natl. Cancer Inst.,* **63**, 367 (1979).

83. M. J. Mastrangelo, R. E. Bellet, and D. Berd, A Phase III comparison of methyl-CCNU + vincristine with or without BCG + allogeneic tumor cells in metastatic melanoma. *Cancer Immunol. Immunother.,* **6**, 231 (1979).

84. D. W. Hedley, T. J. McElwain, and G. A. Currie, Tumour regression and survival of patients with disseminated malignant melanoma treated with chemotherapy and specific active immunotherapy. *Eur. J. Cancer,* **13**, 1169 (1977).

85. D. W. Hedley, T. J. McElwain, and G. A. Currie, Specific active immunotherapy does not prolong survival in surgically treated patients with Stage IIB malignant melanoma and may promote early recurrence. *Br. J. Cancer,* **37**, 491 (1978).

86. W. R. Jewell, J. H. Thomas, P. Morse, and L. J. Humphrey, Comparison of allogeneic tumor vaccine with leukocyte transfer and transfer factor treatment of human cancer. *Ann. N. Y. Acad. Sci.,* **277**, 516 (1976).

87. L. J. Humphrey, B. Boehm, W. R. Jewell, and R. O. Boehm, Immunologic response of cancer patients modified by immunization with tumor vaccine. *Ann. Surg.,* **176**, 554 (1972).

88. J. G. Sinkovics, Immunotherapy with viral oncolysates for sarcoma. *J. Am. Med. Assoc.,* **237**, 869 (1977).

89. M. J. McMurtrey, L. T. Campos, J. G. Sinkovics, J. J. Romero, K. K. Loh, and M. M. Romsdahl, Chemoimmunotherapy for melanoma: Preliminary clinical data and difficulties with *in vitro* monitoring of tumor-specific immune reactions. In M. D. Anderson Hospital and Tumor Institute, Ed., *Neoplasms of the Skin and Malignant Melanoma,* Yearbook Medical Publishers, Chicago, 1976, p. 471.

90. M. Arlen, A. Hollinshead, and F. Scherrer, Tumor-specific immunity in patients with malignant melanoma. *Surg. Forum,* **28**, 168 (1977).

91. F. R. Gerner and G. E. Moore, Feasibility study of immunotherapy in patients with solid tumors. *Cancer,* **38**, 131 (1976).

92. F. R. Eilber and D. L. Morton, Immunologic and immunotherapeutic studies with human sarcomas. *Surg. Forum,* **21**, 127 (1970).

93. F. R. Eilber, C. Townsend, and D. L. Morton, Osteosarcoma. Results of treatment employing adjuvant immunotherapy. *Clin. Orthop.,* **111**, 94 (1975).

94. A. A. Green, C. Pratt, R. G. Webster, and K. Smith, Immunotherapy of osteosarcoma patients with virus-modified tumor cells. *Ann. N. Y. Acad. Sci.,* **277**, 396 (1976).

95. J. G. Sinkovics, L. T. Campos, K. K. Loh, F. Cormia, W. Velasquez, and C. C. Shullenberger, Chemoimmunotherapy for three categories of solid tumors (sarcoma, melanoma, lymphoma): The problem of immunoresistant tumors. In R. G. Cripsen, Ed., *Neoplasm Immunity: Mechanisms* (Proceedings of a Chicago Symposium), ITR Press, Chicago, 1975, p. 193.

96. C. M. Townsend, Jr., F. R. Eilber, and D. L. Morton, Skeletal and soft tissue sarcomas: Treatment with adjuvant immunotherapy. *J. Am. Med. Assoc.,* **236**, 2187 (1976).

97. J. R. Neff and W. F. Enneking, Adoptive immunotherapy in primary osteosarcoma, *J. Bone Joint Surg.,* **57**, 145 (1975).

98. R. C. Marcove, C. M. Southam, A. Levin, V. Miké, and A. Huvos, A clinical trial of autogenous vaccine in osteogenic sarcoma in patients under the age of twenty-five. *Surg. Forum,* **22**, 434 (1971).

99. J. E. Sokal and C. W. Aungst, Immunotherapy with cultured human cells and BCG. *Transplant. Proc.,* **7**, 317 (1975).

100. T. H. Stewart, A. C. Hollinshead, J. E. Harris, S. Raman, R. Belanger, A. Crepeau, A. F. Crook, W. E. Hirte, D. Hooper, D. J. Klaasen, E. F. Rapp, and H. J. Sachs, Specific active immunochemotherapy in lung cancer: A survival study. *Can. J. Surg.,* **20**, 370 (1977).

101. G. Alth, H. Denck, M. Fischer, K. Karrer, O. Kokron, E. Korizek, M. Micksche, E. Ogris, C. Reider, R. Titscher, and H. Wrba, Aspects of the immunologic treatment of lung cancer. *Cancer Chemo. Rep.,* **3**, 271 (1973).

102. H. Takita, M. Takada, J. Minowada, T. Han and F. Edgerton, Adjuvant immunotherapy of Stage III lung carcinoma. In W. D. Terry and D. Windhorst, Eds., *Immunotherapy of Cancer: Present Status of Trials in Man,* Raven, New York, 1978, p. 217.

103. C. M. Southam, Present status of oncolytic virus studies, *Transact. N. Y. Acad. Sci.,* **22**, 657 (1960).

104. D. H. Pardridge, F. C. Sparks, J. E. Goodnight, I. K. Spears, and D. L. Morton, Chemoimmunotherapy of Stage III breast carcinoma with BCG and a live allogeneic tumor cell vaccine. *Cancer Immunol. Immunother.,* **5**, 217 (1979).

105. F. C. Sparks, A. Wile, K. P. Ramming, H. K. Silver, R. W. Wolk, and D. L. Morton, Immunology and adjuvant chemoimmunotherapy of breast cancer. *Arch. Surg.,* **3**, 1057 (1976).

106. J. M. Anderson, F. Kelly, S. E. Wood, K. D. Rodger, and R. I. Freshney, Evaluation of leukocyte functions six years after tumour autograft in human mammary cancer. *Br. J. Cancer,* **28**, 83 (1973).

107. J. M. Anderson, F. Kelly, G. Gettinby, and S. E. Wood, Prolonged survival after immuno-therapy (irradiated cancer autografts) for mammary cancers, assessed by a measure of therapeutic deficiency. *Cancer,* **40**, 30 (1977).

108. J. M. Anderson, F. Kelly, S. E. Wood, and D. E. Halnan, Stimulatory immunotherapy in mammary cancer. *Br. J. Surg.,* **61**, 778 (1974).

109. S. G. Taylor, D. E. Bytell, G. A. Sisson, S. Nisius, and W. D. Dewys, Methotrexate-leu-covorin with immunotherapy as adjuvant to surgery and radiotherapy in Stage III-IV head and neck squamous cancer patients. In S. E. Salmon and S. E. Jones, Eds., *Adjuvant Therapy of Cancer,* Elsevier/North-Holland, Amsterdam, 1977 p. 457.

110. T. J. Cunningham, R. Antemann, D. Paonessa, R. W. Sponzo, and T. Steiner, Adjuvant immuno- and/or chemotherapy with neuraminidase-treated autogenous tumor vaccine and *Bacillus Calmette-Guerin* for head and neck cancers, *Ann. N. Y. Acad. Sci.,* **277**, 339 (1976).

111. W. O. Griffen, Jr. and W. R. Meeker, Colon carcinoma and immunologic phenomena, *Surg. Clin. North Am.,* **52**, 839 (1972).

112. C. N. Hudson, J. E. McHardy, O. M. Curling, P. E. English, L. Levin, T. A. Poulton, M. Crowther, and M. Leighton. Active specific immunotherapy for ovarian cancer. *Lancet,* **2**, 877 (1976).

113. J. J. G. Bloom, M. J. Peckham, A. E. Richardson, P. A. Alexander, and P. M. Payne, Glioblastoma multiforme: A controlled trial to assess the value of specific active immuno-therapy in patients treated by radical surgery and radiotherapy. *Br. J. Cancer,* **27**, 253 (1973).

114. T. Tallberg, H. Tykka, M. K. Halttunen, H. Uusitalo, O. Carlson, B. Sandstedt, K. Ora-visto, T. Lehtonen, S. Sarna, and H. Strandstrom, Cancer immunity. The effect in cancer immunotherapy of polymerised autologous tumour tissue and supportive measures. *Scand. J. Clin. Lab. Invest.,* **39**, 1 (1979).

115. M. K. Wallack, Vaccinia virus-augmented tumor vaccines as a new form of immunother-apy. *GANN Monogr. Cancer Res.,* **23** (1979).

116. J. B. Graham and R. M. Graham, Autogenous vaccine in cancer patients. *Surg. Gynecol. Obstet.,* **114**, 1 (1962).

117. G. Taylor and J. L. Odili, Histological evidence of tumour rejection after active immuno-therapy in human malignant disease. *Br. Med. J.,* **2**, 183 (1972).

118. F. E. Rosato, Active specific immunotherapy of human solid tumors. *Ann. N. Y. Acad. Sci.,* **277**, 332 (1976).

119. L. E. Hughes, R. Kearney, and M. Tully, A study in clinical cancer immunotherapy. *Can-cer,* **26**, 269 (1970).

120. E. E. Miller, A. S. Brown, J. L. Johnson, A. Moskovitz, M. K. Wallack, E. F. Rosato, and F. E. Rosato, Neuraminidase immunotherapy: Serum potentiation of lymphocyte cy-totoxicity related to immunoglobulin levels. *J. Surg. Oncol.,* **8**, 351 (1976).

121. M. Aswaq, V. Richards, and S. McFadden, Immunologic response to autologous cancer vaccine. *Arch. Surg.,* **89**, 485 (1964).

122. N. P. Czajkowski, M. Rosenblatt, P. L. Wolf, and J. Vasquez, A new method of active immunization to autologous human tumour tissue. *Lancet,* **2**, 905 (1967).

123. G. J. F. Juillard, P. J. J. Boyer, and C. H. Yamashiro, A Phase I study of active specific intralymphatic immunotherapy (ASILI). *Cancer,* **41**, 2215 (1978).

124. S. H. Nadler and G. E. Moore, Immunotherapy of malignant disease. *Arch. Surg.,* **99**, 376 (1969).

125. M. Brodie and W. H. Park, Active immunization against poliomyelitis. *Am. J. Pub. Health,* **26**, 119 (1936).

126. J. A. Kolmer, Vaccination against acute anterior poliomyelitis. *Am. J. Pub. Health,* **26**, 126 (1936).

127. J. F. Edners, T. H. Weller, and F. C. Robbins, Cultivation of the Lansing strain of poliomyelitis virus in cultures of various human embryonic tissues. *Science,* **109**, 85 (1949).

128. W. M. Smith, V. C. Chambers, and C. A. Evans, Growth of neutrotropic viruses in extraneural tissues: Preliminary report on propagation of poliomyelitis virus (Lansing and Hof strains) in cultures of human testicular tissue. *Northwest Med.,* **49**, 368 (1950).

129. D. Bodian, J. F. Kessel, and C. Pait, Differentiation of three groups of poliomyelitis virus. *Proc. Soc. Exp. Biol. Med.,* **70**, 315 (1949).

130. J. E. Salk, B. L. Bennett, L. Lewis, E. N. Ward, and J. S. Youngner, Studies in human subjects on active immunization against poliomyelitis: A preliminary report of experiments in progress. *J. Am. Med. Assoc.,* **151**, 1081 (1949).

131. J. E. Salk, Vaccination against paralytic poliomyelitis—Performance and prospects. *Am. J. Pub. Health,* **45**, 575 (1955).

132. P. O. Livingston, H. Shiku, R. Michitsch, H. F. Oettgen, and L. J. Old, Antibody-dependent cell-mediated cytotoxicity for autologous melanoma. *Cellular Immunology,* **64**, 131 (1981).

133. N. A. Mitchison, Immunologic approach to cancer. *Transplant. Proc.,* **2**, 92 (1970).

134. E. M. Fenyö, E. Klein, G. Klein, and K. Sweich, Selection of an immunoresistant Moloney lymphoma subline with decreased concentration of tumor-specific surface antigens. *J. Natl. Cancer Inst.,* **40**, 69 (1968).

135. M. V. Pimm and R. W. Baldwin, Antigenic differences between primary methylcholanthrene-induced rat sarcomas and post surgical recurrences. *Internatl. J. Cancer,* **20**, 37 (1977).

136. K. E. Hellström, I. Hellström, and J. T. Nepom, Specific blocking factors—Are they important? *Biophys. Biochem. Acta,* **473**, 121–148 (1977).

137. S. Bansal and H. O. Sjögren, Correlation between changes in antitumor immune parameters and tumor growth *in vivo* in rats. *Fed. Proc.,* **32**, 165 (1973).

138. F. Lilly, E. A. Boyse, and L. J. Old, Genetic basis for susceptibility to viral leukaemogenesis. *Lancet,* **2**, 1207 (1964).

139. H. O. McDevitt and B. Benacerraf, Genetic control of specific immune responses. *Adv. Immunol.,* **11**, 31 (1969).

140. J. F. Miller, R. C. Ting, and L. W. Law, Influence of thymectomy on tumor induction by polyoma virus in C57BL mice. *Proc. Soc. Exp. Biol. Med.,* **116**, 323 (1964).

141. O. W. Weigle, Cellular events in experimental autoimmune thyroiditis, allergic encephalomyelitis and tolerance to self. In N. Talal, Ed., *Autoimmunity: Genetic, Immunologic, Virologic and Clinical Aspects,* Academic, New York, 1977, p. 141.

142. A. C. Allison, Autoimmune diseases: Concepts of pathogenesis and control. In N. Talal, Ed., *Autoimmunity: Genetic, Immunologic, Virologic and Clinical Aspects,* Academic, New York, 1977, p. 91.

143. T. A. Waldmann and S. Broder, Suppressor cells in the regulation of the immune response. *Prog. Clin. Immunol.,* **3**, 155 (1977).

144. A. C. Allison, A. M. Denman, and R. D. Barnes, Cooperating and controlling functions of thymus-derived lymphocytes in relation to autoimmunity. *Lancet,* **2**, (1971).

145. B. Benacerraf and R. N. Germain, The immune response genes of the major histocompatibility complex. *Immunol. Rev.,* **38**, 70 (1978).

146. M. Pierres, R. N. Germain, M. E. Dorf, and B. Benacerraf, *In vivo* effects of anti-Ia alloantisera. I. Elimination of specific suppression by *in vivo* administration of antisera specific for I-J controlled determinants. *J. Exp. Med.,* **147**, 656 (1978).

147. S. Fujimoto, M. Greene, and A. H. Sehon, Regulation of the immune response to tumor antigens. I. Immunosuppressor cells in tumor-bearing hosts. *J. Immunol.,* **116**, 791 (1976).

148. S. Fujimoto, M. Greene, and A. H. Sehon, Regulation of the immune response to tumor antigens. II. The nature of immunosuppressor cells in tumor-bearing hosts. *J. Immunol.,* **116**, 800 (1976).

149. M. I. Greene, S. Fujimoto, and A. H. Sehon, Regulation of the immune response to tumor antigens. III. Characterization of thymic suppressor factor(s) produced by tumor-bearing hosts. *J. Immunol.,* **119**, 757 (1977).

150. M. I. Greene, M. E. Dorf, M. Pierres, and B. Benacerraf, Reduction of syngeneic tumor growth by an anti-I-J alloantiserum. *Proc. Natl. Acad. Sci. (USA),* **74**, 5118 (1977).

151. H. Cantor, Control of the immune system by inhibitor and inducer T lymphocytes. *Ann. Rev. Med.,* **30**, 169 (1979).

152. E. L. Reinherz and S. F. Schlossman, Characterization of regulatory T cells in man. In B. Pernis and H. J. Vogel, Eds., *Regulatory T Cells,* Arden House, New York (in press).

153. H. Koprowski, R. Love, and I. Koprowski, Enhancement of susceptibility to viruses in neoplastic tissues. *Tex. Rep. Biol. Med.,* **15**, 559 (1957).

154. J. Lindenmann and P. A. Klein, Viral oncolysis: Increased immunogenicity of host cell antigen associated with influenza virus. *J. Exp. Med.,* **126**, 93 (1967).

155. D. A. Axler and A. J. Girardi, SV40 Tumor-specific transplantation antigen (TSTA) in NDV lysates of SV40-transformed cells. *Proc. Am. Assoc. Cancer Res.,* **11**, 4 (1970).

156. C. W. Boone, M. Paranjpe, T. Orme, and R. Gillette, Virus augmented tumor transplantation antigens: Evidence for a helper antigen mechanism. *Internatl. J. Cancer,* **13**, 543 (1974).

157. J. Lindenmann, Viruses as immunologic adjuvants in cancer. *Biochem. Biophys. Acta.* **355**, 49 (1974).

158. C. W. Boone, F. C. Austin, M. Gail, R. Case, and E. Klein, Melanoma skin test antigens of improved sensitivity prepared from vesicular stomatitis virus-infected tumor cells. *Cancer,* **41**, 1781 (1978).

159. M. D. Prager and F. S. Baechtel, Methods for modification of cancer cells to enhance their antigenicity. In H. Busch, Ed., *Methods in Cancer Research,* Academic, New York, 1973 p. 339.

160. O. J. Lachmann and K. Sikora, Coupling PPD to tumor cells enhances their antigenicity in BCG-primed mice. *Nature,* **271**, 463 (1978).

161. G. Klein and E. Klein, Induction of tumor cell rejection in the low responsive YAC-lymphoma strain A host combination by immunization with somatic cell hybrids. *Eur. J. Cancer,* **15**, 551 (1978).

162. T. E. Carey, K. O. Lloyd, T. Takahashi, L. Travassos, and L. J. Old, AU cell surface antigen of human malignant melanoma: Solubilization and partial characterization. *Proc. Natl. Acad. Sci. (USA),* **76**, 2898 (1979).

163. P. O. Livingston, H. Shiku, M. A. Bean, C. M. Pinsky, H. F. Oettgen, and L. J. Old, Cell-mediated cytotoxicity for cultured autologous melanoma cells. *Internatl. J. Cancer,* **24**, 34 (1979).

164. R. M. Zinkernagel and P. C. Doherty, Restriction of *in vitro* T cell-mediated cytotoxicity in lymphocytic choriomeningitis within a syngeneic or allogeneic system. *Nature (Lond.),* **248**, 701 (1974).

165. G. M. Shearer, Cell-mediated cytotoxicity to trinitrophenyl-modified syngeneic lymphocytes. *Eur. J. Immunol.,* **4**, 527 (1974).

166. G. D. Snell, A. M. Cloudman, E. Failor, and P. Douglass, Inhibition and Stimulation of tumor homoio-transplants by prior injections of lyophilized tumor tissue. *J. Natl. Cancer Inst.,* **6**, 303 (1946).

167. N. Kaliss, Immunological enhancement of tumor homografts in mice: A review. *Cancer Res.,* **18**, 992 (1958).

168. R. E. Wilson, E. B. Hager, C. I. Hampers, J. M. Corson, J. P. Merrill, and J. E. Murray, Immunologic rejection of human cancer transplanted with a renal allograft. *New Engl. J. Med.,* **278**, 479 (1968).

169. C. F. Zukoski, D. A. Killen, E. Ginn, B. Matter, D. O. Lucos, and H. F. Seigler, Transplanted carcinoma in immunosuppressed patients. *Transplantation,* **9**, 71 (1970).

13

Modification of Tumor Antigenicity in Therapeutics: Increase in Immunologic Foreignness of Tumor Cells in Experimental Model Systems

HIROSHI KOBAYASHI
Laboratory of Pathology, Cancer Institute
Hokkaido University School of Medicine
Sapporo, Japan

1. INTRODUCTION

There is no conclusive understanding regarding the nature of tumor-specific antigens. The antigenicity of tumor cells is very weak or unrecognizable and in most cases is unable to induce effective immune responses. The existence of antigens specific for cancer cells has not yet been ascertained in humans. Moreover, experimental evidence indicates that antigens are variably expressed and are dependent on the kinds of tumor and on the conditions and stages of tumor growth. The main aims of cancer immunology have been to identify antitumor immune responses of the host and attempt to stimulate them. However, notwithstanding the fundamental urgency of establishing the nature and function of tumor-specific antigens in people, cancer immunology should not be focused only on this aim. It is also extremely important to attempt to increase the immunogenicity of tumor cells. If antigens on tumor cells could be seen and magnified, it might be possible to exploit host defenses against cancer. This chapter is concerned primarily with approaches aimed at increasing therapeutic exploitation of tumor antigenicity.

The subject is considered from two points of view: how to increase existing tumor-associated antigen (TAA) and how to artificially impart new foreign antigens onto tumor cells.

2. INCREASE IN ANTIGENICITY OF TUMOR-ASSOCIATED ANTIGEN (TAA)

Since it is based on the possibility that unique TAA exists in human tumors, similar to what has been shown in animal tumor cells, it may be useful to find out how to increase this antigenicity. Current knowledge of the nature of TAA and various approaches increasing tumor cell antigenicity are discussed here.

2.1. Anitgenicity of Tumor Cells

Variable Expression of TAA.   Central to the study of tumor immunology is the concept that tumor cells have specific and unique antigens not present on normal cells. It is already known that animal tumor cells may express antigens that impart a certain degree of immunogenicity. However, it is also known that antigenicity varies with the cause of the tumor, the organ affected, the stage of the tumor growth, age, sex, and other host factors.

There are major differences in the degree of antigenicity (immunogenicity) of experimental tumors, ranging from extremely high antigenic to nonantigenic tumors in which no tumor-associated antigen can be detected. Extremely high antigenic tumors are unable to grow and kill the syngeneic normal host. For example, rat tumors induced by murine leukemia viruses such as Friend, Gross, and Rauscher viruses are not able to grow in syngeneic rats and regress spontaneously (1). The same is true for tumors induced in mice by SV40 virus and murine sarcoma virus (2,3) and for those induced by ultraviolet irradiation (4). Evidence that these highly antigenic tumors are still neoplastic in nature is provided by the fact that they are all able to grow and kill hosts immunologically suppressed or rendered immunologically tolerant to the specific antigen.

Tumors induced by various chemical carcinogens also show a different degree of antigenicity. For instance, DMBA-induced hepatomas are comparatively highly antigenic, but still grow and kill the hosts (5). Methylcholanthrene-induced sarcomas are moderately antigenic, in general, but their antigenicity ranges from high antigenic to low antigenic and depends on each tumor-host relationship (6). Certain tumors show low antigenicity, such as AAF-induced rat breast carcinomas and hepatomas and urethan-induced tumors (5). Certain tumors have no demonstrable antigenicity; diethylnitrosamine-induced mouse lung cancer (7), celophan-film-induced tumors (8), and some spontaneously developed experimental tumors provide such examples. Hewitt et al. (9) has recently reported that 27 lines of mouse tumors spontaneously developed were nonantigenic by the transplantation test. The existence of such apparently nonantigenic tumors suggests that the presence of TAA is not a prerequisite for the very neoplastic nature of a cell and gives rise to questions concerning the nature of the specific antigen demonstrated for certain tumor cells.

Nature of TAA.   The existence of tumor-specific antigens has not yet been verified in humans (see also Chapters 1 and 12). Indeed, at best it was possible to demonstrate the existence of TAA that appear to be uniquely present on tumor cells in the adult host. Generally, TAA can be divided into two groups: (1) "differentiation-related antigen," including retrograde differentiation antigen and disdifferentiation antigen; and (2) "induced antigen," including virally induced antigen, chemically induced antigen, and possibly tumor-specific antigen in a strict sense.

The retrograde differentiation antigens are antigens that appear in most undifferentiated cells. Thus the retrograde differentiation antigens often appear in some types of tumor consequent to the retrograde differentiation of normal cells to malignant cells. Oncofetal antigens have potential for eliciting rejection of tumors. Alphafetoprotein (AFP) does not have this potential and represents another type of retrograde differentiation antigen.

Antigens such as organ-specific antigen and histocompatibility antigen may also be identified as TAA. In an aminoazobenzene-induced rat liver cancer, Butenandt (10) observed by immunofluorescence a cross-reactivity between antigens on kidney cells and antigens on liver tumors. In other words, some of the antigenic specificities that appeared on liver cancer cells were normally expressed on kidney cells of the host. Thymus leukemia (TL) antigen is another type of organ-specific antigen (11). It originally exists in normal thymus cells of mice and incidentally appears in leukemia cells. In addition, histocompatibility antigen also represents certain types of TAA. For example, fibrosarcoma in the BALB/c mouse may acquire alien histocompatibility antigen of the $H2^k$ haplotype, in addition to its own $H2^d$ antigen characteristic of the BALB/c mouse (12,13). Reticulum cell sarcomas in the SJL/J mouse also acquire alien $H2^d$ antigen, in addition to autochthonous $H2^s$ antigen (14). Alien histocompatibility antigens that appear on tumor cells may sometimes act as rejection antigens. Thus TAA may consist of alien organ-specific or histocompatibility antigen. These antigens are tentatively referred to as *disdifferentiation antigens.*

Antigens induced by oncogenic viruses and chemicals may also represent TAA. Virus-associated antigens (VAA) appear in most virus-induced tumors. They are rarely, if ever, specific for individual tumors, but rather are specific for all the tumors induced by that virus; hence the definition VAA or, briefly, viral antigen. In contrast to the VAA, TAA present on cells of carcinogen-induced tumors are usually specific for the individual tumor; questions are still unanswered as to the role of the chemical carcinogen in TAA induction. It has been observed that the antigenicity of tumor cells induced by a large amount of chemical carcinogen within a short period of time is generally high, whereas the antigenicity of tumor cells induced by a small amount of chemical carcinogen over a comparatively long period of time is generally low. Baldwin (15) has recently shown that animals immunized with normal embryonic cells or fibroblasts exposed to certain chemical carcinogens are capable of rejecting tumor cells induced by the same type of carcinogen. Thus TAA responsible for the rejection of tumors may be produced by a single exposure of normal cells to certain chemicals. These observations are compatible with the suggestion that TAA are coded through the action of causative agents such as viruses or chemicals.

With the acquisition of increasing knowledge of differentiation-related and carcinogen-induced tumor antigens, the initial assumptions about the existence of tumor-specific antigens have been changed and the more conservative concept of TAA has been defined. However, the question has not yet been answered as to whether tumor-specific antigens in a strict sense may nevertheless exist on tumor cells. With the advent of monoclonal antibody methodologies, rapid progress can be reasonably expected toward the clarification of this important question.

Overcoming Escape Mechanisms.   The defenses of the host do not seem capable of inhibiting the ultimate growth of tumor cells. There are a number of possible explanations for the "escape mechanism" of tumor cells (see also Chapter 2). The basic assumption often made is that the antigenicity of tumor cells is too weak to elicit a strong response in the host. In addition, antigenic determinants on the surfaces of tumor cells may be masked by substances such as sialic acid, hyalonic acid, and chondroitin sulfate, which are produced by the tumor cells (16,17). However, it is also apparent that in some cases tumors have self-serving immunosuppressive effects that are based on a variety of mechanisms (18–23). These include the actions of blocking factors (18,19) and the involvement of suppressor T cells, which specifically inhibit the activity of cytotoxic T lymphocytes (20,21) and that of suppressor B cells and suppressor macrophages (22,23). Immunosuppressive soluble factors may also be involved. A number of such factors have been found, particularly in the sera of cancer patients, and are referred to as *serum inhibitors.*

On the basis of knowledge of some of the "escape mechanisms" involved in tumor growth, it may be possible to augment the host response against tumor cells. For example, neuraminidase has been used to take sialic acid off the cell surface (see also Chapter 14), and this has succeeded in heightening the antigenicity of tumor cells (24). However, since surface substances such as sialic acid are continuously produced by live tumor cells, the effectiveness of the removal of these substances from the cell surface may be limited unless the modified cells are metabolically inactive. Other approaches to augment the effectiveness of antitumor host defenses include inhibition of the release of free tumor antigen and the subsequent production of immune complexes in the sera, the production and/or action of suppressor cells (25–29), and the production of the serum suppressive factors. However, only limited success has been achieved as yet in this area.

Purpose of Tumor Cell Modifications.   Active specific immunization with the use of tumor cell vaccine has been tried by many investigators in attempts to kill residual tumor cells through an augmented specific host response. Limited results have been obtained to date with this approach when the vaccine was administered to a tumor-bearing host or after tumor resection. Questions arose as to whether it may be futile to immunize the host with such tumor cell vaccines since the host is operationally tolerant to tumor growth. Attempts have been made to strengthen antitumor immunity by increasing the immunogenicity of tumor cells employing physical and chemical treatments and virus infection. In fact, active immunization with the use of tumor cells modified in their antigenicity may induce effective immune response against the tumor cells.

There is sometimes an element of confusion between the terms "antigenicity" and "immunogenicity." Antigenicity is responsible for both the immunogenic activity and the immunosensitivity of tumor cells. In this article the term "antigenicity" is mainly used to define both of these functions. The term "immunogenicity" is used to define the immunizing activity of the tumors as reflected by the host response against it.

2.2. Immunogenicity of Physically Treated Tumor Cells

Irradiated Tumor Cells.   Irradiated tumor cells may have a comparatively strong immunogenic activity and have been used in the original demonstration of immunity against autochthonous tumors (30). x-Irradiated tumor cells have become a standard against which other antigen-modifying treatments are compared. The strong immunogenicity of irradiated tumor cells may be related to the retention of a degree of viability by the tumor cells that then would be capable of growing during a certain period of time (31,32). The viability of tumor cells depends on the dose of x-irradiation used. Too little irradiation may allow the retention of tumorigenicity with the possible lethal growth of tumors in the host, whereas too extensive an irradiation may destroy tumor cells with loss of immunogenic activity. Therefore, a dose of x-irradiation between 6000 and 12,000 rads to tumor cells is required for effective immunization. Depending on the dose of x-irradiation, one to three cell divisions have been observed before the ultimate death of the tumor cells. The strong immunogenicity of x-irradiated cells seems dependent on the natural state of TAA and may be explained by such phenomena as the continuous release of antigen from viable tumor cells. Binucleated cells are also observed in irradiated tumor cell populations. It is not known whether such binucleated cells have altered immunogenicity. Irradiated tumor cells are also effective stimulator cells in *in vitro* systems. In particular, in tests of mixed lymphocyte tumor cell culture (MLTC), irradiated tumor cells seem to be more suitable than mitomycin C-treated cells in this respect (33). Irradiation with ultraviolet or γ-ray sources has also been used successfully.

Other Physically Treated Tumor Cells.   Treatment of tumor cells with heat usually reduces or abolishes their immunogenicity. Deep-freezing of tumor cells has been widely employed in the preservation of TAA, but in most cases repeated freezing and thawing causes a loss of immunogenic activity.

Cryosurgery of tumor tissues has been used in atempts to increase tumor immunogenicity with consequent inhibition of tumor metastasis by the expected augmented response of host defenses. However, it was found (Yamashita et al., unpublished data) that the sudden release of a large amount of cyronecrotized tissue antigen leads to the formation of antigen-antibody complexes that enhance the development of metastases in both regional lymph nodes and distant organs. Therefore, the value of this approach must be questioned at this time.

2.3.   Immunogenicity of Chemically Treated Tumor Cells

In this section, attempts at chemical modification of tumor cells are classified mainly on the basis of the mechanisms underlying the actual increases in immunogenicity obtained (Table 1).

Chemical Modification of Tumor Cells and Oncogenic Potential of Tumor Cells. Formaldehyde, as a representative chemical, has been used to obtain safe and stable immunogens as tumor cell vaccines. Learning how to preserve tumor cells rather than increase their immunogenicity had been the main aim in early attempts directed toward obtaining efficient antigen for specific immunotherapy. Lin et al. (34) described the optimal method for inactivating tumor cells with exposure to a 1:500 dilution of formaldehyde for 18 hours at 4°C. Oikawa et al. (35) recently reported that paraformaldehyde-fixed tumor cells of BALB/c mice retained tumor-associated transplantation antigen (TATA) activity to a degree comparable to that of x-ray-inactivated tumor cells under the optimal condition of exposure to 1% paraformaldehyde for 30 minutes at 37°C.

Glutaraldehyde has also been used for the chemical modification of tumor cells. Frost and Sanderson (36) described the efficacy of glutaraldehyde-treated Meth A tumor cells in protecting against subsequent challenge with viable tumor cells. Tumor cells treated with such agents as iodoacetate and iodoacetamide have also produced protection against viable tumor cell challenge, as shown by Apffel et al. (37) and Prager et al. (38), and are easy to use and do not require any special equipment. Mitomycin C is also effective for treating tumor cells (39,40), and the immunogenicity of cells so treated seems to be superior to that of cells treated with other chemicals. It may be reasonably assumed that the immunogenicity of chemically modified tumor cells after various chemical treatments may depend on residual metabolic activities, the "viability" of tumor cells and/or the integrity of membrane antigens. When tumor cells are treated with highly concentrated formaldehyde for long periods of time, for example, tumor-associated antigens may be denatured, this resulting in decreased immunogenicity of the cells. On the other hand, the danger is real that local growth occurs with tumor cells treated with too low a concentration of formaldehyde for too short a period of time. The strong immunogenicity of tumor cells treated with mitomycin C (25 mg/ml, 37°C, for 60 minutes) may be explained by the fact that mitomycin C-treated cells can maintain

TABLE 1. Increase in Immunogenicity of TAA by Chemicals

Tumor	Host	Tissue Treatment	Result	Reference
Lymphoma Ib	C58	UV, x-irradiation, formaldehyde, disruption	+ +	34
mKSA	BALB/c	Paraformaldehyde	+ +	35
Spontaneous mammary adenoacanthoma tumor	BALB/c	Glutaraldehyde	+	36
Sarcoma, MCT, EL-4	C57BL (Pondville)	Iodoacetate	+ +	37
Sarcoma 1	A/Jax	Iodoacetate, iodoacetamide	+ +	37
Lymphoma EPF-1, lymphoma 6C3HED	C3H	Iodoacetamide, iodoacetate, N-ethylmaleimide	+ +	38
EL-4, S49A	BALB/c	Mitomycin C	+ +	40
MAC-induced, fibrosarcomas	CBA/H	Mitomycin C	+	39
Mammary carcinoma, hepatoma	Wistar rats	Bovine serum albumin coupled to irradiated cells, 4-acetamido-4'-isothio-cyanatostilbene-2, 2'-disulfonic acid coupled to irradiated cells	–	46
Spontaneous mammary adenocarcinoma MCA-induced squamous cell carcinoma	C3H	Human γ-globulin	+	43
Breast, ovarian, colon prostate tumors, CLL	Human	Rabbit γ-globulin	+	44

412

Tumor	Strain	Agent		Ref.
MCT, EL4, Krebs-2	C57BL Swiss	Sodium iodoacetate	+	37
Melanoma LPC-1, melanoma S-91	(BALB/c × DBA/2)F$_1$	Coupled with keyhole limpet hemocyanin or rabbit γ-globulin	+	42
Breast, stomach, colon, malignant melanoma	Human	Rabbit γ-globulin	−	45
Rauscher leukemia virus-induced ascites tumor (MCDV-12)	BALB/c	DNP Methylated bovine α-globulin, (MBGG)	+	47
MCA-induced tumors	C57BL/10	PPD	+	48
Plasmacytoma	C3H/He	PPD	+	49
YAC tumor	A	TNP	+	50
X5563	C3H/He	TNP	+	51
T-lymphoma, B-lymphoma, primary thymoma, mammary carcinoma	Mice	Cholesterol, cholesteryl hemisuccinate	+	55
P1798 lymphoma	BALB/c	Dimethyldioctadecyl ammonium bromide (DDA)	+	57
P1798 lymphoma	BALB/c	Iodoacetamide (IAd) with dimethydioctadecyl ammonium bromide (DDA)	+	58
MCA-induced tumor	DBA/2J	Acetoacetylation via diketone	+	60
EL-4	C57BL	Concanavalin A	+	63
6C3HED	C3H/He	Concanavalin A	+	38
L1210	BDF$_1$	Concanavalin A	+	64
Melanoma	C57BL/6	5-bromodeoxyuridine	+	67

their metabolic activity for certain periods of time after the treatment (40). This is also the case with irradiated tumor cells, where a high quantity of TAA is produced while the irradiated tumor cells are dividing for a certain number of generations before cell death.

Increase in Immunogenicity by Hapten Carrier Conjugation.

There have been several reports describing attempts to increase the immunogenicity of TAA with the use of helper antigens. The concept is to attach tumor cells to antigenic foreign protein as a "carrier" and to elicit an immune response against weak antigenic TAA. Foreign gamma globulin obtained from hosts of different species were initially used for conjugation of tumor antigen. For example, tumor cells from dogs and mice have been coupled to human or rabbit gamma globulin (41–43), whereas tumor cells from humans have been coupled to rabbit gamma globulin (44,45). The antitumor effects of immunization with such vaccines, however, have not been satisfactory; thus, for example, the host response to rat hepatoma could not be further increased by immunization with irradiated cells coupled to bovine serum albumin (46). Braun et al. (47) complexed tumor cells with methylated proteins and obtained increased immunogenicity of weak antigens in syngeneic hosts, but in his experiments nonimmunized animals were paradoxically more resistant to rechallenge than were immunized animals.

Recent studies of the carrier effect have shown that combining an antigenic determinant which evokes a powerful T-cell response with a weak antigen greatly enhances the immunogenicity of the latter by providing "antigenic help." Lachmann and Sikora (48) and Takatsu et al. (49) clearly demonstrated that purified protein derivative (PPD) is a particularly effective producer of antigenic help in increasing the immunogenicity of tumor-specific transplantation antigens (TSTA) in syngeneic mice. Trinitrophenyl has also been used to increase immunogenicity. Trinitrophenylated and irradiated or mitomycin C-treated Moloney virus-induced YAC cells have been found to induce a higher cytotoxic antibody response and a better protection against viable tumor cells in syngeneic, low responsive strain A mice, whereas irradiated or mitomycin C-treated YAC tumor cells have failed to induce such a response (50). These results suggested that the unresponsiveness of certain host systems can be overcome by antigenic modification, that is, by coupling the nonrecognized moiety to compounds that are immunogenic for the unresponsive genotype. Priming with trinitrophenylated isologous mouse gamma globulin may enhance the immunogenicity of trinitrophenylated tumor cells based on stimulation of reactive T helper cells, with the coexistence of carrier and hapten on the same molecules being required to achieve the previously mentioned hapten carrier effect (51). However, in the case of "helper determinant," which has recently been shown to occur in the virally enhanced immunogenicity of tumor cells, presensitization with modified tumor cells does not increase tumor immunogenicity and the coexistence of carrier and hapten on the same molecules does not seem to be necessary. The differences between hapten carrier effect and helper determinant effect must be studied further. In conclusion, chemically modified tumor cells equipped with new antigenic determinants could become an effective means for stimulating antitumor immunity.

Increase in Immunogenicity Due to Changes in Membrane Function. It is known that the fluidity of the cell membrane is important for the antigenicity of cells. Fluidity is increased in transformed cells consequent to virus infection (52,53), and the immunosensitivity of TAA in tumor cells following artificial infection with nonlytic viruses (54) is also increased as compared to that of noninfected tumor cells. Skornick and Shinitzky (55) have tested the immunogenicity of irradiated tumor cells after alteration of the cell membrane's lipid microviscosity and recognized that enrichment with cholesterol or cholesteryl hemisuccinate (CHS) increased the membrane's lipid microviscosity, affording a marked increase in cell immunogenicity as compared to that obtained with cells that were only irradiated.

Alkylcatechols including pentadecylcatechol (PDC) and natural plant oil urushiol are also lipophilic and are potent hypersensitizing agents. Incorporation of PDC or unrushiol led to changes in membrane fluidity as determined by polarization of fluorescence from a fluorescence probe. Treatment with these agents enhances the capacity of a weakly immunogenic rat hepatoma to induce immunity against transplanted tumor cells (56).

Prager and Gordon (57) used dimethyldioctadecyl ammonium bromide (DDA) as an agent for antigenic modification because of the possibility of complexing the lipophylic cation with negatively charged lymphoma cells. Increasing the lipid content by certain antigen modifiers led to cell-mediated responses to native antigens without a concomitant humoral response. After vaccination with iodoacetamide-treated lymphoma cells plus DDA, there were 71% survivors, compared to 29% for mice similarly vaccinated but without DDA (58). Also, diketene has been shown to selectively induce cellular responses against native antigen (59,60). Perhaps this results from the increased lipophylicity of the antigen (61,62).

Concanavalian A is also capable of increasing the immunogenicity of tumor cells; apparently this increase is related to the clustering of TAA. Concanavalin A treatment of x-irradiated tumor cells was found to enhance immunogenicity (63). The same has been true in tumor cells treated with Con A following glutaraldehyde treatment (64). The mechanism of the increase in immunogenicity caused by Con A treatment has not yet been ascertained. It is conceivable that the lectin might have a carrier activity as well as an adjuvant activity in addition to causing the increased membrane fluidity that results in clustering of tumor cell-surface antigens. Abrin is also capable of inducing strong immunogenicity (65).

Other means to bring about increases in the immunogenicity of tumor cells have been explored. The compounds IUdR and BUdR have been used to accelerate differentiation of tumor cells (66). They may also activate in tumors the production of latent viruses, this resulting in an increase in immunogenicity

(67). The C-type virus possibly induced by methylcholanthrene seems to increase the immunogenicity of TAA and to produce new viral antigen, resulting in an increased foreignness of tumor cells (68).

General Considerations. The increased immunogenicity that may be achieved through chemical modification of tumor cells is still unsatisfactory. There are no certain ways of prohibiting the growth of tumors that have already been established by postvaccination with such weak antigenic tumor cells. Moreover, vaccination with such weak immunogenic tumor cells occasionally enhances the growth of the tumor. The immunogenicity of tumor cells modified by various chemicals is usually weaker than that of irradiated tumor cells. Seeking ways to render tumor cells more immunogenic than irradiated tumor cells has been the main focus of recent studies. There are several ways to further enhance the immunogenicity of irradiated tumor cells. However, the increase in immunogenicity obtained is still poor, and it is still difficult to say which method of chemical modification is the best, since the effectiveness of the various methods may vary with the type of tumor and strain of mouse. New and different conditions should be developed to obtain an efficient protective vaccine. Indeed, increases in the immunogenicity of tumor cells may not be observed even when tumor cells are modified by strongly foreign antigenic chemicals or by large amounts of such chemicals if conditions are not appropriately selected.

The stability of chemically modified tumor cell-immunogenicity is rather poor as compared to that of virally modified tumor cells (next section). Whereas tumor antigens modified by viruses may be maintained as genetically stable markers even after several cell divisions, tumor antigens modified by chemicals do not seem to persist long after cell division.

2.4.   Immunogenicity of Virally Infected Tumor Cells

Immunogenicity of Lytic Virus-Infected Tumor Cell Extracts.   Most types of virus are cytolytic, making it difficult to obtain stable immunogenic TAA from destroyed tumor cells (oncolysate). However, it seems that the immunogenicity of tumor-associated antigen obtained from the oncolysate of tumor cells infected with cytolytic virus is higher than that obtained from oncolysate of non-virus-infected tumor cells (Table 2). Lindenmann (69) and Lindenmann and Klein (70,71) demonstrated that oncolysate obtained from influenza virus-infected Ehrlich tumor cells show a higher immunogenicity (ability to immunize against subsequent challenge with Ehrlich cells) than do lysates from non-infected Ehrlich cells. Eaton et al. (72) and Eaton and Almquist (73) reported that immunization with lymphoma cells that had been infected with Newcastle disease virus in mice caused a stronger inhibition of tumor rechallenge. Boon (74) and Boone and Blackman (75) infected SV40 transformed BALB/3T3 cells (E4 cells) with influenza virus and demonstrated an immunogenicity of homogenates from virus-infected cells higher than those from noninfected

TABLE 2. Increase in Immunogenicity of TAA by Infection with Viruses

Species	Animal Strain	Tumor	Materials and Methods	Note	Reference
Increase in Immunogenicity of Extracts of Tumor Cells by Infection with Lytic Viruses					
Mouse	A2G	Ehrlich	Influenza A virus (oncolysate)	Immunization with oncolysate or crude membrane	71
Mouse	C3H	Lymphoma	Newcastle disease virus (oncolysate)		72
Mouse	BALB/c	SV3T3-E4	Influenza A virus (homogenate)		74
Mouse	CBA BALB/c	337	Newcastle disease virus		77
Mouse	DBA/2J	L1210	Vesicular stomatitis virus (oncolysate)		76
Mouse	BALB/c	E4	Influenza (crude membrane)		78
Increase in Immunogenicity of Intact Tumor Cells by Infection with Nonlytic Budding Viruses					
Rat	WKA Donryu	WST, KMT DLT	Friend virus	Immunization with xenogenized viable tumor cells	86
Rat	BDIX Wistar/Fu	MBDB 290 T PW-41	Mouse endogenous virus (inactivated by x-irradiation) Polyoma virus		90
Mouse	BDF₁	L1210	HVJ-pi		91
Rat	WKA	KMT-17	Friend virus (inactivated by MMC, glutaraldehyde, and formalin)		88

417

cells. The immunogenicity of oncolysates prepared from tumor cells infected with lytic virus has often been weak (76–78). This may be due to the fact that the TAA determinants are quite unstable and that they are frequently destroyed in cell-free preparation. There have been several reports of clinical studies undertaken with lytic virus-infected oncolysate in combination with chemotherapy (79–84). The results of these studies are at present too preliminary or too inadequate to provide definite conclusions.

Immunogenicity of Nonlytic Virus-Infected Intact Tumor Cells. In 1970 the author succeeded in obtaining an experimental model for producing highly immunogenic TAA by infection of rat tumor cells with nonlytic foreign viruses (Table 2). Both viruses and tumor cells grow concurrently without lysis of tumor cells *in vitro* and in immunologically suppressed hosts (85–91). Tumor-associated antigens are comparatively stable in such virus-infected viable tumor cells, and the immunogenicity of such virus-infected viable cells is definitely stronger than that of the oncolysate of virus-infected cells. Roughly speaking, the LTD_{50}—namely, the number of tumor cells following immunization required for lethal tumor growth in 50% of the animals—was increased more than 10,000-fold with such virus-infected intact cells (92), whereas less than a 10-fold increase was seen in the hosts immunized with the viral oncolysate (93). "Viable intact" tumor cells can be used as a vaccine without the danger of progressive tumor growth since regression occurs without the aid of other treatment due to the immunologic mechanism described in the following paragraphs. They may be better immunogens due to a quantitative increase in the amount of tumor antigen as well as to an increase in the overall stability of the TAA. Virus-infected viable tumor cells are an effective means of producing tumor immunity because the TAA complex is left intact and because the presence of the replicating cells allows for a gradual but continual release of natural tumor antigen into the host. The preceding process has been shown to favor the development of the cell-mediated immune responses.

Studies comparing virus-infected and noninfected tumor cell preparations inactivated with x-irradiation, mitomycin C, glutaraldehyde, and formaldehyde have generally shown that infected tumor cell preparations are more immunogenic, but that the increased level of protection is quite low; thus the weakness of such inactivated tumor cell immunogenicity should be noted (93). Again, the effectiveness of "viable" tumor cell vaccine should be emphasized. Irradiated tumor cells have been used in clinical immunotherapy to enhance the antitumor effect of treatments such as chemotherapy and nonspecific immunotherapy (94,95). It should, therefore, be possible to further enhance antitumor effects by the use of "viable" tumor cell vaccine with definitely increased immunogenicity.

Viable tumor cells not infected with virus can be used to immunize the host, but usually they produce a tumor mass that must be amputated. Effective tumor immunity will develop following amputation, but the host may die secondary to recurrence of metastatic tumor. This danger of tumor recurrence does not occur with viable tumor cells when they are infected with nonlytic foreign virus since the host response completely eliminates all such cells. This means that viable tumor cells infected with foreign virus may be effectively used for active immunotherapy of animal tumors.

Mechanism of Increase in Immunogenicity of Tumor Cells.   The mechanism of the increased TAA immunogenicity of virus-infected tumor cells has not been defined. Several possible explanations exist; one may be that there is a quantitative and qualitative change of TAA on the virus-infected cells. The possibility of a qualitative change of TAA still remains, whereas that of a quantitative change of TAA cannot be supported by most experiments on the absorption capability of TAA (54,96). A second possibility regards nonspecific adjuvant activity, but this has not been considered in most cases. A third possibility regards the "hapten carrier effects" of TAA conjugated with the carrier VAA. This possibility has been considered in some cases of chemically modified tumor cells as described in the previous section. The hypothesis, however, has not always been substantiated in the case of virus-induced increases in immunogenicity (77,97). A fourth possible explanation is that the VAA on the surface of the tumor cell has helper activity by which it can cause an increase in the immune responses of the host (75, 98–100). Associative recognition of VAA and TAA as a unit may make possible the development of a stronger level of *in vitro* immunity to the TAA. In other words, VAA may play a role as helper determinants. If this were to occur, it would be important to have the two antigens in the same vicinity (101). A fifth explanation involves the possibility that mobility of TAA is somewhat altered by the presence of the VAA on the cell surface. This, in turn, could have an effect on how the TAA is presented to the intricate immune responses of the tumor-bearing host. From complement-dependent cytotoxicity test (96) and immunoelectron microscopy (102), it has been shown that TAA easily move and cluster with corresponding antibodies on a certain area of the cell surface if the tumor cells are first infected with a virus. The clustering of TAA may produce a better *in vivo* immune response and may also explain the higher immunosensitivity of tumor cells *in vitro*. It is not clear as yet whether the above-mentioned increased mobility of the tumor cell surface is actually associated with the increase in immunogenicity. Further studies are needed to more completely define the mechanisms responsible for the increased immunogenicity seen with virus-infected tumor cells.

Immunosensitivity of Virally Infected Tumor Cells.   Antigenicity is responsible for immunogenicity and immunosensitivity. As already mentioned, immunogenicity in a strict sense involves the immunogenic capability of tumor antigen. Immunosensitivity expresses the sensitivity of tumor cells to immune effectors.

It is possible to measure the immunosensitivity of tumor cells as affected by infection with nonlytic moderate virus, since in this case tumor cells may survive without lysis under certain conditions. The data indicate that the moderate virus-infected tumor cells are more sensitive to complement-dependent cytotoxicity (57,96,103,106) and lymphocyte-mediated cytotoxicity (104,105, 107) as compared to noninfected tumor cells. For example, infection of tumor cells with a nonlytic budding virus can cause the cells to have a higher sensitivity to complement-dependent cytotoxicity and to antitumor lymphocytes. Takeichi et al. (78) reported that MSV-infected E4 cells were much more sensitive to cell-mediated cytotoxicity by immune lymphocytes. Kasai et al. (106) demonstrated that mumps virus-infected human melanoma cells (M14) were more sensitive than noninfected melanoma cells to antibodies against oncofetal antigen, melanoma-associated antigen, and HLA antigen when the antibodies were obtained from melanoma patients. Because of these observations, it is suggested that virus-infected intact tumor cells may be useful for the detection of weaker tumor-associated antigens (TAA) present on tumor cells with the use of either humoral or cellular assay systems. The main reason for the increased immunosensitivity may be the increased fluidity of the tumor cell-membrane that follows infection by the virus (108).

2.5. Immunogenicity of Hybrid Tumor Cells

Hybrid tumor cells fused with normal or tumor cells derived from syngeneic, allogeneic, and xenogeneic hosts are experimentally used for the purpose of increasing the immunogenicity of tumor cells. The main aim of this approach is to increase the expression of TAA by fusing foreign antigen with tumor cells. Klein (109) had already noted that cell hybridization may be one of three possible ways of increasing immunogenicity, with the others being coupled with chemicals and viral xenogenization.

The main characteristic of hybrid tumor cells is that they can be used as a viable cell vaccine for immunization. This is due to the fact that most lines of hybrid tumor cells fused with either normal or malignant cells lose their malignancy and are incapable of growing in the host even if viable hybrid cells are transplanted. For example, Watkins and Chen (110) observed that viable mouse Ehrlich ascitic tumor cells fused with polyoma-transformed baby hamster kidney cells are capable of producing strong resistance against the challenge of Ehrlich ascitic tumor cells without the danger of local growth of viable hybrid tumor cells; in other words, the hybrid cells are analogous to "attenuated" tumor cells. Thus the hybrid formed between a tumor with weak transplantation antigens and a cell line with transplantation antigens that are very strong in the host animal can be used to immunize the host against challenge with the tumor. Such attenuated tumor cells may have immunizing properties superior to those of tumor cells killed by physical or chemical means. Kim (111) also indicated that hybrid cells derived from the fusion of BALB/c plasmacytoma and L cells (C3H origin) could be used to stimulate tumor-specific immunity against the parental plasmacytoma cells since viable hybrid cells induced tumor-specific immunity against BALB/c plasmacytoma more effectively than did mitomycin-C-treated hybrid or parental plasmacytoma cells. Yoshida (112) also observed that immunologic protection against Ehrlich ascitic tumor cell challenge is achieved by preimmunization with viable rat/Ehrlich hybrid cells. Such strong resistance against challenge with parental tumor cells due to hybrid tumor cells sensitization may be obtained as a result of the viability of the cells used for immunization, which may well be preserved without deterioration of TAA in the host. For an objective comparison of immunogenicity, however, both hybrid and parental tumor cells must be inactivated and their immunogenicity compared under the same conditions. Klein (113,114) compared the immunogenicity of a somatic cell hybrid of YAC lymphoma cells fused with some established mouse fibroblasts with that of parental YAC lymphoma cells and observed that hybrid cells induced a more efficient rejection reaction against the challenge of parental YAC in strain A mice than did parental YAC cell immunization under the same conditions of x-irradiation.

There seem to be some difficulties and limitations to the use of cell hybridization in attempting to increase the immunogenicity of tumor cells. First, immunogenicity due to hybrid tumor cells differs in each clone of hybrid tumor cells and varies with each cell-to-cell combination. As Klein (113,114) indicated, immunity against subcutaneously grafted YAC cells varies according to the cells that were fused. They appear to be immunogenic as reflected both by rejection and by antibody titers but to fall in between the low immunogenic YAC and the relatively highly immunogenic YAC IR/A9HT. Lower degrees of immunization have been achieved with other somatic cell hybrids. Murphy et al. (115) have also indicated that immunization with non-pre-treated interspecies of somatic hybrid cells carrying twice the number of parental cell chromosomes was not found to be more efficient than immunization with x-irradiated parental cells in terms of transplantation resistance induction. There have been some cases, as described by Favre et al. (116), where a loss of antitumor immunogenicity occurred in somatic cell hybrid lines. Thus, even if an increase in immunogenicity is observed in somatic hybrid cells, the degree of the increase in general does not seem to be superior to those obtained by x-irradiation and other methods. Another difficulty or limitation of hybrid tumor cells is the time required for obtaining immunogenic hybrid tumor cells.

2.6. Immunogenicity of Tumor Cells When Mixed with Foreign Antigen

Tumor cells mixed with bacteria are sometimes strongly immunogenic. Taking examples from recent experiments, Zbar et al. (117) indicated that tumor cells mixed with live BCG when injected intradermally produced a 500-fold increased resistance to transplantation. Bartlett and Kreider (118) and Titus et al. (119) also observed that LSTRA tumor cells mixed with *C. parvum* produced transplantation resistance even though no resistance was observed when either was used as a single immunizing agent. Baldwin and Byers (120) obtained similar results showing that immunization with irradiated or viable tumor cells mixed with BCG or *C. parvum* enhanced an antitumor effect that had not been observed with either used as a single immunizing agent. In clinical studies, Schapira et al. (121) observed that irradiated autologous renal carcinoma cells mixed with bacterial adjuvant seemed to produce regression of metastatic tumors. Thus immunization with a tumor cell-bacillus mixture is a recently developed way for immunizing the host. The reason for the strong immunity of such mixtures is not related to antigenic changes and thus this immunizing effect cannot be ascribed to "xenogenization" of tumor cells (89).

Regional immunotherapy is actually effective in inhibiting the recurrence of tumor cells and in prolonging the survival of cancer patients. The potential of regional immunotherapy was originally demonstrated in tests indicating that the injection of viable BCG organisms into an intradermal tumor of the guinea pig Line 10 hepatoma induced regression of the local tumor and prevented the development of draining lymph node metastasis (122–124). This approach has subsequently been developed to show that transplanted tumors can regress consequent to the intratumoral injection of bacterial vaccine. Regional immunotherapy may be basically the same as the above-mentioned active immunization with a mixture tumor cells and bacilli.

2.7. Source and Usage of Immunogenic Tumor Cells

The main purpose of increasing the antigenicity of tumor cells is to obtain a vaccine of tumor-specific antigens for potentially active specific immunotherapy. In contrast to nonspecific immunotherapy with a variety of vaccines that possess antigenically unrelated antigen, TAA is restricted to use only as a vaccine for specific immunotherapy. Primary specific immunotherapy with tumor antigen may result in a direct attack on TAA, whereas in the case of nonspecific active immunization with such agents as bacterial products, for example, specific immunity may develop secondarily and may contribute to the therapeutic outcome through an attack on TAA.

Source of Tumor Cells for Specific Immunity. For specific immunotherapy, it is important to decide what tumor cell sources are to be used to immunize the host. A question arises as to what types of tumor cell, allogeneic or autochthonous, are potentially more immunogenic in inhibiting the growth of tumor cells. Basically, the antigenicity of tumor cells used for immunization must be the same as that of the tumor cells in the host. However, there is no definite conclusion at present on the cross-reactivity of TAA among various types of tumor cell. Spontaneously developed tumors are considered to be almost or completely nonantigenic (125). In specific immunotherapy no antitumor effect may be expected when the host is immunized with antigenically unrelated tumors or with nonantigenic tumors. Although there have been been some reports describing human tumors showing specific common antigens, there has been no evidence that the antigen commonly existing on human tumors is capable of eliciting a response that could cause the rejection of the tumor. For this reason, although differences between primary and metastasized tumors have been described even in the autochthonous host (126), it may be presumed that the TAA in autochthonous tumors is more cross-reactive to the antigen residing in the autochthonous host than to allogeneic tumor cells. At present, both allogeneic and autochthonous tumor cells are used as vaccine for active immunotherapy. An advantage in the use of allogeneic tumor cells is that there is little danger of tumor growth, even if they are used as viable cells. In contrast, the converse is a disadvantage of autochthonous tumor cells. The question still remains as to which have more potential as a tumor immunogen.

Normal Cells for Specific Immunity.   Tumor-specific antigen to be used as a vaccine for specific immunotherapy may be obtained not only from allogeneic and autochthonous tumor cells, but also from normal cells containing some parts of the TAA. For example, tumor cells sometimes contain alien histocompatibility antigens developed during carcinogenesis. This alien histocompatibility antigen may be the same as the antigen cross-reactive to allogeneic normal cells. Therefore, there are possibilities for cross-reaction among normal and tumor cells induced by different causes in different individuals. In other words, a newly developed histocompatibility antigen may play a role in rejecting tumor cells that may share some common histocompatability antigen with normal cells. These points have been confirmed by Invernizzi and Parmiani (12), Gibson et al. (13), Martin et al. (127), and Wrathmell et al. (128). The fact that common antigens may be associated with endogenous virus also suggests the possibility that the viral antigen participates in the immunization (129). In fact, some reports have suggested a possible role of endogenous virus in increasing the immunogenicity of tumor cells following some types of chemical treatment that had been employed to increase immunogenicity (67).

Immunization Conditions.   Some other important considerations should be mentioned. These relate to the importance of the route of immunization. Trials to increase the immunogenicity of tumor cells should not be restricted to immunization per se, but should also investigate other factors capable of enhancing immune response.

Experimentally, nonlytic virus-infected xenogenized tumor cells can produce an approximately 10,000-fold increase in immunogenicity when administered intradermally, whereas only a 2000-fold increase is produced when such cells are administered subcutaneously (92). It is generally accepted that intradermal immunization results in a higher immunizing effect, as indicated by the fact that irradiated tumor cells combined with nonspecific immunotherapy are now clinically employed intradermally. The status of the regulation of the immune response and its possible alteration by antitumor treatments may alter the effectiveness of immunization in either direction (26,27,93,130).

3. PRODUCTION OF NEW FOREIGN ANTIGEN IN TUMOR CELLS

Another way to increase the antigenicity of tumor cells is to produce some new foreign antigen on the tumor cells without the involvement of a direct relationship with TAA, since the above-mentioned attempts at increasing the immunogenicity of formerly existing TAA have not always brought about the expected results. Chemicals and viruses have been used for the artificial production of new foreign antigen.

3.1. New Foreign Antigen Due to Chemicals

If new antigen is artifically produced on the cell surface, this new antigen should act as a marker of foreignness to be recognized by the host, leading to the production of immune responses against the new antigen and, in addition, to the weakly antigenic TAA on the tumor cells. It would be of value if immunologically determined regression of tumors could be obtained following production of new foreign antigens with chemicals. However, questions need to be answered as to what kind of chemicals should be used to modify tumor cells.

There have been a number of reports describing antigenic changes of tumor cells following serial passages *in vivo* and *vitro*. Biedler and Riehm (131) reported that a tumor line resistant to actinomycin D and daunorubicin reduced heterotransplantability into the cheek pouch of cortisone-treated weanling Syrian hamsters, this reduction being related to an alteration of surface properties (132). Bonmassar et al. (133) reported that lines of L1210 leukemia cells exposed to 5-(3,3-dimethyl-1-triazine)imidazole-4-carboxamide (DTIC) became unable to grow in normal DCF_1 mice but were able to grow in DTIC-conditioned mice (133). Serial passages of drug-conditioned tumor cells may lead to a higher possibility of selection and mutation, by which antigenical variant lines with different immunogenicity from the original line are often produced (134–137). Most variant cells are unable to grow in animals, and strong antitumor immunity crossing to the original line is observed. Boon et al. have also reported that by treatment with the mutagen N-methyl-N'-nitro-N-nitrosoguanidine (MNNG) (138,139), it is possible to obtain cell variants that are incapable of progressive growth in syngeneic mice. Syngeneic C57B1/6 mice reject these nontumorigenic clones and acquire a strong radioresistant immunity against the immunizing clones. They suggested that the procedure of using a mutagen to generate nontumorigenic variants carrying new transplantation antigens may be generally applicable to cancer cells. However, there have been few studies describing the nature of new transplantation antigen and the comparable strength of TAA immunogenicity in these at random variant tumor cell lines. Reproducibility in obtaining new variant cell lines with a defined degree of TAA immunogenicity is a problem that still must be solved.

3.2. New Foreign Antigen Due to Virus

The acquisition of a new antigen on tumor cells following artificial infection with viruses is rather easily recognized. This new type antigen has been quantitatively detected in mice and hamsters by using the complement-dependent cytotoxicity test (140), transplantation resistance (141–149), and the immunofluorescence technique (148) (Table 3). Stück et al. (140) referred to such phenomena as "antigenic conversion," Svet-Moldavsky and Hamburg (141–144) described it as "heterogenization" and Sjögren and Hellström (145,146) as "acquisition of virus-specific new antigen." Since then, a number of reports describing similar phenomena have appeared.

Immunologic Regression of Tumor Cells Following Nonlytic Virus Infection. If an acquired antigen is extremely foreign to the host, the virus-infected tumor cells will regress in the tumor host without additional therapy. Kobayashi et al. (85) first succeeded in producing immunologic regression of various types of rat tumor by artificial infection with murine leukemia viruses such as Friend and Gross (85–88, 150). Most transplanted tumors in rats were unable to grow in the syngeneic and autochthonous host if the tumors had been surgically removed and artificially infected with the virus either *in vivo* or *in vitro*. Even if the virus-infected tumors grew initially, they eventually regressed without treatment in the normal host (Table 3). It was also observed that rat tumor metastases regressed if the tumor cells were previously infected with murine leukemia virus (149). If the host was made immunologically tolerant through neonatal injection of Friend or Gross virus, or if the host was immunologically suppressed by chemicals or irradiation, then the virus-infected tumor cells would still grow and eventually kill the host. The reason for the regression of rat tumors infected with murine leukemia virus in the normal host is that the newly acquired VAA was recognized as foreign and was rejected by the host even without previous sensitization. The author was the first to refer to this phenomenon as *viral xenogenization* of tumor cells (87,88,150,152).

It is of interest to determine whether the above-mentioned phenomenon could be observed with tumors and viruses other than rat tumors and the murine leukemia virus (Table 3). Holtermann and Majde (153) reported that the lethal growth of adenocarcinoma cells in SWR/J mice decreased by 50% when the tumor was infected with LCM virus. Barbieri et al. (68) and Al-Ghazzouli et al. (154) also reported that the lethal growth of mouse tumors decreased when the tumors were infected with Rauscher leukemia virus. Greenberger and Aaronson (155) reported regression of mouse tumors following infection with Moloney sarcoma virus (MSV) nonproducer and regression of other tumor cells by infection with C-type helper virus. Similar results were demonstrated in mice by Basombrio (156), Kuzumaki et al. (157), and Takeichi et al. (78), by infecting several types of tumor with MSV. Ishimoto et al. (158) demonstrated that a THK tumor in hamster regressed after infection of the tumor

TABLE 3. Production of a Virus-Specific New Antigen in Tumor Cells

Animal					
Species	Strain	Tumor	Virus	Note	Reference
Inhibition of Tumor Growth in Preimmunized Hosts					
Mouse		EL4	Rauscher	Antigenic conversion (cytotoxicity test)	140
Hamster Mouse		Sarcoma Leukemia	Herpes Polyoma SV40 Adeno	Heterogenization (transplantation)	141
Mouse		Lymphoma	Polyoma	Acquisition of virus-specific new antigen	145
Mouse	dd/Om	OMT-6	Friend		147
Mouse		Leukemia		Fluorescence	148
Mouse		Ehrlich	LCM		149
Regression of Tumor in Normal Hosts					
Rat	WKA Donryu	KMT-68 WST-5 (sarcoma) Takeda (sarcoma) DLT (squamous cell carcinoma) AH-109	Friend	Xenogenization (transplantation, cytotoxicity test, etc.)	152
Rat	WKA	MCA-primary	Friend		150
Mouse	SWR/J	Adenocarcinoma (spontaneous)	LCM		153

Species	Strain	Cell line/Tumor	Virus	Assay	Ref.
Mouse	C57BL	P4bic (sarcoma), TBLC2 (MC-sarcoma)	Rauscher		68
Mouse	BALB/c	SS1 (sarcoma)	MSV		156
Mouse	NIH Swiss BALB/c	MSV-tumor	RNA C-type		155
Mouse	BALB/cCr	WM-7, WM-8, WM-211	Rauscher	Transplantation, Cr-release assay, Winn assay	154
Rat	BDIX Wistar/Fu	MBDB (fibro-sarcoma), 290T (neurogenic), PW41 (sarcoma)	Mouse endogenous, Polyoma		157
Mouse	BALB/c	E4 (sarcoma)	MSV		101
Hamster	—	THK	Friend		
Hamster		GM2	HVJ, Rubella		159
Mouse	BDF$_1$	L1210 (lymphoma)	HVJ-pi		
Mouse	Nude	BHK, HeLa	Mumps		160
Rat	WKA	KMT-17	DEAE-D + Friend	Regression of growing tumor	161

with Friend virus. Thus the viral xenogenization phenomenon has been gener-alized. From these results, one can now say that the immunologic regression of tumor cells infected with foreign virus may be observed in many virus-tumor combinations in different species. Two conditions must be satisfied for regression of a tumor to occur. One is that the virus be of the nonlytic surface budding type, and the other is that genetic disparity exist between the host most susceptible to the virus and the host from which the cells originated.

Recently, reports have appeared describing the regression of tumor cells after infection with nononcogenic virus. Lympho choriomeningitis (LCM) virus, as reported by Holterman and Majde (153), was the first nononcogenic virus used for the regression of tumors, although the virus occasionally caused lethal inflammatory changes in the brain of the host. Yamada and Hatano (159) have reported a decrease in the lethal growth of tumor cells in hamsters, following previous infection of the tumor cells with HVJ virus. They have also succeeded in causing the regression of tumors in hamsters by infection with Rubella virus. Takeyama et al. (91) reported that more than half of BDF_1 mice bearing L1210 leukemia cells regressed by infection with HVJ-pi virus, which is a variant of HVJ, and that strong immunity was induced following the re-gression of the tumor. Kuzumaki et al. (90) noted that rat tumor cells regressed after artificial infection with endogenous oncornavirus obtained from nude mice. Reid et al. (160) infected HeLa tumor cells with mumps virus and trans-planted them into nude mice. The mumps virus-infected viable tumor cells grew only if the nude mice were x-irradiated.

Attempts at In Vivo Xenogenization of Tumor Cells.   It is also interesting to speculate whether it would be possible to cause viral infection of an existing tumor to xenogenize it, thereby causing the tumor to undergo regression with-out the surgical removal of the tumor from the host. For this approach to suc-ceed, the nonlytic virus would have to infect the growing tumor cells as ef-ficiently and as quickly as possible, as the virus would be quickly eliminated by the immune response of the host. For this purpose, possible substances producing new foreign antigen must be concentrated into tumor tissues. For example, treatment with angiotensin and hyperthermia might be one way of dilating vessels preferentially in tumor tissues, thus enabling viruses to con-centrate in the tumor. Tumor-specific antibody attached to viruses may also be applied to direct them to the tumor. Diethylaminoethyl-D (DEAE-D) is also useful in attaching a foreign body to the cell surface due to change in the nega-tive charge induced on the tumor cells. Kodama et al. (161) observed that intralesional inoculation of DEAE-D before direct infection of the virus ap-pears to produce a higher rate of regression of primary tumors. Liposomes containing certain substances might also be useful for producing foreign anti-gen in tumor cells.

Mechanisms of Regression of Xenogenized Tumor Cells and Subsequently Produced Antitumor Immunity.   It is most likely that the main reason for the regression of xenogenized tumor cells is the recognition of the VAA as foreign in the host. The initial immune defense of the host against virally xenogenized tumor cells may not be directed against the weak antigenic TAA, but most likely is directed against the strong antigenic VAA. Xenogenized tumor cells infected with foreign budding virus were rejected by humoral immunity, as demonstrated in experiments where the xenogenized tumor cells were placed in a three-layer diffusion chamber inserted into the abdominal cavity of rats. The number of xenogenized tumor cells in the chamber decreased and finally disappeared (162). It has been generally accepted that the rejection of strong foreign antigens is through the humoral response and that weaker foreign antigens are rejected through cell-mediated immune responses. It appears reasonable to say that virally xenogenized tumor cells, when they are highly antigenic, are rejected primarily through the humoral immune response. It is also obvious that the cell-mediated immune response may play a very important role in rejecting xenogenized tumor cells. Evidence that xenogenized tumor cells are destroyed by T lymphocytes from the tumor-bearing host has already been obtained *in vitro* (103,104). No data are yet available with regard to the type or subset of cell responsible for the regression of these cells.

Immunity against both TAA and VAA is produced following the regression of virally xenogenized tumor cells. Anti-TAA immunity is important in inhibiting the growth of corresponding types of tumor whereas anti-VAA immunity is necessary in making the tumor vaccine regress. The strength of immunogenicity caused by virally xenogenized tumor cells depends on the amount of VAA that appears on the cell surface (99).

New Foreign Antigen Due to Hybridization. The somatic cell hybrids formed by fusion of syngeneic tumor cells with either allogeneic or xenogeneic cells are rejected by the host. As discussed previously, a possible basis for rejection of the hybrid is the presence of foreign histocompatibility antigens on the surface of the hybridoma cells.

4. CONCLUDING REMARKS: INCREASE IN TAA VERSUS NEW FOREIGN ANTIGEN

The author has divided the main subject of how to increase the antigenicity of tumor cells into two parts, namely, how to increase formerly existing TAA and how to artificially produce new foreign antigen in tumor cells. Both antigens must be foreign antigens if immune responses to tumor cells are to develop in the host. The only difference between the preceding two objectives is that the first is aimed at increasing the immunogenicity of formerly existing weak-antigenic TAA, whereas the second is aimed at introducing some new foreign antigen into the tumor cell. It is of interest that weakly immunogenic TAA increases following incorporation of new foreign antigen, with both antigens being cooperatively associated.

There are some similarities and differences in the preceding two approaches. The main aim of attempting to increase the immunogenicity of TAA is to use the TAA as a vaccine to immunize the host by which specific immune responses may be enhanced. For example, if the minimum number of residual tumor cells still remaining in the host following surgical removal of the tumor are treated with immunotherapy using TAA modified and/or increased in some way, recurrence and metastasis of cancer should be inhibited. In contrast, the main aim of attempting to produce new foreign antigen is to artificially introduce this new antigen into the tumor cells so that the immune responses of the host will attack the cells. The final goal of producing new foreign antigen on tumor cells is to cause immunologic regression of the tumor cells without any other aids. As long as the new foreign antigen is not antigenically associated with the existing TAA, it cannot be used as an immunogen to kill residual tumor cells in the way TAA can be.

The mechanism for increasing the immunogenicity of TAA may vary with several factors, such as the degree of TAA antigenicity in the tumor cells and the procedures used for increasing immunogenicity. It is suggested that the increase in the immunogenicity of TAA is caused by the "hapten-carrier effect" in cases of attachment of the tumor cells to PPD and TNP (48–51). In contrast, in cases of artificial infection of tumor cells with viruses an increase in the immunogenicity of TAA is caused by the "helper activity" of VAA produced on the cell surface (100). In addition, it is noteworthy that the immunosensitivity of TAA also increases following the production of new foreign antigen. The mechanism causing the increase in immunosensitivity may perhaps be explained by an increase in "antigenic mobility" on the cell surface due to virus infection. Therefore, it may be concluded that an increase in the antigenicity of TAA caused by a virus infection must be explained separately in the case of immunogenicity and immunosensitivity. Thus both the hapten carrier effect and helper activity are of considerable importance in explaining the mechanism of increase in immunogenicity, as is the increased mobility of the cell membrane in explaining the mechanism of increase in immunosensitivity. In other words, the increased antigenicity of TAA may reflect various mechanisms, depending on conditions.

There are several difficult problems involved in finding ways to increase the antigenicity of TAA. Irradiated tumor cells can produce a standard level of immunogenicity, whereas tumor cells modified with certain chemical and biological products can also produce increased immunogenicity of tumor cells. However, there are limits to the application of this approach to clinical treatment due to the weakness of the host response obtained. As previously noted, viable tumor cells and irradiated tumor cells infected with moderate foreign viruses can produce a higher antitumor effect experimentally. However, this effect depends on the kinds of virus used for the experiment and the amounts of new foreign antigen appearing on the cell surface. Variant tumor cells obtained by the treatment with mutagenic chemicals are also capable of inhibiting the growth of remaining tumor cells of the original lines. The use of such viable tumor cells previously xenogenized with chemicals and viruses involves problems still unsolved regarding the safety of growing tumor cell vaccine in the clinical setting. The cross-reactivity of TAA is another problem still unsolved. In some tumor systems the TAA antigenicity of metastatic tumor differs from that of primary tumor (126). Therefore, the former might not be responsive to immunization with the TAA of primary tumor cells even if the latter could be potentially immunogenic. However, the strengthened immunogenic tumor cells might cause wider cross-reactivity even if the original tumor cells are individually weak immunogenic.

The artificially produced new antigen on human cells are expected to act as new markers. New foreign antigens often result in an increase in formerly existing TAA immunogenicity in viral xenogenization and produce an alternative new antigen on the cell surface in chemical (or mutagenic) xenogenization. These newly appearing antigens may be easily recognized as foreign and be rejected by the host. A number of reports have, in fact, described the immunologic regression of tumors following xenogenization by infection with virus or by exposure of tumor cells to mutagenic chemicals.

REFERENCES

1. H. Kobayashi, N. Kuzumaki, E. Gotohda, N. Takeichi, F. Sendo, M. Hosokawa, and T. Kodama, Specific antigenicity of tumors and immunological tolerance in the rat induced by Friend, Gross and Rauscher viruses. *Cancer Res., 33,* 1598 (1973).

2. K. K. Takemoto, R. C. Y. Ting, H. L. Ozer, and P. Fabisch, Establishment of a cell line from an inbred mouse strain for transformation studies: Simian virus 40 transformation and tumor production. *J. Natl. Cancer Inst., 41,* 1401 (1969).

3. J. B. Moloney, A virus-induced rhabdomyosarcoma of mice. *Natl. Cancer Inst. Monogr., 22,* 139 (1966).

4. M. L. Kripke and M. S. Fischer, Immunologic responses of the autochthonous host against tumors induced by ultraviolet light. *Adv. Exp. Med. Biol., 66,* 445 (1976).

5. R. W. Baldwin, Immunological aspects of chemical carcinogenesis. In G. Klein and S. Weinhouse, Eds., *Advances in Cancer Research,* Vol. 18, Academic, New York, 1973, p. 1.

6. K. Takeda, Y. Kikuchi, S. Yamawaki, T. Ueda, and T. Yoshiki, Treatment of artificial metastasis of methylcholanthrene-induced rat sarcoma by autoimmunization of the autochthonous host. *Cancer Res., 28,* 2149 (1968).

7. R. W. Baldwin, Tumor associated antigens, *Z. Krebsforsch., 89,* 1 (1977).

8. G. Klein, H. O. Sjögren, and E. Klein, Demonstration of host resistance against sarcomas induced by implantation of cellophane films in isologous recipients. *Cancer Res., 23,* 84 (1963).

9. H. B. Hewitt, E. R. Blake, and A. S. Walder, A critique of the evidence for active host defence against cancer, based on personal studies of 27 murine tumors of spontaneous origin. *Br. J. Cancer, 33,* 241 (1976).

10. K. E. Butenandt, personal communication.

11. L. J. Old, E. A. Boyse, and E. Stockert, Antigenic properties of experimental leukemias. 1. Serological studies *in vitro* with spontaneous and radiation-induced leukemias. *J. Natl. Cancer Inst., 31,* 977 (1963).

12. G. Invernizzi and G. Parmiani, Tumor-associated transplantation antigens of chemically induced sarcomata cross-reacting with allogeneic histocompatibility antigens. *Nature,* **254,** 713 (1975).

13. T. G. Gibson, M. Imamura, H. A. Conliffe, and W. J. Martin, Lung tumor-associated depressed alloantigen coded for by the K region of the H-2 major histocompatibility complex. *J. Exp. Med.,* **147,** 1363 (1978).

14. B. Bonavida, J. Roman, and I. V. Hutchison, In appropriate alloantigen-like specificities detected on reticulum cell sarcomas of SJL/J mice: Characterization and biological role. *Proc. AACR and ASCO.,* **20,** 264 (1979).

15. R. W. Baldwin, personal communication.

16. B. H. Sanford, An alteration in tumor histocompatibility induced by neuraminidase. *Transplantation,* **5,** 1273 (1967).

17. G. A. Currie and K. D. Bagshawe, The role of sialic acid in antigenic expression: Further studies of the Landschutz ascites tumor. *Br. J. Cancer,* **22,** 843 (1968).

18. K. E. Hellström and I. Hellström, Immunological enhancement as studied by cell culture techniques. *Annu. Rev. Microbiol.,* **24,** 373 (1970).

19. R. W. Baldwin, M. R. Price, and R. A. Robins, Inhibition of hepatoma-immune lymph-node cell cytotoxicity by tumor-bearer serum, and solubilized hepatoma antigen. *Internatl. J. Cancer,* **11,** 527 (1973).

20. S. Fujimoto, M. J. Greene, and A. H. Sehon, Regulation of the immune response to tumor antigens. I. Immunosuppressor cells in tumor-bearing hosts. *J. Immunol.,* **116,** 791 (1976).

21. D. Naor, Suppressor cells: Permitters and promoters of malignancy? In G. Klein and S. Weinhouse, Eds., *Advances in Cancer Research,* Vol. 29, Academic, New York, 1979, p. 45.

22. H. Kirchner, A. V. Muchmore, T. M. Chused, H. T. Holden, and R. B. Herberman, Inhibition of proliferation of lymphoma cells and T lymphocyte by suppressor cells from spleens of tumor-bearing mice. *J. Immunol.,* **114,** 206 (1975).

23. R. B. Herberman, A. C. Hollinshead, T. C. Alford, J. L. McCoy, R. H. Halterman, and B. G. Leventhal, Delayed cutaneous hypersensitivity reactions to extracts of human tumors, *Natl. Cancer Inst. Monogr.,* **37,** 189 (1973).

24. J. G. Bekesi and J. F. Holland, Active immunotherapy in leukemia with neuraminidase-modified leukemic cells. In G. Mathe, Ed., *Tactics and Strategy in Cancer Treatment* (*Recent Results in Cancer Research,* Vol. 62), Springer-Verlag, Berlin, 1979, p. 78.

25. R. Netas, A. Winkelstein, S. B. Salvin, and H. Mendelow, The effect of cyclophosphamide on suppressor cells in guinea pigs. *Cell. Immunol.,* **33,** 403 (1977).

26. Y. Mizushima, F. Sendo, T. Miyake, and H. Kobayashi, Augmentation of specific cell-mediated immune responses to tumor cells in tumor-bearing rats pretreated with the anti-leukemia drug busulfan. *J. Natl. Cancer Inst.,* **66,** 659 (1981).

27. Y. Mizushima, F. Sendo, N. Takeichi, M. Hosokawa, and H. Kobayashi, Enhancement of antitumor transplantation resistance in rats by appropriately timed administration of busulfan. *Cancer Res.,* **41,** 2917 (1981).

28. M. Zembala and G. L. Asherson, The effect of cyclophosphamide and irradiation on cells which suppress contact sensitivity in the mouse. *Clin., Exp. Immunol.,* **23,** 554 (1976).

29. Y. Z. Patt, M. Washington, and R. Goldman, A radio-sensitive, thymic hormone sensitive suppressor cells. *Proc. AACR and ASCO,* **40,** 139 (1979).

30. G. Klein, H. O. Sjögren, and E. Klein, Demonstration of resistance against methylcholanthrene-induced sarcoma in the primary autochthonous host. *Cancer Res.,* **20,** 1561 (1960).

31. R. B. Herberman, Immunogenicity of tumor antigens. *Biochim Biophys. Acta,* **437,** 93 (1977).

32. D. A. Campbell, Jr., R. K. Oldham, and J. Ortaldo, Effect of X-irradiation on tumor

associated antigens. In H. E. Nieburgs, Ed., *High Risk Markers: Detection Methods and Management (Prevention and Detection of Cancer,* Part II, Vol. 1), Dekker, New York, 1978, p. 447.

33. G. M. Mavligit, J. U. Gutterman, C. M. McBride, and E. M. Hersh, Cell method immunity to human solid tumors: *In vitro* detection by lymphocytes blastogenic responses to cell-associated and solubilized tumor antigens. *Natl. Cancer Inst. Monogr.,* **37,** 167 (1972).

34. J. S. L. Lin, N. Huber, and W. H. Murphy, Immunization of C58 mice to line Ib leukemia. *Cancer Res.,* **29,** 2157 (1969).

35. T. Oikawa, E. Gotohda, F. C. Austin, N. Takeichi, and C. W. Boone, Temperature-dependent alteration in immunogenicity of tumor-associated transplantation antigen monitored via paraformaldehyde fixation. *Cancer Res.,* **39,** 3519 (1979).

36. P. Frost and C. J. Sanderson, Tumor immunoprophylaxis in mice using glutaraldehyde-treated syngeneic tumor cells. *Cancer Res.,* **35,** 2646 (1975).

37. C. A. Apffel, B. G. Arnason, and J. H. Peters, Induction of tumour immunity with tumour cells treated with iodoacetate. *Nature,* **209,** 694 (1966).

38. M. D. Prager, F. S. Baechtel, R. J. Ribble, C. M. Ludden, and J. M. Mehta, Immunological stimulation with modified lymphoma cells in a minimally responsive tumor-host system. *Cancer Res.,* **34,** 3203 (1974).

39. R. L. Wu and R. Kearney, Specific tumor immunity induced with mitomycin C-treated sygeneic tumor cells (MCT). Effects of carrageenan and trypan blue on MCT-induced immunity in mice. *J. Natl. Cancer Inst.,* **64,** 81 (1980).

40. E. Benjamini, S. Fong, C. Erickson, C. Y. Leung, D. Rennick, and R. J. Scibiensky, Immunity to lymphoid tumors induced in syngeneic mice by immunization with mitomycin C-treated cells. *J. Immunol.,* **118,** 685 (1977).

41. M. Rosenblatt, C. Chiba, T. Motoyoshi, A. Morris, V. Zuehlke, P. Wolf, and R. J. Bing, The production of a state of active immunity to isologous and autologous serum protein. *Am. J. Clin. Pathol.,* **46,** 362 (1966).

42. M. T. McEnany, M. G. Kelly, and J. L. Fahey, Effects of immunization with tumor cell-foreign protein conjugates on growth of syngeneic tumor grafts. *Proc. AACR and ASCO,* **9,** 46 (1968).

43. N. P. Czajkowski, M. Rosenblatt, F. R. Cushing, J. Vazquez, and P. L. Wolf, Production of active immunity to malignant neoplastic tissue, chemical coupling to an antigenic protein carrier. *Cancer,* **19,** 739 (1966).

44. N. P. Czajkowski, M. Rosenblatt, P. L. Wolf, and J. Vazquez, A new method of active immunization to autologous human tumor tissue. *Lancet,* **II,** 905 (1967).

45. T. J. Cunningham, K. B. Olson, R. Laffin, J. Horton, and J. Sullivan, Treatment of advanced cancer with active immunization. *Cancer,* **24,** 932 (1969).

46. R. W. Baldwin and C. R. Barker, Immunization against human tumours. *Lancet,* **II,** 1090 (1967).

47. W. Braun, O. L. Plescia, J. Paskova, and D. Webb, Basic proteins and synthetic polynucleotides as modifiers of immunogenicity of syngeneic tumor cells. *Isr. J. Med. Sci.,* **7,** 72 (1971).

48. P. J. Lachmann and K. Sikora, Coupling PPD to tumour cells enhances their antigenicity in BCG-primed mice. *Nature,* **271,** 463 (1978).

49. K. Takatsu, A. Tominaga, and Late M. Kitagawa, Induction of antitumor activity in mice presensitized with Mycobacterium by immunization with tuberculin-coated tumor. *Gann,* **69,** 597 (1978).

50. N. Galili, D. Naor, B. Asjo, and G. Klein, Induction of immune responsiveness in a genetically low responsive tumor-host combination by chemical modification of the immunogen. *Eur. J. Immunol.,* **6,** 473 (1976).

51. T. Hamaoka, H. Fujiwara, T. Tsuchida, T. Konouchi, and H. Aoki, Induction of immune resistance against tumor by immunization with hapten-modified tumor cells in the presence of hapten-reactive helper T cells. In H. Kobayashi, Ed., *Immunological Xenogenization of Tumor Cells* (*GANN Monograph on Cancer Research,* No. 23), Japan Scientific Societies Press, Tokyo, University Park Press, Baltimore, 1979, p. 123.

52. G. Poste and P. Reeve, Agglutination of normal cells by plant lectins following infection with non-oncogenic viruses. *Nature New Biol.,* **237,** 113 (1972).

53. J. M. Zarling and S. S. Tevethia, Expression of concanavalin A binding sites in rabbit kidney cells infected with vaccinia virus. *Virology,* **45,** 313 (1971).

54. E. Gotohda, T. Moriuchi, T. Kodama, and H. Kobayashi, Stabilized expression of tumor-associated antigen in xenogenized tumor cells to complement-dependent cytotoxicity. In H. Kobayashi, Ed., *Immunological Xenogenization of Tumor Cells* (*GANN Monograph on Cancer Research,* No. 23), Japan Scientific Societies Press, Tokyo, University Park Press, Baltimore, 1979, p. 47.

55. Y. Skornick and M. Shinitzky, Effective tumor immunization induced by cells of elevated membrane microviscosity, *Abstract of Meeting on Immunological Aspects of Experimental and Clinical Cancer,* Tel Aviv, Israel, 1979, p. 153.

56. V. S. Byers and R. W. Baldwin, personal communication.

57. M. D. Prager and W. C. Gordon, Enhanced response to chemoimmunotherapy and immunoprophylaxis using tumor associated antigens with a lipophylic agent, *Cancer Res.,* **38,** 2052 (1978).

58. M. D. Prager and W. C. Gordon, Immunoprophylasix and therapy with lipid conjugated lymphoma cells. In H. Kobayashi, Ed., *Immunological Xenogenization of Tumor Cells* (*GANN Monograph on Cancer Research,* No. 23), Japan Scientific Societies Press, Tokyo, University Park Press, Baltimore, 1979, p. 143.

59. H. Chao, S. C. Peiper, R. D. Aach, and C. W. Parker, Introduction of cellular immunity to a chemically altered tumor antigen, *J. Immunol.,* **111,** 1800 (1973).

60. J. G. Levy, R. B. Whitney, A. G. Smith, and L. Panno, The relationship of immune status to the efficacy of immunotherapy in preventing tumour recurrence in mice, *Br. J. Cancer,* **30,** 269 (1974).

61. C. R. Parish, Immune response to chemically modified flagellin. II. Evidence for a fundamental relationship between humoral and cell-mediated immunity. *J. Exp. Med.,* **134,** 21 (1971).

62. C. R. Parish, Preferential induction of cell-mediated immunity by chemically modified sheep erythrocytes. *Eur. J. Immunol.,* **2,** 143 (1972).

63. W. J. Martin, J. R. Wunderlich, F. Fletcher, and J. K. Inman, Enhanced immunogenicity of chemically-coated syngeneic tumor cells. *Proc. Natl. Acad. Sci.* (*USA*), **68,** 469 (1971).

64. T. Kataoka, H. Kobayashi, and Y. Sakurai, Potentiation of concanavalin A-bound L1210 vaccine *in vivo* by chemotherapeutic agents. *Cancer Res.,* **38,** 1202 (1978).

65. H. Shionoya, M. Arai, N. Koyanagi, S. Ohtake, H. Kato, T. Kodama, and H. Kobayashi, Immunogenicity of abrin treated tumor cells (2). *Proc. Jap. Cancer Assoc.,* **38,** 115 (1979) (in Japanese).

66. D. Schubert and F. Jacob, 5-Bromodeoxyuridine-induced differentiation of a neuroblastoma. *Proc. Natl. Acad. Sci.* (*USA*), **67,** 247 (1970).

67. S. Silagi, D. Beju J. Wrathall, and D. de Harven, Tumorigenicity, immunogenicity, and virus production in mouse melanoma cells treated with 5-bromodeoxyuridine. *Proc. Natl. Acad. Sci.* (*USA*), **69,** 3443 (1972).

68. D. Barbieri, J. Belehradek, Jr., and G. Barski, Decrease in tumor-producing capacity of mouse cell lines following infection with mouse leukemia viruses. *Internatl. J. Cancer,* **7,** 364 (1971).

69. J. Lindenmann, Immunity to transplantable tumors following viral oncolysis. 1. Mechanism of immunity to Ehrlich ascites tumor. *J. Immunol.,* **92**, 912 (1964).

70. J. Lindenmann and P. A. Klein, *Immunological Aspects of Viral Oncolysis, Recent Results in Cancer Research,* Vol. 9, Springer-Verlag, Berlin, Heidelberg, New York, 1967, pp. 1–84.

71. J. Lindenmann and P. A. Klein, Viral oncolysis: Increased immunogenicity of tumor cell antigen associated with influenza virus. *J. Exp. Med.,* **126**, 93 (1967).

72. M. D. Eaton, J. D. Lerinthal, A. R. Scala, and M. L. Jewell, Immunity and antibody formation induced in intraperitoneal or subcutaneous injection of Krebs 2 ascites tumor cells treated with influenza virus. *J. Natl. Cancer Inst.,* **39**, 1089 (1967).

73. M. D. Eaton and S. J. P. Almquist, Antibody response of syngeneic mice to membrane antigens from NDV-infected lymphoma. *Proc. Soc. Exp. Biol. Med.,* **148**, 1090 (1974).

74. C. W. Boone, Augmented immunogenicity of tumor cell homogenates produced by infection with influenza virus. *Natl. Cancer Inst. Monogr.,* **35**, 301 (1972).

75. C. W. Boone and K. Blackman, Augmented immunogenicity of tumor homogenates infected with influenza virus. *Cancer Res.,* **32**, 1018 (1972).

76. K. S. Wise, Vesicular stomatitis virus-infected L1210 murine leukemia cells: Increased immunogenicity and altered surface antigens. *J. Natl. Cancer Inst.,* **58**, 83 (1977).

77. P. C. L. Beverley, R. M. Lowenthal, and D. A. J. Tyrrell, Immune responses in mice to tumor challenge after immunization with Newcastle disease virus-infected or X-irradiated tumor cells or cell fractions. *Internatl. J. Cancer,* **11**, 212 (1973).

78. N. Takeichi, F. C. Austin, T. Oikawa, and C. W. Boone, Augmented immunogenicity of tumor cell membranes produced by infection with influenza virus as compared to Moloney sarcoma virus. *Cancer Res.,* **38**, 4580 (1978).

79. D. R. Murray, W. A. Cassel, A. H. Torbin, A. L. Olkowski, and M. E. Moore, Viral oncolysate in the management of malignant melanoma. II. Clinical studies. *Cancer,* **40**, 680 (1977).

80. M. K. Wallack, Z. Steplewski, H. Koprowski, E. Rosoto, J. Geroge, B. Hulihan, and J. Johnson, A new approach in specific, active immunotherapy. *Cancer,* **39**, 560 (1977).

81. C. Sauter, J. Lindenmann, J. P. Gmur, W. Berchtold, P. Alerto, P. Obrecht, and H. J. Senn, Viral oncolysis: Its application in maintenance treatment of acute myelogenous leukemia. In W. D. Terry and D. Windhorst, Ed., *Immunotherapy of Cancer: Present Status of Trials in Man (Progress in Cancer Research and Therapy,* Vol. 6), Raven, New York, 1978, p. 355.

82. J. G. Sinkovics, C. Plager, M. J. McMurtrey, J. J. Remero, and M. M. Romsdohl, Viral oncolysates for the immunotherapy of human tumors. *Proc. ACCR and ASCO,* **18**, 86 (1977).

83. K. Burdick, R. St. Jacques, S. Deodhar, and H. Roening, Immunotherapy of malignant melanoma with vaccinia virus. *Arch. Dermatol.,* **109**, 668 (1973).

84. R. Freedman, J. M. Bowen, J. Herson, A. Hamberger, J. T. Wharton, and F. Rutledge, Adjunctive virus-modified extracts in invasive vulva carcinoma. *Proc. AACR and ASCO,* **21**, 217 (1980).

85. H. Kobayashi, F. Sendo, T. Shirai, H. Kaji, T. Kodama, and H. Saito, Modification in growth of transplantable rat tumors exposed to Friend virus. *J. Natl. Cancer Inst.,* **42**, 413 (1969).

86. H. Kobayashi, F. Sendo, H. Kaji, T. Shirai, H. Saito, N. Takeichi, M. Hosokawa, and T. Kodama, Inhibition of transplanted rat tumors by immunization with identical tumor cells infected with Friend virus. *J. Natl. Cancer Inst.,* **44**, 11 (1970).

87. H. Kobayashi, T. Kodama, and E. Gotohda, *Xenogenization of Tumor Cells (Hokkaido University Medical Library Series,* Vol. 9), Hokkaido University School of Medicine, Sapporo, 1977, pp. 1–124.

88. H. Kobayashi, N. Takeichi, and N. Kuzumaki, *Xenogenization of Lymphocytes, Erythroblasts, and Tumor Cells* (*Hokkaido University Medical Library Series*, Vol. 10), Hokkaido University School of Medicine, Sapporo, 1978, pp. 1–174.

89. H. Kobayashi, Viral xenogenization of intact tumor cells. In G. Klein and S. Weinhouse, Eds., *Advances in Cancer Research*, Vol. 30, Academic, New York, 1979, p. 279.

90. N. Kuzumaki, E. M. Fenyö, B. C. Giovanella, and G. Klein, Increased immunogenicity of low-antigenic rat tumors after superinfection with endogenous murine C-type virus in nude mice. *Internatl. J. Cancer,* **21**, 62 (1978).

91. H. Takeyama, K. Kawashima, K. Yamada, and Y. Ito, Induction of tumor resistance in mice by L1210 leukemia cells persistently infected with HVJ (Sendai virus). *Gann,* **70**, 493 (1979).

92. K. Okayasu, H. Katoh, M. Hosokawa, and H. Kobayashi, Study on methods to augment the immunogenicity of viable xenogenized tumor cells (in preparation).

93. H. Kobayashi and F. Sendo, Immunogenicity of viable xenogenized tumor cells. In H. Kobayashi, Ed., *Immunological Xenogenization of Tumor Cells* (*GANN Monograph on Cancer Research,* No. 23), Japan Scientific Societies Press, Tokyo, University Park Press, Baltimore, 1979, p. 27.

94. P. Reizenstein, G. Brenning, L. Engstedt, S. Franzén, G. Gahrton, B. Gullbring, G. Holm, P. Höocker, S. Höglund, P. Hörnsten, S. Jameson, A. Killander, D. Killander, E. Klein, B. Lantz, Ch. Lindemalm, D. Lockner, B. Lönnqvist, H. Mellstedt, J. Palmblad, C. Pauli, K. O. Skärberg, A.-M. Udén, F. Vánky, and B. Wadman, Effect of immunotherapy on survival and remission duration in acute nonlymphatic leukemia. In W. D. Terry and D. Windhorst, Eds., *Immunotherapy of Cancer: Present Status of Trials in Man* (*Progress in Cancer Research and Therapy,* Vol. 6), Raven, New York, 1978, p. 329.

95. J. F. Holland and J. G. Bekesi, Comparison of chemotherapy with chemotherapy plus VCN-treated cells in acute myelocytic leukemia. In W. D. Terry and D. Windhorst, Eds., *Immunotherapy of Cancer: Present Status of Trials in Man* (*Progress in Cancer Research and Therapy,* Vol. 6), Raven, New York, 1978, p. 347.

96. T. Moriuchi and H. Kobayashi, Role of virus-associated antigen on xenogenized tumor cell surface in production of antibody against tumor-associated antigen. In H. Kobayashi, Ed., *Immunological Xenogenization of Tumor Cells* (*GANN Monograph on Cancer Research,* No. 23), Japan Scientific Societies Press, Tokyo, University Park Press, Baltimore, 1979, p. 65.

97. J. F. Evermann and T. Burnstein, Immune enhancement of the tumorigenicity of hamster brain tumor cells persistently infected with measles virus. *Internatl. J. Cancer,* **16**, 861 (1975).

98. J. Lindenmann, Viruses as immunological adjuvants in cancer. *Biochim. Biophys. Acta,* **355**, 49 (1974).

99. H. Yamaguchi, T. Moriuchi, M. Hosokawa, and H. Kobayashi, Relationship between expression of virus-associated antigen and immunogenicity of tumor-associated antigen in Friend virus-infected rat fibrosarcoma cells. *Cancer Immunol. Immunother.* (in press).

100. J. Bromberg, M. Brenan, E. A. Clark, P. Lake, N. A. Mitchison, I. Nakashima, and K. B. Sainis, Associative recognition in the response to alloantigens (and xenogenization of alloantigens). In H. Kobayashi, Ed., *Immunological Xenogenization of Tumor Cells* (*GANN Monograph on Cancer Research,* No. 23), Japan Scientific Societies Press, Tokyo, University Park Press, Baltimore, 1979, p. 185.

101. C. W. Boone, N. Takeichi, F. C. Austin, E. Gotohda, T. Oikawa, and R. Gillette, Virus augmentation: Increased immunogenicity of tumor-associated transplantation antigens in tumor cell extracts after infection with surface budding viruses. In H. Kobayashi, Ed., *Immunological Xenogenization of Tumor Cells* (*GANN Monograph on Cancer Research,*

No. 23), Japan Scientific Societies Press, Tokyo, University Park Press, Baltimore, 1979, p. 7.

102. T. Kodama, Lateral mobility and stabilized expression of tumor-associated surface antigen in xenogenized tumor cells. In H. Kobayashi, Ed., *Immunological Xenogenization of Tumor Cells* (*GANN Monograph on Cancer Research*, No. 23), Japan Scientific Societies Press, Tokyo, University Park Press, Baltimore, 1979, p. 57.

103. T. Shirai, H. Kaji, N. Takeichi, F. Sendo, H. Saito, M. Hosokawa, and H. Kobayashi, Cell surface antigens detectable by cytotoxic test on Friend virus-induced and Friend virus-infected tumors in the rat. *J. Natl. Cancer Inst., 46,* 449 (1971).

104. M. Hosokawa, M. Kasai, H. Yamaguchi, and H. Kobayashi, Increased sensitivity to cell-mediated cytotoxicity of murine leukemia virus-infected rat tumor cells. *Gann, 70,* 131 (1979).

105. M. Hosokawa, M. Kasai, H. Yamaguchi, and H. Kobayashi, Increased immunosensitivity of xenogenized tumor cells to lymphocyte cytotoxicity. In H. Kobayashi, Ed., *Immunological Xenogenization of Tumor Cells* (*GANN Monograph on Cancer Research,* No. 23), Japan Scientific Societies Press, Tokyo, University Park Press, Baltimore, 1979, p. 73.

106. M. Kasai, R. F. Irie, E. C. Holmes, and K. Irie, Increased cytotoxic sensitivity of mumps virus-infected melanoma cells to antibody from melanoma patients. *Proc. AACR and ASCO, 21,* 220 (1980).

107. M. Kasai, H. Yamaguchi, M. Hosokawa, Y. Mizushima, and H. Kobayashi, Increased sensitivity of murine leukemia virus-infected tumor cells to lymphocyte-mediated cytotoxicity. *J. Natl. Cancer Inst., 67,* 417 (1981).

108. T. Moriuchi, E. Gotohda, T. Kodama, M. Hosokawa, and H. Kobayashi, Correlation between concanavalin A agglutinability and cytotoxic sensitivity to antiserum against tumor-associated antigen in rat fibrosarcoma cells. *J. Natl. Cancer Inst., 62,* 579 (1979).

109. G. Klein and E. Klein, Immune surveillance against virus-induced tumors and nonrejectability of spontaneous tumors: Contrasting consequences of host *versus* tumor evolution. *Proc. Natl. Acad. Sci. (USA), 74,* 2121 (1977).

110. J. F. Watkins and L. Chen, Immunization of mice against Ehrlich ascites tumour using a hamster/Ehrlich ascites tumour hybrid cell lines, *Nature, 223,* 1018 (1969).

111. B. S. Kim, Tumor-specific immunity induced by somatic hybrids. II. Elicitation of enhanced immunity against the parent plasmacytoma. *J. Immunol., 123,* 739 (1979).

112. M. C. Yoshida, Regression of Ehrlich ascites tumor in mice immunized by interspecific hybrid cells. *Proc. Jap. Acad., 55,* 238 (1979).

113. G. Klein and E. Klein, Induction of tumor cell rejection in the low responsive YAC-lymphoma strain A host combination by immunization with somatic cell hybrids. *Eur. J. Cancer, 15,* 551 (1979).

114. G. Klein, Antigenic expression in somatic hybrids and the use of fusion in tumor xenogenization. In H. Kobayashi, Ed., *Immunological Xenogenization of Tumor Cells* (*GANN Monograph on Cancer Research,* No. 23), Japan Scientific Societies, Tokyo, University Park Press, Baltimore, 1979, p. 225.

115. M. S. Murphy, J. Belehradek, Jr., and G. Barski, Interspecies mouse x Akodon urichi somatic cell hybrids: Comparative immunogenicity of parental and hybrid cells. *Eur. J. Cancer, 12,* 33 (1976).

116. R. Favre, Y. Carcassonne, and G. Meyer, Loss of antitumour immunogenicity of a somatic cell hybrid line with increasing subculture, *Br. J. Cancer, 32,* 10 (1975).

117. B. Zbar, S. Sukurmar, and H. J. Rapp, Immunoprophyloxis of syngeneic murine sarcomas with BCG and tumor cells. *Proc. AACR and ASCO, 20,* 55 (1979).

118. G. L. Bartlett and J. W. Kreider, Active, tumor-specific immunotherapy of LSTRA murine

leukemia using irradiated tumor cells and *Corynebacterium parvum. Proc. AACR and ASCO,* **20,** 189 (1979).

119. M. J. Titus, G. L. Bartlett, and J. W. Kreider, Local effects in the prevention of tumor cell immunization by supraoptimal doses of admixed *Corynebacterium parvum. Proc. AACR and ASCO,* **21,** 217 (1980).

120. R. W. Baldwin and V. S. Byers, Immunoregulation by bacterial organisms and their role in the immunotherapy of cancer. *Springer Semin. Immunopathol.* **2,** 79 (1979).

121. D. V. Schapira, C. S. McCune, and E. C. Henshaw, Treatment of advanced renal cell carcinoma with specific immunotherapy of autologous tumor cells and *C. parvum. Proc. AACR and ASCO,* **20,** 348 (1979).

122. B. Zbar and T. Tanaka, Immunotherapy of cancer: regression of tumors after intralesional injection of living *Mycobacterium bovis. Science,* **172,** 271 (1971).

123. B. Zbar, I. D. Bernstein, G. L. Bartlett, M. G. Hanna, Jr., and H. J. Rapp, Immunotherapy of cancer: regression of intradermal tumors and prevention of growth of lymph node metastases after intralesional injection of living *Mycobacterium bovis. J. Natl. Cancer Inst.,* **49,** 119 (1972).

124. B. Zbar, Tumor regression mediated by *Mycobacterium bovis* (strain BCG). *Natl. Cancer Inst. Monogr.,* **35,** 341 (1972).

125. H. B. Hewitt, The choice of animal tumors for experimental studies of cancer therapy. In G. Klein and S. Weinhouse, Ed., *Advances in Cancer Research,* Vol. 27, Academic, New York, 1979, p. 149.

126. M. V. Pimm, M. J. Embleton, and R. W. Baldwin, Multiple antigenic specificities within primary 3-methylcholanthrene-induced rat sarcomas and metastases. *Internatl. J. Cancer,* **25,** 621 (1980).

127. W. J. Martin, J. G. Gipson, and J. M. Rice, H-2^a associated alloantigen expressed by several transplantally induced lung tumor of C3Hf mice. *Nature,* **26,** 738 (1977).

128. A. B. Wrathmell, C. L. Gauci, and P. Alexander, Cross reactivity of an alloantigen present on normal cells with the tumour-specific transplantation-type antigen of the acute myeloid leukemia (SAL) of rats. *Br. J. Cancer,* **33,** 187 (1976).

129. C. E. Whitmire and R. J. Huebner, Inhibition of chemical carcinogenesis by viral vaccines. *Science,* **177,** 60 (1972).

130. F. Sendo, T. Miyake, S. Fuyama, and S. Arai, Spontaneous regression of syngeneic transplanted tumor in rats pretreated with the antileukemia drug busulfan. *J. Natl. Cancer Inst.,* **60,** 385 (1978).

131. J. L. Biedler and H. Riehm, Reduced tumor producing capacity of Chinese hamster cells resistant to actinomycin D and daunomycin. *Proc. AACR and ASCO,* **11,** 8 (1970).

132. J. L. Biedler and R. H. F. Peterson, Reduced tumorigenicity of syngeneic mouse sarcoma cells resistant to actinomycin D and ethidium bromide. *Proc. AACR and ASCO,* **14,** 72 (1973).

133. E. Bonmassar, A. Bonmassar, S. Vadlamudi, and A. Goldin, Immunological alteration of leukemic cells *in vivo* after treatment with an antitumor drug. *Proc. Natl. Acad. Sci. (USA),* **66,** 1089 (1970).

134. E. Mihich, Tumor immunogenicity in therapeutics. In E. Mihich, Ed., *Drug Resistance and Selectivity: Biochemical and Cellular Basis,* Academic, New York, 1973, pp. 413–452.

135. A. Nicolin, S. Vadlamudi, and A. Goldin, Antigenicity of L1210 leukemic sublines induced by drugs. *Cancer Res.,* **32,** 653 (1972).

136. E. Bonmassar, A. Bonmassar, S. Vadlamudi, and A. Goldin, Antigenic changes of L1210 leukemia in mice treated with 5-(3, 3-dimethyl-1-triazeno) imidazole-4-carboxamide. *Cancer Res.,* **32,** 1446 (1972).

137. M. C. Fioretti, Immunopharmacology of 5-(3, 3-diethyl-1-triazeno)-imidazole-4-carboxamide (DTIC), *Pharmacological Research Communications,* **7**, 481 (1975).

138. T. Boon and A. Van Pel, Teratocarcinoma cell variants rejected by syngeneic mice: Protection of mice immunized with these variants against other variants and against the original malignant cell line. *Proc. Natl. Acad. Sci. (USA),* **75**, 1519 (1978).

139. A. Van Pel, M. Georlette, and T. Boon, Tumor cell variants obtained by mutagenesis of a Lewis lung carcinoma cell line: Immune rejection by syngeneic mice. *Proc. Natl. Acad. Sci. (USA),* **76**, 5282 (1979).

140. B. Stück, L. J. Old, and E. A. Boyse, Antigenic conversion of established leukemias by an unrelated leukemogenic virus. *Nature,* **202**, 1016 (1964).

141. V. P. Hamburg and G. J. Svet-Moldavsky, Artificial heterogenization of tumors by means of herpes simplex and polyoma virus. *Nature,* **203**, 772 (1964).

142. V. P. Hamburg and G. J. Svet-Moldavsky, Suppression of viral and chemical carcinogenesis by means of artifical heterogenization. *Nature,* **215**, 1300 (1967).

143. G. J. Svet-Moldavsky and V. P. Hamburg, Quantitative relationship in viral oncolysis and the possibility of artificial heterogenization of tumors. *Nature,* **8**, 303 (1964).

144. G. J Svet-Moldavsky and V. P. Hamburg, An approach to the immunological treatment of tumors by artificial heterogenization. *Specific Tumor Antigens,* **2**, 323 (1967).

145. H. O. Sjögren and I. Hellström, Induction of polyoma specific transplantation antigenicity in Moloney leukemic cells. *Exp. Cell. Res.,* **40**, 208 (1965).

146. H. O. Sjögren and I. Hellström, *In vivo* and *in vitro* demonstration of the polyoma specific transplantation antigen induced in polyoma infected Moloney lymphoma cells. *Specific Tumor Antigens,* **2**, 162 (1967).

147. M. Hosokawa, T. Kodama, F. Sendo, N. Takeichi, and H. Kobayashi, Immunological characteristics of methylcholanthrene-induced tumors exposed to Friend virus, *J. Cancer Immunopathol.,* **3**, 42 (1967).

148. G. Pasternak and L. Pasternak, Demonstration of Graffi leukemia virus and virus-induced antigens in leukemic and nonleukemic tissues of mice. *J. Natl. Cancer Inst.,* **38**, 157 (1967).

149. J. Eiselein and M. W. Biggs, Observations with a variant of lymphocytic choriomeningitis virus in mouse tumors, *Cancer Res.,* **30**, 1953 (1970).

150. F. Sendo, H. Kaji, H. Saito, and H. Kobayashi, Antigenic modification of rat tumor cells artificially infected with Friend virus in the primary autochthonous host. *Gann,* **61**, 223 (1970).

151. T. Kodama, E. Gotohda, N. Takeichi, N. Kuzumaki, and H. Kobayashi, Histopathology of immunologic regression of tumor metastasis. *J. Natl. Cancer Inst.,* **52**, 931 (1979).

152. H. Kobayashi, T. Kodama, T. Shirai, H. Kaji, M. Hosokawa, F. Sendo, H. Saito, and N. Takeichi, Artificial regression of rat tumors infected with Friend virus (xenogenization): An effect produced by acquired antigen. *Hokkaido J. Med. Sci.,* **44**, 133 (1969).

153. O. A. Holterman and J. A. Majde, Rejection of skin and tumor grafts from mice chronically infected with lymphocytic choriomeningitis virus by non-infected syngeneic recipients. *Nature,* **223**, 624 (1969).

154. I. K. Al-Ghazzouli, R. M. Donahoe, K.-Y. Huang, B. Sass, R. L. Peters, and G. J. Kelloff, Immunity to virus-free syngeneic tumor cell transplantation in the BALB/c mouse after immunization with homologous tumor cells infected with type C virus. *J. Immunol.,* **117**, 2239 (1976).

155. J. S. Greenberger and S. A. Aaronson, *In vivo* inoculation of RNA C-type viruses inducing regression of experimental solid tumors, *J. Natl. Cancer Inst.,* **51**, 1935 (1973).

156. M. A. Basombrio, Antigenic conversion of established tumors with the Moloney sarcoma virus. *Proc. AACR and ASCO,* **13**, 74 (1972).

157. N. Kuzumaki, E. M. Fenyö, E. Klein, and G. Klein, Protective effect of murine sarcoma virus (MSV)-superinfected mouse tumor cells against the outgrowth of the corresponding non-infected tumor. *Transplantation,* **26**, 304 (1978).

158. A. Ishimoto, J. Hartley, and W. Rowe, Infection of hamster cells with Friend virus, *J. Virology* (in press).

159. K. Yamada and M. Hatano, Lowered transplantability of cultured tumor cells by persistent infection with paramyxovirus (HVJ). *Gann,* **63**, 647 (1972).

160. L. M. Reid, C. L. Jones, and J. Holland, Virus carrier state suppresses tumorigenicity of tumor cells in athymic (nude) mice. *J. Gen. Virol.,* **42**, 609 (1979).

161. T. Kodama, H. Kato, E. Gotohda, H. Kobayashi, and F. Sendo, Regression of established tumors in rats by injection of diethylaminoethyl-dextran and Friend murine leukemia virus. *J. Natl. Cancer Inst.,* **61**, 403 (1978).

162. T. Itaya, T. Moriuchi, T. Kodama, and H. Kobayashi, Regression mechanism of xenogenized tumor cells in the view point of humoral immunity. *Proc. Jap. Cancer Assoc.,* **37**, 85 (1978) (in Japanese).

14

Immunotherapy Trials with Neuraminidase-Modified Tumor Cells

J. GEORGE BEKESI
JAMES F. HOLLAND
JULIA P. ROBOZ
Department of Neoplastic Diseases
The Mount Sinai School of Medicine and Hospital
New York, New York

This work was supported in part by grant No. CA-1-5936-02, NCI Immunotherapy Program No. 1-CO-43225, and the T. J. Martell Memorial fund for Leukemia Research.

We express our appreciation to the Behring Institute, Behringwerek AG, Marburg, Federal Republic of Germany, for supplying the highly purified neuraminidase for this study. We also thank Ms. Diane Andujar for the excellent secretarial assistance.

441

1. INTRODUCTION

The possibility of utilizing modified tumor cells as immunogen is a potentially significant application of immunotherapy in the treatment of human neoplastic diseases.

Varying degrees of immunity have been achieved by immunization of experimental animals with x-irradiated tumor cells (1–5), tumor cells modified with iodoacetamide, iodoacetate or *N*-ethylmaleimide (5–10), cultured nontumorigenic ascites tissue culture cells (11), and concanavalin A (Con A)-treated tumor cells (12).

Immunotherapy has been actively persued in human cancer since the original observations of Mathe et al. (13–17), who used allogeneic irradiated myeloblasts and BCG as specific and nonspecific immunostimulants in human leukemia. In 1971 the British Medical Research Council (18) was unable to corroborate Mathe's findings. This was in part ascribed to immunosuppression due to vincristine or adamantine treatment. Similar studies were subsequently undertaken by Crowther et al. (19), Powles et al. (20,21), Powles (22), Gutterman et al. (23), Vogler and Chan (24) and reviewed by Hersh et al. (25) and Mastrangelo et al. (26). These investigators reported possible differences in remission duration between groups of patients who received chemotherapy alone or those who received immunotherapy in addition. Relapsed patients were reported to have higher frequency and greater "ease" of reinduction. Bacillus Calmette-Guerin (BCG) has been used in conjunction with cultured leukemic cells in the immunization of patients with chronic myelocytic leukemia by Sokal et al. (27–29). Under optimal conditions prolonged survival of chronic myelogenous leukemia (CML) patients was achieved as compared to the chemotherapy control group. Effectiveness of immunotherapy with BCG plus cultured irradiated melanoma cells was reported by Morton et al. (30,31) in Stages II and III melanoma patients. Although results reported by Morton et al. (30, 31) and Goodnight and Morton (32) have been encouraging, their control patient group was historical, and thus no definite conclusion can be derived from their study.

Increased immunogenicity of human and experimental tumors following treatment with neuraminidase of *Vibrio cholerae* origin has been shown in

TABLE 1. Successful Immunization with Neuraminidase-Modified Experimental Tumor Cells

Host	Tumor	Reference
Mouse	TA3 carcinoma	101–103
Mouse	Landschutz ascites tumor	99,104
Mouse	Leukemia L1210	39,40,45,46 49, 53–56, 105,106
Mouse	Ehrlich ascites carcinoma	101
Mouse	MC-induced fibrosarcoma	51,52 107–110, 112,132
Mouse	Squamous cell carcinoma	111
Mouse	B-16 melanoma	52
Guinea pig	Melanoma	113
Mouse	Lewis adenocarcinoma	111
Rat	Rhabdomyosarcoma	114
Mice	Yoshida sarcoma	115
Rat	WFCC-3 adenocarcinoma of colon	116
Mouse	Dunn osterosarcoma	117
Mouse	Mammary adenocarcinoma	118
Mouse	AKR leukemia	39,40,105,119
Dog	Mammary tumor	120–124
Mouse	6C3HED-lymphosarcoma	125

animal (Table 1) and clinical studies (33–42) to have practical value in the treatment of neoplastic diseases. The observed increase in tumor immunogenicity can be attributed exclusively to the enzymatic release of N-acetylneuraminic acid (sialic acid) (NANA) from the surface of tumor cells (43–56). The objectives of this chapter are to examine (1) the biological role of NANA in glycoproteins and changes induced by treatment with neuraminidase, (2) the effectiveness of neuraminidase-modified spontaneous and transplantable tumor cells as immunogen in both immunoprophylaxis and immunotherapeutic experiments in experimental animals, (3) the nature and specificity of immunity induced by neuraminidase-modified tumor cells, and (4) therapeutic advantage of combining neuraminidase-treated allogeneic myeloblasts with a highly effective remission inducing and sustaining chemotherapy protocol in humans for treatment of acute myelocytic leukemia as compared to the use of chemotherapy alone.

Hirst (57) and Burnet (58) made the pioneering observation that red blood cells (RBC) were irreversibly agglutinated by fluids containing infectious influenza virus. Later, Burnet (58) and Gottschalk (59) demonstrated that agglutination can be prevented by addition of a mucoproteinlike substance. The inhibitory property of these mucoproteins was lost, however, when treated with living influenza virus or *V. cholerae* culture filtrate. Blix et al. (60) and Suttajit and Winzler (61) reported that all virus hemagglutinin inhibitors are glycoproteins containing sialic acid. Sialic acid, in turn, is the constituent cleaved off by virus particles and *V. cholerae* filtrate enzyme in the inactivation reaction. The enzyme embedded in the influenza virus surface and present in the *V. cholerae* filtrate was termed *neuraminidase* (EC3.2.1.18), and its action was defined as a hydrolytic cleavage of the glycosidic link between the keto group of the NANA to the D-galactose, the penultimate carbohydrate of the oligosaccharide chain (59,62,63). Different types of neuraminidase have been found in myxoviruses (64–66), various bacteria, protozoa, and different vertebrate organs (65, 66). The various enzymes differ in their substrate specificities. It is now well established that the neuraminidase of *V. cholerae* splits the 2-3, 2-4, 2-6, and 2-8 glycosidic linkages (Figure 1) with different reaction rates. Newcastle disease-virus and influenza virus neuraminidase split only the 2-3 and 2-8 glycosidic linkages (66). Most of the work related to glycoproteins in cell biology and tumor immunotherapy has been performed with *V. cholerae* neuraminidase because this enzyme cleaves a broad range of α-O-ketosidically linked *N*-acetylneuraminic acid (Figure 1).

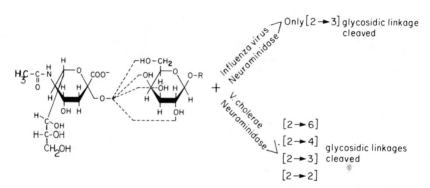

Figure 1. Action of neuraminidase on the possible glycosidic linkages between NANA and the penultimate sugar residue of glycoproteins.

Recently, considerable effort has been devoted to elucidate the biological role of sialic acid in normal and neoplastic tissues (45,47,48,50,53,54, 67–70). A possible structure of the polysaccharide portion of the plasma membrane of normal and neoplastic cell is presented in Figure 2. Mucins, which serve as protective coat and lubricant, contain closely spaced sialic acid moieties that, because of their mutual electrostatic repulsion, cause expansion and rigidity to the molecule (71). Removal of NANA by N'ase causes a marked decrease in viscosity and concomitant loss of biological activity of this glycoprotein.

Morell et al. (72) demonstrated that intravenous injection of desialylated glycoproteins (orosomucoid, fetuin, ceruloplasmin, haptoglobulin, and β_2-macroglobulin) into rats resulted in their prompt removal from the circulation and concomitant accumulation within the parenchymal cells of the liver. Pricer and Ashwell (73) have shown that NANA plays a major role in determining

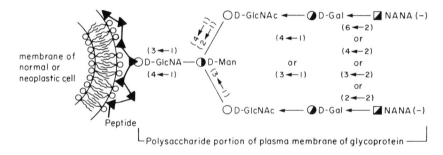

Figure 2. Possible structure for the polysaccharide portion of the plasma membrane glyco-protein.

the fate of serum glycoproteins in circulation. Enzymatic removal of this sugar residue results in exposure of the penultimate galactosyl residues, which, in turn, serves as a recognition signal for prompt hepatic binding and transport of the NANA-deficient molecules. Treatment of asialocaeruloplasmin with galactose oxidase or with galactosidase produced striking changes in the normal survival time of these serum glycoproteins. This led to the realization that the viability of many of the serum glycoproteins, including biologically potent glycoproteins, such as human chorionic gonadotropin and follicle-stimulating hormones, depend on the presence of normal complement of NANA (74). In addition, NANA is involved in the migration of transfused lympho-cytes and peritoneal macrophages (75,76). Treatment of normal or neoplastic cells with neuraminidase yielded reduction of negative cell-surface charge and decreased the electrophoretic mobility of the cells and caused an increase in cellular deformability (77–81). Removal of the NANA residue reduced the energy barriers that hindered cell-to-cell interaction (78–81), increased cell adherence (82,83) and aggregation (84,85), facilitated macrophage phagocyto-sis (78,86), opsonization of neuraminidase-treated sheep red blood cells (87), and increased macrophage cytotoxicity (88). Enhanced lymphocyte function was observed in one-way MLC when the target lymphocytes were pretreated with neuraminidase (89–92). Similarly, an increase in blastogenic response to Con A and pokeweed mitogens was noted with treated peripheral blood lymph-ocytes (93–95). In addition, NANA is directly involved in the inhibition of sperm penetration of rabbit ova (96) and in determining the transport of po-tassium and protein across the membrane of leukemia L1210 tumor cells (97,98).

2. THERAPEUTIC EFFECTIVENESS OF NEURAMINIDASE-TREATED TUMOR CELLS IN EXPERIMENTAL-ANIMAL TUMOR SYSTEMS

The immune surveillance system of animals bearing experimental tumors has been the subject of intensive investigation. Currie and Bagshawe (43,99), Sanford (100), and Lindemann (101) investigated the role of the terminal sugar residue, NANA acid in determining the antigenicity of neoplastic cells. The following tumor systems were used by these investigators: Landschutz ascites tumor, chemically induced fibrosarcoma, leukemia L1210, TA3 ascites tumor, and Ehrlich ascites carcinoma. It was consistently observed that under optimal conditions, *V. cholerae* neuraminidase treatment, by exposing the penultimate galactosyl residues, increased the immunogenicity of experimental tumors and protected against untreated, viable syngeneic tumor challenge. Table 1 summarizes studies that were performed since 1967 in a variety of experimental tumor systems. By causing major alteration in the self-expression of tumor cells, treatment with neuraminidase of *V. cholerae* origin induced tumor specific immunity in syngeneic and autochthonous host. However, certain systems, as a consequence of tumor enhancement elicited by antigenic excess and immunotherapy with neuraminidase-treated tumor cells alone or in combination with chemotherapy and/or adjuvant immunotherapy proved to be ineffectual (Table 2). Unfortunately, in most cases, even where successful immunotherapy was ultimately introduced, little attempt was made to establish optimal conditions such as total NANA content of tumor cells, enzyme concentration needed for cleavage of NANA, kinetics of NANA release, awareness of allosteric inhibitory property of NANA during incubation, dose and frequency of immunization, immunologic status of host (particularly when chemotherapy is also used), combination of chemotherapy with specific and/or adjuvant (BCG, MER, *C. parvum*) immunotherapy, and nature of immunity induced by the neuraminidase-treated cells alone or with immunoadjuvants. To establish baseline conditions for human immunotherapeutic investigations, these parameters must be defined and the various therapeutic modalities integrated. A summary of experience with murine leukemias as a basis for the treatment of human AML is presented in the following paragraphs.

The kinetics of NANA release from a variety of tumor cells have been studied. The quantitation of total and neuraminidase-susceptible NANA in tu-

TABLE 2.   Unsuccessful Immunization with Neuraminidase-Modified Experimental Tumor Cells

Host	Tumor	Reference
Mouse	TA3 carcinoma	127
Mouse	Leukemia L1210	54
Mouse	AKR leukemia	126,128
Mouse	B-16 melanoma	129
Rat	Fibrosarcoma,	
	Mammary carcinoma	130
Mouse	Fibrosarcoma	112,131,132
Mouse	Glioma	133
Dog	Mammary tumor	120
Mouse	6C3HED-lymphosarcoma	125

mor cells must be established to ensure the reproducibility of immunogen for immunotherapy. A specific and sensitive mass spectrometric procedure was developed by Roboz et al. (134,135), and the well-known colorimetric method was modified to provide the needed specificity for determination of NANA in biological samples (136). Data obtained in analytical studies (134,136) indicate that the total covalently bound NANA varies significantly in various tumors: for mouse lymphocytes, 0.37 μmoles; for AKR spontaneous leukemia, 0.25 μmoles; for E2G leukemia, 0.41 μmoles; for leukemia L1210, 0.68 μmoles; and for sarcoma 180, 1.86 μmoles. For solid tumors, MTV induced mammary carcinoma, 0.28 μmoles; for 6C3HED lymphosarcoma, 0.63 μmoles; for Walker-256 carcinosarcoma, 3.01 μmoles; and for B-16 melanoma, 12.9 μmoles per 10^9 tumor cells.

Incubation of tumor cells without *V. cholerae* neuraminidase released negligible quantity of bound NANA and the cells produced tumor in syngeneic host. Incubation with various concentrations of *V. cholerae* neuraminidase can result in the following changes of antigenicity of tumor cells in leukemia L1210, 6C3HED lymphosarcoma, AKR leukemia and E2G leukemia:

1. At low enzyme concentration, cleavage of neuraminidase-susceptible NANA is incomplete and all recipients die from tumor after being injected with neuraminidase-treated tumor cells.

2. At optimal enzyme concentration, which is fifteen- to thirtyfold excess of enzyme to susceptible NANA molecules, about 70% of total NANA is cleaved in 45 minutes. The treated leukemic cells remained morphologically intact with no marked change in their permeability to trypan blue (70 to 90%) but could not initiate tumor growth in syngeneic host injected i.p. or intradermally (i.d.) (39,40,43,46,49,53, 54–56 106,125).

3. Despite the absence of any detectable proteolytic activity in neuraminidase preparation, use of greater than fiftyfold excess to NANA available on the cell surface rapidly increased the permeability of tumor cells to trypan blue and at the same time decreased their immunogenicity as evidenced by decreased refractoriness to subsequent challenge of the immunized host (45,46,49,53,135).

To prove that the increased immunogenicity of tumor cells was attributable to the release of bound NANA by neuraminidase, tumor cells were incubated in the presence or absence of *V. cholerae* neuraminidase. No measurable low-molecular-weight substance was detectable in the incubate with buffer alone. In the incubates that contained tumor cells with neuraminidase, significant quantities of low-molecular-weight substances were found. They were identified as *N*-acetylneuraminic acid and *N*-glycolylneuraminic acid in a ratio of 20:1. Thus the increased immunogenicity of the neuraminidase-treated tumor cells is most likely attributable to the enzymatic removal of NANA rather than to the release of a nonspecific protein (45,48,103). Furthermore, treating the tumor cells with neuraminidase and then with α and β-galactosidase or periodate oxidation abrogated their immunogenicity (Figure 3). Loss of immunogenicity of tumor cells appears to indicate that the unmasked penultimate sugar residue D-galactose may be the tumor-specific transplantation antigenic (TSTA) determinant in the plasma membrane of the tumor cells, and this constitutes a recognition signal for the immune surveillance of the challenged host.

Neuraminidase from other sources, such as influenza virus or *Clostridium perfringens*, released significantly less measurable NANA from the tumor cells than did *V. cholerae* neuraminidase, and all recipient mice inoculated with influenza virus or *C. perfringens* neuraminidase died from tumor (43, 44–46, 47,50). *Vibrio cholerae* neuraminidase was also ineffective when the incubation was performed at pH 7.4 or in the absence of Ca^{2+} (46,137,138). Treatment of leukemia L1210 or Landschutz ascites tumor cells with proteolytic enzymes, such as trypsin, ribonuclease, deoxribonuclease, collagenase, and hyaluronidase, did not change the lethality of the tumor in syngeneic mice (43–45, 99,104).

3. IMMUNOGENICITY OF SPONTANEOUS AND TRANSPLANTABLE TUMOR CELLS FOLLOWING NEURAMINIDASE TREATMENT

The effect of treatment with varying concentrations of neuraminidase on the immunogenicity of leukemia L1210, Gross leukemia virus-induced leukemia,

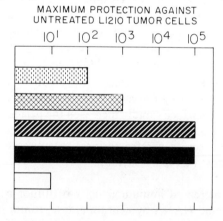

Figure 3. Effect of various treatments on the immunogenicity of leukemia L1210 in DBA/2 Ha mice. From left to right: (*a*) 10^7 formaldehyde-fixed L1210 cells were injected i.p.; (*b*) L1210 cells were exposed to 10,000-R x-irradiation and then 10^7 cells injected i.p.; (*c*) L1210 cells incubated with neuraminidase and then 10^7 cells were injected i.p. per mouse; (*d*) L1210 treated first with neuraminidase followed by trypsin and then 10^7 cells were injected i.p. per mouse; and (*e*) leukemia L1210 cells first treated with neuraminidase followed by α- and β-galactosidase and then 10^7 treated washed cells were injected i.p. per mouse. Challenge of the immunized DBA/2 mice was made 30 days after immunization by inoculating various challenge doses of untreated L1210 tumor cells.

and 6C3HED lymphosarcoma were tested in DBA2/BDF1, AKR, and C3H mice, respectively (39,40, 43–46, 49, 53–56, 105,106,125,138). In experiments with L1210 leukemia where low concentration of neuraminidase was used (less than number of NANA sites available) or where tumor cells were incubated in incubation media alone, DBA2 or BDF1 mice died from tumor after being injected with the treated cells. The immunogenicity of cells significantly increased after treatment with optimal concentration of neuraminidase (fifteen- to twentyfold excess of neuraminidase with respect to receptor sites), and all immunized animals were refractory to a challenge of 10^5 untreated L1210 cells. The LD_{100} in the DBA2/BDF animal system was one viable L1210 cell; thus the increase in resistance was about 100,000-fold (Figure 3). Refractoriness of mice to untreated leukemia L1210 cells, immunized once or at weekly intervals four times, was directly proportional to the number of neuraminidase-treated L1210 cells used as immunogen. However, mice whose immune status was impaired by prior treatment with x-irradiation or cytoxan succumbed to death by progressive growth of neuraminidase treated leukemic cells (44–46 49, 53). Whereas neuraminidase-treated leukemia L1210 cells under optimal condition significantly increased tumor immunogenicity, incubation performed in the presence of fiftyfold excess of neuraminidase gradually decreased immunogenicity of the cells, as manifested by decreased refractoriness of the immunized hosts toward untreated L1210 cell challenge (45,46,49,53). When a 200-fold excess of enzyme was used Bagshawe and Currie (43) failed to achieve protection of mice that under optimal conditions survived a primary injection of neuraminidase-treated L1210 cells against challenge doses higher than 8×10^3 viable untreated L1210 cells.

To compare the immunogenicity of formalin fixed, x-irradiated and neuraminidase-treated leukemia L1210 cells, DBA/2 mice were immunized with single or multiple doses of such cells. Figure 3 shows that when the resistance to leukomogenic challenge was measured, the neuraminidase-treated L1210 cells appeared to be 3 and 2 logs more immunogenic than formalin or x-irradiated L1210 cells, respectively (43, 44–46). Data presented in Table 3 show that leukemia L1210 cells exposed to 5000-R radiation before or after neuraminidase treatment or leukemic cells treated with neuraminidase in the presence of mitomycin C were as effective immunogen as leukemic cells treated with neuraminidase alone. This mode of combination treatment of tumor cells has practical significance in both clinical and experimental protocols where cytoreductive therapy is applied in conjunction with active immunotherapy to circumvent possible initiation of tumor growth in the immunosuppressed host, attributable to the resynthesis of surface membrane NANA (48).

Studies on the kinetics of host response after vaccination with neuraminidase-treated leukemia L1210 cells indicate measurable immunity against untreated L1210 cells as early as 5 days after immunization; reaching a peak in about 30 to 60 days when all mice became refractory to 10^5 untreated L1210 tumor cells. Even at 90 to 150 days after immunization, most challenged mice resisted 10^4 to 10^5 untreated L1210 cells (40,44,46,49,138). Immunity induced

TABLE 3.   Immunogenicity of Leukemia L1210 Cells After Treatment with Neuraminidase, x-Irradiation, or Trypsin in DBA/2 Mice

Treatment of Leukemia L1210 cells	Challenge Dose[a]	[51]Cr Cytotoxicity Assay[b]	
		Antibody Titer	Cellular Cytotoxicity (0/0 ± SE)
Neuraminidase	10^7	1024	28.1 ± 2.9
x-Irradiated (5000 R)	10^4	512	3.3 ± 0.5
x-Irradiated (5000 R) then neuraminidase	10^7	1024	22.5 ± 3.6
Neuraminidase then x-Irradiated (5000 R)	10^7	1024	26.1 ± 3.2
Neuraminidase plus mitomycin C	10^7	1024	27.9 ± 4.1
Trypsin followed by neuraminidase	10^6	512	20.3 ± 2.2
Neuraminidase followed by trypsin	—	—	—
Neuraminidase plus MER[c]	10^5	1024	2.5 ± 0.3

[a]Mice were immunized with 10^7-treated leukemia L1210 cells on days, 0, 7, 14, and 21. Challenge with untreated L1210 cells was done 21 days after the last immunization i.p.

[b]For the ^{51}Cr cytotoxicity assay sera and lymphocytes were obtained 15 days after a challenge with untreated leukemia L1210 cells.

[c]Mice were immunized with 10^7 neuraminidase-treated L1210 cells (i.p.) and 0.1 mg MER (s.c.) on days 0, 7, 14, and 21. Challenge with untreated L1210 cells was done 21 days after the last immunization (i.p.).

by neuraminidase-treated L1210 cells is specific, the immunized mice were refractory to challenge with untreated L1210 cells but remained as susceptible as the controls to sarcoma 180, Ehrlich ascites carcinoma, Krebs-2 tumor, or transplant of spontaneous mammary tumor (44–46, 49). Because of the etiologic difference between transplantable tumor and virally induced neoplasia, a great deal of attention has been directed to the study of the response to immunotherapy of three experimental animal systems: (1) AKR mice where the vertically transmitted Gross leukemia virus (MuLV) is the etiologic agent of the spontaneous leukemia/lymphoma (139–145); (2) mammary tumor virus (MTV)-free (MTV–) C3H mice; and (3) MTV-infected (MTV+) C3H mice.

The immunoprotection of young AKR mice was investigated in a manner similar to that of the L1210/DBA2 system. The use of both neuraminidase-treated spontaneous leukemic thymocytes and allogeneic E2G leukemic cells resulted in a significant delay of the appearance of the primary lymphoma in AKR mice (105,119,138). This observation is consistent with the findings by Oldstone et al. (142) that MuLV-infected AKR mice manifest no immunologic tolerance against MuLV-induced leukemia but lack the complement C5 fraction, thus leading to renal deposit of IgG-antigen complex. Immunization performed with untreated E2G ♀ leukemic cells or neuraminidase-treated leukemia L1210 cells, or normal (AKR) thymocytes was ineffectual, and the treated mice died at about the same rate as did the control animals (Figure 4). It is particularly significant that the allogeneic MuLV induced E2G♀ leukemic cells used as immunogen were as effective in delaying the appearance of primary lymphoma as were the syngeneic AKR leukemic thymocytes (119,138). This system may, therefore, represent the best model for working out optimal conditions for chemoimmunotherapy with the use of allogeneic leukemic blast cells as immunogen in human leukemia.

The effectiveness of neuraminidase-treated 6C3HED lymphosarcoma, which is syngeneic in both MTV-free and MTV-infected C3H mice, was tested in an immunoprophylactic therapy protocol. Mammary tumor virus-free C3H mice that have been repeatedly immunized with neuraminidase-treated 6C3HED tumor cells resisted a challenge of 10^6 untreated 6C3HED tumor cells inoculated i.p., whereas all control animals died after injection with less than 10 cells. In contrast, there was no increase in the refractoriness to challenge when MTV-infected C3H mice were immunized (125). Failure of the immune system in the "immunized" MTV-infected C3H mice to cope with the challenging lymphosarcoma, even at low numbers, was reflected not in the absence of humoral response, but in relatively poor cell-mediated immunity (125,146, 147).

This apparent immunologic deficiency observed in the MTV-infected C3H mice could be obviated by the transfer of lymphocytes from MTV-free C3H mice that have been immunized with neuraminidase-treated cells. The recipient MTV-infected mice were then able to reject a subsequent challenge with lymphosarcoma tumor grafts.

Increase in immunogenicity of experimental tumors, as a direct consequence of neuraminidase-treatment, has been reported in a variety of other tumor-host systems (Tables 1 and 2). However, the mechanism(s) that plays (play) central role(s) for the inhibition of neuraminidase-treated tumor cells to induce tumor in a syngeneic host is still not well understood. One hypothesis, namely, that neuraminidase treatment increases the immunogenicity of treated tumor cells by unmasking the penultimate galactose residue, thus sending specific recognition signals to the host immune surveillance system, appears to have gained general acceptance (43,45,46,49, 53–56, 88,100,102,104,108,109,118, 125). In support of this theory is the fact that the neuraminidase-treated tumor cells in the immunosuppressed hosts are able to restore the neuraminidase-cleaved NANA within 16 to 18 hours and thus to commence uninhibited tumor growth (48,49,53). This supports the view that neuraminidase treatment does not influence cell viability or the malignant state of tumor growth. Data in Figure 5 indicate that the galactose residue on the surface of neuraminidase-treated tumor cells renders the treated L1210 tumor cells to be receptive to factor(s) that appears (appear) to be essential for the selective processing of

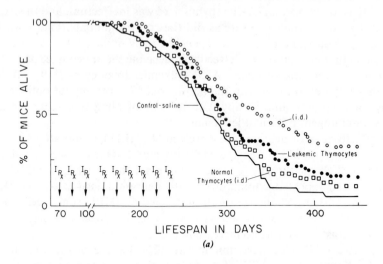

EFFECT OF PREIMMUNIZATION WITH NEURAMINIDASE
TREATED NORMAL OR LEUKEMIC THYMOCYTES ON THE
APPEARANCE OF SPONTANEOUS LEUKEMIA IN AKR MICE

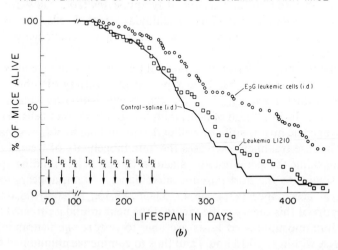

EFFECT OF PREIMMUNIZATION WITH NEURAMINIDASE
TREATED ALLOGENEIC E_2G OR L1210 LEUKEMIC CELLS ON
THE APPEARANCE OF SPONTANEOUS LEUKEMIA IN AKR MICE

Figure 4. Effect of immunotherapy with neuraminidase-treated normal and leukemic thymocytes on the appearance of primary leukemia in AKR mice. (*a*) Mice were immunized
at days indicated with 2×10^7 cells with normal thymocytes ($\square$), leukemic thymocytes
injected i.p. ($\bullet$), leukemic thymocytes injected i.d. ($\bigcirc$), control—saline, control—
0.9% NaCl; (*b*) AKR mice were preimmunized with neuraminidase-treated E2G or
L1210 tumor cells as in group *a* experiments.

tumor antigen(s) (102,103). Sanford and Codington (102), Sethi and Brandis (49,88) and Schlesinger and Bekesi (148) indeed demonstrated the existence of a heat-labile factor present in normal mouse sera capable of exerting cytotoxic effects on neuraminidase-treated, but not non-neuraminidase-treated, tumor cells. On injection into the peritoneal cavity of normal DBA/2 mice, the neuraminidase-treated L1210 cells rapidly disappeared ($T_{1/2}$ 20 hours). This process was inoperable, however, if the neuraminidase-treated tumor cells were treated with α- and β-galactosidase, the galactose residue were oxidized by periodate, or L1210 cells were treated with formalin or x-irradiation.

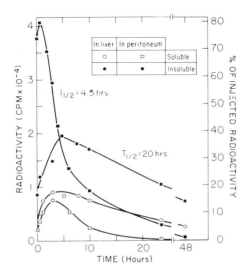

Figure 5. Fate of neuraminidase-treated ^{14}C-labeled leukemia L1210 cells in normal DBA/2 Ha mice. The L1210 cells were labeled *in vivo* with glucosamine ^{14}C followed by treatment with neuraminidase and then 5×10^7 L1210 tumor cells injected i.p. per mouse. At preselected time intervals a group of mice were killed and the soluble and insoluble radioactivity in each organ determined.

4. CHARACTERISTICS OF IMMUNITY INDUCED BY NEURAMINIDASE-TREATED TUMOR CELLS IN EXPERIMENTAL ANIMALS

Neutralization and passive immunity experiments were performed to test the ability of serum and splenic lymphocytes of DBA/2 mice immunized against leukemia L1210 to transfer resistance against the disease (40,44,49,53,88,105, 125,138,149). Similar studies were done in MTV-free and (MTV)-infected C3H mice that had been immunized against 6C3HED lymphosarcoma (125). Table 4 illustrates that L1210 cells incubated *in vitro* with nonabsorbed anti-L1210 serum, or with serum repeatedly absorbed with normal or neuraminidase-treated splenic lymphocytes, produced no tumor when inoculated into normal DBA/2 mice. Tumor growth was evident when injected L1210 cells were preincubated with serum from nonimmune DBA/2 mice or from DBA/2 mice repeatedly immunized with neuraminidase-treated syngeneic lymphocytes or with anti-L1210 serum extensively absorbed with neuraminidase-treated L1210 cells, but not with sarcoma 180, P388, K36, and E2G leukemic cells. All these animals died as the controls when challenged with untreated leukemia L1210 cells.

Cell-mediated immunity has a central role in the rejection of tumor cells in experimental animals immunized with neuraminidase-treated tumor cells (40,44,49,53,125,149). Mice inoculated with 100,000 leukemia L1210 cells preincubated with immune lymphocytes (100:1 immune lymphocyte:tumor cell ratio or higher) failed to develop tumors in DBA/2 mice (Table 5). Ani-

TABLE 4. Neutralization of Leukemia L1210 Cells *in Vitro* with Sera from Immunized DBA/2 Mice

		Serum Dilution[e]			
		Undiluted		1:5	
Source of Sera	L1210 cells with	TF/T[f]	Survival Time (in Days)	TF/T[f]	Survival Time (in Days)
Normal DBA/2 mice	Unabsorbed sera	0/20	9.3 ± 1.1	0/20	9.2 ± 0.8
Mice immunized with splenic lymphocytes[a]	Unabsorbed sera	0/20	9.0 ± 1.0	0/20	9.5 ± 1.4
Mice immunized with leukemia L1210 cells[b]	Unabsorbed sera	20/20		8/20	18.2 ± 2.4
	Sera absorbed with L1210[c]	0/10	9.2 ± 1.2	0/20	8.9 ± 1.5
	Sera absorbed with lymphocytes[c]	20/20		6/20	17.9 ± 1.5
	Sera absorbed with lymphocytes[d]	20/20		8/20	18.1 ± 1.9

[a]DBA/2 mice were immunized with 10^6 neuraminidase-treated normal spleen cells on days 0, 7, 14, and 21. Mice were challenged with 10^5 untreated normal spleen cells 21 days after the last immunization. Sera were obtained 14 days after challenge.

[b]DBA/2 mice were immunized with 10^6 neuraminidase-treated leukemia L1210 cells on days, 0, 7, 14, and 21. Mice were then challenged with untreated L1210 tumor cells 21 days after the last immunization. Sera were obtained 15 days after the challenge.

[c]Treated with neuraminidase.

[d]Treated with deactivated neuraminidase.

[e]Preincubation: to 5 ml of unabsorbed or absorbed sera or diluted to 1:5 or 1:10 with PBS, 10^7 leukemia L1210 tumor cells were added, mixed, and then incubated at 37 °C. After 30 minutes of incubation, 0.5 ml of this cell suspension (containing 10^5 L1210 tumor cells) was inoculated i.p. in each of the 10 mice.

[f]Number of mice free of tumor at day 30 per number of mice receiving 10^5 leukemia L1210 transplant.

mals remaining free of tumor were refractory to subsequent challenge with 100,000 untreated leukemia L1210 cells. Preincubation of L1210 cells with splenic lymphocytes from DBA/2 mice immunized with neuraminidase-treated normal splenic lymphocytes, or lymphocytes from nonimmunized DBA/2 mice in a ratio of 300:1 lymphocytes to tumor cells did not prevent tumor growth, and as in the control group, all animals died from tumors. These observations provided convincing evidence that neuraminidase treated tumor cells induce strong humoral and cellular immunity (40,44,49,53,149), and this immunity can successfully be transferred to normal nonimmunized mice.

The participation of the T-cell subpopulation of splenic lymphocytes in cell-mediated immunity induced by neuraminidase-treated L1210 cells was

TABLE 5. Neutralization of Leukemia L1210 Cells *in Vitro* by Immune Lymphocytes

| | | Ratio of Spleen Cells to Tumor Cells | | | |
| | | 100:1 | | 300:1 | |
	Source of Spleen Cells	TF/T[c]	Challenge[d]	TF/T[c]	Challenge[d]
L1210 tumor cells were preincubated with spleen cells for 30 minutes at 37 °C prior to inoculation of tumor cells i.p.[a]	Normal DBA/2 mice	0/20		0/20	
	Mice immunized with splenic lymphocytes[b]	0/20		0/20	
	Mice immunized with leukemia L1210 cells[b]	14/20	12/14	20/20	20/20
	Immune spleen cells pretreated with normal AKR mouse sera + complement	13/20	12/13	20/20	20/20
	Immune spleen cells pretreated with antithymocyte sera + complement	0/20		0/20	
10⁵ L1210 tumor cells were transplanted i.p. 24 hours prior to the injection of splenic lymphocytes	Normal DBA/2 mice	0/20		0/20	
	Mice immunized with splenic lymphocytes[b]	0/20		0/20	
	Mice immunized with leukemia L1210 cells[b]	4/20	4/4	12/20	12/12

[a] 10^5 preincubated leukemia L1210 cells were injected intraperitoneally per each mouse.

[b] DBA/2 Ha mice were immunized with either neuraminidase-treated normal splenic lymphocytes or L1210 tumor cells as indicated in Table 4.

[c] Number of mice free of tumor at day 30 per number of mice inoculated with tumor.

[d] Number of mice free of tumor at day 30 per number of mice challenged with 10^5 untreated L1210 cells.

demonstrated. Immune lymphocytes pretreated with anti-θ serum plus rabbit complement lost their ability to neutralize the tumorigenicity of leukemia L1210 cells (Table 5). Similarly, immune lymphocytes pretreated with anti-θ serum and then cultured with specific T-cell mitogens demonstrated complete lack of stimulation by PHA and Con A. These pretreated immune lymphocytes failed to achieve cytolysis of leukemia L1210 or lymphosarcoma cells (40,44, 125,138,149). Participation of B lymphocytes in the immune lysis or their synergism with T lymphocytes in cell-mediated immunity reactions could not be conclusively established in these experiments (40,44,125,138,149,151).

To gain additional information on the nature of immunity, antibody titers and cellular immunity were examined *in vitro* following immunization with neuraminidase-treated tumor cells. Chromium-51 microcytotoxicity assays were performed to test the cell-mediated and humoral immunity in mice that were repeatedly immunized with neuraminidase-treated leukemia L1210 cells and challenged 21 days after the last immunization. Although no measurable humoral or cell-mediated immunity could be detected in DBA/2 mice immunized with neuraminidase-treated leukemia L1210 cells or in C3H mice (40,44,125,138,149) immunized with the lymphosarcoma at the time of the first challenge, the target cells preincubated with such sera or splenic lymphocytes lost their ability to produce tumor when inoculated in nonimmune mice (40,44,138,149). A challenge dose-dependent antibody titer and cell-mediated immunity were observed 15 days after the first challenge with viable leukemia L1210 cells. The data in Table 6 show the presence of a strong humoral and cellular immunity in mice immunized with neuraminidase-treated tumor cells. Extensive absorption with large numbers of syngeneic or allogeneic splenic lymphocytes, spontanous mammary carcinoma, or allogeneic K36 and E2G leukemic cells did not reduce the titer of anti-L1210 antiserum against leukemia L1210 antigen. These findings appear to indicate the specificity of immunity against leukemia antigens, and not against the histocompatibility or other tumor antigens.

It is noteworthy that mice that received multiple immunizations with x-irradiated leukemic cells or neuraminidase-treated L1210 cells plus MER showed strong antibody titer against L1210 tumor cells but virtually no cell-mediated immunity (Table 3). These observations appear to suggest that the mechanism by which the injected host processes the neuraminidase-treated or x-irradiated leukemic cells may be distinctly different.

Preventive immunotherapy has little usefulness to humans or to experimental animals with diagnosed neoplasia. For this reason it was of considerable importance to establish whether chemotherapy, which reduces the number of tumor cells to below the maximal tumor burden, thereby rendering the host's immune mechanism approachable, combined with active immunotherapy, might provide a better therapeutic approach in the tumor-bearing host.

To perform successful immunotherapy with the use of neuraminidase-treated syngeneic, autologous, or allogeneic tumor cells in tumor bearing mice after cytoreductive therapy, it was imperative to (1) establish the host immunocom-

TABLE 6. Increased Immunogenicity of Leukemia L1210 Cells After Neuraminidase Treatment[a]

Number of Leukemia L1210 Cells Used for Multiple Immunization	^{51}Cr Microcytotoxicity Assay[c]		
	Challenge Dose[b]	Antibody Titer	Cellular Cytotoxicity (% ± SE)
10^4	10^2	16	1.6 ± 0.5
10^5	10^4	64	8.2 ± 2.1
10^6	10^5	256	14.9 ± 3.6
10^7	10^7	1024	28.1 ± 2.9
10^7	10^7	8[d]	2.6 ± 0.9[e]
10^8	10^8	4096	43.5 ± 5.1
10^8	10^8	8[d]	1.9 ± 0.4[e]

[a] For each cell dose, 20 DBA/2 Ha mice were immunized with neuraminidase-treated leukemia L1210 cells on days 0, 7, 14, and 21.

[b] Immunized mice were challenged with the maximum tolerable dose of untreated leukemia L1210 cells 21 days after the last immunization.

[c] For the *in vitro* determination of immunity, sera and splenic lymphocytes were obtained 15 days after challenge of the immunized mice with untreated leukemia L1210 cells.

[d] Serum was absorbed with neuraminidase-treated leukemia L1210 cells.

[e] Effector cells pretreated with anti-(−) serum plus complement.

petence after cytoreductive therapy and (2) determine the susceptibility of the sensitized lymphocytes to various chemotherapeutic agents. Prednisone and cytoxan, at the optimal dose for complete eradication or marked reduction of tumor burden, caused long-lasting immunosuppression with slow recovery of immune function in tumor-bearing mice. Mice treated with these two therapeutic agents responded poorly to immunization with neuraminidase-treated L1210 cells (Figure 6). Methyl CCNU and methotrexate caused only moderate changes in the host immune system, and the treated mice responded quite well to immunization with neuraminidase-treated L1210 cells and to subsequent challenge with untreated L1210 cells. Susceptibility of sensitized lymphocytes in mice immunized with neuraminidase-treated L1210 cells was dependent on the chemotherapeutic agent as well as time elapsed after immunization (Figure 7). The use of prednisone, cytoxan, and methotrexate in treatment of "immunized" host resulted in almost complete abrogation of sensitized lymphocyte population, particularly if the treatment commenced during the first 15 days after immunotherapy. All such treated animals manifested minimal resistance against subsequent challenge with untreated leukemia L1210 cells. Methyl CCNU treatment produced the least change in the response of the sensitized lymphocyte subpopulation but still reduced the refractoriness of immunized DBA/2 mice to challenge by 2 logs as compared to the untreated im-

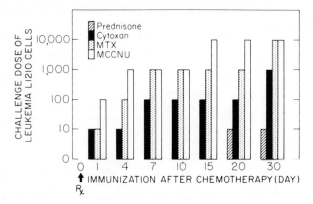

Figure 6.   Selective immunosuppression induced by various chemotherapeutic agents in DBA/2 mice. Chemotherapy: prednisone (45 mg/kg); cytoxan (135 mg/kg; methyl CCNU (20 mg/kg); methotrexate (45 mg/kg). At days indicated DBA/2 Ha mice were immunized with 10⁷ neuraminidase-treated L1210 tumor cells i.p. per mouse. Challenge of the immunized DBA/2 Ha mice was made 30 days after immunization by inoculating various challenge doses of L1210 cells.

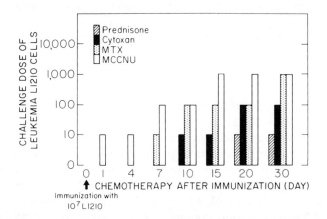

Figure 7.   Chemotherapy reduces the refractoriness of immunized DBA/2 mice to leukemia L1210 challenge. Mice were immunized with 10⁷ neuraminidase-treated L1210 cell i.p. per mouse. At days indicated mice were treated with one of the chemotherapeutic agents and challenged with untreated leukemia L1210 cells as described in the legend to Figure 5.

munized host. Thus chemotherapy significantly impaired the host ability to respond to immunization and significantly reduced the response to tumor challenge of the immunized animals. These observations were further substantiated by the assessment of the functional integrity of lymphocytes *in vitro* obtained from mice treated with various chemotherapeutic agents. Prednisone and cytoxan at the optimal dose for reduction of tumor burden caused significant reduction in blastogenesis by T-cell-specific mitogens (PHA and Con A) reflecting severe immunosuppression. Lymphocytes obtained from mice treated with methyl CCNU and BCNU showed only moderate changes in blastogenesis, and such mice responded well to specific immunization as early as 3 days after chemotherapy (40,44, 54–56, 105,138,149). These findings were further tested in a chemotherapeutic model by using DBA/2 mice with leukemia L1210.

All DBA/2 mice inoculated with 10 million leukemia L1210 cells died within 7 days. Figure 8 shows that when methyl CCNU, cytoxan, or methotrexate was injected within 2 days after the L1210 graft, survival increased, but only 10% of mice were cured (Figure 8). However, after a single dose of cytoxan, methyl CCNU, methotrexate, or BCNU plus immunization with neuraminidase-treated leukemia L1210 cells on day 4 after cytoreductive therapy, cure resulted in 20, 55, 40, and 40% of the immunized mice, respectively (40, 54–56, 105,138). If chemotherapy was delayed 3 to 5 days after tumor inoculation, the effect of immunotherapy was significantly reduced or completely eliminated due to the large tumor burden.

Immunization of mice with the nonspecific adjuvants BCG or MER augmented survival after chemotherapy, but to a significantly lesser degree. Combination of specific and nonspecific immunization after chemotherapy produced indefinite survival in a larger percentage of DBA/2 mice than either treatment alone (40, 54–56).

Immunotherapy of established leukemia L1210 with neuraminidase-treated L1210 cells or with MER alone without prior cytoreductive therapy did not significantly improve survival of the tumor-bearing host (40).

Mice that survived free of tumor after chemoimmunotherapy were refractory for up to 10^5 untreated leukemia L1210 cells and showed strong complement-dependent antibody titer and cell-mediated immunity, as determined by the ^{51}Cr microcytotoxicity assay. These observations led to study of chemoimmunotherapy in AKR mice with spontaneous leukemia (40,105,138,149).

5. CHEMOIMMUNOTHERAPY IN AKR MICE WITH SPONTANEOUS LEUKEMIA

The vertically transmitted Gross leukemia virus is the etiologic agent for leukemia in the AKR strain of mice. The time lapse between the first appearance of the viable leukemia cells in the thymus and the clinical diagnosis is about 30 days. The spontaneous leukemia in AKR mice has several characteristics similar to those of the human leukemias (139,145 152–158).

At the time of clinical diagnosis there are about 0.8 to 1.5 × 10^9 widely disseminated lymphoma cells in AKR mice. The average thymus weighs 680 mg, the spleen weighs 450 mg, and the leukocyte count is approximately 27,000 mm^{-3}. All tissues tested in leukemic AKR mice yielded transplantable leukemic cells. Without cytoreductive therapy, AKR mice died after diagnosis of

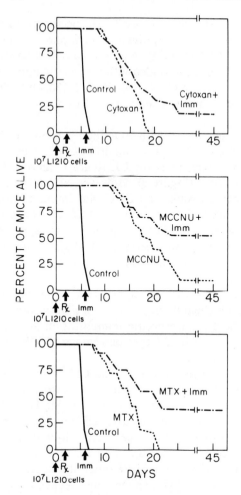

Figure 8. Effectiveness of chemoimmunotherapy on the survival of leukemic DBA/2 Ha mice. Mice were inoculated with 10^7 leukemia L1210 cells i.p. on day 0. Chemotherapy: methyl CCNU (20 mg/kg), or cytoxan (135 mg/kg), or methotrexate (45 mg/kg) on day 2 after tumor inoculation. Immunotherapy: immunization with a single dose of 2×10^7 neuraminidase-treated L1210 tumor cells i.p. 6 days after transplantation of L1210 tumor grafts.

spontaneous leukemia at a rate of 50% by 14 days, 90% by 33 days, and 96% by 56 days. Thus it is not surprising that with such a tumor load, immunization alone has no therapeutic value to the tumor-bearing host (105,119,137, 138,149). Combined chemotherapy with immunotherapy might offer the best potential for the treatment of leukemia. Combination chemotherapy with vincristine, dexamethasone, or vincristine plus prednisone were good remission inducer treatment but provided short remission (105). The median survival time after the cessation of treatment was 90 to 100%, but none of the treated mice survived 100 days. Immunization of AKR mice treated with vincristine plus dexamethasone showed essentially the same survival pattern as the control groups where the immunogen was neuraminidase-treated normal thymocytes or leukemia L1210 cells. The combination of vincristine and steroid with immunization using 2×10^7 neuraminidase-treated leukemic thymocytes injected intradermally at multiple sites allowed 15 to 29% of the mice to survive 100 days without incidence of the disease to relapse by 130 days from a presumptively new leukemogenic event (105,119,138). Spontaneous leukemic AKR mice treated with vincristine plus cytoxan followed by methyl CCNU sustained an increase in life-span of about 180%, but fewer than 5% of the animals survived beyond 100 days. Quantitative splenomegaly assay indicated an apparent cell cure in these mice, but reappearance of leukemia inevitably followed. This recurrence can be ascribed to viral reinduction (105,119,137, 138,149,152,153,156,157). Figure 9 shows that combination drug therapy plus intradermal immunization with neuraminidase-treated spontaneous leukemic thymocytes or with allogeneic E2G leukemia, but not leukemia L1210 or normal thymocytes, resulted in survival of 30 to 35% of animals beyond 150 days without evidence of disease. It is particularly significant that neuraminidase-

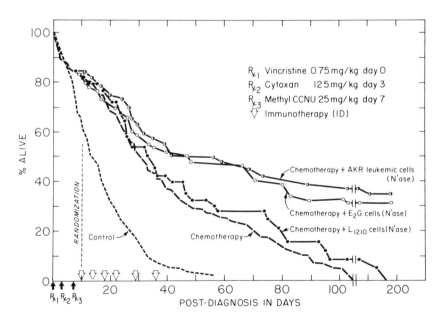

Figure 9. Effect of chemoimmunotherapy with syngeneic and allogeneic leukemic cells on the survival of AKR mice with spontaneous leukemia. Animals were randomized into five equal groups: control; chemotherapy alone; chemotherapy plus neuraminidase-treated L1210-cells; chemotherapy plus neuraminidase-treated E2G leukemia cells; and chemotherapy plus neuraminidase-treated leukemic thymocytes. Animals were immunized intradermally at multiple sites with 2×10^7 neuraminidase-treated tumor cells at days indicated by the arrows.

treated allogeneic E2G leukemic cells that, as the AKR leukemia, are Gross virus induced but are completely different at the H2 genetic locus from AKR mice, were as effective as the syngeneic leukemic cells in prolonging the survival of leukemic AKR mice. This suggests the existence of a cross-reacting common viral membrane antigen and would suggest that if similar etiology existed for human acute leukemia, it would not be essential to use autologous leukemia cells for immunization. These data provided the basis for using neuraminidase-treated allogeneic myeloblasts as immunogen in patients with acute myelocytic leukemia.

6. IMMUNOTHERAPY OF PATIENTS WITH ACUTE MYELOCYTIC LEUKEMIA

Our total experience in a systematic randomized chemoimmunotherapy program began in 1973 at Roswell Park Memorial Institute with five control patients and nine patients immunized with neuraminidase-treated allogeneic myeloblasts. The second study was initiated in 1974 at the Mount Sinai Medical School, using a three-way deliberately unbalanced randomization: 11 AML patients served as controls, 21 were immunized with neuraminidase-treated myeloblasts, and 21 were immunized with neuraminidase-treated myeloblasts plus MER (the methanol extraction residue of BCG). In the third, current investigation 86 patients have been studied in a two-way randomized protocol: 45 patients have been randomized to control and 41 to chemotherapy plus neuraminidase-treated myeloblasts.

6.1. Collection of Allogeneic Myeloblasts for Immunotherapy

Patients become eligible for collection of myeloblasts after satisfying the following criteria: negative HA-A as determined by radioimmunoassay (RIA), no previous chemotherapy, total WBC higher than 25,000/ μl, and more than 70% myeloblasts in the peripheral blood. The myeloblasts were obtained by leukophoresis. In the last 5 years we have collected myeloblasts from 93 patients between the ages of 14 and 72 years and have not encountered any important side effects during the 2- to 4-hour procedure. After leukophoresis, the myeloblasts were separated from contaminating red blood cells by sedimentation at 37 °C. After sedimentation leukemia cells were mixed with special freezing media (free of calcium and magnesium) containing 15% autologous or AB plasma and 10% DMSO. Myeloblasts were frozen by programmed freezing and were immediately stored in the vapor phase of liquid nitrogen. The quantification of the total neuraminidase-susceptible and total cellular NANA of myeloblasts used as immunogen was performed as described by Roboz et al. (134). Total NANA content of myeloblasts ranges from 0.3 to 0.6 μ mole per 10^9 cells. Under optimal conditions, with about ten- to twentyfold excess neuraminidase (e.g., 300 units per 10^9 cells), 68 to 75% of bound NANA was cleaved by the enzyme. Presently there is no information available concerning the relationship between the total sialic acid content of the myeloblasts and the delayed hypersensitivity reactions evoked in patients immunized with neuraminidase-treated myeloblasts.

To avoid using nonantigenic myeloblasts for immunotherapy, fresh myeloblasts from all donors were tested in mixed lymphocyte tumor cell culture against a pool of lymphocytes from normal subjects as well as against remission lymphocytes of AML patients randomized to receive neuraminidase-treated cells. The delayed-type hypersensitivity (DTH) response to neuraminidase-treated myeloblasts was tested in designated recipients. Myeloblasts from 11 donors elicited poor MLTC response and DTH reaction with normal and remission lymphocytes and thus were not used for immunization.

6.2. Treatment of Myeloblasts with Neuraminidase for Immunotherapy

On the day of immunotherapy, myeloblasts were removed rapidly thawed and purified on 22% human albumin gradient supported by 45% sucrose (1:3) to separate the viable from nonviable cells. Yields ranged from 15 to 90% with a viability of 90 to 98%. After purification, myeloblasts were incubated with neuraminidase. The enzyme used throughout this study has been purified 2500- to 3000-fold and was free of other enzymes and bacterial endotoxins. The incubation media contained 15 units of enzyme per 5×10^7 myeloblasts/ml, in sodium acetate buffer at pH 5.6 for 60 minutes at 37 °C. Under these conditions 65 to 75% of bound NANA was cleaved by neuraminidase, with no harmful effects to the cells. However, a 75-fold excess of enzyme in relation to the sialic acid residue or prolonged incubation (>90 minutes) resulted in pronounced alteration in the morphological integrity and antigenicity of the myeloblasts. Similarly, the effectiveness of neuraminidase-modified myeloblasts as immunogen can be significantly reduced by using less units of enzyme than available sialic acid residue. After washing, myeloblasts were suspended in physiological saline to give a final cell concentration of 0.8 to 1×10^9 cells/ml and were used as immunogen within 60 minutes.

6.3. Immunization with Allogeneic Myeloblasts and MER

Immunization with neuraminidase-treated allogeneic myeloblasts was performed by intradermal injections. To provide maximum exposure to the immunogen, sites were widely spread in the supraclavicular, infraclavicular, arm, forearm, parasternal, thoracic, suprainguinal, and femoral regions draining into several node-bearing areas.

A dose-dependent cellular titration was performed with each immunization with 0.5, 1.5, and 2.0×10^8 and 0 cells. The total immunization load was about 10^{10} cells at 48 body sites. In addition, as control injections, heat-denatured neuraminidase, x-irradiated myeloblasts, and the supernatant of the incubation fluid were also injected. Reaction to neuraminidase-treated cells at 48 hours as measured by the induration at the injection sites was proportional to the number of cells injected per site and increased with the frequency of administration (40–42, 149). In most patients, despite the monthly sustaining chemotherapy, the delayed cutaneous hypersensitivity (DCH) response is prolonged and may persist for several week. The injections of neuraminidase-treated myeloblasts produced no local lesions other than the DCH reaction, and none of the patients developed chills, fever, or adenopathy. The biopsies of cutaneous reactions induced by neuraminidase-treated myeloblasts showed immunoblastic infiltration. No hypersensitivity reaction was apparent at the site of injection of physiological saline, heat-denatured neuraminidase, or the supernatant of cell incubation media. In patients randomized to receive MER too, 10 intradermal sites of 100 μg/0.1 ml, each totaling 1.0 mg, of MER was used. In patients who received immunization with neuraminidase-treated myeloblasts plus MER, the DCH reaction to the specific immunogen was reduced rather than increased, when compared to the induration in patients immunized with neuraminidase-treated cells only from the same donor (Table 7).

TABLE 7.   Effect of MER on DCH[a] Response to Neuraminidase-Treated Allogeneic Myeloblasts in AML Patients

Immunization Cycles	Immunotherapy		
	Cells[b]	Cells[c] +	MER[c]
1	13.2 ± 3.5	9.3 ± 2.7	10.3 ± 3.0
3	16.9 ± 4.1	10.4 ± 2.0	13.9 ± 3.4
6	18.7 ± 4.6	7.1 ± 2.3	21.8 ± 5.1
12	21.6 ± 5.1	6.8 ± 1.7	26.7 ± 5.9
Patients tested	4	5	

[a] Delayed cutaneous hypersensitivity response was measured 48 hours after injection.

[b] Mean induration ± SD in millimeters obtained from 48 sites injected with neuraminidase-treated myeloblasts, using the same donor's myeloblasts.

[c] Mean induration ± SD in millimeters obtained from 10 sites injected with 100 μg of MER per site.

7. CHEMOIMMUNOTHERAPY IN PREVIOUSLY UNTREATED PATIENTS WITH ACUTE MYELOCYTIC LEUKEMIA

The chemoimmunotherapy protocol is predicated on the maximal chemotherapeutic reduction of leukemic burden. This is achieved by induction therapy with a regimen of cytosine arabinoside continuously administered intravenously for 7 days at 100 mg/(m² · day) and by direct injection of daunorubicin at 45 mg/(m² · day) on days 1, 2, and 3. This regimen has induced approximately 70% of patients into remission. All patients were between the ages of 15 and 70. Initially, maintenance chemotherapy consisted of rotational cycles of cytosine arabinoside at 100 mg administered i.v. every 12 hours in 10 doses, daunorubicin at 45 mg/m^2 in two doses, cytosine arabinoside as previously, cyclophosphamide 1000 mg/m^2 i.v. in one dose, cytosine arabinoside as previously, and thioquanine 100 mg/m^2 every 12 hours orally in 10 doses. All patients received cyclical maintenance chemotherapy every 6 weeks. Beginning on day 15 after the first sustaining course of chemotherapy, to be continued monthly, patients were randomly allocated to receive either chemotherapy alone or chemotherapy plus neuraminidase-treated allogeneic myeloblasts. This rotational cycle of chemotherapy was continued until relapse or a maximum of 4 years, whereas immunotherapy was administered for up to 5 years. In the second series of patients, from 1974 to 1977, identical chemotherapy was practiced except that an additional maintenance cycle of cytosine arabinoside for 5 days and CCNU were added.

All patients received cyclical maintenance chemotherapy every 4 weeks. On day 8 after the first sustaining course of chemotherapy, to be continued on day 15 of each cycle thereafter, patients were randomly allocated to receive chemotherapy alone, or chemotherapy plus neuraminidase-treated myeloblasts plus MER. During this study when evidence of MER-related immunodepression occurred, MER was significantly reduced or omitted.

In the current investigation, which commenced in 1977, the induction chemotherapy remained identical to that employed throughout the previous two studies. On attaining complete remission, patients are randomized to chemotherapy or chemotherapy plus neuraminidase-treated myeloblasts. The current maintenance therapy consists of the following regimen: cytosine arabinoside 100 mg/m^2 every 12 hours subcutaneously administered plus thioquanine at 100 mg/m^2 every 12 hours orally for 10 doses each, followed in monthly cycles with cytosine arabinoside at the same dose; vincristine 2 mg i.v. in a single dose; and dexamethasone 8 mg/m^2 in two doses. In the group randomized to receive neuraminidase-treated myeloblasts, immunization is given every 28 days, mid-way between the maintenance cycles of chemotherapy.

Analysis of remission and survival data were carried out by using the Kaplan-Meier method. Remission and survival curves were also compared by using Breslow's extension of Beham's generalized Wilcoxon test, the Logrank procedure, and the Cox regression analysis.

From our first study (1973), four of nine patients who received chemotherapy plus neuraminidase-treated myeloblasts are still in their first remission in excess of 7 years. One immunized patient died of myocardial infarction (MI) in complete clinical remission on day 1941. All patients who were treated with chemotherapy alone relapsed within the first 14 months.

Data presented in Table 8 summarize the impact of neuraminidase-treated myeloblasts with/without MER on the remission and survival times of AML patients as compared to the chemotherapy control in the second study. Comparison of remission and survival times among the three groups show statistically significant difference ($p = .0001$). Between the two immunotherapy groups the level of difference is $p = .004$. Five of 21 patients from the group who received neuraminidase-treated cells are still in their first remission, and six are

TABLE 8. Effect of Immunotherapy on Remission and Survival of AML Patients

	Treatment Group		
	Control	Specific Immunotherapy	Specific Immunotherapy plus MER
Remission (in Days)			
Seventy-fifth percentile	125	351	198
Median	198	641	318
Twenty-fifth percentile	285	Not yet reached	522
Survival (in Days)			
Seventy-fifth percentile	180	449	360
Median	319	748	416
Twenty-fifth percentile	384	Not yet reached	558

alive in excess of 5 years after randomization. Combination of specific plus adjuvant immunotherapy with MER did not act synergistically in treatment of AML patients. All patients treated with this combination relapsed by 3.5 years after randomization. Despite the poor performance of patients who received this mode of immunotherapy, the difference between the control versus this immunotherapy regimen is still significant at $p = .04$.

In the current chemoimmunotherapy study so far 41 patients have been randomized to receive immunotherapy and 45 patients were treated with chemotherapy alone. Table 9 shows the remission and survival times of patients in the immunotherapy protocol. In the chemotherapy group 11 of 45 (24%) patients are in complete remission as well as 20 of 41 (49%) in the group who received

TABLE 9. Effect of Immunotherapy on Remission and Survival of AML Patients

	Treatment Group	
	Chemotherapy	Chemoimmunotherapy
Remission (in Days)		
Seventy-fifth percentile	155	236
Median	280	605
Twenty-fifth percentile	662	Not yet reached
Survival (in Days)		
Seventy-fifth percentile	204	374
Median	398	736
Twenty-fifth percentile	766	Not yet reached

neuraminidase-treated myeloblasts. Thirteen of 45 (29%) patients are alive in the chemotherapy group, as compared to 24 of 41 (58%) of the immunotherapy group. Comparison of remission curves at this early stage of observation period yielded $p = .09$, and .06 by the Breslow, Logrank, and Cox regression analyses, respectively. An additional 2 years of follow-up is needed to provide a better assessment of the effectiveness of this combination chemoimmunotherapy, taking into consideration the inclusion of steroids in the maintenance therapy.

Figures 10 and 11 show the total entries into the chemoimmunotherapy study, with 61 patients for chemotherapy alone, 71 patients treated with chemotherapy plus neuraminidase-treated myeloblasts and 21 patients who received chemotherapy plus neuraminidase-treated myeloblasts plus MER. By each of the three methods of statistical analysis, a signficant ($p = .001$) prolongation of remission and survival time was noted in the group of patients receiving the combination of cytoreductive therapy with active immunization with neuraminidase-treated allogeneic myeloblasts. The use of MER in addition to neuraminidase-treated myeloblasts eliminated the plateau phase of continuing remission duration observed in patients who received neuraminidase-treated myeloblasts alone. There is no evidence from a large clinical study conducted by Cancer Acute Leukemia Group B (CALGB) that MER is an effective adjuvant (159). Although BCG has shown positive results in controlled trials by several investigators (20–23, 25,26), the magnitude of the effect is low and the plateau is substantially below that of the present investigation.

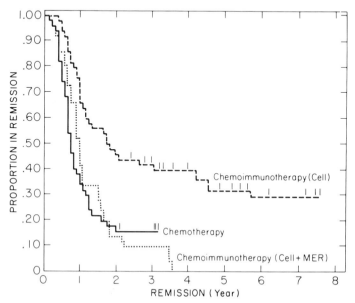

Figure 10.   Duration of remission in previously untreated patients with acute myelocytic leukemia immunized with neuraminidase treated myeloglasts.

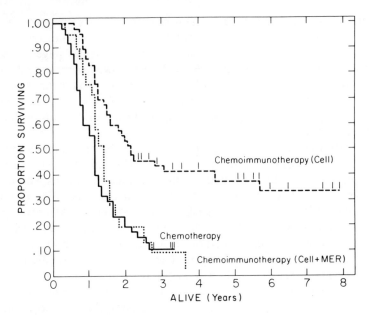

Figure 11. Impact of active immunotherapy on the life-span of untreated patients with acute myelocytic leukemia.

8. IMMUNOLOGIC STATUS OF AML PATIENTS IN THE CHEMOIMMUNOTHERAPY PROTOCOL

The *in vivo* immunologic status of AML patients randomized in the immunotherapy protocol was measured by DCH response to five recall antigens: PPD, mumps, candida, varidase, and dermatophytin. The initial skin testing was performed at the time of randomization into the protocol. Subsequent skin tests were administered at every third cycle of the therapy, at least 48 hours prior to each immunization.

Data summarized in Figure 12 show that there was considerable improvement in cell-mediated immunity among AML patients immunized with neuraminidase-treated myeloblasts as measured in conversion to positive to at least three recall antigens: mumps, candida, and varidase. However, all patients immunized with neuraminidase-treated cells plus MER showed a decline and most showed complete loss of DCH response to recall antigens after the sixth treatment cycle, with the exception of three patients whose MER dose was attenuated from the onset. The decline or complete loss in response to recall antigens preceded subsequent relapse.

The *in vitro* immunocompetence of AML patients was determined by monitoring lymphocyte subpopulations, the lymphocyte blastogenesis induced by selected T- and B-cell mitogens, and lymphocyte transformation induced by allogeneic myeloblasts in MLTC reaction. At the time of randomization, patients showed a low number of mononuclear cell population and within that, a high percentage of lymphocytes without any detectable surface markers, that is, "null cells," as compared to healthy subjects. It was of considerable im-

IN VIVO RESPONSE TO RECALL ANTIGENS IN AML

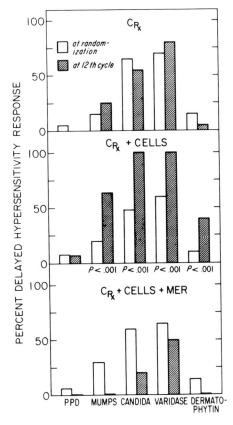

Figure 12. Change of delayed hypersensitivity response to recall antigens during the course of chemoimmunotherapy.

portance, therefore, to determine whether systematic immunotherapy regimen, in spite of concomitant chemotherapy, affected the restoration and maintenance of mononuclear cell population.

Although the quantification of WBC, total mononuclear cells, and T and B lymphocytes were performed monthly on all patients in the chemoimmunotherapy protocol, Table 10 summarizes only three test periods: (1) at the time of randomization; (2) at 12 months; and (3) at 24 months of chemotherapy-chemoimmunotherapy. The median values for total mononuclear cells of 75 healthy donors are $2589 \pm 357/ \mu$l, in which 70 to 75% are T cells, 18 to 23% B cells, and 3 to 12% "null cells." Patients at the time of randomization, still under recovery from induction and consolidating chemotherapy, have shown significantly lower total mononuclear cells (837–981), lower percentage (49.2 to 53) and absolute number (412 to 519) of T-cells, lower percentage (18.2 to 19.8) and absolute number (152 to 186) of B lymphocytes, and higher percentage (27.2 to 32.6) of "null cells." It is clearly demonstrated that patients who have received this mode of immunotherapy showed continuous improvement despite the monthly maintenance chemotherapy. At the twenty-third immunotherapy cycle the number of mononuclear cells increased to 837 to 1601, the percentage from 49.2 to 71, and the absolute number of T lymphocytes from

TABLE 10. Lymphocyte Subpopulations in AML Patients in Chemoimmunotherapy

| | Treatment Group | | | | | | | | |
| | Chemotherapy | | | Chemotherapy + Neuraminidase Cells | | | Chemotherapy + Neuraminidase + MER | | |
	At Randomization	At 12 months	At 24 months	At Randomization	At 12 months	At 24 months	At Randomization	At 12 months	At 23 months
Total mononuclear cells (number/mm)	981 ±78[a]	1153 ±128		837 ±72	1283 ±91	1601[b] ±129	941 ±112	1297 ±89	1307 ±102
T Cells									
Percentage	53	65.2		49.2	69.3	70.7	51.7	70.1	72.3
Absolute number	519 ±47	752 ±63		412 ±35	889[b] ±95	1132[b] ±129	487 ±45	909[b] ±101	945[b] ±93
B Cells									
Percentage	18.3	21.9		18.2	21.6	21.2	19.8	22.3	20.3
Absolute number	180 ±21	253 ±25		152 ±13	277 ±41	337[a] ±35	146 ±17	289 ±13	263 ±28
Patients tested[c]	11	4	0[c]	21	14	11	19	7	3

[a]Mean ± standard deviation.
[b]Statistical significance between absolute T or B lymphocytes at the time of randomization vs. during therapy of AML $p = .0001$.
[c]All control group patients relapsed in this study prior to the twenty-fourth course of chemotherapy treatment.

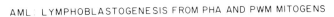

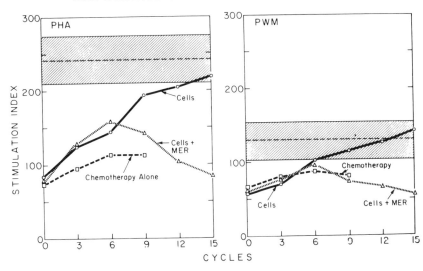

Figure 13. Lymphoblastogenesis of remission lymphocytes induced by PHA and PWM mitogens obtained in AML patients in the chemoimmunotherapy study.

412 to 1200. At the same time the percentage of "null cells" returned to the range of that of healthy subjects. Similar improvement of mononuclear cells, percentage, and absolute number of T and B lymphocytes was apparent in the first 12 cycles of immunotherapy when MER was used in addition to neuraminidase-treated myeloblasts. Patients randomized to receive chemotherapy alone showed no substantial restoration of mononuclear cells or T and B lymphocytes as compared to values at the time of randomization.

The functional integrity of the lymphocytes of AML patients in each arm of the study was assessed by lymphocyte blastogenesis induced by selected T-cell and B-cell mitogens and by monitoring the response of remission lymphocytes to autologous myeloblasts. Phytohemagglutinin (PHA) was used for T cells and pokeweed mitogen (PWM) for B cells. The mitogen concentration that yielded maximum stimulation was established. Results of these studies are summarized in Figure 13 and Table 11. A progressive restoration of lymphocyte function in AML patients receiving neuraminidase-treated myeloblasts as immunogen is apparent. Both mitogens show depressed stimulation of lymphocytes at the time of randomization as compared to normal subjects, and there was no apparent improvement in patients who received chemotherapy alone. It is noteworthy that lymphoblastogenesis approached the normal range by the twelfth course of chemoimmunotherapy for remission lymphocytes of patients who were treated with cyclic maintenance chemotherapy and immunization with neuraminidase-treated allogeneic myeloblasts as immunogen.

Most of the AML patients immunized with neuraminidase-treated myeloblasts plus MER showed, during the first four to eight immunotherapy cycles, improvement in their response to recall antigens, number of mononuclear

TABLE 11.   Lymphocyte Function of Chemoimmunotherapy Patients

	No.	PHA Maximum Stimulation cpm $\times$ 10^3	ConA Maximum Stimulation cpm $\times$ 10^3	MLTC[a] Maximum Stimulation cpm $\times$ 10^3	MLTC[b] Maximum Stimulation cpm $\times$ 10^3
		Chemotherapy			
At randomization	28	42.1 ±6.4	39.3 ±4.8	15.2 ±2.4	18.6 ±3.1
Twelfth course	9	61.2 ±9.3	60.3 ±7.5	15.3 ±2.3	19.7 ±3.7
Twenty-fourth course	5	62.9 ±7.2	64.0 ±5.2	17.5 ±2.9	24.2 ±2.9
		Immunotherapy			
At randomization	31	39.7 ±4.7	40.6 ±3.1	16.4 ±3.8	20.1 ±1.9
Twelfth course	16	81.6* ±4.5	78.2* ±4.1	29.7* ±2.9	27.6* ±2.2
Twenty-fourth course	11	85.3* ±4.9	79.7* ±3.8	33.9* ±3.1	26.1* ±2.7

Allogeneic myeloblasts used[a] for immunotherapy or not used[b] for immunotherapy. The following mixed tumor-leukocyte culture was performed. Myeloblasts incubated with mitomycin C at 30 μ g/ml of 2 $\times$ 10^6 cell suspension for 30 minutes at 37 °C. after washing 2 $\times$ 10^5 myeloblasts were distributed in each of the replicate wells of the Falcon microplates containing 10^5 responding lymphocytes per well in RPMI 1640 media supplemented with 20% heat-inactivated autologous plasma. After 90 hours of incubation 1 μ Ci of ^{3}H-TdR was added per well. Cultures were harvested for 18 hours with the addition of excess cold thymidine.
*p = < .01

cells, and T lymphocytes (Table 10) to synthetic mitogens (Figure 13). Inevitably, however, a decline of *in vivo* and *in vitro* cell-mediated immunity ensued. Figures 14 and 15 show typical examples of clinical and laboratory data obtained. Lymphocyte blastogenesis induced by PHA and DCH response to recall antigens and MER were in the normal range in this patient (Figure 14) in the first eight cycles of immunotherapy. A decline in response to PHA and a marked increase in DCH response to MER followed. In the next cycle of immunotherapy the dose of MER was attenuated; nonetheless, there was no rebound in the cell-mediated immunity, and the patient relapsed soon thereafter. A similar rapid decline of lymphocyte function, loss of response to recall antigens, and increased sensitivity to MER was noted in another patient as early as the fourth immunotherapy cycle (Figure 15). Despite reduction of MER dose, further decline of *in vitro* and *in vivo* immune response continued and was followed by relapse. Similar biphasic effect of MER on the *in vivo* and *in vitro* cell-mediated immunity was noted in all AML patients receiving this form of immunotherapy, but not among those AML patients who were immunized with neuraminidase-treated myeloblasts alone.

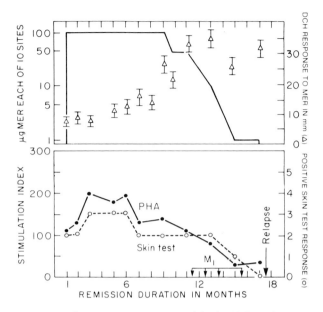

Figure 14. Appearances of suppressor monocyte activity in AML patients treated with neura-minidase-modified myeloblasts plus MER.

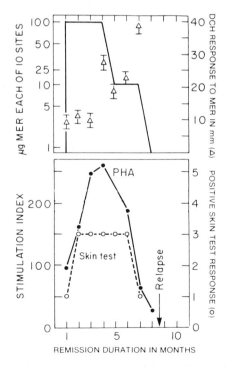

Figure 15. Appearances of suppressor monocyte activity in AML patients treated with neura-minidase-modified myeloblasts plus MER.

The fact that patients treated with neuraminidase-treated myeloblasts plus MER have similar number of mononuclear cells and T lymphocytes as patients immunized with neuraminidase-treated myeloblasts alone, but have significantly altered *in vivo* and *in vitro* immune function, raised the possibility of the presence of an inhibitory mononuclear cell population in the blood of such immunized AML patients. This hypothesis was tested and the data are summarized in Figure 16. Isolated enriched T-lymphocyte fraction from normal donors or from AML patients immunized with neuraminidase-modified myeloblasts gave similar incorporation of H³TdR into DNA as the unseparated peripheral blood lymphocytes. However, T lymphocytes obtained from AML patients who received neuraminidase-treated myeloblasts plus MER and have shown declining *in vivo* and *in vitro* immunologic responses gave 3 to 7 times greater H³TdR incorporation than unseparated mononuclear cells. The response of the T lymphocytes was strongly inhibited by addition of autologous macrophages or B lymphocytes. This was not the case with macrophages or B cells of normal donors. These findings appear to suggest that depression of cell-mediated immunity is seen in all the tested AML patients who received treated myeloblasts plus MER, but not in the patients immunized with neuraminidase-treated myeloblasts as immunogen. This suppression of T-lymphocyte function might be attributed to circulating "suppressor macrophages" induced by MER. The time of occurrence of the apparent "suppressor macrophage" activity differed from patient to patient. Omission of MER from the treatment prompted recovery of the patient's *in vivo* and *in vitro* immunologic

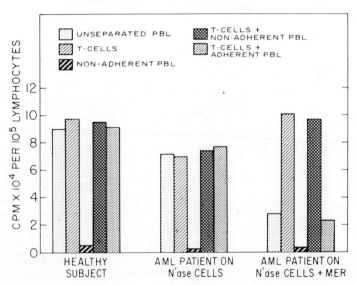

Figure 16. Impact of neuraminidase-treated myeloblasts plus MER on the functional integrity of remission lymphocytes.

parameters and a gradual decrease of "suppressor macrophage" population in only one of 21 patients. Clinical and laboratory data leave little doubt that addition of MER to specific immunotherapy abolished the therapeutic activity of neuraminidase-modified myeloblasts as immunogen.

It was of considerable importance to determine whether active immunotherapy with the use of neuraminidase-treated allogeneic myeloblasts would increase lymphocyte response to autologous myeloblasts and whether lymphoblastogenesis induced by autologous myeloblasts in MLTC could be correlated with the performance of the AML patients in the chemoimmunotherapy programs. From the onset of this study (1973) attempt was made to obtain and store myeloblasts from all AML patients after clinical diagnosis of the disease. Myeloblasts were collected after the clinical diagnosis as well as remission lymphocytes at specific time intervals during the treatment program and were then frozen and stored in liquid nitrogen. Both myeloblasts and lymphocytes retained—with only minor loss up to 24 months—their original activity, an observation that is in an agreement with the findings of Holden et al. (160) and Golub (161).

Results shown in Figure 17 summarize lymphocyte transformation induced by autologous myeloblasts of the following AML patients: 12 who received

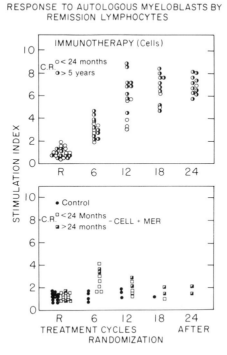

Figure 17.   Responses to autologous myeloblasts by remission lymphocytes in AML patients immunized with neuraminidase-treated allogeneic myeloblasts.

chemotherapy; 20 who were treated with chemotherapy plus neuraminidase-modified myeloblasts; and 13 who received chemotherapy plus modified myeloblasts plus MER. Patients recipient of chemotherapy, neuraminidase-treated myeloblasts, and MER or chemotherapy treatment alone did not respond in MLTC to their leukemic cells and had shorter disease free intervals and none of them survived beyond 3.6 years. Similar observations were reported by other laboratories concerning the lack of reactivity of ALL and AML patients' remission lymphocytes to autochthonous myeloblasts in individuals treated with chemotherapy (150, 162–167). Positive response to autologous myeloblasts by the patients' own remission lymphocytes was achieved only in those AML patients who received chemotherapy plus neuraminidase-modified myeloblasts as immunogen. The majority of these patients' lymphocytes showed progressively stronger response in MLTC against their leukemic cells. Nine of 11 patients immunized with myeloblasts and who responded to their autologous myeloblasts are still in first remissions, ranging from 4 to 7.5 years. Positive reaction in MLTC to autochthonous myeloblasts correlated with the length of remission and survival of the immunotherapy patients. This appears to indicate that patients with AML have improved cell-mediated immune reaction to leukemia-associated antigens as a direct consequence of immunotherapy with neuraminidase-treated allogeneic myeloblasts. Serum samples obtained serially from 63 AML patients who have been receiving modified cells (20) or cells plus MER (19) or treated with chemotherapy (25) alone were tested against HLA-typed untreated lymphocytes of 25 selected donors who cover the spectrum of 32 well-defined antigens of the HLA A, B, and C series. Nine out of the 63 patients' sera showed cytotoxic activity in the presence of rabbit complement at the time of randomization and remained unchanged during the course of therapy. In the course of immunotherapy with neuraminidase-treated myeloblasts, but not with neuraminidase-treated myeloblasts plus MER, 11 (55%) of the patients developed strong complement-dependent cytotoxic antibodies against neuraminidase-treated lymphocytes, and fifteen (75%) of 20 patients developed cytotoxic antibodies against neuraminidase-treated allogeneic myeloblasts but showed no activity against ALL, CLL, or CML. Sera of individuals with measurable autoantibodies to neuraminidase-treated lymphcytes also showed a stronger level of cytotoxic activity for myeloblasts. It is significant from the point of view of clinical status of immunotherapy patients that both antibodies rapidly disappeared 4 to 8 weeks prior to clinical relapse. Thus monitoring these two distinct autoantibodies has potential value in monitoring the clinical status of AML patients in the immunotherapy protocol.

REFERENCES

1. P. Alexander, D. I. Connell, and Z. B. Mikulska, Treatment of a murine leukemia with spleen cells or sera from allogeneic mice immunized against the tumor. *Cancer Res.*, **26**, 1508 (1966).

2. R. Laterjet, Action inhibitrice d'extraits leucemiques isologues irradies sur la leucemo-genese spontanee de la souris AKR. *Ann Inst. Pasteur Lille,* **107**, 1 (1964).

3. L. Revesz, Detection of antigenic differences in isologous host-tumor systems by pre-treatment with heavily irradiated tumor cells. *Cancer Res.,* **20**, 443 (1960).

4. A. Wolf, D. M. Parry, and R. K. Barfoot, Loss of weak antigenicity of lymphoma cells following treatment with difluorodinitrobenzene. *Transplantation,* **10**, 340 (1970).

5. M. D. Parger, Vaccination and immunotherapy with chemically modified cancer cells. *Bibl. Haematol.,* **39**, 706 (1973).

6. M. D. Parger, F. S. Baechtel, R. J. Ribble, C. M. Ludden, and J. M. Mehta, Immuno-logical stimulation with modified lymphoma cells in minimally responsive tumor-host sys-tem. *Cancer Res.,* **34**, 3203 (1974).

7. C. Z. Apffel, B. C. Arnanson, and J. H. Peters, Induction of tumor immunity with tumor cells treated with iodoacetate, *Nature (Lond.),* **209**, 694 (1966).

8. C. Jasmin, C. Piton, and C. Rosenfeld, Effects de l'iodoacetamide sur les cellules de la leucemie virale de Rauscher. *Internatl. J. Cancer,* **3**, 254 (1968).

9. M. D. Prager and F. S. Baechtel, Methods for modification of cancer cells to enhance their antigenicity, *Meth. Cancer Res.,* **9**, 339 (1973).

10. M. D. Prager, I. Derr, A. Swann, and J. Cotropia, Immunization with chemically modified lymphoma cells. *Cancer Res.,* **31**, 1488 (1971).

11. C. P. Eng, L. P. Kleine, and J. F. Morgan, Tumor-specific immunity induced by non-tumor-igeneic 6C3HED ascites tissue culture cells. *J. Natl. Cancer Inst.,* **45**, 235 (1970).

12. W. J. Martin, J. R. Wunderlich, R. Flether, and J. K. Inman, Enhanced immunogeni-city of chemically coated syngeneic tumor cells. *Proc. Natl. Acad. Sci. (USA),* **68**, 469 (1971).

13. G. Mathe, F. Facy, F. Hatton and O. Halle-Pannenko, BCG vaccination and acute leu-kemia. *Biomed. Express,* **21**, 132 (1974).

14. G. Mathe, J. L. Amiel, L. Schwarzenberg, M. Schneider, A. Cattan, J. R. Schulmberger, M. Hayat, and F. DeVassal, Active immunotherapy for acute lymphoblastic leukemia. *Lancet,* **1**, 697 (1969).

15. G. Mathe, L. Schwarzenberg, J. L. Ameil, P. Pouillart, M. Hayat, F. De Vassal, C. Rosen-feld, and E. Jasmin, New experimental and clinical data on leukemia immunotherapy. *Proc. Roy. Soc. Med.,* **68**, 211 (1973).

16. G. Mathe, J. L. Amiel, L. Schwarzenberg, M. Schneider, M. Hayat, F. De Vassal, C. Jasmin, C. Rosenfeld, and P. Pouillart, 1971. Preliminary results of a new protocol for the active immunotherapy of acute lymphoblastic leukemia: Inhibition of the immuno-therapeutic effect by vincristine or adamantadine. *Rev. Eur. Etudes Clin. Biol.,* **16**, 216 (1971).

17. G. Mathe, J. L. Amiel, L. Schwarzenbert, P. Pouillart, D. Belpomme, C. Jasmin, and J. L. Misset, Ten years of immunotherapy for acute lymphoblastic leukemia. Prognostic factor—other than cytological in acute lymphocytic leukemia. *Bull. Cancer,* **61**, 377 (1974).

18. Medical Research Council, Treatment of acute lymphoblastic leukemia. Comparison of immunotherapy (BCG), intermittent methotrexate and no therapy after a five month in-tensive cytotoxic regimen (Concord Trial). Preliminary Report to the Medical Research Council by the Leukaemia Committee and the Working Party on Leukaemia in Childhood. *Br. Med. J.,* **4**, 189 (1971).

19. C. Crowther, R. L. Powles, C. J. T. Bateman, M. E. J. Beard, C. J. Gauci, P. F. M. Wrig-ley, J. S. Malpas, G. Hamilton-Fairley, and R. B. Scott, Management of adult acute myelo-genous leukemia. *Br. Med. J.,* **1**, 131 (1973).

20. R. Powles, Immunotherapy of acute myelogenous leukemia in man. *Natl. Cancer Inst. Monogr.,* **39**, 243 (1973).

21. R. L. Powles, D. Crowther, C. J. T. Bateman, M. E. J. Beard, T. J. McElwain, J. Russell, T. A. Lister, J. M. A. Whitehouse, P. F. M. Wrigley, M. Pike, P. Alexander, and G. Hamilton-Fairley, Immunotherapy for acute myelogenous leukemia. *Br. J. Cancer,* **28,** 365 (1973).

22. R. Powles, Immunotherapy for acute myelogenous leukemia. *Br. J. Cancer,* **28,** (Suppl. 1), 262 (1973).

23. J. U. Gutterman, E. M. Hersh, V. Rodriguez, K. B. McCredie, G. Mavligit, R. Red, M. A. Burgess, T. Smith, E. Gehan, G. P. Bodey, Jr., and E. J. Freirech, Chemoimmunotherapy of adult acute leukemia. Prolongation of remission in myeloblastic leukemia with BCG. *Lancet,* **2,** 1405 (1974).

24. W. R. Vogler and Y. K. Chan, Prolonging remission in myeloblastic leukemia by Tice-strain Bacillus Calmette-Guerin. *Lancet,* **2,** 128 (1974).

25. E. M. Hersh, J. U. Gutterman, G. M. Mavligit, C. H. Granatek, R. D. Rosen, A. Rios, A. A. Goldstein, Y. Z. Patt, E. Rivera, S. P. Richman, J. C. Bottino, D. Farguhar, D. Morris, and K. Ezaki, Clinical rationale for immunotherapy and its role in cancer treatment. In The University of Texas System Cancer Center, *Immunotherapy of Human Cancer,* Raven, New York, 1978, p. 83.

26. M. J. Mastrangelo, D. Berd, and R. E. Bellet, Limitations, obstacles, and controversies in the optimal development of immunotherapy. In The University of Texas System Cancer Center, *Immunotherapy of Human Cancer,* Raven, New York, 1978, p. 375.

27. J. E. Sokal and J. T. Grace, An attempt to protect patients with chronic myelocytic leukemia (CML) against blastic transformation. *Proc. Am. Assoc. Cancer Res.,* **10,** 85 (1969).

28. J. E. Sokal, C. W. Aungst, and J. T. Grace, Immunotherapy of myeloid leukemia. *Ann. Int. Med.,* **76,** 878 (1972).

29. J. E. Sokal and C. W. Aungst, Immunotherapy with cultured human cells and BCG. *Transplant. Proc.,* **7,** 317 (1975).

30. D. L. Morton and F. R. Eilber, E. C. Holmes, J. S. Hunt, A. S. Ketcham, M. S. Silverstein, and F. C. Sparks, BCG immunotherapy of malignant melanoma: Summary of a seven year experience. *Ann. Surg.,* **180,** 635 (1974).

31. D. L. Morton, Cancer immunotherapy: An overview. *Semin. Oncol.,* **1,** 297 (1974).

32. J. E. Goodnight and D. L. Morton, Adjuvant immunotherapy. *Internatl. Adv. Surg. Oncol.,* **1,** 53 (1978).

33. H. F. Seigler, E. Cox, F. Mutzner, L. Shepherd, E. Nicholson, and W. W. Shingleton, Specific active immunotherapy for melanoma. *Ann. Surg.,* **190,** 336 (1979).

34. H. Takita, J. Minowada, T. Han, M. Takada, and W. W. Lane, Adjuvant immunotherapy in bronchogenic carcinoma. *Ann. N. Y. Acad. Sci.,* **277,** 345 (1976).

35. H. Takita, M. Takada, J. Minowada, T. Han, and F. Edgerton, Adjuvant immunotherapy in stage III lung carcinoma. In W. D. Terry and D. Windhorst, Eds., *Immunotherapy of Cancer: Present Status of Trials in Man,* Vol. 6, Raven, New York, 1978, p. 696.

36. T. J. Cunningham, R. Antemann, D. Paonessa, R. W. Sponzo, and D. Steiner, Adjuvant immuno- and/or chemotherapy with neuraminidase-treated autogenous tumor vaccine and Bacillus Calmette-Guerin for head and neck cancers. *Ann. N. Y. Acad. Sci.,* **277,** 339 (1976).

37. F. E. Rosato, E. Miller, E. F. Rosato, A. Brown, M. K. Wallach, J. Johnson, and E. Moskowitz, Active specific immunotherapy of human solid tumors. *Ann. N. Y. Acad. Sci.,* **277,** 332 (1976).

38. F. E. Rosato, E. Miller, and E. F. Rosato, Active specific immunotherapy of human solid tumors. *Va. Med.,* **105,** 221 (1978).

39. J. F. Holland and J. G. Bekesi, Immunotherapy of human leukemia with neuraminidase

modified cells. In W. Terry, Ed., *Medical Clinics Symposium on Immunotherapy in Malignant Disease,* Vol. 60, Saunders, Philadelphia, 1976, p. 539.

40. J. G. Bekesi, J. P. Roboz, and J. F. Holland, Therapeutic effectiveness of neuraminidase-treated leukemia cells as immunogen in man and experimental animals with leukemia. *Ann. N. Y. Acad. Sci.,* **277,** 313 (1976).

41. J. F. Holland and J. G. Bekesi, Comparison of chemotherapy with chemotherapy plus VCN-treated cells in acute myelocytic leukemia. In W. D. Terry and D. Windhorst, Eds., *Immunotherapy of Cancer: Present Status of Trials in Man,* Vol. 6, Raven, New York, 1978, pp. 347.

42. J. G. Bekesi and J. F. Holland, Impact of specific immunotherapy in acute myelocytic leukemia. In R. Neth, Ed., *Modern Trends in Human Leukemia III,* Springer-Verlag, New York, 1979, p. 74.

43. K. D. Bagshawe and G. Currie, Immunogenicity of L1210 murine leukemia cells after treatment with neuraminidase. *Nature (Lond.),* **218,** 1254 (1968).

44. J. G. Bekesi, J. P. Roboz, L. Walter, and J. F. Holland, Stimulation of specific immunity against cancer by neuraminidase-treated tumor cells. *Behring Inst. Mitt.,* **55,** 309 (1974).

45. J. G. Bekesi, G. St-Arneault, and J. F. Holland, Increase of leukemia L1210 immunogenicity by Vibrio cholerae neuraminidase treatment. *Cancer Res,* **31,** 2130, (1971).

46. J. G. Bekesi, G. St-Arneault, L. Walter, and J. F. Holland, Immunogenicity of leukemia L1210 cells after neuraminidase treatment. *J. Natl. Cancer Inst.,* **49,** 107 (1972).

47. G. A. Currie and K. D. Bagshawe, The role of sialic acid in antigenic expression: Further studies of the Landschutz ascites tumor. *Br. J. Cancer,* **22,** 843 (1968).

48. R. C. Hughes, B. Sanford, and R. W. Jeanloz, Regeneration of the surface glycoproteins of a transplantable mouse tumor cell after treatment with neuraminidase. *Proc. Natl. Acad. Sci. (USA),* **69,** 842 (1972).

49. K. K. Sethi and H. Brandis, Neuraminidase induced loss in the transplantability of murine leukemia L1210 induction of immuno-protection and the transfer of induced immunity to normal DBA/2 mice by serum and peritoneal cells. *Br. J. Cancer,* **27,** 106 (1973).

50. P. K. Ray and R. L. Simmons, Differential release of sialic acid from normal and malignant cells by vibrio cholerae neuraminidase or influenza virus neuraminidase. *Cancer Res.,* **33,** 936 (1973).

51. A. Rios and R. L. Simmons, Active specific immunotherapy of minimal residual tumor: Excision plus neuraminidase-treated tumor cells. *Internatl. J. Cancer,* **13,** 71 (1974).

52. A. Rios and R. L. Simmons, Immunospecific regression of various syngeneic mouse tumors in response to neuraminidase treated tumor cells. *J. Natl. Cancer Inst.,* **51,** 637 (1973).

53. K. K. Sethi and M. Teschner, Neuraminidase induced immunospecific destruction of transplantable experimental tumors. *Post Hig. Med. Dosw.,* **28,** 103 (1974).

54. J. J. Killion, The immunotherapeutic value of a L1210 tumor cell vaccine depends upon the expression of cell-surface carbohydrates. *Cancer Immunol. Immunother.,* **3,** 87 (1977).

55. J. J. Killion, Immunotherapy with tumor cell subpopulations. I. Active, specific immunotherapy of L1210 leukemia. *Cancer Immunol. Immunother.,* **4,** 115 (1978).

56. J. J. Killion, M. A. Wallenbrock, J. A. Rogers, G. M. Kollmorgen, W. A. Sansing, and J. L. Cantrell, Tumorigenicity and the expression of cell-surface carbohydrates. *Nature,* **261,** 54 (1976).

57. G. K. Hirst, Adsorption of influenza hemagglutinins and virus by red blood cells. *J. Exp. Med.,* **76,** 195 (1942).

58. F. M. Burnet, Mucoproteins in relation to virus action. *Physiol. Rev.* **31,** 131 (1951).

59. A. Gottschalk, Neuraminidase: The specific enzyme of influenza virus and Vibrio cholerae. *Biochem. Biophys. Acta,* **23,** 646 (1957).

60. G. Blix, A. Gottschalk, and E. Klenk, Proposed nomenclature in the field of neuraminic and sialic acids. *Nature (Lond.)*, **197**, 1088 (1957).

61. M. Suttajit and R. J. Winzler, Effect of modification N-acetylneuraminic acid on the binding of glycoprotein to influenza virus and on susceptibility to cleavage by neuraminidase. *J. Biol. Chem.*, **246**, 3398 (1971).

62. G. Blix, The carbohydrate groups of the submaxillary mucin. *Z. Physiol. Chem.*, **240**, 43 (1936).

63. A. Gottschalk, *The Chemistry and Biology of Sialic Acids and Related Substances,* Cambridge Univ. Press, London, 1960.

64. R. Drzeniek, Differences in splitting capacity of virus and Vibrio cholerae neuraminidases on sialic acid type substrates. *Biochem. Biophys. Res. Commun.*, **26**, 631 (1967).

65. R. Drzeniek and A. Gaube, Differences in substrate specificity of myxovirus neuraminidase. *Biochem. Biophys. Res. Commun.*, **38**, 651 (1970).

66. R. Drzeniek, Viral and bacterial neuraminidases. *Top. Microbiol. Immunol.*, **59**, 35 (1972).

67. N. Sharon, *Complex Carbohydrates: Their Chemistry, Biosynthesis and Functions,* Addison-Wesley, Reading, Mass., 1975.

68. E. F. Walborg, Glycoproteins and glycolipids in disease processes. In American Cancer Society Symposium No. 80, 1978.

69. R. L. Juliano and A. Rothstein, Cell surface glycoproteins: Structure, biosynthesis and biological functions. In F. Bronner and A. Kleinzeller, Eds., *Current Topics in Membranes and Transport,* Academic, New York, 1978.

70. W. J. Lennarz, *The Biochemistry of Glycoproteins and Proteoglycans,* Plenum, New York (1980).

71. W. Pigman and A. Gottschalk, Submaxillary Gland Glycoproteins. Vol. 5, *Glycoproteins,* Elsevier, Amsterdam, 1966, pp. 434–435.

72. A. G. Morell, G. Gregoriadis, and H. I. Scheinberg, The role of sialic acid in determining the survival of glycoproteins in the circulation. *J. Biol. Chem.*, **246**, 1461 (1967).

73. W. E. Pricer and G. Ashwell, The binding of desialylated glycoproteins by plasma membranes of rat liver. *J. Biol. Chem.*, **246**, 4825 (1967).

74. G. Ashwell and A. Morell, The dual role of sialic acid in the hepatic recognition and catabolism of serum glycoproteins. *Biochem. Soc. Symp.*, **40**, 117 (1974).

75. J. Woodruff and B. M. Gesner, The effect of neuraminidase on the fate of transfused lymphocytes. *J. Exp. Med.*, **129**, 551 (1969).

76. H. G. Remold and J. R. David, Further studies on migration inhibitory factor (MIF): Evidence for its glycoprotein nature. *J. Immunol.*, **107**, 1090 (1971).

77. L. Weiss, Studies on cell deformability. I. Effect of surface charge. *J. Cell. Biol.*, **26**, 735 (1965).

78. L. Weiss, E. Mayhew, and K. Ulrich, The effect of neuraminidase on the phagocytic process in human monocytes. *Lab. Invest.*, **15**, 1304 (1966).

79. L. Weiss, Studies on cell adhesion in tissue culture. IX. Electrophoretic mobility and contact phenomena. *Exp. Cell. Res.*, **51**, 609 (1968).

80. L. Weiss, Studies on cell deformability. V. Some effects of ribonuclease. *J. Theor. Biol.*, **18**, 9 (1968).

81. L. Weiss and L. F. Sinc, The electrokinetic surface of human cells of lymphoid origin and their ribonuclease susceptibility. *Cancer Res.*, **30**, 90 (1970).

82. P. K. Ray and S. Challerjee, Neuraminidase treatment enhances the lysolecithin induced intercellular adhesion of Amoeba proteus. *Z. Naturforsch.*, **30c**, 551 (1975).

83. D. Cormak, Effect of enzymatic removal of cell surface sialic acid on the adherence of Walker 256 tumor cells to mesothelial membrane. *Cancer Res.*, **30**, 1459 (1970).

84. R. B. Kemp, Effect of the removal of cell surface sialic acids on cell aggregation *in vitro*. *Nature (Lond.)*, **218**, 1255 (1968).

85. C. Sauter, J. Lindenmann, and A. Gerber, Agglutination of leukemic myeloblasts by neuraminidase. *Eur. J. Cancer*, **8**, 451 (1972).

86. A. Lee, Effect of neuraminidase on the phagocytosis of heterologous red cells by mouse peripheral macrophages. *Proc. Soc. Exp. Biol. Med.*, **128**, 891 (1968).

87. J. R. Schmidtke and R. L. Simmons, Augmented uptake neuraminidase-treated sheep red blood cells: Participation of Opsonic Factors. *J. Natl. Cancer Inst.*, **54**, 1379 (1975).

88. K. K. Sethi and H. Brandis, Synergistic cytotoxic effect of macrophages and normal mouse serum on neuraminidase-treated murine leukaemia cells. *Eur. J. Cancer*, **9**, 809 (1973).

89. T. Han, Enhancement of mixed lymphocyte reactivity by neuraminidase. *Transplantation*, **14**, 515 (1972).

90. T. Han, Enchancement of mixed lymphocyte reactivity by neuraminidase. *Transplantation*, **14**, 515 (1972).

91. G. Lundgreen, L. Jeitz, L. Lundin, and R. L. Simmons, Increased stimulation by neuraminidase-treated cells in mixed lymphocyte cultures. *Fed. Proc.*, **30**, 395 (1971).

92. G. Lundgreen and R. L. Simmons, Effect of neuraminidase on the stimulatory capacity of cells in mixed lymphocyte cultures. *Clin. Exp. Immunol.*, **9**, 915 (1971).

93. K. Lindahl-Kiessline and R. D. A. Peterson, The mechanism of phytohemmagglutinin action. III. Stimulation of lymphocytes by allogeneic lymphocytes and phytohemagglutinin. *Exp. Cell. Res.*, **55**, 85 (1969).

94. T. Han, Enhancement of *in vitro* lymphocyte response by neuraminidase. *Clin. Exp. Immunol.*, **13**, 165 (1973).

95. T. Han, Specific effect of neuraminidase on blastogenic response of sensitized lymphocytes. *Immunology*, **28**, 283 (1975).

96. P. S. Soupart and T. H. Clewe, Sperm penetration of rabbit zona pellucida inhibited by treatment of ova with neuraminidase. *Fertil. Steril.*, **16**, 677 (1965).

97. J. L. Glick and S. Githens, The role of sialic acid in potassium transport of L1210 leukemia cells. *Nature (Lond.)*, **208**, 88 (1965).

98. J. L. Glick, A. R. Goldberg, and A. B. Pardee, The role of sialic acid in the release of proteins from L1210 leukemia cells. *Cancer Res.*, **26**, 1774 (1966).

99. G. A. Currie and K. D. Bagshawe, The effect of neuraminidase on the immunogenicity of the Landschutz ascites tumor: Site and mode of action. *Br. J. Cancer*, **22**, 588 (1968).

100. B. H. Sanford, An alteration in tumor histocompatibility induced by neuraminidase. *Transplantation*, **5**, 1273 (1967).

101. J. Lindenmann and P. A. Klein, *Immunological Aspects of Viral Oncolysis*, Springer-Verlag, Berlin, 1967 p. 63.

102. B. H. Sanford and J. F. Codington, Further studies on the effect of neuraminidase on tumor cell transplantability. *Tissue Antigens*, **1**, 153 (1971).

103. J. F. Codington, B. H. Sanford, and R. W. Jeanloz, Glycoprotein coat of the TA3 cell. I. Removal of carbohydrate and protein material from viable cells. *J. Natl. Cancer Inst.*, **45**, 637 (1970).

104. G. A. Currie, Masking of antigens on the Landschutz ascites tumor. *Lancet*, **II**, 1336 (1967).

105. J. G. Bekesi and J. F. Holland, Combined chemotherapy and immunotherapy of transplantable and spontaneous murine leukemia in DBA/2 and AKR mice. In G. Mathe, Ed., *Recent Results in Cancer Research*, Vol. 47, Springer-Verlag, Berlin, 1974, p. 357.

106. A. V. LeFever, J. J. Killion, and G. M. Kollmorgen, Active immunotherapy of L1210 leukemia with nueraminidase-treated, drug-resistant L1210 sublines. *Cancer Immunol. Immunother.*, **1**, 211 (1976).

107. G. A. Currie and K. D. Bagshawe, Tumor specific immunogenicity of methylcholanthrene-induced sarcoma cells after incubation in neuraminidase. *Br. J. Cancer,* **23**, 141 (1969).

108. P. K. Ray, V. S. Thakur, and K. Sundaram, Antitumor immunity. I. Differential response of neuraminidase-treated and x-irradiated tumor vaccine. *Eur. J. Cancer,* **11**, 1 (1975).

109. P. K. Ray, V. S. Thakur, and K. Sundaram, Antitumor immunity. II. Viability, tumorigenicity, and immunogenicity of neuraminidase-treated tumor cells: Effective immunization of animals with a tumor vaccine. *J. Natl. Cancer Inst.,* **56**, 83 (1976).

110. R. L. Simmons, A. Rios, and G. Lundgren, Immunospecific regression of methylcholanthrene fibrosarcoma with the use of neuraminidase. *Surgery,* **70**, 38 (1971).

111. C. D. Alley and M. J. Snodgrass, Effectiveness of neuraminidase in experimental immunotherapy of two murine pulmonary carcinomas. *Cancer Res.,* **37**, 95 (1977).

112. R. E. Wilson, S. T. Sonis, and E. A. Godrick, Neuraminidase as an adjunct in the treatment of residual systemic tumor with specific immune therapy. *Behring Inst. Mitt.,* **55**, 334 (1974).

113. J. Egeberg and O. A. Jensen, The effect of neuraminidase-treated tumor cells on the growth of transplantable malignant melanoma of the Syrian golden hamster (mesocricetus auratus). *Internatl. Rev. Cytol. (Suppl.)* **2**, 1573 (1974).

114. D. T. Gia and F. Loisillier, Effect of immunotherapy on the kinetics of proliferation of a transplanted rat rhabdomyosarcoma. *Eur. J. Cancer,* **14**, 1085 (1978).

115. P. K. Ray and M. Seshadri, Inhibition of growth of rat Yoshida sarcoma using neuraminidase-treated tumor vaccine. *Indian J. Exp. Biol.,* **17**, 36 (1979).

116. W. E. Enker, J. L. Jacobitz, K. Craft, and R. W. Wissler, Surgical adjuvant immunotherapy for colorectal cancer. *J. Surg. Oncol.,* **10**, 389 (1978).

117. C. W. Miller, R. F. DeBlasi, and S. J. Fisher, Immunological studies in murine osteosarcoma. *J. Bone Joint Surg.,* **58**, 312 (1976).

118. R. L. Simmons and A. Rios, Differential effect of neuraminidase on the immunogenicity of viral associated and private antigens of mammary carcinomas. *J. Immunol.,* **3**, 1820 (1973).

119. J. G. Bekesi, J. P. Roboz, E. Zimmerman, and J. F. Holland, Treatment of spontaneous leukemia in AKR mice with chemotherapy, immunotherapy, interferon and virazole. *Cancer Res.,* **36**, 631 (1976).

120. H. H. Sedlacek and F. R. Seiler, Demonstration of Vibrio cholerae neuraminidase (VCN) on the surface of VCN-treated cells. *Behring Inst. Mitt.,* **55**, 254 (1974).

121. H. H. Sedlacek and F. R. Seiler, Effect of Vibrio cholerae neuraminidase on the cellular immune response *in vivo.* In *Proceedings of the Symposium "Immunotherapy of Malignant Diseases,"* Schattauer, and Stuttgart, New York, 1978, p. 268.

122. H. H. Sedlacek and F. R. Seiler, Spontaneous mammary tumors in mongrel dogs: A relevant model to demonstrate tumor therapeutical success by application of neuraminidase. *Dev. Biol. Stand.,* **38**, 399 (1978).

123. H. H. Sedlacek and F. R. Seiler, Neuraminidase immunotherapy of spontaneous canine mammary tumors. In *Proceedings of the Symposium "Immunotherapy of Malignant Diseases,"* Schattauer and Stuttgart, New York, 1978, p. 227.

124. H. H. Sedlacek, H. Meesmann, and F. R. Seiler, Regression of spontaneous mammary tumors in dogs after infection of neuraminidase-treated tumor cells. *Internatl. J. Cancer,* **15**, 409 (1975).

125. J. G. Bekesi, J. P. Roboz, and J. F. Holland, Characteristics of immunity induced by neuraminidase-treated lymphosarcoma cells in C3H (MTV +) mice and C3H (MTV −) mice. *Isr. J. Med.,* **12**, 288 (1976).

126. G. Mathe, O. Halle-Pannenko, and C. Bourut, Active immunotherapy of AKR mice with spontaneous leukemia. *Rev. Eur. Études Clin. Biol.,* **17**, 997 (1973).

127. L. Weiss, Neuraminidase, sialic acids, and cell interactions. *J. Natl. Cancer Inst.,* **50**, 3 (1973).

128. J. F. Dore, M. J. Hadjiyannakis, C. Guibout, A. Coudert, L. Marholev, and K. Imai, Use of enzyme-treated cell in immunotherapy of a murine leukemia. *Lancet,* **17**, 600 (1973).

129. G. Froese, I. Berczi, and A. H. Sehon, Brief communication: Neuraminidase-induced enhancement of tumor growth in mice. *J. Natl. Cancer Inst.,* **52**, 1905 (1974).

130. M. V. Pimm, A. J. Cook, and R. W. Baldwin, Failure of neuraminidase treatment to influence tumorigenicity or immunogenicity of syngeneically transplanted rat tumor cells. *Eur. J. Cancer,* **14**, 869 (1978).

131. R. J. Spence, R. M. Simon, and A. R. Baker, Failure of immunotherapy with neuraminidase-treated tumor cell vaccine in mice bearing established 3-methylcholanthrene-induced sarcomas. *J. Natl. Cancer Inst.,* **60**, 451 (1978).

132. F. C. Sparks and J. H. Breeding, Tumor regression and enhancement resulting from immunotherapy with Bacillus Calmette-Guerin and neuraminidase. *Cancer Res.,* **34**, 3262 (1974).

133. L. Albright, J. C. Madigan, M. R. Gaston, and D. P. Houchens, Therapy in an intracerebral murine glioma model, using Bacillus Calmette-Guerin, neuraminidase-treated tumor cells, and 1-(2-chloroethyl)-3-cyclohexyl-1-nitrosourea. *Cancer Res.,* **35**, 658 (1975).

134. J. P. Roboz, R. Suzuki, and J. G. Bekesi, Determination of neuraminidase-susceptible and total *N*-acetylneuraminic acid in normal and neoplastic cells by selected ion monitoring. *Anal. Biochem.,* **87**, 195 (1978).

135. J. P. Roboz, R. Suzuki, and J. G. Bekesi, Mass spectrometric quantification of *N*-acetylneuraminic acid in correlation to immunogenicity of leukemia cells. *Quant. Mass Spectr. Life Sci.,* **2**, 191 (1978).

136. J. P. Roboz, M. Suttajit, and J. G. Bekesi, Elimination of 2-deoxyribase interference in the thiobarbitine acid determination of *N*-acetylneuraminic acid in tumor cells by pH-dependent extraction with cyclohexamone. *Anal. Biochem.,* **110**, 380 (1981).

137. J. G. Bekesi, J. F. Holland, and J. P. Roboz, Immunotherapeutic efficacy of neuraminidase-treated allogeneic myeloblasts in patients with acute myelocytic leukemia. In M. A. Chirigos, Ed., *Control of Neoplasia by Modulation of the Immune System,* Raven, New York, 1977, p. 573.

138. J. G. Bekesi, J. P. Roboz, and J. F. Holland, Immunotherapy with neuraminidase-treated murine leukemia cells after cytoreductive therapy in leukemic mice. *Modulation of host immune resistance.* In M. C. Chirigos, Ed., Fogarty International Center Proceedings, Vol. 28, 1977, p. 219.

139. L. Gross, *"Mouse leukemia" in Oncogenic Viruses.* Vol. 24, Pergamon, New York, 1970, p. 286.

140. J. N. Ihle, M. Yurconic, Jr., and M. G. Hanna, Jr., Autogenous immunity to endogenous RNA tumor virus: Radioimmune precipitation assay of mouse serum antibody levels. *J. Exp. Med.,* **38**, 194 (1973).

141. L. W. Law, Increase in incidence of leukemia in hybrid mice bearing thymic transplants from a high leukemic strain. *J. Natl. Cancer Inst.,* **12**, 789 (1952).

142. M. B. Oldstone, T. Aoki, and F. J. Dixon, The antibody response of mice to murine leukemia virus in spontaneous infection: Absence of classical immunological tolerance. *Proc. Natl. Acad. Sci. (USA),* **69**, 134 (1972).

143. J. F. Miller, Studies on mouse leukemia. The fate of thymus homografts in immunologically tolerant mice. *Br. J. Cancer,* **14**, 244 (1960).

144. K. Nakakuki and Y. Nichizuka, Effect of adult thymectomy on lymphoid tissues and the pathology of leukemia in mice of high leukemia strains. *Gann,* **55**, 509 (1964).

145. R. V. Markham, Jr., J. C. Sutherland, E. F. Cimino, W. P. Drake, and M. R. Hardindy, Immune complexes localized in the renal glomeruli of AKR mice: the presence of MuLV gs-1 and C-type RNA tumor virus gs-3 determinants. *Rev. Eur. Etude Clin. Biology,* **17**, 690 (1972).

146. D. L. Morton, Acquired immunological tolerance and carcinogenesis by the mammary tumor virus. I. Effect of neonatal infection with the mammary tumor virus on the growth of spontaneous mammary adenocarcinoma. *J. Natl. Cancer Inst.,* **42**, 311 (1969).

147. D. L. Morton, L. Goldman, and D. A. Wood. Acquired immunological tolerance and carcinogenesis by the mammary tumor virus. II. Immune responses influencing growth of spontaneous mammary adenocarcinomas. *J. Natl. Cancer Inst.,* **42**, 321 (1969).

148. M. Schlesinger and J. G. Bekesi, Natural autoantibodies for thymus cells and for neuraminidase treated leukemia cells in the sera of normal AKR mice. *J. Natl. Cancer Inst.,* **59**, 1945 (1977).

149. J. G. Bekesi, J. F. Holland, and J. P. Roboz, Specific immunotherapy with neuraminidase-modified leukemic cells. *Med. Clin. Symp. Adv. Treat. Cancer,* **61**, 1083 (1977).

150. J. L. McCoy, J. H. Dean, and L. W. Law, Immunogenicity, antigenicity and mechanism of tumor rejection of mineral-oil induced plasmacytomas in syngeneic BALB/c mice. *Internatl. J. Cancer,* **14**, 264 (1974).

151. B. T. Rouse, M. Röllinghoff, and N. L. Warner, Anti-theta serum-induced suppression of the cellular transfer of tumour-specific immunity to a syngeneic plasma cell tumour. *Nature (New Biol.),* **238**, 116 (1972).

152. M. Omine and S. Perry, Perturbation of leukemic cell population in AKR mice due to chemotherapy. *Cancer Res.,* **33**, 2596 (1973).

153. M. Omine, G. P. Sarha, and S. Perry, Composition of leukemic cell populations in AKR leukemia and effects of chemotherapy. *Eur. J. Cancer,* **9**, 557 (1973).

154. M. Pollard and N. Sharon, Prevention and treatment of spontaneous leukemia in germ free AKR mice. *Proc. Soc. Exp. Biol. Med.,* **137**, 1494 (1971).

155. F. M. Schabel, H. E. Skipper, M. W. Trader, W. R. Laster, and L. Simpson-Herren, Spontaneous AKR leukemia (lymphoma) as a model system. *Cancer Chemother. Rep.,* **53**, 329 (1969).

156. H. E. Skipper, F. M. Schabel, and M. W. Trader, Basic and therapeutic trial results obtained in the spontaneous AKR leukemia (lymphoma) model end of 1971. *Cancer Chemother. Rep.,* **56**, 273 (1972).

157. H. E. Skipper, F. M. Schabel, M. W. Trader, and W. R. Lester, Response to therapy of spontaneous, first passage, and long passage lines of AKR leukemia. *Cancer Chemother. Rep.,* **53**, 345 (1969).

158. M. J. Straus, S. C. Choi, and A. Goldin, Increased lifespan in AKR leukemia mice treated with prophylactin chemotherapy. *Cancer Res.,* **33**, 1724 (1973).

159. J. Cuttner, O. Glidewell, J. G. Bekesi, and J. F. Holland, Chemoimmunotherapy of leukemia: MER in acute myelocytic leukemia. In W. D. Terry and D. Windhorst, Eds., *Immunotherapy of Cancer: Present Status of Trials in Man,* Raven, New York, 1978, p. 369.

160. H. T. Holden, R. K. Oldham, J. R. Ortaldo, and R. B. Herberman, Cryopreservation of the functional reactivity of normal and immune leukocytes and of tumor cells. In B. R. Bloom and J. R. David, Eds., *In Vitro Methods in Cell-Mediated and Tumor Immunity,* Academic, New York, 1976, p. 273.

161. S. H. Golub, Cryopreservation of human lymphocytes. In B. R. Bloom and J. R. David, Eds., *In Vitro Methods in Cell-Mediated and Tumor Immunity,* Academic, New York, 1976, p. 731.

162. M. E. Oren and R. B. Herberman, Delayed cutaneous hypersensitivity reactions to membrane extracts of human tumor cells. *Clin. Exp. Immunol.,* **9**, 45 (1971).

163. B. G. Leventhal, R. H. Halterman, E. B. Rosenberg, and R. B. Herberman, Immune reactivity of leukemia patients autologous blast cells. *Cancer Res.,* **32**, 1820 (1972).

164. W. H. Fridman and F. M. Kourilsky, Stimulation of lymphocytes by autologous leukemic cells in acute leukemia. *Nature (Lond.),* **224**, 277 (1969).

165. R. L. Powles, L. A. Balchin, and G. Hamilton-Fairley, Recognition of leukemia cells as foreign before and after autoimmunization. *Br. Med. J.,* **1**, 486 (1971).

166. M. L. Bach, F. H. Bach, and P. Joo, Leukemia associated antigens in the mixed lymphocyte culture test. *Science,* **166**, 1520 (1969).

167. A. R. Cheema and E. M. Hersh, Patient survival after chemotherapy and its relationship to *in vitro* lymphocyte blastogenesis. *Cancer,* **28**, 851 (1971).

15

Influences of
Nutrition on Immunity

ROBERT A. GOOD
ANNE WEST
GABRIEL FERNANDES
Memorial Sloan-Kettering Cancer Center
New York, New York

1. INTRODUCTION

The importance of proper nutrition in achieving a long and healthy life has been recognized throughout history. However, the precise relationships between specific nutritional elements, specific immunologic functions, and disease are only beginning to be identified. There are now studies in progress all over the world on both the sociocultural dimensions of the malnutrition-infection complex (1), which accounts for the majority of deaths in developing countries, and the biomedical particulars of this relationship (2–5). To understand exact-

The original work described in this review has been aided by grants CA-17404, CA-19267, CA-08748, AI-11843, AG-00541, AG-02247, and NS-11457 from the National Institutes of Health; the National Foundation-March of Dimes; the Special Projects Committee of Memorial Sloan-Kettering Cancer Center; the Joe Brooks Fund for the Advanced Study of Cancer; the Richard Molin Memorial Foundation; the Earl M. Coleman Laboratory; the Sherman Fairchild Foundation New Frontiers Fund; the Neil A. McConnell Foundation; the Paul Lane and Nat Peters Research Fund; the Pew Memorial Trust; and the Zelda R. Weintraub Cancer Fund.

ly how dietary factors correlate with health and disease, investigators are calling on our expanding knowledge of the immunity system for perspectives on how the constituents of this system interact with one another and also on how the entire immunologic network interacts with the rest of the body economy. We have learned, for instance, that even a single nutrient—the trace metal zinc— is essential to immunologic functions and that deficiency of this one substance can be lethal to both humans and animals (6). We have also seen that overfeeding, as well as underfeeding, may be associated with morbidity in several experimental models and that it is possible with those animals to inhibit or even prevent disease development by restricting protein, calories, or fat in the diet (7). Through sufficiently detailed knowledge of these biological relationships, we hope it may become possible to manipulate nutritional variables for the treatment or even the prevention of diseases associated with declined immunologic effectiveness, including all of the major diseases of aging; such as arteriosclerosis and other vascular diseases, atherosclerosis, amyloidosis, renal disease, autoimmune diseases such as arthritis, infectious diseases, and cancer. Such a resource might enable us to realize the rich genetic potential of human beings for a fully extended and healthy life.

2. MALNUTRITION: CLINICAL AND EXPERIMENTAL OBSERVATIONS

Studies on nutrition and immunity were carried out principally in field situations in the developing countries for a number of years (in reference 8). Protein-calorie malnutrition was virtually always linked with heightened susceptibility to infection. These infections, frequently accompanied by parasitic infestation, further damaged the immunologic functioning of individuals suffering from multiple dietary deficiencies, associated in severe cases with marasmus or even kwashiorkor. In contrast, studies of Australian aboriginal school children on a moderately protein-deficient diet showed that whereas these children's antibody production was impaired, several aspects of their cellular immunity, including proliferative responses of lymphocytes to certain T-cell mitogens, were enhanced (9).

When controlled laboratory studies were conducted to analyze this apparent paradox, a dramatic discrepancy emerged between the effects of protein or protein-calorie malnutrition on antibody production, largely a function of B lymphocytes, and on several T-cell functions including proliferative responses to mitogens, rate of allograft rejection, development of delayed allergy, and formation of migration inhibition factor (reviewed in reference 10). Although B-cell function was impaired in proportion to the degree of dietary restriction (Figure 1), T-cell functions were unaffected or actually enhanced in several experimental systems, including those of mice, rats, guinea pigs, and even a few monkeys (10). Tumor immunity was preserved or enhanced in nutritionally deprived animals. When mice and rats on restricted diets were immunized with syngeneic, allogeneic, or xenogeneic tumors, they responded with normal or increased cell-mediated cytotoxicity, even when protein was reduced from 28% to as low as 5% of the diet (Table 1).

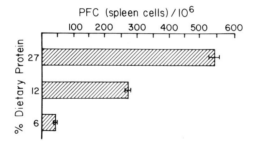

Figure 1.   Effect of protein deprivation on antibody production. (See reference 11.)

TABLE 1.   Cellular Immune Response to Allogeneic and Syngeneic Tumor Challenge in Protein-Restricted Animals

Intake cal/day	Percent protein	Percent Cell-Mediated Lysis of Tumor Cells	
		Allogeneic Challenge[a]	Syngeneic Challenge[b]
21	28	54	78
20	11	52	68
18	8	58	67
18	5	63	72
15	3	10	12

Source: Good et al. (10).

[a] C57B1/6J mice were immunized with DBA/2 mastocytoma cells; the standard Cr-release test was performed on day 11.

[b] C3Hf/Umc mice were immunized with C3H/B1 mammary tumor cells; the assay was performed on day 12.

Moreover, the ability of these animals to resist different kinds of infection depended on whether the immune response necessary to control the challenging pathogen was primarily mediated by the B- or the T-cell system. Protein-deprived mice were nearly 2 logs more sensitive than were controls to streptococci, an encapsulated pathogen defended against principally by antibody. However, this group showed a greater resistance than did controls to the pseudorabies virus, presumably because their cellular immunity was enhanced. Figure 2 shows that less than 20% the number of bacteria necessary to kill 50% of normal animals will kill 50% of protein-deprived animals (LD_{50}). By contrast, 100 times more pseudorabies virus is required to kill protein-deprived animals than to kill animals in the control group (11).

This paradox between the effects of nutritional deprivation on humans and on experimental animal models may be interpreted in several ways. Given our growing recognition of different immunoregulatory cell subpopulations, especially within the T-cell system, it is not surprising that different types of dietary change have different effects on specific types of cells or cellular interaction. We also now know that the entire T-cell system is uniquely sensitive to

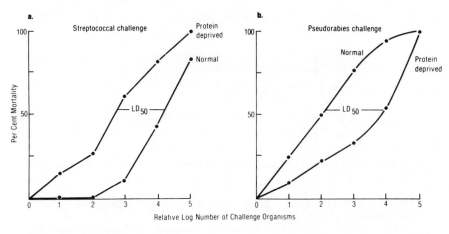

Figure 2. Effect of protein deprivation on survival of pathogen-challenged mice. (See reference 11.)

the trace metal zinc (as we discuss later), a nutrient usually is not available to human populations with multiple dietary deficiencies, although it is present in the standard food given to experimental animals. Morever, we may anticipate that other specific nutrients will, like zinc, prove to be crucial to normal immunoregulation in ways that we have not yet analyzed and that could play a part in the wide-ranging immunologic deficiencies of malnourished humans.

3. ZINC AND THYMUS

Zinc has been shown to exert powerful and apparently specific influences on the thymus, T lymphocytes, and cellular immunity in humans and in several animal systems (6). A dramatic illustration of this effect is in the A-46 mutant of black, pied, Danish cattle, a variant of the Holstein-Friesian line, which is genetically unable to absorb zinc normally through the gastrointestinal tract. Extensively studied by the Danish investigators Brummerstedt and colleagues (12), animals with this defect have a severely hypoplastic thymus and profoundly impaired thymus-derived immunity. Calves are stunted and lethargic, develop a number of skin disorders, and are vulnerable to a variety of infections, which are frequently fatal. However, administration of sufficient zinc either orally or parenterally cures this entire syndrome. Calves are immunologically reconstituted, and their symptoms disappear (Figure 3).

The human disease acrodermatitis enteropathica (AE), defined as a clinical entity for the first time in 1942 (13), represents a human counterpart of the zinc-deficiency syndrome in A-46 Friesian cattle. This disorder, also transmitted as an autosomal recessive trait, features malabsorption of zinc, severe skin lesions, gastrointestinal malfunction, and central nervous system disturbances among other symptoms, as well as extreme susceptibility to infections, especially with fungi, and often profound immunodeficiency (14–16).

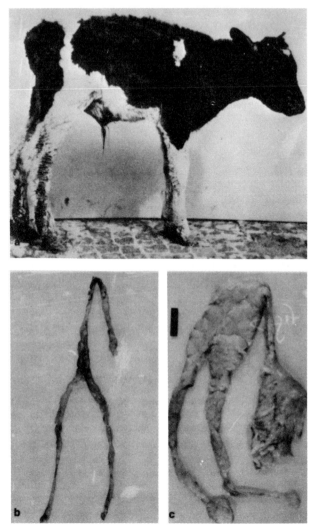

Figure 3. (*a*) Calf with hereditary thymus hypoplasia (lethal trait A-46) showing typical late lesions. (*b*) Hypoplastic thymus (9.5 g) from affected calf. (*c*) Normal-sized thymus (372 g) from a reconstituted calf. (Reprinted from reference 12. Illustrations courtesy of the authors and the *American Journal of Pathology.*)

Fortunately, a physician managing one such child who was also lactase-deficient became concerned that his patient's lactose-free diet might be deficient in zinc. He administered a zinc supplement and completely cured his patient (17). This case firmly established the association between zinc deficiency and immunodeficiency disease.

Studies of the biological role of zinc in both human and animal systems have revealed that more than 90 metalloenzymes, including several necessary for the synthesis of DNA and RNA (i.e., thymidine kinase, DNA polymerase, and DNA-dependent RNA polymerase), require zinc for proper functioning (18). It is logical to expect, therefore, that the availability of zinc is crucial for biological processes that involve rapid growth and division of cells. Cell proliferation is, of course, essential to immunologic vigor. Zinc might in fact be characterized as the only lymphocyte mitogen that occurs naturally in the body (reviewed, 7). Deoxyribonucleic acid synthesis, blast transformation, and mitosis of lymphocytes in response to zinc occur over a narrow range of zinc concentrations (0.1 to 0.15 mM) and are comparable to those of phytohemagglutinin but somewhat slower (reviewed in reference 19) (Figure 4).

In experimentally zinc-deprived mice, the thymus and T-cell numbers and functions become severely involuted (20,21). The growth of deprived animals is not only stunted; animals lose weight beginning with the second week of deprivation (Figure 5). Acrodermatitis enteropathica and lymphoid system abnormalities develop in these animals, and there is a dramatic breakdown in their immunity function, particularly the functions of helper T cells (21) and killer T cells *in vivo* (20) (Table 2). By contrast, *in vitro* immunization of spleen cells with either sheep red blood cells (SRBC) or EL-4 tumor cells in the presence of adequate zinc reveals no defect in the intrinsic ability of cells from zinc-deficient animals to mount specific immune response. Thymus-dependent humoral immunity, such as the ability to mount a plaque-forming cell (PFC) response to *in vivo* challenge with SRBC, also deteriorates in zinc-deficient animals (Table 3). Whereas the primary antibody response drops substantially,

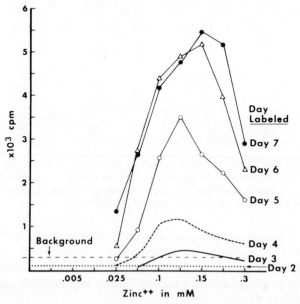

Figure 4. Time-dose response of human peripheral lymphocytes to zinc. (Reprinted from reference 6.)

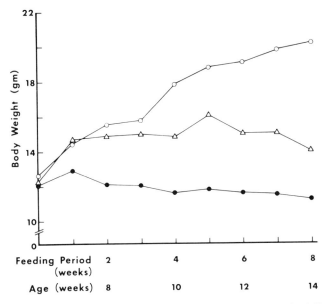

Figure 5. Effects of Zn(−) (filled circles) pair-fed Zn(+) (triangles) and *ad lib* Zn(+) (open circles) diets on growth of C57BL/Ks female mice. (Reprinted from reference 15.)

the secondary response, which requires helper T lymphocytes, essentially disappears. Again, when cells are challenged *in vitro* in the presence of zinc, they show normal PFC-forming capacity. The direct influence of zinc on lymphocyte functions has been established by *in vitro* analyses in which the proliferative responses of T lymphocytes to phytomitogens were observed after dialysis with the chelator EDTA. Removal of zinc and other cations by this means com-

TABLE 2. Cytotoxic T Killer Cell Activity After *in Vivo* Immunization of Zn⁻ CBA/H Mice

	Percent ⁵¹Cr release at 4 hours[b]		
Diet[a]	1:100[c]	1:50	1:25
Zn⁻	26.6 ± 2.3	20.7 ± 2.4	13.4 ± 2.0
Zn⁺ PF	65.5 ± 9.9	56.5 ± 10.6	43.1 ± 9.6
Lab chow[d]	66.1 ± 6.3	63.1 ± 6.3	47.5 ± 3.4

Source: Fernandes et al. (20).

[a] In each dietary group, four or five individual spleens were tested (PF, pair-fed).

[b] After 8 weeks on diets, mice were immunized *in vivo* with 10⁷ EL4 cells i.p., and cytotoxicity testing was carried out *in vitro* 12 days after immunization. Data are shown as mean ± SEM.

[c] Target: lymphocyte ratios.

[d] Standard laboratory food.

TABLE 3. PFC Response in C57BL/Ks Mice Maintained on Different Diets[a]

Diet	Duration (Weeks)	Direct PFC per Spleen	Indirect PFC per Spleen
Zn⁻	2	29,127 ± 9,682	23,149 ± 8,402
Zn⁺ PF[b]	2	25,428 ± 1,276	19,699 ± 920
Zn⁻	4	18,502 ± 5,606	14,913 ± 5,466
Zn⁺ PF[b]	4	38,392 ± 9,902	31,934 ± 8,549
Lab chow	6	64,281 ± 7,152	53,294 ± 3,144
Zn⁻	6	8,278 ± 2,651	5,128 ± 2,312
Zn⁺ PF	6	80,983 ± 2,772	69,071 ± 6,749
Zn⁺ *ad lib*	6	117,968 ± 15,858	95,446 ± 7,393
Lab chow	8	104,662 ± 18,937	74,647 ± 6,202

Source: Fernandes et al. (20).

[a] At least four mice were immunized with SRBC (0.2 ml of 10% cell suspension) in each group. Data are shown as mean ± SEM. For secondary responses, a second immunization was carried out on day 7. The assays were carried out on day 4 (primary response) or on day 11 (secondary response).

[b] Pair-fed.

pletely abrogated lymphocyte proliferation. When zinc alone was returned to the culture medium after EDTA treatment, responses of the T cells were fully restored. Returning other divalent cations in the absence of Zn^{2+} failed to correct the deficient responsiveness of the T lymphocytes (22).

This unique sensitivity of the thymus and thymocytes to the presence or absence of zinc may be related to the fact that terminal deoxyribonucleotidyl transferase (TdT), a zinc-containing DNA polymerase, is present almost exclusively in the thymus and immature thymocytes, but not in mature T cells (23). In zinc deficiency the DNA content of the thymus is depressed (24), as a result of which one might expect to observe an arrest in the differentiation of T-cell precursors to become immunocompetent thymocytes. It is interesting to note, however, that two functionally distinct populations of cells are differently affected by zinc deficiency: whereas natural killer (NK) activity toward lymphoma cells drops substantially in zinc-deficient animals, one form of antibody-dependent cell-mediated cytotoxicity is actually slightly increased (20). This observation is consistent with those by Fraker et al. (21) and Chvapil (25), who found that different constituents of the immunity network are differently affected by zinc deficiency.

Levels of the thymic hormone facteur thymique serique (FTS) described by Bach and colleagues (26) are also drastically reduced in zinc-deficient mice (27). This hormone is also involved in the induction of precursor cells to differentiate into θ-positive lymphocytes. In mice and humans, levels of FTS usually decline rapidly after the onset of sexual maturation (26). Administration of zinc actually delays the apparent age dependent thymic involution.

Several clinical situations have proved to be associated with zinc deficiency (19). Both the present authors and others (28,29) have found that certain patients with common variable immunodeficiency disease may have low levels of serum zinc, in some cases clearly caused by inadequate diet. Sufficient supplements of dietary zinc led to improvement of clinical symptoms and reconstitution of some immunologic functions in several cases (28,29).

Other clinical studies showed that the proliferative responses of peripheral blood lymphocytes to *in vitro* stimulation with either zinc or the mitogen phytohemagglutinin (PHA) were depressed to similar degrees in patients with several forms of cancer, including adenocarcinoma of the breast, epidermal carcinoma of the head and neck region, and lymphoma (30). Low serum zinc levels coupled with cellular immunodeficiency were observed in patients with epidermoid cancer of the head and neck region, especially when these lesions involved the mouth. This abnormality also was related to inadequate diet (31). Surgical treatment itself may be followed by prolonged or permanent zinc deficiency, especially in patients who had low serum zinc levels prior to surgery (32). Zinc deficiency and resulting immunodeficiencies are particularly likely to develop in individuals who have undergone intestinal bypass surgery or are subjected to tube feedings during the postoperative period (32).

A number of striking similarities can be observed between zinc deficiency and protein-calorie malnutrition in humans, including skin lesions, diarrhea, and anorexia among many other symptoms, as well as seriously compromised immunity function and several biochemical abnormalities (reviewed in reference 8). Indeed, zinc deficiency has been identified as a frequent concomitant of protein-calorie malnutrition (33,34), a fact that may largely account for why protein-calorie malnourished children suffer from wide-ranging immunologic deficits, including deficiencies of the T-cell system, whereas laboratory animals on calorie-restricted diets, which contain a standard quota of zinc, do not. The altered overall state of the body's functioning under circumstances either of severe malnutrition or of other debilitating diseases may also exacerbate the individual's condition; diarrhea, vomiting, impaired absorption, and a variety of metabolic changes caused by generalized infection may contribute further to the breakdown of the undernourished person's nutritional status and of normal immunologic functioning (1).

4. NUTRITION, THYMUS-DERIVED IMMUNITY AND THE DISEASES OF AGING

Now that sanitation, effective immunizations, antibiotics, and chemotherapies have minimized the threat of infectious diseases in the developed countries, we can afford the relative luxury of addressing the diseases of aging. Paradoxically, there is now substantial evidence that dietary excess may also lead to diseases that shorten and lower the quality of life.

We have seen from the studies reviewed above in the previous sections the thymus may be the single biological component of the greatest importance in translating nutritional causes into immunologic effects. Nutritional deficiencies, including the striking example of zinc deficiency, may severely impair thymic immunity function and lead to serious morbidity and high mortality. On the other hand, excessive dietary intake associated with full development and vigorous activity of the thymus very early in life in several strains of short-lived, autoimmune-prone mice has been strongly implicated in the early disorganization of their immunity functions and the development of the sets of diseases that characterize these strains (35). Studies in our own (reviewed in reference 7) and other (36) laboratories over the past several years have clearly shown that even genetically determined involution of the immunologic apparatus in such models may be modified by diet, with striking inhibitory effects on the development of disease. Taken as a group, the characteristic diseases of these experimental strains of mice are analogous to all the major diseases of aging in humans: arteriosclerosis and other vascular diseases; atherosclerosis; amyloidosis; renal disease; autoimmune diseases such as arthritis; infectious diseases; and cancer.

The NZB mouse typically develops disorders analogous to virtually all the diseases of aging in humans: atherosclerosis; hyalinizing renal disease correlated with autoimmune phenomena; Coombs-positive hemolytic anemia with autoantibodies against red blood cells; several kinds of cancer including leukemia, sarcoma, and hepatoma; amyloid deposits; cardiovascular disease; and splenomegaly. Mice of this strain frequently develop autoantibodies to immunologically active cells and consequently tend to develop increasingly severe immunodeficiency. Lowering the fat component in the diet of these animals caused their disease to occur significantly later and to be less severe, and mice lived correspondingly longer (37). Lower titers of autoantibodies and increased cellular cytotoxicity after tumor immunization were associated with the low-fat diet (38). When the same strain of mice was chronically deprived of protein, thymic involution was delayed, splenomegaly was inhibited, and cellular immunities were more vigorous than in controls receiving conventional diets (39).

Even more dramatic studies that used hybrid (NZB × NZW)F$_1$ (B/W) mice, which under normal feeding conditions develop rampant autoimmune renal disease and die between 8 and 14 months of age, showed that these animals' life-spans could be literally doubled in some instances when total food intake was decreased (40,41). Every aspect of the disorganization of immunologic function normally seen in this strain can be modified simply by limiting calorie intake. Moreover, it seemed that fat was the most critical dietary variable in the development of disease by these animals as well as by NZB mice. When calories were restricted while a high proportion of fat was included in the diet, mice developed their characteristic autoimmune and immunodestructive pathology at an early age. However, when the diet was low in both calories and fat, disease development was prevented and life-span greatly prolonged in these animals (42).

Studies of other immunologic parameters, including generation of killer cells in response to stimulation with allogeneic tumor cells, proliferative responses of spleen cells to T-cell mitogens and allogeneic cells, and the PFC response to SRBC showed that these functions are all much better preserved in animals fed 10 instead of 20 cal/day. Autoimmune activity is also much lower in animals fed low-calorie diets. Anti-DNA antibody levels in the serum, which increase rapidly in normally fed mice, are elevated less than 50% as much in mice from the low-calorie group at the same age (41) (see Table 4). Circulating immune complex levels in the blood and immune complex deposition in the kidneys was also much less extensive in the animals subjected to dietary restriction (Figure 6).

TABLE 4. Changes in Binding of ^{125}I-labeled DNA by Sera from Normal and Calorie Restricted B/W Mice[a]

Intake (cal/day)	Percent DNA Binding		
	3 Months	6 Months	9 Months
20	8.4 ± 2.7	18.1 ± 4.7	53.2 ± 6.0
10	5.2 ± 0.7	11.6 ± 6.9	21.9 ± 2.8
P	NS	NS	< 0.001

Source: Fernandes et al. (41).

[a]DNA-binding capacity of the serum of individual mice was measured by a micro method assaying the amount of labeled DNA precipitable by ammonium sulfate.

It was even possible to inhibit the development of renal disease and to prolong the life-span of these animals when dietary restriction was imposed after the disease process had already begun (43). Conversely, overfeeding facilitated development of autoimmune disease, hastened involution of the thymus and T-cell system, and shortened life in both NZB and B/W strains. Recent work in our laboratories has shown that the dietary intake of B/W mice may be correlated with their characteristic hypertension and with serum cholesterol levels, as well as with renal disease. Certain B/W mice on high-calorie, high-fat diets (20 cal/day, 20% fat) have developed enlarged hearts as well as myocardial and arteriosclerotic lesions and increased levels of serum cholesterol. When the fat component is lowered to 5%, these abnormal features are less pronounced, but when the fat component remains at 5% while total calories are reduced to 10, there is no evidence of cardiovascular disease (44).

Calorie restriction also dramatically prolongs life in the *kd/kd* mutant mouse, inhibiting the development of autoimmune interstitial nephritis and progressive tubular damage (45). In MRL/1 mice the characteristic extraordinary lymphoproliferative disease is dramatically reduced by controlling the diet, and life may be prolonged to as much as three times the normal length (46).

We have also found, confirming the work of early investigators (47–50), that severe restriction of calorie intake can inhibit or even completely prevent

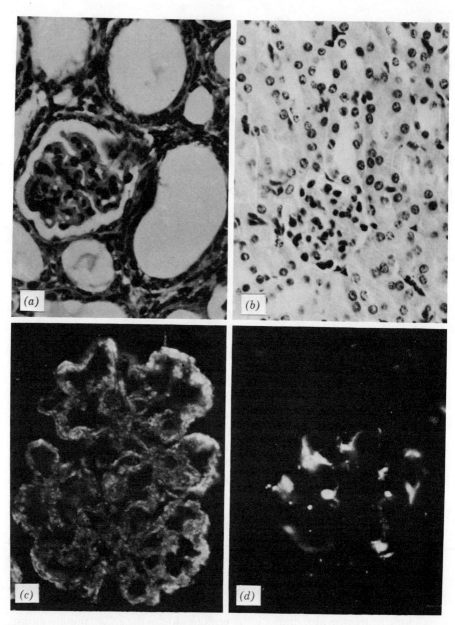

Figure 6. Comparison of kidneys from (NZB × NZW)F₁ mice on high (20-cal/day)- and low (10-cal/day)-calorie diets. (*a*) High-power view showing tubular dilation, tubular cell atrophy, and glomerulosclerosis of 10-month-old B/W mouse on high-calorie diet (400×). (*b*) High-power view showing normal tubules and glomeruli of 10-month-old B/W mouse on low calorie diet (400×). (*c*) Immunofluorescence microscopy showing glomerulus of 10-month-old B/W mouse fed 20 cal/day, stained with fluorescent anti-serum specific for IgG. Note irregular granular deposits of IgG lining cell capillaries of

mammary adenocarcinoma in female C3H/Bi mice (51), of which 70 to 80% normally develop tumors by 16 months of age (Figure 7). Tucker in England has found in several systems that even restricting total food intake by as little as 20% results in significantly reduced incidence and delayed onset of tumor growth and increased longevity (52). She also noted that whereas this restriction affected the most common tumors in both rats and mice, other tumors were unaffected, suggesting that this latter group had a different etiology, possibly viral. In collaborative studies with Sarkar et al. (53) of the murine mammary tumor virus (MuMTV) in female C3H mice, we have seen that both the presence and maturity of virus particles may be substantially diminished by diet. When C3H female mice are fed 16 cal/day, they show evidence of well-developed MuMTV particles in most cells of the mammary glands examined. By contrast, mammary tissue sections taken from mice on 10 cal/day contain fewer or less mature virus particles (Figure 8). At the same time, restricted animals have normal estrous cycles and are apparently healthy, with even better development of the mammary glands than is seen in the unrestricted mice. Again, as in studies of NZB and B/W mice, the proportion of fat in the diet has emerged as the crucial nutritional variable in the development of disease in this strain (54). When total calories are kept low but the proportion of fat is raised, C3H mice develop as many tumors as animals on the high-calorie regimens. We have also seen that animals on the higher fat diet show signs of tumor development earlier, as well as having higher cholesterol levels (54). Saturated and unsaturated fats are equally highly correlated with serum cholesterol and tumor growth.

Other immunologic interactions in the C3H mouse model, particularly those involving distinct subpopulations of T cells, will be important subjects for study in the near future, particularly in light of the possibility that dietary restriction may have different effects on their functions. We have already observed that reduced food intake in hybrid B/W mice has different effects on two distinct types of suppressor T cell. Older B/W mice with active autoimmune disease, on a normal *ad libitum* diet, spontaneously develop cells that suppress PFC formation. However, a population of mitogen-inducible suppressors present in young animals is lost as their disease progresses. When total food intake is reduced, the precursors of inducible suppressors are apparently maintained, whereas development of spontaneous suppressor activity seems to be inhibited (41). Decreased expression of the xenotropic viruses described by Levy and associates (55) has been shown not to be responsible for

the glomerulus. Every glomerulus of the kidneys from these 10-month-old B/W mice showed these characteristics (500×). (*d*) Immunofluorescence microscopy showing glomerulus of 10-month-old B/W mouse fed 10 cal/day. Note that glomerular capillaries are completely free of IgG deposits. The only IgG demonstrable appeared in the mesangium of the glomerular tuft (650×). (Parts *a* and *b* reprinted from reference 45; parts *c* and *d* reprinted from reference 41.)

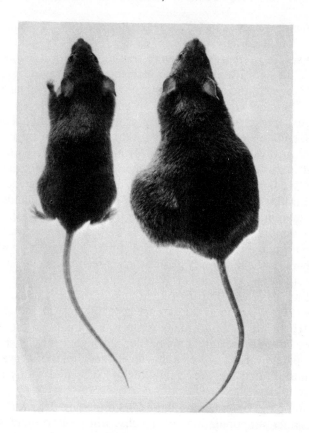

Figure 7. Ten-month-old C3H virgin female mice fed 10 cal/day (left) and 20 cal/day (right). Mammary tumor development is prominently visible on mouse maintained on the high-calorie diet. (Reprinted from reference 7.)

the preserved immunologic and physical vigor of these moderately deprived animals (56). Zinc deprivation also has different effects on different immunologic functions in mice, substantially inhibiting natural killer (NK) cell activity while slightly enhancing antibody-dependent cell-mediated cytotoxicity (ADCC) (20). Examination of these immunologic parameters in the C3H mouse model, as well as other mammary tumor-prone strains of mice maintained on different diets and exposed to viral, hormonal, or chemical carcinogens, may lead to important new information on precisely how dietary factors affect the immunologic circumstances that prevent or permit the development of cancer. The approach to questions of pathogenesis in human breast cancer should be substantially aided by such additions to our understanding of the cellular and molecular mechanisms involved in tumorigenesis.

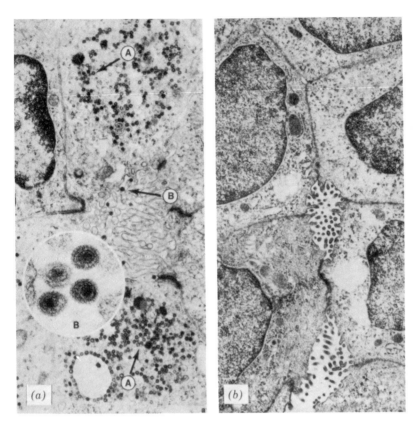

Figure 8. (*a*) Electron micrograph of mammary epithelial cells from C3H mice on a normal diet (16 cal/day). Note the large number of MuMTV A particles (A) at the apical part of the cells and some budding and mature B particles (900×). Inset shows higher magnification of MuMTV B particles (105,000×). (*b*) Electron micrograph of mammary epithelial cells from C3H mice on a low-calorie diet (10 cal/day). None of the cells contain A or B particles. Only a few MuMTV particles were observed in a large number of cell sections examined (900×). (Reprinted from reference 7. Photographs courtesy of Nurul H. Sarkar, Ph.D., and the *Clinical Bulletin of Memorial Sloan-Kettering Cancer Center.*)

5.   COMMENTS AND CONCLUSIONS

Our knowledge of the relationships between nutrition, immunity, and disease is now being rapidly expanded by clinical and experimental studies such as those described previously. We now know that deficiencies or excesses of each major dietary component, including proteins, fats, total calories, and vitamins or minerals, may profoundly affect diseases development and longevity. This research also suggests many areas for related investigations. Physiological and endocrine mechanisms and their interactions with the central nervous system are very likely to participate in the processes by which diet alters immunologic functions. Future inquiries into the nature of these biological events are likely to focus on altered immunoregulation involving distinct subpopulations of lymphoid cells and the molecular mediators they release, as well as the DNA, RNA, and protein content of these cellular elements.

Great care must certainly be exercised before extending any of these experimental findings, which are highlighted by some fairly drastic dietary manipulations, to human beings. However, our growing ability to address both normal and pathogenetic immunologic processes in terms of cells and molecules gives us cause for optimism about future applications of the knowledge being generated. We may begin to anticipate a time when the therapeutic potential of a scientifically modified diet will be realized and made deliverable.

REFERENCES

1. L. Mata, The malnutrition-infection complex and its environment factors. *Proc. Nutr. Soc.,* **38**, 29 (1979).

2. R. E. Olson, Ed., *Protein-Calorie Malnutrition,* Academic, New York, 1975.

3. R. K. Chandra and P. M. Newberne, Eds., *Nutrition, Immunity and Infection. Mechanisms of Interactions,* Plenum, New York, 1977.

4. R. R. Suskind, Ed., *Malnutrition and the Immune Response,* Raven, New York, 1977.

5. R. A. Good, G. Fernandes, and A. West, Nutrition, immunity, and cancer—A Review. Part I. Influence of protein or protein-calorie malnutrition and zinc deficiency on immunity. *Clin. Bull. MSKCC,* **9**, 63.

6. L. H. Schloen, G. Fernandes, J. A. Garofalo, and R. A. Good, Nutrition, immunity, and cancer—A Review. Part II. Zinc, immune function and cancer. *Clin. Bull. MSKCC,* **9**, 63.

7. G. Fernandes, A. West, and R. A. Good, Nutrition, immunity, and cancer—A Review. Part III. Effects of diet on the diseases of aging. *Clin. Bull. MSKCC,* **9**, 91 (1979).

8. M. A. Hansen, G. Fernandes, and R. A. Good, Infection in the special host: The severely malnourished host. In A. J. Nahmias and R. J. O'Reilly, Eds., *Immunology of Human Infection,* Vol. 10, *Comprehensive Immunology,* Plenum, New York (in press).

9. D. G. Jose, J. S. Welch, and R. L. Doherty, Humoral and cellular immune responses to streptococci, influenza, and other antigens in Australian aboriginal school children. *Aust. Pediatr. J.,* **6**, 192 (1970).

10. R. A. Good, G. Fernandes, E. J. Yunis, W. C. Cooper, D. G. Jose, T. R. Kramer, and M. A. Hansen, Nutritional deficiency, immunological function, and disease. *Am. J. Pathol.,* **84**, 599 (1976).

11. W. C. Cooper, R. A. Good, and T. Mariani, Effects of protein insufficiency on immune responsiveness. *Am. J. Clin. Nutr.,* **27**, 647 (1974).

12. E. Brummerstedt, A. Basse, T. Flagstad, and E. Andresen, Animal model of human disease: Acrodermatitis enteropathica, zinc malabsorption. *Am. J. Pathol.,* **87** (3), 725 (1977).

13. N. Danbolt and K. Closs, Acrodermatitis enteropathica. *Acta. Derm. Venereol. (Stockh.),* **23**, 127 (1942).

14. A. E. Rodin and A. S. Goldman, Autopsy findings in acrodermatitis enteropathica. *Am. J. Clin. Pathol.,* **51**, 315 (1969).

15. R. Julius, M. Schilkind, T. Sprinkle, and O. Bennert, Acrodermatitis enteropathica with immune deficiency. *J. Pediatr.,* **83**, 1007 (1973).

16. R. A. Good, unpublished observations.

17. E. J. Moynahan and P. M. Barnes, Zinc deficiency and a synthetic diet for lactose intolerance. *Lancet,* **1**, 676 (1973).

18. J. F. Riordan and B. L. Vallee, Structure and function of zinc metalloenzymes. In A. S. Prasad, Ed., *Trace Elements in Human Health and Disease,* Vol. 1, *Zinc and Copper,* Academic, New York, 1976, p. 227.

19. R. A. Good, G. Fernandes, C. Cunningham-Rundles, S. Cunningham-Rundles, J. A. Garofalo, K. M. K. Rao, G. S. Incefy, and T. Iwata, The relation of zinc deficiency to immunologic function in animals and man. In M. Seligmann, Ed., *Primary Immunodeficiencies: Proceedings of the Symposium on Primary Immunodeficiencies,* Royamont, France, 1980 (also Elsevier/North Holland Biomedical Press, Amsterdam, 1981).

20. G. Fernandes, M. Nair, K. Onoe, T. Tanaka, R. Floyd, and R. A. Good, Impairment of cell-mediated immunity functions by dietary zinc deficiency in mice. *Proc. Natl. Acad. Sci. (USA),* **76**, 457 (1979).

21. P. J. Fraker, S. M. Haas, and R. W. Luecke, Effect of zinc deficiency on the immune response of the young adult A/J mouse. *J. Nutr.,* **197**, 1889 (1997).

22. P. Zanzanico, G. Fernandes, and R. A. Good, The differential sensitivity of T cell and B cell mitogenesis to *in vitro* zinc deficiency. *Cell. Immunol.,* **60**, 203 (1981).

23. R. McCaffrey, D. F. Smoler, and D. Baltimore, Terminal deoxyribonucleotidyl transferase in a case of childhood lymphoblastic leukemia. *Proc. Natl. Acad. Sci. (USA),* **70**, 521 (1973).

24. P. K. Ku, D. E. Ullery, and E. R. Miller, Zinc deficiency and tissue nucleic acid and protein concentration. In C. F. Mills, Ed., *Trace Element Metabolism in Animals,* Livingston, London, 1970.

25. M. Chvapil, The role of zinc in the function of some inflammatory cells. *Progr. Clin. Biol. Res.,* **4**, 103 (1977).

26. J. F. Bach, M. A. Bach, J. Charreire, M. Dardenne, C. Fournier, M. Papiernik, and J. M. Pleau, The circulating thymic factor (TF). Biochemistry, physiology, biological activities and clinical applications. A summary. In D. W. van Bekkum, Ed., *The Biological Activity of Thymic Hormones,* Kooyker Scientific Publications, Rotterdam, 1979, p. 145.

27. T. Iwata, G. S. Incefy, T. Tanaka, G. Fernandes, C. J. Menendez-Botet, K. Pih, and R. A. Good, Circulating thymic hormone levels in zinc deficiency. *Cell. Immunol.,* **47**, 100 (1979).

28. C. Cunningham-Rundles, S. Cunningham-Rundles, J. A. Garofalo, T. Iwata, G. Incefy, J. Twomey, and R. A. Good, Increased T lymphocyte function and thymopoietin following zinc repletion in man. *Fed. Proc. Fed. Am. Soc. Exp. Biol.,* **38**, 1222 (1979). (abstr.)

29. J. M. Oleske, M. L. Westphal, S. Shore, D. Gorden, J. Bogden, and A. Nahmias, Correction with zinc therapy of depressed cellular immunity in acrodermatitis enterophatica. *Am. J. Dis. Childh.,* **133**, 915 (1979).

30. J. A. Garofalo, S. Cunningham-Rundles, D. W. Braun, and R. A. Good, *In vitro* mitogenic effect of Zn^{++} on peripheral blood lymphocytes in patients with cancer. *Internatl. J. Immunopharmacol.,* **2**, 37 (1980).

31. J. A. Garofalo, E. Erlandson, E. W. Strong, M. Lesser, F. Gerold, R. Spiro, M. Schwartz, and R. A. Good, Serum zinc, serum copper and the Cu/Zn ratio in patients with epidermoid cancers of the head and neck. *J. Surg. Oncol.,* **15**, 381 (1980).

32. J. A. Garofalo, E. W. Strong, and R. A. Good, Zinc deficiency and intestinal bypass procedures. *Ann. Int. Med.,* **90**, 990 (1979).

33. M. Khalid, A. Kabiel, S. El-Khateeb, K. Aref, M. El-Lozy, S. Jahin, and F. Nasr, Plasma

and red cell water and elements in protein-calorie malnutrition. *Am. J. Clin. Nutr.,* **27**, 260 (1974).

34. M. H. N. Golden, B. E. Golden, P. S. E. G. Harland, and A. A. Jackson, Zinc and immuno-competence in protein-energy malnutrition. *Lancet,* **1**, 1226 (1978).

35. R. L. Walford, R. K. Liu, M. Gerbase-Delima, M. Mathies, and G. S. Smith, Longterm dietary restriction and immune function in mice: Response to sheep red blood cells and to mitogenic agents. *Mech. Aging Devel.,* **2**, 447 (1974).

36. R. H. Weindruch, J. A. Kristie, K. E. Cheney, and R. L. Walford, Influence of controlled dietary restriction on immunologic function and aging. *Fed. Proc.,* **38**, 2007 (1979).

37. G. Fernandes, E. J. Yunis, J. Smith, and R. A. Good, Dietary influence on breeding behavior, hemolytic anemia and longevity in NZB mice. *Proc. Soc. Exp. Biol. Med.,* **139**, 1189 (1972).

38. G. Fernandes, E. J. Yunis, D. G. Jose, and R. A. Good, Dietary influence on antinuclear antibodies and cell-mediated immunity in NZB mice. *Internatl. Arch. Allergy,* **44**, 770 (1973).

39. G. Fernandes, E. J. Yunis, and R. A. Good, Influence of protein restriction on immune function in NZB mice. *J. Immunol.,* **116**, 782 (1976).

40. G. Fernandes, E. J. Yunis, and R. A. Good, Influence of diet on survival of mice. *Proc. Natl. Acad. Sci. (USA),* **73**, 1279 (1976).

41. G. Fernandes, P. Friend, E. J. Yunis, and R. A. Good, Influence of dietary restriction on immunologic function and renal disease in (NZB × NZW)F$_1$ mice. *Proc. Natl. Acad. Sci. (USA),* **75**, 1500 (1978).

42. G. Fernandes and R. A. Good, unpublished observations.

43. P. S. Friend, G. Fernandes, R. A. Good, A. F. Michael, and E. J. Yunis, Dietary restriction early and late: Effects on the nephropathy of the NZB × NZW mouse. *Lab Invest.,* **38**, 629 (1978).

44. G. Fernandes, T. Tanaka, and R. A. Good, manuscript in preparation.

45. G. Fernandes, E. J. Yunis, M. Miranda, J. Smith, and R. A. Good, Nutritional inhibition of genetically determined renal disease and autoimmunity with prolongation of life in *kd/kd* mice. *Proc. Natl. Acad. Sci. (USA),* **75**, 2888 (1978).

46. G. Fernandes and R. A. Good, Alterations of longevity and immune function of B/W and MRL/1 mice by restriction of dietary intake. *Fed. Proc.,* **38**, 1370, 197.

47. P. Rous, The influence of diet on transplanted and spontaneous mouse tumors. *J. Exp. Med.,* **14**, 433 (1914).

48. C. M. McCay, L. A. Maynard, G. Sperling, and L. L. Barnes, Retarded growth, life span, ultimate body size and age changes in albino rats after feeding diets restricted in calories. *J. Nutr.,* **18**, 1 (1939).

49. A. Tannenbaum, The initiation and growth of tumors. Introduction, I. Effects of underfeeding. *Am. J. Cancer,* **38**, 335 (1940).

50. M. B. Visscher, Z. B. Ball, R. H. Barnes, and I. Sivertsen, The influence of calorie restriction upon the incidence of spontaneous mammary carcinoma in mice. *Surgery,* **11**, 48 (1942).

51. G. Fernandes, E. J. Yunis, and R. A. Good, Suppression of adenocarcinoma by the immunological consequences of calorie restriction. *Nature,* **263**, 504 (1976).

52. M. J. Tucker, the effect of long-term food restriction on tumors in rodents. *Internatl. J. Cancer,* **23**, 803 (1979).

53. N. K. Sarkar, G. Fernandes, K. Karande, and R. A. Good, manuscript in preparation.

54. G. Fernandes and R. A. Good, unpublished observations.

55. M. B. Gardner, J. N. Ihle, R. J. Pillarisetty, N. Talal, E. L. Dubois, and J. A. Levy, Type C virus expression and host response in diet-cured NZB/W mice. *Nature,* **268**, 341 (1977).

56. E. L. Dubois and L. Strain, Effect of diet on survival and nephropathy of NZB/NZW hybrid mice. *Biochem. Med.,* **7**, 336 (1973).

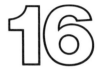

16

Perspectives for Immunological and Biological Therapeutic Intervention in Human Cancer

EVAN HERSH
University of Texas
M. D. Anderson Hospital
Houston, Texas

1. INTRODUCTION

The concept of cancer immunotherapy is an old one dating back to the original observations of Paul Ehrlich (1). Many attempts were made during the first half of the twentieth century to immunize patients against their own tumors, in general without striking success. After it was established in animal systems that certain syngeneic tumors contained tumor-specific antigens and induced a tumor-specific immune response in the tumor-bearing host and after it was established that immunotherapy could prevent or delay the development of experimental tumors in animal models, there was a strong impetus to explore it in both animal models and humans.

The immunologic basis for human cancer immunotherapy is now relatively well established. Thus both animal and human tumors do indeed contain tumor-associated or tumor-specific antigens and can be demonstrated to elicit a specific antitumor immune response (2). Evidence for tumor immunity in humans includes the demonstration of lymphocyte, macrophage, and plasma cell infiltration of primary and metastatic tumors and the observation that such infiltration is often associated with a better prognosis. Spontaneous regression of tumors has been observed and has been attributed to immunologic mechanisms (3). There is a higher incidence of *in situ* tumors of various primary sites discovered at autopsy than the clinical incidence of these tumors in living subjects (4). General immunocompetence has also been related to tumor prognosis; thus immunocompetent patients with cancer usually have a better prognosis than do immunoincompetent patients (5). Furthermore, the immunologic basis of this immunoincompetence has been discovered in many cases.

During the last decade a variety of laboratory studies have demonstrated tumor antigens and tumor immunity in humans. These include studies of cell-mediated immunity such as lymphocyte blastogenic response to tumor cells and tumor antigens (6) and lymphocyte- and macrophage-mediated cytotoxicity to tumor cells containing tumor antigens (7). The detection of circulating tumors antigens (8) and circulating antitumor antibodies and immune complexes (9) in cancer patients has also contributed useful information. The observation that microbial adjuvants such as Bacillus Calmette Guerin (BCG) and *Corynebacterium parvum* (*C. parvum*) can prevent development of both viral and carcinogen induced tumors (10) and can cause regression of these tumors or prevent their recurrence after surgery (11) prompted the initial clinical trials of immunotherapy in the modern era.

Three clinical studies conducted approximately a decade ago prompted a large number of immunotherapy trials in humans. These were the report by Mathe et al. (12) that BCG, tumor cell vaccine, or the combination of prolonged remission duration and survival in patients with acute lymphocytic leukemia (ALL) after chemotherapy, the report by Morton et al. (13) that the intralesional injection of BCG caused the regression of metastatic nodules of malignant melanoma in immunocompetent patients, and the report by Klein (14) that the injection of dinitrochlorobenzine (DNCB) into primary or metastatic cutaneous tumors of DNCB sensitized patients resulted not only in regression of their tumors, but slowing in the rate of new tumor development. Subsequent to these observations, in the last decade there has been a great effort to investigate the immunotherapy of human cancer in a variety of clinical circumstances. These have included studies in patients with primary and metastatic solid tumors as well as leukemias and lymphomas, therapy applied as an adjuvant after surgery or radiation and therapy applied after chemotherapy or intermittently between courses of chemotherapy.

The approaches used have involved mainly active nonspecific immunotherapy with microbial adjuvants such as BCG, *C. parvum,* and the methanol extraction residue of BCG (MER) and have involved active specific immunotherapy with tumor cell vaccines, or immunorestorative immunotherapy with levamisole. However, some attempts at immunotherapy have been made with all major classes of immunotherapy, including active specific immunotherapy, active nonspecific immunotherapy, adoptive immunotherapy, passive immunotherapy, and immunorestorative immunotherapy. In general, the results can be summarized as follows: immunotherapy as used to date does not generally increase the remission rate or itself induce remission. Immunotherapy induces a modest prolongation of remission duration and survival, but does not affect the long-term remission rate or survival as induced by conventional therapy. Negative as well as positive immunotherapy trials have been reported. The toxicity of immunotherapy is usually mild to moderate. Immunotherapy generally has not resulted in tumor enhancement.

More recently, a number of major developments in science have stimulated a great resurgence of interest in the field of immunotherapy and expanded the concept to include the broader area of biological therapy. First have been the newer developments in immunology. These are exemplified by the discovery of suppressor cell mechanisms. Thus lymphocyte proliferation and lymphocyte-mediated antitumor effector mechanisms can be inhibited by both suppressor lymphocytes (15) and suppressor monocytes and macrophages (16). In animal models these have been demonstrated to impair host control of tumor growth. Increased suppressor cell activity has been identified in cancer patients and pharmacological regulation of suppressor cell activity with H2 receptor antagonists (17) and cyclooxygenase inhibitors (18) has been demonstrated. This suggests that immunomodulation, directed toward reduction in suppressor cell activity, may benefit patients with malignancy. Related to this are recent developments in our understanding of thymic hormones and their role in immunobiology. It now appears that the status of the lymphoid organ and the expression of its activity is regulated by a group of thymic hormones, that this regulation is disturbed in cancer patients and can be restored to normal by the administration of xenogeneic thymic extracts (19). This also offers the possibility of clinically useful immunotherapy.

Another major new development relates to interferons. This antiviral and antiproliferative group of glycopeptides has recently been shown to inhibit tumor growth in animal models (20) and to induce remissions in a number of human malignancies including breast cancer, malignant lymphoma, and multiple myeloma (21). This finding is extremely important because it is one of the first demonstrations that natural host defense molecules, produced in response to a viral challenge, can have meaningful tumor regressive activity. This finding opens the entire field of cytokine therapy to intensive investigation.

From studies with immunorestorative agents such as the thymic hormones and the sulfur-containing compounds such as levamisole, the concept of immunomodulation has developed. The fundamental observation is that if T-cell number and function are depressed, they are restored into the normal range by these agents, whereas if they are normal, they may be depressed (22). The latter can be due to a direct effect on the functional cells or through activation of suppressor mechanisms. The important concept is that these agents are immunomodulatory rather than only immunostimulatory and their effects depend on the resting state of host defense function. If the disease state is related to immunodeficiency, immunorestoration can be achieved; if the disease state is due to hyperactive immune mechanisms such as hyperactive suppressor mechanisms, these may be suppressed. However, if the object of therapy is immunologic stimulation and the resting state of the immune system is normal, a detrimental immunosuppressive effect may be achieved. This concept of immunomodulation will be important in the development of immunotherapy in the future.

The development of recombinant DNA methodology (23) is also likely to have a major impact on immunotherapy in the future. As effector molecules with potential therapeutic value are detected (interferon, lymphotoxin, and maturation and differentiation factors), they can be synthesized in large amounts and in high degrees of purity by the recombinant DNA methodology. This finding will allow the use of natural regulatory molecules in the biological therapy of cancer.

Finally, the development of hybridoma methodology, through which extremely high-titer monoclonal antibodies directed at specific antigenic moieties can be produced in large amounts, will have a profound impact on the field of immunotherapy as well as other areas of medicine (24). The availability of these antibodies, directed against tumor antigens, will permit the antibody-mediated targeting of cytotoxic therapy. The direct use of these antibodies as antitumor agents will also be possible. They can also be used as immunoabsorbants for the purification of tumor antigens for use in immunotherapy.

From some of these developments, and from the results with immunotherapy to date, the concept of biological response modifiers has been developed. A biological response modifier may be defined as an agent or therapy that modifies either the host or the tumor, thus causing the occurrence of a host-tumor interaction that favors the host and produces toxic effects against the tumor. These may be direct effects or may be indirect, mediated through changes in other organs, such as bone marrow. Biological response modifiers include the classical immunotherapeutic agents, immunomodulators, cytokines, maturation and differentiation factors, and metabolic therapy. Thus it can be seen that although the effects of immunotherapy have been modest to the present time, there is every reason to believe that the future of this field is bright and that biological therapy of cancer will become the fourth major modality of cancer treatment. A classification of biological therapy agents is given in the following outline:

A. Augmenting agents
    I. Intact microbial organisms
        a. BCG
        b. *C. parvum*
        c. OK 432
    II. Microbial fractions
        a. Staph phage lysate
        b. Methanol extraction residue of BCG (MER)
        c. Brucella abortus extraction residue (BRU-PEL)
        d. Cell-wall fractions of various organisms
        e. Cell-wall skeleton fractions of various organisms
        f. Peptidoglycans (MDP and analogues)
        g. Glycolipids (trehalose dimycolate and analogues)
        h. Glucans and other polysaccharides
            1. Glucan
            2. Lentinan
            3. Schizophyllan
            4. Krestin (PSK)
            5. Mannosym
        i. Lipopolysaccharide (endotoxin)
    III. Synthetic macrophage activators and interferon inducers
        a. High-molecular-weight compounds
            1. Pyran copolymer
            2. MVE series (1 to 5)
            3. Poly IC, poly ICLC, poly IC with mismatched bases
            4. Poly AU

      b. Low-molecular-weight compounds
         1. Pyrimidinoles
         2. Lysolecithin analogues
         3. Lipoidal amines

B. Cytokines
    I. Interferons
       a. Human leukocyte interferon
       b. Human lymphoblastoid interferon
       c. Human fibroblast interferon
       d. Human immune interferon
   II. Transfer factor
  III. Lymphokine (1788 cell-line supernatant)
  IV. Tumor necrosis factor (TNF)

C. Immunomodulators
    I. Thymic hormones
       a. Thymosin F5
       b. Thymosin α1
       c. Facteur thymique serique [serum thymic factor (FTS)]
       d. Thymic humoral factor (THF)
       e. Thymopoetin (Pentapeptide)
       f. Thymostimulin (TS[1] or TP-1)
   II. Thiol compounds
       a. Levamisole
       b. Thiazolbenzimidazole (Wy 40453)
       c. Diethyldithiocarbamate (DTC)
       d. 2-Mercapto-2-methylpropanoly-L-cysteine (SA96)
  III. Other compounds
       a. Isoprinosine
       b. Inosine analogues (NPT 15392)
       c. Bestatin
       d. Cyclomunine
       e. NED 137
       f. BAY i7433
       g. Azimexon
       h. Imexon
       i. Indomethacin and other PGE synthetase inhibitors
       j. Cimetidine
       k. Lynestrenol

D. Active specific immunotherapy
    I. Tumor cell vaccine
   II. Tumor factor
  III. Viral oncolysate of tumor cells

E. Adoptive immunotherapy
- I.   Immune RNA
- II. Transfer factor
- III. Immune leukocyte infusions

F. Passive immunotherapy
- I.   Antitumor antibody
- II. Antitumor antibody—coupled cytotoxic agent
  - a. Radioisotope (^{131}I)
  - b. Drugs

G. Depletive therapy
- I.   Plasmapheresis
- II. Plasma exchange
- III. Immunoabsorbtion

H. Nutritional therapy
- I.   Vitamin A and analogues
- II. Vitamin C
- III. Hyperalimentation

I . Metabolic therapy
- I. Cyclic nucleotide analogues
- II. Chemotherapeutic agents

Although specific aspects of immunotherapy are reviewed in detail elsewhere in this volume, a brief critique of the development of clinical immunotherapy is presented here as a direct introduction to the discussion of future perspectives in this area.

2. THE DEVELOPMENT OF IMMUNOTHERAPY

2.1. Bacillus Calmette-Guerin (BCG)

As noted in Section 1, the modern era of immunotherapy research at the clinical level began with the studies of Mathe et al. (12), Morton et al. (13), and Klein (14). The majority of immunotherapy trials have been conducted with microbial adjuvants and mainly with BCG, *C. parvum,* and MER (25). Fairly extensive studies with the use of BCG intralesionally have been reported. Response depends on the immunocompetence of the patient, and 80% of patients who are immunocompetent show regression of metastatic cutaneous tumor nodules when injected with BCG. In addition, about 20% of noninjected nodules in the treated patients show some regression suggesting the activation of systemic host defense mechanisms. Most studies of intralesional immunotherapy have been confined to metastatic nodules in two malignances, malignant melanoma and breast cancer. In melanoma it has been demonstrated that local-regional disease (local recurrence and in transit metastasis) can be effectively controlled by BCG injections (26). Very few other malignant disease entities have been treated with intralesional BCG, and only one subgroup of melanoma can be considered controllable with this approach at this time.

Based on the guinea pig hepatoma model of Rapp and Zbar and their coworkers (27) in which the primary tumor is treated with an intralesional injection of BCG and both the primary tumor and the metastatic regional lymph nodes regress, it has been suggested that intralesional immunotherapy of primary malignancies be studied in humans. Preliminary studies in malignant melanoma by Rosenberg et al. (28) and in lung cancer by Holmes et al. (29) suggest that this approach is feasible and may lead to improved survival. However, only small numbers of patients have been treated to date, and extensive clinical trials will be necessary to unequivocally document this effect.

Mathe's work with BCG administered by scarification as well as the results of intralesional immunotherapy of metastatic tumor nodules have led to extensive studies of both local-regional immunotherapy with BCG and BCG administered into the skin for either local-regional or systemic effects. Local-regional immunotherapy has been carried out with BCG administered into the extremities to control regional recurrence of melanoma in lymph nodes (30), with BCG administered by intrapleural injection after surgical removal of Stage I lung cancer (31) and has been used intravesically to prevent recurrence and development of new lesions in superficial bladder carcinoma (32). In melanoma for patients with less than five positive lymph nodes, there is evidence in some studies that the disease-free interval and survival are increased by BCG administration (30). However, this has not been confirmed in every study (33). In lung cancer intrapleural BCG in Stage I disease has shown unequivocal prolongation of disease-free interval and survival in one study (31), equivocal improvement in disease-free interval and survival in a second study (34), and no effect in two other studies (35, 36). Thus, the activity of intrapleural BCG must be considered unproved at this time. In contrast, intravesical BCG immunotherapy combined with concurrent cutaneous administration of BCG into the lower extremities has shown marked reduction in the recurrence rate in three studies (32,37,38) and can be considered to be documented as effective at this time.

The results with BCG administered by the scarification technique or one of its modifications for a systemic effect has in general produced equivocal results. The experiment is the removal of a primary tumor such as breast, lung, colon, or head and neck cancer, and the repeated application of BCG into multiple cutaneous sites. Another setting is the treatment of metastatic or disseminated disease by intermittent cycles of chemotherapy and the administration of BCG between cycles. Virtually no studies have shown that BCG improves the response rate to chemotherapy. However, a number of studies have demonstrated prolongation of remission duration and survival by the administration of BCG. However, the majority have not been confirmed; therefore, the effectiveness of BCG in this setting is equivocal. In contrast, in adult AML most studies of BCG therapy administered alone or with an allogeneic irradiated tumor cell vaccine have shown either prolongation of survival or prolongation of remission duration and survival (39,40).

Many problems are associated with BCG immunotherapy. The therapeutic activity is minimal in terms of the percent improvement in remission duration and survival. The effect is often transient. After 2 to 5 years of follow-up there is usually no difference in the disease-free or overall survival of treated and control groups. Bacillus Calmette-Guerin is difficult to administer, causes moderate to severe local cutaneous reaction, and is associated with the danger of systemic BCG disease. Furthermore, strains of BCG vary in their biological and immunologic activity. No standard strain has been accepted or has been used in comparative studies. Bacillus Calmette-Guerin is a complex organism with complex and as yet poorly understood biological activities. In animal models it may have detrimental effects such as the induction of suppressor cells (41).

Furthermore, many studies utilizing BCG have had certain defects that preclude definitive analysis: (1) most studies have been done with small numbers of patients; and (2) the dose, route, and schedule of BCG administration have been arbitrary and have not been based on animal model studies or sound Phase I trials. Indeed, there has not been a single well-designed complete Phase I dose response and toxicity study of BCG in humans. In view of these deficiencies, it is surprising that any therapeutic activity for BCG has been demonstrated. Finally, these two problems are relevant to microbial adjuvant immunotherapy in general and, indeed, to all immunotherapy. Only recently has the concept developed that careful Phase I dose response studies must be done with immunotherapeutic agents before they are applied broadly in Phase II clinical trials.

2.2. Other Microbial Adjuvants

The second most extensively studied intact microbial adjuvant for human cancer immunotherapy has been *C. parvum*. *Corynebacterium parvum* had antitumor activity in animal models at least equivalent to that manifested by BCG. In addition, the *C. parvum* had the potential advantage of being a killed rather than a viable microbial adjuvant. Thus it could be used in a high dose by the intravenous route. *Corynebacterium parvum* like BCG has been utilized intralesionally, intradermally, subcutaneously, and intravenously. By the intradermal and subcutaneous route, doses of up to 5 mg/m^2 are reasonably well tolerated, although they do produce moderate to severe local reactions and can produce ulceration in rare cases. By the intravenous route, *C. parvum* produces severe toxicity in the average patients including shaking chills, high fever, prostration, and acute respiratory symptoms (42). The results with *C. parvum* are analogous to those with BCG, except that fewer positive studies have been reported. However, *C. parvum* can cause regression of tumor on intralesional injection. Also, daily intravenous *C. parvum* injection can induce regression of metastatic tumor nodules at diverse sites, particularly in the lung in up to 40% of cases (43). However, the toxicity and lack of major activity in most studies would preclude further use of *C. parvum*.

The third microbial adjuvant preparation that has been used fairly extensively has been the methanol extraction residue of BCG (MER). This agent has been demonstrated to have antitumor activity in animal models, and because it was a nonviable, particulate, cell-wall extract of BCG, it was thought to possibly retain the desired activity and not be associated with systemic BCG disease or other toxic side effects (44). Extensive studies of MER immunotherapy by the intradermal route have been carried out in patients with solid tumors and acute leukemia. These have been included adjuvant studies after surgery (45) and also studies in which MER was administered between courses of chemotherapy for metastatic or disseminated disease (46). Recently, several groups have begun Phase I studies of MER by the intravenous route (47). In general, MER has not proved useful when administered by the intradermal route. Almost all the studies have shown no difference between treated and control groups in remission rate or remission duration or survival. In addition, the toxicity of MER by the intradermal route is severe, with painful draining ulcers as the usual result. Finally, there are several instances in which the MER patient group has shown a worse prognosis than the control group, and it has been suggested that this is related to suppressor cell activiation (48).

Methanol extraction residue does have some activity when administered intralesionally, approximately the same as that of BCG (49). Recent studies of MER have focused on treatment by the intravenous route. Several groups have conducted studies of intravenous MER and partial or complete remissions have been noted in rare cases of lymphoma, gastrointestinal cancer, and smoldering acute leukemia (47,50). It was also demonstrated that MER by the intravenous route activated cell-mediated cytotoxicity mechanisms, including ADCC and NK and did not activate prostaglandin-producing suppressor cells (50). The limitation of intravenous MER is that it produces a diffuse interstitial pneumonitis in 10 to 40% of patients after a mean of four doses, particularly in patients who are PPD positive or who have received prior BCG (50). This limitation will preclude its widespread use, but it is suggested that synthetic nontoxic augmenting agents with analogous immunologic activity may be quite useful in cancer immunotherapy in the future.

Current work on the microbial adjuvants is focused on more purified subcomponents. These include pseudomonas vaccine, BCG cell-wall skeleton preparations (peptidoglycans), cell-wall skeleton preparations of other microorganisms such as Nocardia, and other more defined BCG derivatives such as trehalose dimycolate (P3) and muramyl dipeptide and their analogues. Extensive studies of these have been done in animal models demonstrating that selected components or combinations of components retain the antitumor activity of the intact microbial organisms. However, only very limited studies have yet been undertaken in humans. Bacillus Calmette-Guerin cell-wall skeleton plus P3 causes regression of cutaneous melanoma nodules equivalent to that produced by BCG (51). Intrapleural or intraperitoneal BCG cell-wall skeleton plus P3 can cause regression or stabilization of malignant effusions (52). Intravenous cell-wall skeleton is fairly well tolerated in cancer patients (51), and Phase I studies to identify the optimal doses are continuing. Extensive studies of Nocardia cell-wall skeleton have been done by Japanese workers for lung cancer, and tumor regression after intralesional injection as well as prolongation of remission duration and survival have been reported (53). Muramyl dipeptide derivatives as well as cell-wall skeleton plus trehalose dimycolate coated onto oil droplets have not been used systemically in humans. There has been one clinical trial with pseudomonas vaccine in acute leukemia, suggesting prolongation of remission duration and survival when the vaccine was administered during remission induction (54). This is now undergoing a repeat trial. The hope for the future in this area is that chemically defined components of microbial adjuvants with activity limited to the desired immunologic or host defense effects will be developed and will be moved into clinical trials through careful animal model studies and through careful dose and schedule Phase I studies in humans.

2.3. Active Specific Immunotherapy

Immunotherapy with tumor cells and tumor antigen either alone or administered with adjuvants has been explored to only a very limited extent in clinical immunotherapy trials. Although it seems logical that induction of active tumor-specific immunity is desirable and certainly is effective in highly antigenic animal tumors, there are many reasons why this approach has not moved forward vigorously in humans. In general, viable human tumor cells are not readily accessible in sufficient quantities for repeated immunization. Allogeneic, fresh, or cultured tumor cells have been used, but these may lack relevant tumor antigens or may contain undesired components such as those that may activate suppressor cells or mechanisms. Careful dose response studies have not been done, in part because of a lack of appropriate monitoring methodology. Monitoring is also limited because of a lack of adequate numbers of target tumor cells.

The most extensive studies of active specific immunotherapy have been done in acute leukemia in which patients have received repeated immunizations with either viable, irradiated, or neuraminidase-treated, usually allogeneic tumor cells mixed with or administered simultaneously with adjuvant (e.g., BCG or Freund's adjuvant). Immunotherapy is given between courses of remission induction and maintenance chemotherapy or after remission had been induced. The overall results of this approach have been mentioned previously and generally have been limited to a modest, temporary prolongation of survival (48). No increase in remission rate has been observed. Tumor antigen immunization in complete Freund's adjuvant has been utilized in patients surgically cured of Stage I or Stage II resectable lung cancer (55). Prolongation of disease-free interval and survival has been reported. However, it is not clear at this time whether the results are related to patient selection, the Freund's adjuvant, or the tumor antigen. Active specific immunotherapy has also been utilized in renal carcinoma in patients with pulmonary metastases (56). Anecdotal reports involving few patients suggest that this approach results in regression of pulmonary metastases. The regression is usually partial or transient, but it does confirm the presence of tumor antigens and inducible, effective, tumor immunity in this disease.

The future of active specific immunotherapy will depend on the characterization, isolation, and purification of those tumor cell-surface antigens that can be subject to effective immunologic attack. It will also depend on the preparation of sufficient quantities of these antigens for immunotherapy and monitoring. Finally, it will depend on an increased understanding of the mechanisms of tumor immunity and their potential effectiveness and on whether the relevant antigens are individual-specific, tumor-type-specific, or common tumor-associated antigens.

2.4. Immunorestoration

The only other approach to immunotherapy of human cancer that has been investigated extensively is the so-called immunorestorative immunotherapy. As noted previously, thinking about this approach has now been modified, and we consider the so-called immunorestorative agents to be immunomodulatory. Thus these agents can either augment or suppress various T-cell-mediated and other immune responses, depending on the status of activity of the immune system at a given time, and the balance between suppressor and helper T cells in a given individual. Therefore, ultimate utility of this approach will depend on an improved understanding of T-cell-mediated immunity in cancer, the role of T effector and pre-T effector cells in host control of tumor growth, and an understanding of the balance between suppressor and helper cells and its effect, if any, on the biology of cancer.

In spite of these considerations, extensive work has been done with the immunomodulatory agent levamisole. Most of this work has involved Phases II and III clinical trials at an arbitrarily determined dose and schedule of approximately 100 mg/m^2 daily for 2 or 3 days, repeated every 1 to 3 weeks. As was the case with BCG, no careful dose-response studies have been conducted to determine the optimal dose and schedule of this agent. Studies have been carried out for leukemia, lymphoma, and various solid tumors, both in the adjuvant setting, after the patient has been rendered free of disease, and in concurrence with the administration of chemotherapy. There are conflicting data regarding the efficacy of levamisole; however, the bulk of the data suggests that the agent can increase the remission rate, the remission duration, and the survival in patients with limited or extensive disease in the categories of acute leukemia (57), malignant lymphoma (58), breast cancer (59), lung cancer (60), colon cancer (61), and head and neck cancer (62). In several of the above-mentioned categories of these diseases, however, studies showing no effect and studies actually showing a detrimental effect of levamisole have been reported (34,63). It is speculated that in these circumstances the investigators were dealing with a relatively immunocompetent patient population, where the immunomodulatory effect was thus negative rather than positive. If this modality of treatment is to become well established, it is essential that the characteristics of suitable candidates be determined and the optimal doses and schedules of therapy be established by appropriate Phase I studies. This is particularly important since a large number of immunomodulatory agents are becoming available for clinical trials. These include the thymic hormones and other sulfur-containing compounds and a number of other compounds including isoprinosine and inosine analogues, various low-molecular-weight peptides, azimexon and related aziridine dye compounds, and pharmacological agents that can affect suppressor cell activity (indomethacin and cimetidine).

A variety of other approaches to immunotherapy have been utilized to a limited extent in clinical trials. These include adoptive immunotherapy with transfer factor and immune RNA, passive immunotherapy with antibody, delivery of cytoxic agents to tumor sites with drug or radioisotope attached to antibody, and depletive therapy with approaches such as plasma exchange. Because of the very limited number of clinical studies done with these approaches, they have not had a significant impact on the current status of immunotherapy, but they offer leads for the future and are discussed in detail in Section 3.

3. BIOLOGICAL RESPONSE MODIFIERS

3.1. Introduction

The major approaches to cancer therapy currently consist of surgery, radiation, and chemotherapy. Immunotherapy has yielded some encouraging results, but not sufficient to indicate that it will become the fourth major modality of cancer treatment. Certain scientific and clinical developments have suggested that immunotherapy be placed in a broader context of biological therapy of cancer. The observations that have suggested this include the finding that interferons can cause the regression of both animal (20) and human (21) tumors at least in part by a direct antiproliferative effect. Various other cellular mediators are being defined that can either accelerate or stop the proliferation of both malignant and normal cells. These are exemplified by mediators that affect the proliferation and differentiation of bone marrow components (64). Certain nutritional factors such as the retinoids can prevent or reverse malignant transformation of cells *in vitro* and in animal models (65). Agents that affect cell metabolism through the cyclic nucleotide system such as dibutyrl cyclic AMP can cause cessation of tumor growth or tumor regression in animals (66). From these observations, the concept of biological response modifiers has been developed.

A biological response modifier may be defined as an agent or approach that will modify the relationship between tumor and host, thus modifying the host's biological response to tumor cells with resultant therapeutic benefit. The modification may boost specific tumor immunity or nonspecific effector mechanisms such as macrophage cytotoxicity to tumor cells. It may also render the tumor susceptible to host defense effects. It may change the microenvironment in which the tumor cells reside so that their proliferation, invasion, or metastasis potential are reduced. It may cause the tumor cells to differentiate so that they are no longer malignant or do not behave in a malignant fashion. Finally, it may increase the host's ability to tolerate or recover more rapidly from tissue damage by other modalities of cancer therapy, such as bone marrow protection from the cytotoxic effects of chemotherapy or radiotherapy.

3.2. Interferon

A major impetus to the development of biological response modifier therapy has been observations made over the last 20 years on interferon (67). Interferons are inducible glycoproteins produced by various cells of the body in response to various stimuli. These include natural stimuli such as viruses and bacteria and chemical stimuli such as high-molecular-weight anionic polymers and certain low-molecular-weight agents. Interferons are relatively species specific. There are three major types of interferon: (1) leukocyte interferon; (2) fibroblast interferon; and (3) immune or Type 2 interferon. Leukocyte and fibroblast interferon are pH stable and are produced by leukocytes and fibroblast respectively. They differ in the nature of their glycosilation, in their pharmacology, and in the sensitivity of various tissues to their antiviral and antiproliferative effects. Immune or Type 2 interferon is produced by lymphocytes in response to mitogen stimulation or stimulation with antigens to which the lymphocytes are sensitive. A fourth type of interferon, lymphoblastoid interferon, is produced by B lymphocyte cell lines on *in vitro* viral stimulation and is very closely related antigenically and physicochemically to leukocyte interferon. Animal interferon has been demonstrated to have modest to moderate tumor regressive activity in both virus-induced and non-virus-induced primary and transplantable animal tumors (20). This was the basis for the introduction into human studies.

After a few anecdotal observations that interferon could cause regression of a number of tumors such as breast cancer and Hodgkin's disease, a major study was undertaken in 1975 by Strander et al. (68). Based on the assumption that human osteogenic sarcoma was a virus-induced tumor, they treated a series of patients who had been freed of disease by surgery with partially purified human leukocyte interferon at a dose of 3×10^6 units per day, with therapy extending over a period of 2 years. Their survival was compared to that of a group of nonrandomized concurrent and a group of historical controls. A significant prolongation in disease-free survival was noted in the treated patients. This observation stimulated a number of studies by various groups. Strander and co-workers demonstrated that human leukocyte interferon can cause complete or partial remissions in multiple myeloma (69), Merigan et al. (70) demonstrated that it could produce remissions in patients with lymphocytic lymphoma, whereas Gutterman et al. (71) demonstrated that there was about a 30% complete and partial remission rate in patients with metastatic breast cancer, non-Hodgkin's lymphoma, and multiple myeloma. More recently, the American Cancer Society has sponsored broad Phase II trials of partially purified human leukocyte interferon in a number of disease categories. Five of 23 patients with metastatic breast cancer have shown significant tumor reduction (72). Studies in melanoma and lymphoma are pending. Krown and colleagues recently studied 19 patients with non-oat cell lung cancer and observed 0 of 19 responses (73). Some patients stabilized during the month of treatment, but there were no tumor regressions.

The major problem with studies of human leukocyte interferon therapy have related to (1) the impurity of the product, (2) batch-to-batch variations in antiviral and antiproliferative activity, and (3) the relative unavailability and the high cost, which have limited the number of patients studied during the last 3 years to a few hundred throughout the world. The partial sequencing of leukocyte and fibroblast interferon and the production of interferon through recombinant DNA technology suggests that adequate supplies will be available within the next year or so for definitive large-scale clinical trials.

Studies are just beginning with human lymphoblastoid interferon and with fibroblast interferon. Priestman (74) and co-workers have recently demonstrated that lymphoblastoid interferon 20 to 50 times more pure than the currently available leukocyte interferon is tolerated up to doses of 6×10^6 units/m^2 of body surface daily (74). In the Phase I study they observed partial regression of a malignant melanoma and a gastric carcinoma. Human fibroblast interferon has been studied in a preliminary fashion by the intralesional route and has been shown to cause an inflammatory response in and regression of various tumors metastatic to the skin (75). It is currently undergoing more extensive study in Germany, administered by the intravenous route. Its tolerance and toxicity were similar to that observed for leukocyte interferon. Several responses were noted, including two in patients with nasopharyngeal carcinoma (76).

The pharmacology of fibroblast and leukocyte interferon are quite different. Blood levels after intramuscular injection are regularly detected with leukocyte interferon and never detected with fibroblast interferon (77). After intravenous administration, fibroblast interferon is rapidly cleared from the blood. How these pharmacological differences relate to efficacy will be the subject of future studies. Immunologic observations on animal and human recipients of interferon have shown activation of natural killer cells, and this seems to be a reasonable approach to monitoring in addition to the measurement of serum interferon levels.

The importance of these observations relates to the fact that this is one of the first times that a natural mediator molecule has produced a response to exogenous stimulation and has been known to activate certain host-defense mechanisms that have been demonstrated to have antitumor activity in humans. The other mediator, of course, was corticosteroids. This opens the whole area of cytokine therapy to extensive preclinical and clinical research and places the field of biological response modifier therapy on a firm footing. The ultimate clinical utility of interferon, and related cytokines and other biological approaches must await future preclinical and clinical therapy studies.

4. FUTURE PROSPECTS FOR BIOLOGICAL THERAPY OF CANCER

4.1. Introduction

Future developments in the field of biological therapy of cancer will depend on three factors: (1) the development of agents with greater activity and more tumor specificity; (2) the development of adequate monitoring methodology specific for the new agents, so that optimal doses and schedules of therapy can be developed; and (3) an improved understanding of the various components of host-tumor cell interaction that will permit the development of better therapeutic and monitoring approaches and also permit a prediction of the ultimate degree of therapeutic benefit to be expected from biological therapy. In this section we review the future prospects for a number of the biological therapy approaches including microbial augmenting agents; macrophage activators and interferon inducers; cytokines; maturation and differentiation factors; immunomodulators; active specific, adoptive, and passive immunotherapy; and depletive therapy, nutritional therapy, and metabolic therapy.

4.2. Microbial Augmenting Agents

Because of the limitations and toxicity associated with immunotherapy with intact BCG organisms and because of the interests in the mechanism of action of BCG and other related agents, an extensive effort has been made by Ribi et al. (78,79) and Chedid and co-workers (see Chapter 4) to define the active components and to develop more potent less toxic fractions. Utilizing the guinea pig hepatoma model outlined previously, Ribi has demonstrated that BCG cell-wall skeleton with trehalose dimycolate attached to oil droplets is as or more potent than intact BCG in the guinea pig hepatoma model. Virtually 100% of the animals can be cured with the proper balance between the three components (78). There is an interesting interaction between trehalose dimycolate and another bacterial extract, endotoxin in this therapy model (79). Endotoxin alone can cure only 14% of animals, whereas endotoxin plus trehalose demycolate cures approximately 90%. Cure rates in this range can also be achieved with purified nontoxic fractions of endotoxin from such organisms as Salmonella. The individual components are minimally active, and hence there is a true synergistic effect seen in the combination. Another active component of the BCG cell-wall skeleton has been shown to be muramyl dipeptide (MDP), and a number of muramyl dipeptides analogues are currently under study. In all these experiments intralesional treatment into the primary tumor and attachment of the components to oil droplets are essential.

Clinical studies of these purified subcomponents are beginning. Richman et al. (52) and Vosika et al. (51) have both demonstrated that intrapleural or intralesional therapy of metastatic nodules or disease with BCG cell-wall skeleton or cell-wall skeleton plus P3 can cause regression of injected tumors or disease and also occasionally regression of noninjected nodules. Phase I studies on intradermal cell-wall skeleton plus P3 on oil droplets of intravenous cell-wall skeleton and of intravenous cell-wall skeleton plus P3 have been conducted for assessment of toxicity. These are tolerable, although fever, chills, leukocytosis, and hepatocellular toxicity have been observed (51). The use of these agents systemically, attached to oil droplets, will await the development of an acceptable, metabolizable oil carrier.

In Japan, Yamamura (53) and co-workers have done extensive studies of immunotherapy in animal models and more recently in humans with *Nocarida rubra* cell-wall skeleton (53). They have reported that this material is more active than BCG cell-wall skeleton in animal models. Clinically, they have used *N. rubra* cell-wall skeleton to control malignant pleural effusions with considerable effectiveness and have conducted a randomized trial in patients with lung cancer showing that *N. rubra* cell-wall skeleton can prolong remission duration with serious side effects.

Fractionation studies on *C. parvum* are at an earlier stage of development. However, Cantrell (80) and co-workers have demonstrated recently that a pyridine extract of *C. parvum* combined with P3 and MDP was very active in a number of animal tumor models and yet did not induce splenomegaly, hepatomegaly, or liver necrosis as does the native *C. parvum*. This material is a macrophage and natural killer (NK) cell activator and also induces interferon. Thus an active component with less toxicity has been identified. Extensive studies of various natural polysaccharides have been carried out by DiLuzio (81) for the glucans and for others such as lentinan by Japanese workers. These agents, which are potent macrophage activators, can now be produced at defined molecular weights, and improved materials may be developed by the addition of acetic or lipophylic groups. Extensive clinical trials have not been conducted except in Japan, and the potential of this group of microbial augmenting agents awaits further study.

In summary, the active molecular components of the microbial adjuvants are being defined at present. Active components and their interrelationships have been identified. Clinical trials are beginning. Whether they will have more activity at less toxic doses and will be useful for systemic therapy as defined previously must await careful, well-monitored clinical investigations.

4.3. Synthetic Macrophage Activators and Interferon Inducers

One of the major mechanisms of action of the microbial adjuvants is activation
of effector cells such as macrophages, natural killer cells, and cells that mediate
ADCC. These activities are induced, at least in part, by the generation of interferon. Because of the promising clinical results with interferon, considerable
effort has focused on synthetic interferon inducers and other synthetic polymers with the capacity to activate macrophages. In addition, certain low-molecular-weight compounds with interferon-inducing capacity have been identified.

A class of polymers that mimic viruses and are potent interferon inducers include the synthetic double-stranded RNA group based on poly I-poly C (poly
IC). They include poly IC, poly IC stabilized with poly L lysine (poly ICLC),
and poly IC with mismatched bases. These in general induce interferon, activate macrophages and NK cells in a variety of species and have viral protective and antitumor activities. Poly IC is not a good interferon inducer in humans, whereas poly ICLC, which is less subject to serum nuclease degradation,
is an excellent inducer. Both have been subjected to fairly extensive Phase I
clinical trials. They are highly toxic, producing fever, chills, and prostration,
as well as hematologic and hepatic toxicity and have yet to be shown to have
clear-cut clinical activity (82,83). Poly IC with mismatched bases is rapidly
degraded by serum nucleases, but in animal systems it is a relatively effective
interferon inducer (84). It has the potential advantage of inducing interferon
without toxicity or other unwanted biological effects. It has not yet been subjected to clinical trials.

Another interesting group of polymers consists of the MVE series of maleic-
anhydride divinyl-ether polymers of defined molecular weight based on the
original, anionic, pyran copolymer. These polymers are weak interferon inducers but potent macrophage activators and have potent viral protective and
antitumor activity (85). The biological effects vary with molecular weight and
dose in terms of interferon induction, antitumor activity and toxicity. The low-
er-molecular-weight fractions are less toxic but can still activate macrophages
and exert antitumor activity *in vivo*. The 15,000-molecular-weight fraction
MVE-2 is just being entered into clinical trials at present.

A number of low-molecular-weight substances have also been shown to be
inducers of interferon. These include the heterocyclic bases such as acridine
orange, methylene blue, and a number of quinolines and anthroquinones;
the fluorenones such as tilorone; the lipoidal amines; the pyrimidine derivatives; and certain thiols. None of these have been subjected to major clinical
trials, but for some, such as the pyrimidine derivatives, there is evidence that
there are potent interferon inducers and potent macrophage and NK cell activators with potent antiviral and antitumor activity in animal systems at essentially nontoxic doses (86). Indeed, serum levels of interferon of up to 10,000
units/ml can be induced, making them very promising agents for future clinical trials.

There are several major problems associated with the development of this group of compounds: (1) toxicity—the higher-molecular-weight compounds are toxic in their potent dose range; (2) tolerance development—after a single dose of an interferon inducer, there is often a refractory period of 3 to 4 days before another dose will induce interferon; and (3) other unwanted side effects such as the induction of splenomegaly and the development of immunosuppression. Hopefully, these problems can be overcome, and if so, interferon inducers may be useful therapeutic agents for nonmalignant as well as malignant diseases in humans.

Another group of agents related to the macrophage activators are the lysolecithin analogues (87). Lysolecithin is known to be increased in activated macrophages and can stimulate phagocytosis. The hemolytic activity released into the supernatant after phagocytosis by macrophages apparently is lysolecithin. The increase in lysolecithin is apparently related to the increased activity of phospholipase A, which occurs during phagocytosis. Because lysolecithin is hemolytic, Modolell et. al. (88) began to investigate the activity of relatively nonhemolytic lysolecithin analogues. These were found to be potent macrophage activators, to boost the immune response against sheep red blood cells, and to boost cellular immunity. *In vivo* they have been observed to retard the growth of a number of animal tumors. Further studies showed that the analogues not only activated macrophages, but also had a direct, although slow lethal effect against tumor cells *in vitro* (89). These effects were observed on both animals and human tumor cells. The lethal effect is mediated through cell-surface damage due to the lack of the *O*-alkyl-cleavage enzyme in the malignant cell that is present in normal cells and that is responsible for the continuous renewal of important membrane components. The approach of administering an agent that is relatively nontoxic and both activates host defense mechanisms and is directly cytotoxic to target tumor cells is particularly appealing. The lysolecithin analogues are currently being introduced into clinical trials.

4.4. Cytokines

Cytokines may be defined as effector or regulatory molecules normally released from activated cells that affect the behavior of other cells in the immediate environment or at a distance. They may affect cells of the same or of a different tissue. They are usually glycoproteins and interact with cell-surface receptors, resulting in changes in cyclic nucleotide metabolism, electrolyte flux, and so on. Cytokines that are relevant to the biological therapy of cancer fall into three broad categories: those with direct antitumor activity, those that stimulate or regulate the immune response (e.g., the antitumor immune response), and those that stimulate or regulate other tissues of importance to the management of cancer. An example of the latter would be those cytokines that affect bone marrow proliferation and differentiation. The chalones, which are tissue-specific products that regulate proliferation of the same tissue as that of their origin, may also be considered cytokines. Many cytokine activities have been identified, but purification is proceeding slowly, and individual cytokine molecules may be responsible for multiple activities.

Cytokines with antitumor activity include the interferons, which have already been discussed; the chalones, which are beyond the scope of this review; lymphotoxin, which is included in the crude or partially purified lymphokine preparations derived from continuous proliferating B cell lines; and tumor necrosis factor. Extensive work has been done by Papermaster et al. (90) and to a lesser extent by other investigators on the lymphotoxin activity of preparations derived from the supernatant of the 1788, continuously proliferating B-cell line. This line was demonstrated to have both MAF and MIF and chemotactic and lymphotoxin activity and not to contain interferon. It was shown to produce a reproducible inflammatory reaction in the skin of both experimental animals and cancer patients consisting of mixed infiltration of lymphocytes, macrophages, granulocytes, and eosinophils (91). Preliminary studies in mice have shown that this preparation can produce regression of L1210 leukemia and prolongation of survival in tumor-bearing animals (92). In addition, it can produce regression of human tumors after intralesional injection (93). Major efforts are now under way to purify the active components of this crude preparation and to use these in the appropriate animal and clinical studies.

Another important antitumor cytokine is tumor necrosis factor, a glycoprotein with a molecular weight of under 70,000, that can be obtained from the serum of endotoxin treated mice, previously immunized with BCG (94). It is produced by monocytes and thus may be referred to as a *monokine.* Tumor necrosis factor can cause the *in vivo* necrosis of animal tumors and *in vitro* is toxic to animal and human tumor cells, but not to normal cells. The activity of tumor necrosis factor containing sera is not due to endotoxin interferon, or lysozyme. Currently, adequate amounts of this cytokine are being prepared to conduct more extensive preclinical and ultimately clinical trials.

A number of cytokine activities, most of which are lymphokine activities, play an important role in the expression and regulation of the inflammatory and immune responses. In regard to the inflammatory response, migration inhibitory factor, macrophage activating factor, and chemotactic factor are all lymphokines that play an important role in the migration, accumulation, and activity of macrophages at delayed hypersensitivity and at other immune response sites (95). These lymphokines are present in the supernatant 1788 cell line. Whether they will play a role in antitumor therapy or in immunomodulation remains to be seen. Lymphocyte activating factor (LAF) is a monokine produced by activated monocytes (96). Its activity is to augment the short-term T-cell proliferation in response to PHA and Con A and to augment the antigen-dependent cell-mediated and humoral immune responses. Its current name is *Interleukin 1.*

Of more importance is T-cell growth factor, now referred to as *Interleukin 2* (97). This lymphokine is derived from PHA and Con A-stimulated lymphocyte culture supernatants and more recently from certain lymphoid cell lines. Depending on the species, it has a molecular weight of 15,000 to 30,000. It is absorbed to specific receptors on T cells, can stimulate continuous T-cell proliferation after mitogen or antigen stimulation, and stimulates the production of specific cytotoxic T lymphocytes to cells containing the inducing antigen on their surface. In the continuous presence of T-cell growth factor, clones of specific T lymphocytes can be produced. The importance of these is that they could be produced for antitumor therapy and the T cells could also be cultured for the production of other relevant T-cell lymphokines. The potential of this approach for human anticancer therapy has not yet been explored, but there is considerable enthusiasm for it at the present time.

In addition to the immunoregulatory cytokines just mentioned, there are a number of helper and suppressor factors that operate during the immune response and its regulation have been identified. Considerable work is yet to be done on these, but they may ultimately play a role in immunomodulatory immunotherapy.

Finally, a few words must be said about those lymphokines or cytokines that could play a role in stimulation of bone marrow proliferation. These include colony stimulating factor and other colony stimulating or differentiating activities (98) that could be utilized to protect the bone marrow from the damaging effects of chemotherapy or restore bone marrow function after it had been damaged by chemotherapy, radiotherapy, and so on.

In summary, there is exciting new work in the area of cytokines that indicates that cytokines with antitumor activity, immunomodulating activity, and proliferation regulatory activity on other tissues are available for preclinical or even clinical research. The availability of purified cytokine molecules will allow circumvention of several steps that have been classically required for immunotherapy, that is, the stimulations with exogenous agents of activity in the patient's cells themselves. This will allow for effective biological therapy of cancer even in the presence of severe tissue and cellular deficiency in the host. It will also allow for the highly selective utilization of certain mechanisms rather than the broad cascade of activated mechanisms seen after active stimulation of the host.

4.5. Immunomodulators

The term "immunomodulator" refers to agents that have a biphasic effect on the immune response. They can either stimulate or inhibit the immune response and other host defense mechanisms and parameters depending on the dose and on the baseline status of the immunologic reactivity of a given individual. Immunomodulators are often immunostimulatory at low doses and immunosuppressive at higher doses. They tend to stimulate individuals whose host defense parameters are deficient or low and inhibit host defense parameters in individuals in whom they are normal or already activated. Many of the biological therapy agents in other classes, such as augmenting agents and cytokines, may also exhibit this biphasic function. However, for the purposes of this review, we include the thymic hormones, the sulfur-containing immunomodulators, and a heterogenous group of other compounds in this category.

Extensive work has been conducted on the thymic hormones over the last two decades (see also Chapter 5). The thymic factors that have been studied most extensively include thymosin fraction 5 and its subcomponents studied by Allan Goldstein et al. (99), FTS characterized by Bach et al. (100), THF characterized by Trainin et al. (101), thymopoiten and particularly the thymopoiten pentapeptide characterized by Gideon Goldstein (102), and thymostimulin (TS1 or TP1) studied by a group of Italian investigators (103). These preparations are mainly soluble extracts derived from calf thymus. They do not show species specificity.

The most extensive work has been done with thymosin fraction 5, which has now been demonstrated to contain approximately 20 peptides, some of which have been sequenced and synthesized and for some of which a more defined biological activity has been demonstrated. Thymic serum factor and thymopoietin have also been synthesized. In animal systems and *in vitro* the thymic hormones can be demonstrated to induce activity of specific lymphocyte subpopulations such as helper, suppressor, and killer cell activity; can induce certain cellular markers, such as TdT and the thymus-associated differentiation antigens; and can be demonstrated to increase the percentage of T cells and augment T-lymphocyte proliferative responses, particularly the MLC. In *in vivo* animal systems some of these hormones can be immunorestorative in animals rendered immunodeficient by certain maneuvers such as thymectomy or the induction of a tumor-bearing state. In humans thymic hormones can be demonstrated to carry out similar functions in immunodeficient patients when administered *in vivo*. For example, the percentage of T cells can be elevated or depressed, depending on their baseline state of activity (104). Thymosin fraction 5 has been demonstrated to have therapeutic activity in such T-cell deficiency diseases as the DiGeorge syndrome, the Nezaloff syndrome, and the Wiscott Aldrich syndrome (105). Both TP1 and THF have been shown to have therapeutic activity in patients with underlying malignancy who have T-cell deficiency and disseminated viral infection (106). Extensive anecdotal data now suggest that these modalities of treatment may be life saving.

Only a few trials of the role of thymic hormones as adjuncts to cancer therapy have been reported. Chretien et al. (107) have reported that the addition of a high dose of thymosin (60 mg/m²) has prolonged the remission duration and survival of patients receiving chemotherapy for oat cell carcinoma of the lung (107). Patt et al. (108) demonstrated that immunodeficient patients with malignant melanoma had an apparent lengthening of disease-free survival whereas immunocompetent patients had an apparent decrease in survival when thymosin fraction 5 was added to BCG therapy. In another study, as yet unpublished, Patt and co-workers have demonstrated that the addition of 60 mg/m² of thymosin fraction 5 reduced the response rate and shortened the survival of patients with non-oat cell carcinoma of the lung. These disparate results are what would be expected with an immunomodulator as defined earlier, used on all patients in a class rather than on those with a demonstrable T-cell deficiency.

Efforts to bring thymic hormones to clinical utility in cancer therapy will require several steps. First, it will be essential that all the active thymic hormone components be sequenced and synthesized and that careful *in vivo* and *in vitro* animal model studies be done to characterize the activity of each component. The current data suggest that there may be separate helper and suppressor activities. Second, Phase I studies must be done in immunoincompetent patients who would be the ones expected to benefit. Third, it would be essential to carry out Phases II and III clinical trials sufficiently large to permit clear definition of the activity. These must be done with drug administered only to those with a defined and thymic hormone responsive defect. Fourth, the studies would require appropriate monitoring, with particular reference to the newly identified T-lymphocyte subpopulations that can now be clearly characterized and enumerated with the appropriate monoclonal antibody preparations. Finally, since the extent to which imbalance or deficiency in T-lymphocyte number or function contributes to the progression of cancer is not clearly understood as yet, the extent to which thymic hormone therapy would contribute to conventional anticancer treatment is not yet clearly evident.

4.6. Active Specific Immunotherapy

Active specific immunotherapy is defined as immunization of a subject with tumor cells or tumor antigen preparations, the objective of which is to boost tumor-specific immunity and to allow the generated antibody or effector lymphocytes to kill tumor cells. The concept of active specific immunotherapy is almost 100 years old. However, it is safe to say that this is not, at this time, an established approach to immunotherapy. There are both scientific and practical reasons for this.

Scientifically, it has been difficult to establish that there are indeed tumor-specific antigens and tumor-specific immune responses associated with human malignancies. However, the recent work of Pfreundschuh et al. (109) with natural antibody and of several investigators with monoclonal antibody (110) are correcting this deficiency and have indeed identified these antigens. However, the presences of common tumor antigen for a given histologic type of cancer that are on the cell surface and could be or are the object of an immune attack is questionable. Compelling data are being generated that individual-specific antigens may be more important than common histological-type-specific antigens in host control tumor growth. From the practical point of view, except in the leukemias, the availability of large numbers of tumor cells or large amounts of tumor antigen is greatly restricted. Cultured tumor cells have been proposed as an alternative, but they undergo major antigenic modulation and may prove unsuitable for active immunization. Another possible limitation is that immunization with either whole tumor cells or even tumor antigen may result in activation of an undesired component of the immune system such as specific suppressor cell activiation. There is, however, some evidence that active specific immunization has improved prognosis in terms of remission duration and survival in a number of human malignancies, including acute myelogenous leukemia (48) and lung cancer (111). In none of the studies can a nonspecific immunoadjuvant or immune augmenting effects be ruled out.

In spite of these limitations, the prospects for this area of therapeutic research remain high. Theoretically, if the appropriate tumor-specific immunity could be generated, effective control of tumor growth should be achieved. This is clearly demonstrated by the appropriate animal model studies (112). Moreover, there are major advances in tumor antigen purification that are in part related to the availability of hybridoma antibody that should resolve the problems related to tumor antigen specificity cited previously and that may allow for the production of adequate amounts of tumor antigen for active specific immunization. It is speculated that active specific immunotherapy for at least some types of tumor will become a reality within the next decade.

4.7. Adoptive Immunotherapy

The term "adoptive immunotherapy" (see Chapter 11) implies the transfer of immunocompetence or specific tumor immunity from one individual to another. Transfer can be xenogeneic, allogeneic, or syngeneic and can involve intact cells or subcellular fractions. Bone marrow transplantation as a treatment for malignancy can be considered an approach to adoptive immunotherapy (see Chapter 10). Classically, adoptive immunotherapy in humans has included the transfer from one human to another of leukocytes, lymphocytes, or transfer factor. There are no clear-cut data indicating that leukocyte transfer as previously conducted had any therapeutic benefit. Transfer factor (see Chapter 8), the low-molecular-weight dializable extract of peripheral blood lymphocytes whose structure is as yet undefined, probably consists of a complex of peptides, and nucleic acid; this factor has shown some interesting immunologic and therapeutic activity (113). Transfer factor can, indeed, transfer specific microbial immunity from an immune to a nonimmune subject (114). In addition, it has nonspecific T-cell boosting activities (115). Finally, there is clear-cut evidence that transfer factor can have protective and/or therapeutic activity in a variety of human viral and fungal infections such as herpes zoster (116) and mucocutaneous candidiasis. Fairly extensive studies of transfer factor immunotherapy adjuvant to conventional therapy have been conducted in human cancer. There is currently no evidence that transfer factor has therapeutic activity in human malignancy.

The other approach to adoptive immunotherapy that has received extensive previous investigation is immune RNA (see Chapter 8). It has been demonstrated unequivocally that immune RNA can transfer various types of immunity, including tumor immunity from the lymphoid cells of immunized allogeneic or xenogeneic subjects to nonimmune subjects (117). Tumor immunity transferred with immune RNA in animal models can be tumor preventive and can have true immunotherapeutic activity, causing either tumor regression or prevention of tumor recurrence after surgical extirpation of disease (118). Several groups of investigators have now demonstrated that immune RNA can cause the regression of pulmonary metastasis in renal cell carcinoma (119), and thus it is suggested that this approach to adoptive immunotherapy is ready for more broad clinical development.

The most exciting prospect for the future of adoptive immunotherapy in humans is through cell cloning methodology. Through the use of Interleukin 2 (T-cell growth factor), continuously proliferating clones of cytotoxic T cells can be generated (97). This suggests the possibility that clones of these cells that are cytotoxic to a patient's tumor could be generated. Since they would be autologous cells, they could be administered repeatedly for therapeutic benefit. This has already been achieved to a limited extent in animal models. It offers an enormous potential for the future development of adoptive immunotherapy.

4.8. Passive Immunotherapy

Passive immunotherapy or serotherapy may be defined as the administration of antitumor antibody to cancer patients, generated in a variety of fashions with the intent of causing tumor regression or preventing tumor recurrence. At present, essentially all data regarding serotherapy are anecdotal. Most involve the administration of natural antisera from recovered cancer patients or relatives of cancer patients to patients with active disease. There is some evidence for regression of tumor in leukemias and lymphomas, in Burkitts lymphoma, renal carcinoma, and malignant melanoma (120). In appropriate experimental animal models serotherapy can clearly be active, particularly in preventing recurrence after tumor burden reduction (121). More recently, several investigators have used partially purified xenogeneic antibody, generated by immunization of animals, to deliver drug and/or radioactive isotope to tumor. Some success has been observed with malignant melanoma with the use of antibodies coupled to chlorambucil (122) and in hepatoma using antiferritin antibody coupled to ^{131}I (123). The development of cloned B-cell populations producing highly specific high-titer monoclonal antibody and the potential for developing human myeloma-lymphocyte hybridomas makes the prospects for passive immunotherapy promising at this time.

4.9. Depletive Immunotherapy

Certain circulating serum factors produced by or related to tumors are immunosuppressive and are thought to play a role in the inhibition of effective tumor immunity in humans. These include nonspecific factors such as immunoregulatory globulin and its components (124), prostaglandins (125), suppressor cell activating factors (126), and various factors relating to natural antibody.

These would include both antitumor antibody that might play a blocking role and antitumor or antiidiotype antibody involved in antigen-antibody complexes (127). The observations that these factors can impair antitumor host defenses in animal systems and in human *in vitro* systems has suggested that depletion of these factors could play an important therapeutic role. Indeed, plasmapheresis has been shown to increase tumor-specific immunity in human malignant melanoma (128), and plasmapheresis has been demonstrated by at least one clinic to result in measurable tumor regression in a fraction of treated patients (129). Recently, Terman et al. (130) and subsequently other groups (131) have demonstrated that immunoabsorbtion of plasma in a continuous flow system utilizing protein A or other solid immunoabsorbants, with some selectivity for immune complexes, can activate tumor-associated host defense factors and result in necrosis and regression of mammary carcinoma in dogs. This approach is now ready for Phase I development in human clinical trials.

4.10. Nutritional Therapy

The role of nutrition and nutritional manipulation in cancer, from the point of view of etiology, pathogenesis, natural history, and so on is a broad one and well beyond the scope of this review (see Chapter 15). In this section we focus on two areas: (1) adequacy of nutrition and hyperalimentation therapy and (2) use of vitamins and their analogues, particularly the retinoids.

Malnutrition has been recognized as a concomitant of progressive malignancy for many years. More recently weight loss has been shown to be an important poor prognostic factor in a number of malignancies. Hyperalimentation has been demonstrated to be capable of reversing this immunologic deficiency (132). This is true in both noncancer and cancer patients. It is speculated that hyperalimentation therapy would improve immunologic function, performance status, and marrow resistance to chemotherapy and could conceivably improve the prognosis of cancer patients receiving conventional therapy. Hyperalimentation is currently under investigation as a modality of adjunctive cancer treatment, although clear-cut data indicating the degree of efficacy, if any, is still lacking.

Considerable attention has been focused in recent years on the potential role of vitamins and their analogues in anticancer treatment. The best developed of these is vitamin A and the group of related compounds, the retinoids. Interest in this area arose because it was demonstrated that vitamin A deficiency resulted in increased gastric carcinoma in rats (133) and a decreased incidence of lung cancer in humans who had a high intake of vitamin A (134). Vitamin A and its analogues have been shown to prevent carcinogenesis, including chemically induced breast cancer (135), bladder cancer (136), and skin cancer (137) in animals. In some experimental systems *in vivo* and *in vitro* malignant transformation can be reversed by retinoids (138). Only very limited studies have been conducted in humans. However, basal cell carcinoma (139) and bladder papillomata (140) both regress with topical or systemic retinoid treatment. A number of extensive clinical trials are now under way in such diseases as recurrent bladder cancer. The mechanism of the retinoid action is not completely understood, but may include direct effects on mechanisms of cell differentiation as well as indirect effects mediated through the immunoadjuvant activity of the agents (141). If relatively nontoxic retinoids with the ability to produce high tissue levels can be developed, this will be a very promising approach to cancer prevention and perhaps also an adjunctive approach to cancer treatment.

4.11. Metabolic Therapy

For the purposes of this review, we define metabolic therapy as those therapeutic manipulations that can directly or indirectly effect tumor cell growth and differentiation through the cyclic nucleotide system. It has been recognized for some time, utilizing *in vitro* systems, that increased cyclic AMP (cAMP) can cause cessation of tumor cell proliferation and can cause malignant tumor cells to exhibit characteristics of normal *in vitro* behavior. Human neuroblastoma cells differentiate in the presence of dibutyril cAMP *in vitro* (142); rat uterine adenocarcinoma cells cease proliferating; and differentiating and growth-inhibiting effects have also been demonstrated on three T3 cells, SV40 transform cells, and the Cloudman melanoma cell line with dibutyril cAMP (143). *In vivo* dibutyril cAMP has been demonstrated to cause inhibition of growth and differentiation of a hormone-dependent rat mammary adenocarcinoma (144) and to cause several mouse tumors to regress significantly (145). A negative aspect of this potential approach is that increased levels of cAMP or the administration of cAMP analogues markedly suppress both the afferent and efferent limbs of the cellular and humoral immune response (146). However, the antitumor activity suggests that careful Phase I and possibly Phase II studies should be done with this group of agents in humans.

5. CONCLUSIONS

In this review we have attempted to outline the future prospective of human cancer immunotherapy and biological therapy. During the modern era, immunotherapy has been investigated for over a decade in humans and has yielded intriguing and somewhat promising results. However, much conflicting data, as well as relatively weak and transient effects, have indicated that immunotherapy as currently constituted will not be a major contributor to the treatment of most malignancies. However, several recent advances in science and medicine have suggested that the broader group of therapeutic approaches included in the concept of biological response modifier therapy may achieve this objective. Some of the new agents or classes of treatment approaches include purified microbial adjuvants, synthetic macrophage activators and augmenting agents, cytokines such as interferon, maturation and differentiation factors, immunomodulators, depletive therapy, retinoids, and metabolic therapy. Concepts of the therapeutic utility of these agents have been modified extensively. For example, the concept of an immunomodulator that may either stimulate or depress host defense mechanisms depending on their baseline status has had a profound influence on theories regarding biological therapy of cancer. This, in turn, has markedly influenced the concepts regarding experimental design and the course and objectives of Phases I and II clinical trials. Finally, there have been major developments in science that will influence the course of not only biological response modifer therapy, but medicine in general. These include a markedly improved knowledge and understanding of the immune system and its subcompotents and their interaction with malignant disease and the development of special methodologies such as hybridoma and recombinant DNA methodology, which will have a profound influence on diagnostic and therapeutic agent development. All these observations and considerations taken together strongly suggest that biological response modifier therapy of cancer may, indeed, become the fourth major modality of cancer treatment in the next decade.

REFERENCES

1. P. Ehrlich, Uber den jetzigen Stand der Karzinomforschung. In F. Himmelweit, Ed., *The Collected Papers of Paul Ehrlich,* Vol. 2, Pergamon Press, London, 1957, pp. 550–562.

2. A. Fefer, Immunotherapy and chemotherapy of Moloney sarcoma virus-induced tumors in mice. *Cancer Res., 29,* 2177 (1969).

3. T. C. Everson, Spontaneous regression of cancer. *Ann. New York Acad. Sci.,* **114,** 721 (1964).

4. F. M. Burnet, The concept of immunological surveillance. In F. Hamburger, Ed., *Progress in Experimental Tumor Research,* Vol. 13, Karger, Basel, 1970, p. 1.

5. F. R. Eilber and D. L. Morton, Impaired immunologic reactivity and recurrence following cancer surgery. *Cancer, 25,* 362 (1970).

6. J. U. Gutterman, E. M. Hersh, K. B. McCredie, G. P. Bodey, Sr., V. Rodriguez, and E. J. Freireich, Lymphocyte blastogenesis to human leukemia cell and their relationship to serum factors, immunocompetence and prognosis. *Cancer Res., 32,* 2524 (1972).

7. G. Trinchieri, D. P. Aden, and B. B. Knowles, Cell-mediated cytotoxicity to SV40-specific tumor associated antigens. *Nature, 261,* 312 (1976).

8. D. M. P. Thompson, V. Sellens, S. Eccles, and P. Alexander, Radioimmunoassay of tumour specific transplantation antigen of a chemically induced rat sarcoma: Circulating soluble tumour antigen in tumour bearers. *Br. J. Cancer,* **28,** 377 (1973).

9. R. D. Rossen, M. A. Reisberg, D. Singer, W. N. Suki, E. M. Hersh, G. Eknoyan, F. X. Schloeder, and L. L. Hill, The effect of age on the character of immune complex disease: A comparison of the incidence and relative size of materials reactive with Clq in sera of patients with glomerulonephritis and cancer. *Medicinal, 58,* 65 (1979).

10. L. J. Old, B. Benacerraf, D. Clarke, E. A. Karrswell, and E. Stockert, The role of the reticuloendothelial system in the host reaction to neoplasia. *Cancer Res., 21,* 1281 (1961).

11. M. Woodruff and J. L. Boak, Inhibitory effect of injection of corynebacterium parvum on the growth of tumor transplants in isogenic hosts. *Br. J. Cancer,* **20,** 345 (1966).

12. G. Mathe, J. L. Amiel, L. Schwarzenberg, et al. Active immunotherapy for acute lymphoblastic leukemia. *Lancet,* **2,** 697 (1969).

13. D. L. Morton, E. C. Holmes, F. Eilber, and W. Wood, Immunological aspects of neoplasia; A rational basis for immunotherapy. *Ann. Int. Med.,* **74,** 587 (1971).

14. E. Klein, Tumors of the skin. X. Immunotherapy of cutaneous and mucosal neoplasma. *N. Y. State J. Med.,* **68,** 900 (1968).

15. E. L. Reinherz, A. Rubinstein, R. S. Geha, A. J. Strelkauskas, F. S. Rosen, and S. F. Schlossman, Abnormalities of immunoregulatory T cells in disorders of immune function. *New Engl. J. Med.,* **301,** 1018 (1979).

16. A. E. Eggers and J. R. Wunderlich, Suppressor cells in tumor-bearing mice capable of nonspecific blocking of *in vitro* immunization against transplant antigens. *J. Immunol.,* **114,** 1554 (1975).

17. R. E. Rocklin, Modulation of cellular-immune responses *in vivo* and *in vitro* by histamine receptor-bearing lymphocytes. *J. Clin. Invest.,* **57,** 1051 (1976).

18. J. S. Goodwin, R. P. Messner, A. D. Bankhurst, G. T. Peake, J. H. Saiki, and R. F. Williams, Prostaglandin-producing suppressor cells in Hodgkin's disease. *New Engl. J. Med.,* **297,** 963 (1977).

19. A. L. Goldstein, G. H. Cohen, J. L. Rossio, G. B. Thurman, C. N. Brown and J. T. Ulrich, Use of thymosin in the treatment of primary immunodeficiency diseases and cancer. *Med. Clin. N. Am.,* **60,** 591 (1976).

20. I. Gresser and M. C. Bourali, Inhibition by interferon preparations of a solid malignant tumor and pulmonary metastases in mice. *Nature (New Biol.),* **236,** 78 (1972).

21. J. U. Gutterman, G. R. Blumenschein, R. Alexanian, H. Yap, A. U. Buzdar, F. Cabanillas, G. N. Hortobagyi, A. Distefano, E. M. Hersh, S. Rasmussen, M. Harmon, M. Kramer, and S. Pestka, Leukocyte interferon induced tumor regression in human breast cancer and B cell neoplasms. *Ann. Int. Med.* (in press).

22. J. Symoens, M. Rosenthal, M. DeBrabander, and G. Goldstein, Immunoregulation with levamisole. *Springer Semin. Immunopathol.,* **2,** 49 (1979).

23. M. G. Masucci, R. Szigeti, E. Klein, G. Klein, J. Gruest, L. Montagnier, H. Taira, A. Hall, S. Nagata, and C. Weissmann, Effect of interferon-a-1 from *E. Coli* on some cell functions. *Science,* **209,** 1431 (1980).

24. R. Levy and J. Dilley, The *in vitro* antibody response to cell surface antigens. II. Monoclonal antibodies to human leukemia cells. *J. Immunol.,* **119,** 394 (1977).

25. E. M. Hersh, G. M. Mavligit, J. U. Gutterman, and S. P. Richman, Immunotherapy of Human Cancer. In F. F. Becker, Ed., *Cancer, A Comprehensive Treatise.* Vol. 119, Plenum, New York, 1977, pp. 394–400.

26. M. J. Mastrangelo, H. L. Sulit, L. M. Prehn, R. S. Bornstein, J. W. Yarbro, and R. T. Prehn, Intralesional BCG in the treatment of metastatic malignant melanoma. *Cancer,* **37,** 684 (1976).

27. B. Zbar, I. D. Bernstein, G. L. Bartlett, M. G. Hanna, Jr. and H. J. Rapp, Immunotherapy of cancer: Regression of intradermal tumors and prevention of growth of lymph node metastases after intralesional injection of living mycobacterium bovis (Bacillus Calmette-Guerin). *J. Natl. Cancer Inst.,* **49,** 113 (1976).

28. S. A. Rosenberg, H. Rapp, W. Terry, and B. Zbar, Intralesional BCG therapy of patients with primary stage I melanoma. In W. D. Terry, Ed., *Immunotherapy of Cancer: Present Status of Trials in Man,* Raven, New York (in press).

29. E. C. Holmes, K. P. Rummey, M. E. Bein, and W. F. Coulson, Intralesional BCG immunotherapy of pulmonary tumors. *J. Thor. Card. Surg.,* **77,** 362 (1979).

30. D. L. Morton, F. R. Eilber, E. C. Holmes, and K. P. Rabbing, Preliminary results of a randomized trial of adjuvant immunotherapy in patients with malignant melanoma who have lymph node metastases. *Aust. New Zeal. J. Surg.,* **48,** 49 (1978).

31. M. F. McKneally, C. Maver, and H. W. Kausel, Regional immunotherapy of lung cancer with intrapleural BCG. *Lancet,* **I**, 377 (1976).

32. A. Morales, D. Eidinger, and A. W. Bruce, Adjuvant BCG immunotherapy in recurrent superficial bladder cancer. In W. D. Terry, and D. Windhorst, Eds., *Immunotherapy of Cancer: Current Status of Trials in Man,* Raven, New York, 1978, pp. 225–230.

33. G. Beretta, Controlled study for prolonged chemotherapy, immunotherapy and chemotherapy plus immunotherapy as an adjuvant to surgery in stage I–II malignant melanoma: Preliminary report. In W. D. Terry, and D. Windhorst, Eds., *Immunotherapy of Cancer: Current Status of Trials in Man,* Raven, New York, 1978, pp. 65–72.

34. P. W. Wright, L. D. Hill, A. V. Peterson, R. P. Anderson, S. P. Hammer, L. P. Johnson, E. H. Morgan, and R. D. Pinkham, Adjuvant immunotherapy with intrapleural BCG (IP-BCG) and levamisole in patients with resected, non-small cell lung cancer. In W. D. Terry, Ed., *Immunotherapy of Cancer: Current Status of Trials in Man,* Raven, New York (in press).

35. Lung Cancer Study Group, unpublished observations.

36. J. Lowe, P. B. Iles, D. R. Shore, M. J. S. Langman, and R. W. Baldwin, Intrapleural BCG in operable lung cancer. In W. D. Terry, Ed., *Immunotherapy of Cancer: Current Status of Trials in Man,* Raven, New York (in press).

37. D. L. Lamm, D. E. Thor, S. C. Harris, V. D. Stogdill, and H. M. Radwin, Intravesical and percutaneous BCG immunotherapy of recurrent superficial bladder cancer. In W. D. Terry, Ed., *Immunotherapy of Cancer: Current Status of Trials in Man,* Raven, New York (in press).

38. F. Camacho, C. Pinsky, D. Kerr, W. Whitmore, and H. Oettgen, Treatment of superficial bladder cancer with intravesical BCG. In W. D. Terry, Ed., *Immunotherapy of Cancer: Current Status of Trials in Man,* Raven, New York (in press).

39. P. G. Reizenstein, BCG plus leukemic cell therapy of patients with acute myeloid leukemia. Leukemia Group of Central Sweden. In W. D. Terry, Ed., *Immunotherapy of Cancer: Current Status of Trials in Man,* Raven, New York (in press).

40. R. L. Powles, Immunotherapy for acute myelogenous leukaemia using irradiated and unirradiated leukaemia cells. *Cancer,* **34**, 1558 (1974).

41. M. S. Mitchell, D. Kirpatrick, M. B. Mokyr, and I. Gery, On the mode of action of BCG. *Nature,* **243**, 316 (1973).

42. R. C. Reed, J. U. Gutterman, G. M. Mavligit, A. A. Burgess, and E. M. Hersh, Corynebacterium parvum: Preliminary report of a phase I clinical and immunological study in cancer patients. In B. Halpern, Ed., *Corynebacterium Parvum. Applications in Experimental and Clinical Oncology,* Plenum, New York, 1975, pp. 349–366.

43. L. Israel, R. Edelstein, A. Depierre, and N. Dimitrov, Brief communication: daily intravenous infusions with corynebacterium parvum in twenty patients with disseminated cancer: A preliminary report of clinical and biological findings. *J. Natl. Cancer Inst.,* **55**, 29 (1975).

44. D. W. Weiss, MER and other mycobacterial fractions in the immunotherapy of cancer. *Med. Clin. N. Am.,* **60**, 473 (1976).

45. E. Robinson, A. Bartal, Y. Cohen, D. Milstein, and T. Mekori, Adjuvant therapy in colorectal cancer—a randomized trial comparing radiochemotherapy and radiochemotherapy combined with the methanol extraction residue of BCG, MER. *Biomed. Exp.,* **31**, 8 (1979).

46. J. C. Britell, H. Bisel, D. L. Ahmann, and S. Frytak, Cytoxan, 5-fluorouracil, and predisone therapy in advanced breast cancer. *Proc. Am. Assoc. Cancer Res.,* **20**, 396 (1979).

47. E. Robinson, A. Bartal, J. Honigman, and Y. Cohen, A preliminary study of intravenous methanol extraction residue of BCG intreatment of advanced cancer. *Br. J. Cancer,* **36**, 341 (1977).

48. J. G. Bekesi and J. F. Holland, Impact of specific immunotherapy in acute myelocytic leukemia. *Haematol. Blood Transfus.*, **23**, 79 (1979).

49. J. J. Lokich, M. B. Garnick, and M. Legg, Intralesional immune therapy: Methanol extraction residue of BCG or purified protein derivative. *Oncology*, **36**, 236 (1979).

50. E. M. Hersh, S. Murphy, J. Quesada, J. U. Gutterman, G. M. Mavligit, C. R. Gschwind, and J. Morgan, Effect of immunotherapy with *Corynecbacterium parvum* and methalon extraction residue of BCG administered intravenously on host defense function in cancer patients. *J. Natl. Cancer Inst.*, **66**, 993 (1981).

51. G. J. Vosika, J. R. Schmidtke, A. Goldman, R. Parker, E. Ribi, and G. R. Gray, Phase I study of intravenous mycobacterial cell wall skeleton (CWS). *Proc. Am. Assoc. Cancer Res.*, **21**, 207 (1980).

52. S. P. Richman, J. U. Gutterman, E. M. Hersh, and E. E. Ribi, Phase I-II study of intratumor immunotherapy with BCG cell wall skeleton plus P_3. *Cancer Immunol. Immunother.*, **5**, 41 (1978).

53. Y. Yamamura, Adjuvant immunotherapy of lung cancer with BCG cell wall skeleton. In W. D. Terry, Ed., *Immunotherapy of Cancer: Current Status of Trials in Man,* Raven, New York (in press).

54. B. D. Clarkson, M. D. Dowling, T. S. Gee, I. B. Cunningham, and J. H. Burchenal, Treatment of acute leukemia in adults. *Cancer,* **36**, 775 (1975).

55. T. H. M. Stewart, A. C. Hollinshead, J. E. Harris, S. Raman, R. Belanger, A. Crepeau, A. E. Crook, W E. Hirte, D. Hooper, D. J. Klaassen, E. F. Rapp, and H. J. Sachs, Survival study of immuno-chemotherapy in lung cancer. In W. D. Terry and D. Windhorst, Eds., *Immunotherapy of Cancer: Present Status of Trials in Man,* Raven, New York, 1978, p. 203.

56. H. Tykka, L. Hjelt, K. J. Oravisto, M. Turunen, and T. Tallberg, Disappearance of lung metastases during immunotherapy in five patients suffering from renal carcinoma. *Scand. J. Resp. Dis.,* **89**, 123 (1974).

57. S. Pavlovsky, G. Garay, F. S. Muriel, L. Braier, and E. Svarch, Chemoimmunotherapy with levamisole during maintenance of remission in acute lymphoblastic leukemia. A four year report. *Proc. Am. Soc. Clin. Oncol.,* **21**, 436 (1980).

58. F. Cabanillas, V. Rodriguez, E. M. Hersh, G. M. Mavligit, G. P. Bodey, and E. L. Middleman, Chemoimmunotherapy of advanced non-Hodgkin's lymphoma with CHOP-BLEO + levamisole. *Proc. Am. Soc. Clin Oncol.,* **18**, 328 (1977).

59. E. J. W. Stephens, H. F. Wood, and B. Mason, Levamisole as an adjuvant to cyclic chemotherapy in breast cancer. *Recent Results Cancer Res.,* **68**, 139 (1979).

60. W. K. Amery, Final results of a multicenter placebo-controlled levamisole study of resectable lung cancer. *Cancer Treat. Rep.,* **62**, 1677 (1978).

61. E. C. Broden, J. Crowley, T. E. Davis, W. H. Wolberg, and D. Groveman, Levamisole, effects in primary and recurrent colorectal carcinoma. In W. D. Terry, Ed., *Immunotherapy of Cancer: Current Status of Trials in Man,* Raven, New York (in press).

62. C. M. Pinsky, H. J. Wanebo, E. Y. Hilal, E. W. Strong, and H. F. Oettgen, Randomized trial of levamisole in patients with squamous cancer of the head and neck. In W. D. Terry, Ed., *Immunotherapy of Cancer: Current Status of Trials in Man,* Raven, New York (in press).

63. H. M. Anthony, A. J. Mearns, M. K. Mason, D. G. Scott, K. Moghissi, P. B. Deverall, Z. J. Rozycki, and D. A. Watson, Levamisole and surgery in bronchial carcinoma patients: Increase in deaths from cardiorespiratory failure. *Thorax,* **34**, 4 (1979).

64. D. S. Verma, G. Spitzer, A. R. Zander, M. Beran, K. A. Dicke, and K. B. McCredie, The kinetics of colony-stimulating activity elaboration from human bone marrow cells by immunoadjuvants. Interactions between light density adherent and nonadherent cells *in vitro.* *Leukemla Res.,* **4**, 371 (1980).

65. M. B. Sporn, Approaches to prevention of epithelial cancer during the preneoplastic period. *Cancer Res., 36,* 2699 (1976).

66. M. J. Tisdale, The significance of cyclic AMP and cyclic GMP in cancer treatment. *Cancer Treat. Rev., 6,* 1 (1979).

67. G. Sonnenfeld and T. C. Merigan, The role of interferon in viral infections. *Springer Semin. Immunopathol., 2,* 311 (1979).

68. H. Strander, Interferons: Antineoplastic drugs? *Blut, 35,* 277 (1977).

69. H. Mellstedt, M. Bjorkholm, B. Johansson, A. Ahre, G. Holm, and H. Strander, Interferon therapy in myelomatosis. *Lancet,* I, 245 (1979).

70. T. C. Merigan, K. Sikora, J. H. Breeden, R. Levy, and S. A. Rosenberg, Preliminary observations on the effect of human leukocyte interferon in nonHodgkin's lymphoma. *New Engl. J. Med., 299,* 1449 (1979).

71. J. Gutterman, Y. Yap, A. Buzdar, R. Alexanian, E. M. Hersh, F. Cadanillas, S. Greenberg, Leukocyte interferon (IF) induced tumor regression in patients with breast cancer and B cell neoplasms. *Proc. Am. Assoc. Cancer Res., 20,* 167 (1979).

72. E. Borden, T. Dao, J. Holland, J. Gutterman, and T. Merigan, Interferon in recurrent breast carcinoma: Preliminary report of the American Cancer Society Clinical Trials Program. *Proc. Am. Assoc. Cancer Res., 21,* 187 (1980).

73. S. Krown, M. Stoopler, R. Gralla, S. Cunningham-Rundles, W. Stewart, M. Pollack, and H. Oettgen, Phase II trial of human leukocyte interferon in non-small cell lung cancer. In W. D. Terry, Ed., *Immunotherapy of Cancer: Present Status of Trials in Man,* Raven, New York (in press).

74. T. J. Priestman, Initial evaluation of human lymphoblastoid interferon in patients with advanced malignant disease. *Lancet, 2,* 113 (1980).

75. T. Memoto, W. A. Carter, J. G. Dolen, D. Holyoke, and J. S. Horoszewica, Human interferons and intralesional therapy of melanoma and breast carcinoma. *Proc. Am. Assoc. Cancer Res., 20,* 246 (1979).

76. J. Treuner, D. Niethammer, G. Dannecker, R. Hagmann, V. Neef, and P. H. Hofschneider, Successful treatment of nasopharyngeal carcinoma with interferon. *Lancet,* 1 817 (1980).

77. M. Ho, Pharmacokinetics of interferon. In N. B. Finter, Ed., *Interferons and Interferon Inducers.* American Elsevier, New York, 1973, pp. 241–249.

78. E. Ribi, C. A. McLaughlin, J. L. Cantrell, W. Brehmer, I. Azuma, Y. Yamamura, S. M. Strain, K. B. Hwang, and R. Toubiana, Immunotherapy for tumors with microbial constituents or their synthetic analogues. A review. In *Immunotherapy of Human Cancer, 22nd Annual Clinical Conference on Cancer,* Raven, New York, pp. 131–154.

79. E. Ribi, J. Cantrell, S. Schwartzman, and R. Parker, BCG cell wall skeleton, P3, MDP and other microbial components, structure activity studies in animal models. In Evan Hersh, Michael A. Chirigos and Michael Mastrangelo, Eds., *Augmenting Agents in Cancer Therapy,* Raven, New York, 1981, pp. 15–31.

80. J. L Cantrell, Antitumor activity of a soluble component isolated from C. parvum. *Proc. Am. Assoc. Cancer Res., 21,* 225 (1980).

81. R. Bomford and C. Moreno, Critical overview of the potential of various microbial polysaccharides for cancer immunotherapy. In Evan Hersh, Michael A. Chirigos, and Michael Mastrangelo, Eds., *Augmenting Agents in Cancer Therapy,* Raven, New York, 1981, pp. 91–99.

82. S. E. Krown, D. Kerr, W. E. Stewart, M. S. Pollack, S. C. Rundles, Y. Hirshaut, C. Pinsky, H. B. Levy, and H. F. Oettgen, Phase I trial of poly ICLC in patients with advanced cancer. In Evan Hersh, Michael A. Chirigos, and Michael Mastrangelo, Eds., *Augmenting Agents of Cancer Therapy,* Raven, New York, 1981, pp. 165–176.

83. A. S. Levine, B. Durie, B. Lampkin, B. G. Leventhal, and H. B. Levy, Poly (ICLC) interferon induction, toxicity, and clinical efficacy in leukemia, lymphoma, solid tumors, mye-

loma and laryngeal papillomatosis. In Evan Hersh, Michael A. Chirigos, and Michael Mastrangelo, Eds., *Augmenting Agents in Cancer Therapy*, Raven, New York, 1981, pp. 151–163.

84. P. O. P. Tso, J. L. Alderfer, and J. Levy, An integrated and comparative study of the antiviral effects and other biological properties of the polyinosinic acid-polycytidylic acid and its mismatched analogues. *Molec. Pharmacol.*, **12**, 299 (1976).

85. D. S. Breslow, Biologically active synthetic polymers. *Pure Appl. Chem.*, **46**, 103 (1976).

86. D. A. Stringfellow, H. C. Vanderberg, and S. D. Weed, Interferon induction by 5-Halo-6-Phenyl Pyrimidines. In J. D. Nelson and C. Grassi, Eds., *Current Chemotherapy and Infectious Disease*. American Society for Microbiology, Boston, Mass., 1980, pp. 1406–1408.

87. P. G. Munder, M. Modolell, R. Andreesen, H. U. Weltzien, and O. Westphal, Lysophosphatidylcholine (lysolecithin) and its synthetic analogues. Immune modulating and other biologic effects. *Springer Semin. Immunopathol.*, **2**, 187 (1979).

88. M. Modolell, R. Andreesen, W. Pahlke, U. Brugger, and P. G. Munder, Disturbance of phospholipid metabolism during the selective destruction of tumor cells induced by alkyl-lysophospholipids. *Cancer Res.*, **39**, 4681 (1979).

89. R. Andreesen, M. Modolell, and P. G. Munder, Selective sensitivity of chronic myelogenous leukemia cell populations to alkyl-lysophospholipids. *Blood,* **54**, 519 (1979).

90. B. W. Papermaster, O. A. Holtermann, E. Klein, S. Parmett, D. Dobkin, R. Laudico, and I. Djerassi, Lymphokine properties of a lymphoid cultured cell supernatant fraction active in promoting tumor regression. *Clin. Immunol. Immunopathol.*, **5**, 48 (1976).

91. A. Rios, E. M. Hersh, J. U. Gutterman, M. Mavligit, M. Schimek, J. E. McEntire, and B. W. Papermaster, The use of a leukocyte cell line culture supernatant for skin reaction testing in malignant melanoma. *Cancer*, **44**, 1615 (1979).

92. B. W. Papermaster, C. D. Gilliland, M. Smith, S. Buchok, and J. E. McEntire, Tumor regression induced in mice by partially purified lymphokine fractions. *N. Y. Acad. Sci.,* **332**, 451 (1979).

93. T. Dao and J. J. Costanzi, Preliminary observations on tumor regressions induced by local administration of a lymphoid cell culture supernatant fraction in patients with cutaneous metastatic lesions. *Clin. Immunol., Immunopathol.*, **5**, 31 (1976).

94. E. A. Carswell, L. J. Old, R. L. Kassel, S. Green, N. Fiore, and B. Williamson, An endotoxin-induced serum factor that causes necrosis of tumors. *Proc. Natl. Acad. Sci.*, **72**, 3666 (1975).

95. B. H. Waksman, Modulation of immunity by soluble mediators. *Pharm. Thera.*, **2**, 623 (1978).

96. I. Gery and B. H. Waksman, Potentiation of the T cell response to mitogens. II. The cellular source of potentiating mediator(s). *J. Exp. Med.*, **136**, 143 (1972).

97. S. Gillis, K. A. Smith, and J. Watson, Biochemical and biological characterization of lymphocyte regulatory molecules. II. Purification of a class of rat and human lymphokines. *J. Immunol.*, **124**, 1954 (1980).

98. D. Metcalf, M. A. S. Moore, J. W. Sheridan, and G. Spitzer, Responsiveness of human granulocytic leukemic cells to colony-stimulating factor. *Blood,* **43**, 847 (1974).

99. A. L. Goldstein, A. Guha, M. M. Zatz, A. Hardy, and A. White, Purification and biological activity of thymosin, a hormone of the thymus gland. *Proc. Natl. Acad. Sci.,* **69**, 1800 (1972).

100. J. F. Bach, M. Dardenne, J. M. Pleau, and M. A. Mach, Isolation biochemical characteristics and biological activity of a circulating thymic hormone in the mouse and in the human. *Ann. N. Y. Acad. Sci.,* **249**, 186 (1975).

101. N. Trainin, M. Small, D. Zipori, T. Umiel, A. I. Kook, and V. Rotter, Characteristics of THF, a thymic hormone. In D. K. Van Bekkum, Ed., *The Biological Activity of Thymic Hormones,* Kooyker Scientific Publishers, Rotterdam, 1975, p. 117.

102. G. Goldstein, M. P. Scheid, E. A. Boyse, D. H. Schlesinger, and J. V. Wauwe, A synthetic pentapeptide with biological activity characteristic of the thymic hormone thymopoietin. *Science,* **204**, 1309 (1979).

103. F. Anti, *In vivo* and *in vitro* effect of a thymic extract in patients with primary T cell deficiencies and cancer. In B. Serrou and C. Rosenfeld, Eds., *New Trends in Human Immunology and Cancer Immunotherapy.*

104. B. Serrous, C. Rosenfeld, J. Caraux, C. Thierry, D. Cupissol, and A. L. Goldstein, Thymosin modulation of suppressor function in mice and man. *Ann. N. Y. Acad. Sci.,* **332**, 95 (1979).

105. D. W. Wara, D. J. Barrett, A. J. Ammann, and M. J. Cowan, *In vitro* and *in vivo* enhancement of mixed lymphocyte culture reactivity by thymosin in patients with primary immunodeficiency disease. *Ann. N. Y. Acad. Sci.,* **332**, 128 (1979).

106. R. Zaizov, R. Vogel, B. Wolach, I. J. Cohen, I. Varsano, B. Shohat, Z. Handzel, V. Rotter, Y. Yakir, and N. Trainin, The effect of THF in lymphoproliferative and myeloproliferative diseases in children. *Ann. N. Y. Acad. Sci.,* **332**, 172 (1980).

107. P. B. Chretien, S. D. Lipson, R. W. Makuch, D. E. Kenady, and M. H. Coehn, Effects of thymosin *in vitro* in cancer patients and correlation with clinical course after thymosin immunotherapy. *Ann. N. Y. Acad. Sci.,* **332**, 148 (1979).

108. Y. Z. Patt, E. M. Hersh, L. A. Schafer, T. L. Smith, M. A. Burgess, J. U. Gutterman, A. L. Goldstein, and G. M. Mavligit, The need for immune evaluation prior to thymosin containing chemoimmunotherapy for melanoma. *Cancer Immunol. Immunother.,* **7**, 131 (1979).

109. M. Pfreundschuh, H. Shiku, T. Takahashi, R. Ueda, J. Ransohoff, H. F. Oettgen, and L. J. Old, Serological analysis of cell surface antigens of malignant human brain tumors. *Proc. Natl. Acad. Sci.,* **75**, 5122 (1978).

110. G. Kohler and C. Milstein, Continuous cultures of perfused cells secreting antibody of predefined specificity. *Nature,* **256**, 495 (1975).

111. T. H. M. Stewart, A. C. Hollinshead, J. E. Harris, R. Belanger, A. Crepeau, G. D. Hooper, H. J. Sachs, D. J. Klaassen, W. Hirte, E. Rapp, A. F. Crook, M. Orizaga, D. P. S. Sengar, and S. Raman, Immunochemotherapy of lung cancer. *Ann. N. Y. Acad. Sci.,* **277**, 436 (1976).

112. R. L. Simmons, A. Rios, and P. Trites, Modified tumor cells in the immunotherapy of solid mammary tumors. *Med. Clin. N. Am.,* **60**, 551 (1976).

113. H. S. Lawrence, Transfer factor in cellular immunity. *Harvey Lect.,* **68**, 239 (1974).

114. H. S. Lawrence, *Adv. Immunol.,* **11**, 195 (1969).

115. A. Khan, A. Antonetti, S. L. Burt, J. M. Hill, Induction of cortisone resistance and increased mitogen responsiveness in thymocytes by transfer factor. *J. Clin. Hematol. Oncol.,* **8**, 109 (1978).

116. R. W. Steele, M. G. Myers, and M. M. Vincent Monroe, Transfer factor for the prevention of varicella-zoster infection in childhood leukemia. *New Engl. J. Med.,* **303**, 355 (1980).

117. Y. H. Pilch, K. P. Ramming and P. J. Deckers, Induction of anti-cancer immunity with RNA. *Ann. N. Y. Acad. Sci.,* **207**, 409 (1973).

118. B. S. Wang, S. R. Onikul, and J. A. Mannick, Prevention of death from metastases by immune RNA therapy. *Science,* **202**, 59 (1978).

119. J. B. deKernion and K. P. Ramming, Treatment of hypernephroma with xenogeneic immune RNA. *Natl. Cancer Inst. Monogr.,* **49**, 347 (1978).

120. P. W. Wright, K. E. Hellström, I. E. Hellström, and I. D. Bernstein, Serotherapy of malignant disease. *Med. Clin. N. Am.,* **60**, 607 (1976).

121. E. Mihich, Combined effects of chemotherapy and immunity against leukemia L1210 in DBA/2 mice. *Cancer Res.,* **29**, 848 (1979).

122. T. Ghose, S. T. Norvell, and A. Guclu, Immunochemotherapy of cancer with chlorambucil carrying antibody. *Br. Med. J., 3*, 495 (1972).

123. S. E. Order, J. L. Klein, E. Ettinger, P. Alderson, S. Siegelman, and P. Leichner, Phase I–II study of radiolabeled antibody integrated in the treatment of primary hepatic malignancies. *Internatl. J. Rad. Oncol. Bio. Phys., 6*, 703 (1978).

124. R. W. Baldwin and R. A. Bobins, Humoral factors abrogating cell-mediated immunity in the tumor bearing host. *Curr. Top. Microbiol. Immunol., 72*, 21 (1975).

125. J. S. Goodwin, A. D. Bankhurst, and R. P. Messner, Suppression of human T-cell mitogenesis by prostaglandin. Existence of prostaglandin-producing suppressor cell. *J. Exp. Med., 146*, 1719 (1977).

126. B. Bonavida, Antigen induced cyclophosphamide-resistant suppressor T cells inhibit the *in vitro* generation of cytotoxic cells from one-way mixed leukocyte reactions. *J. Immunol., 119*, 1530 (1977).

127. D. Hartman and M. G. Lewis, Presence and possible role of anti-IgG antibodies in human malignancy. *Lancet,* 1318 (1974).

128. P. Hersey, A. Edwards, E. Adams, J. Isbister, E. Murray, J. Biggs, and G. W. Milton, Antibody dependent cell mediated cytotoxicity against melanoma cells induced by plasmapheresis. *Lancet, I*, 825 (1976).

129. L. Israel, R. Edelstein, P. Mannoni, and E. Radot, Plasmapheresis and immunological control of cancer. *Lancet, 2*, 642 (1976).

130. D. S. Terman, T. Yamamoto, M. Mattioli, G. Cook, R. Tillquist, J. Henry, R. Poser, and Y. Daskal, Extensive necrosis of spontaneous canine mammary adenocarcinoma after extracorporeal perfusion over staphylococcus aureus cowans. I. *J. Immunol., 124*, 795 (1980).

131. T. Holohan, C. Bowles, and A. Deisseroth, Extracorporeal immunoadsorption therapy in spontaneous canine neoplasms. *Proc. Am. Assoc. Cancer Res., 21*, 241 (1980).

132. V. C. Lanzotti, E. M. Copeland, S. L. George, S. J. Dudrick, and M. L. Samuels, Cancer chemotherapeutic response and hyperalimentation. *Cancer Chemother. Rep., 59*, 437 (1975).

133. T. Moore, Effects of vitamin deficiency in animals: Pharmacology and toxicology of vitamin A. In W. H. Sebrill and R. S. Harris, Eds., *The Vitamins,* Academic, 2nd ed., Vol. 1, New York, 1967, pp. 245–266.

134. E. Bjelke, Dietary vitamin A and lung cancer. *Internatl. J. Cancer, 15*, 561 (1975).

135. C. J. Grubbs, R. C. Moon, M. B. Sporn, and D. L. Newton, Inhibition of mammary cancer by retinyl methyl ether. *Cancer Res., 27*, 599 (1977).

136. C. C. Brown and M. B. Sporn, 13-*cis*-Retinoic acid: Inhibition of bladder carcinogenesis induced in rats by *N*-butyl-*N*-(4-hydroxybutyl)nitrosamine. *Science, 198*, 743 (1977).

137. R. E. Davies, Effect of viatmin A on 7,12-Dimethylbenz(a)anthracene-induced papillomas in rhino mouse skin. *Cancer Res., 27*, 237 (1967).

138. I. Lasnitzki and S. D. Goodman, Inhibition of the effects of methylcholanthrene on mouse prostate in organ culture by vitamin A and its analogs. *Cancer Res., 34*, 1564 (1974).

139. W. Bollag, Therapy of epithelial tumors with an aromatic retinoic acid analog. *Chemotherapy, (Basel), 21*, 236 (1975).

140. J. P. Evard and W. Bollag, Conservative treatment of recurrent urinary bladder papillomas with vitamin A acid. *Schweiz. Med. Wochenschr., 102*, 1880 (1972).

141. I. F. Tannock, H. D. Suit, and N. Marshall, Vitamin A and the radiation response of experimental tumors: An immune-mediated effect. *J. Natl. Cancer Inst., 48*, 731 (1972).

142. S. Ishikawa, Differentiation of human neuroblastoma cells *in vitro.* Morphological changes induced by dibutryl cyclic AMP. *Acta. Pathol. Jap., 27*, 697 (1977).

143. A. DiPasquale and J. McGuire, Dibutyrl cyclic AMP arrests the growth of cultivated

Cloudman melanoma cells in the last S and G2 phases of the cell cycle. *J. Cell. Physiol.,* **93**, 395 (1977).

144.   Y. S. Cho-Chung and P. M. Gullino, *Science,* **183**, 87 (1974).

145.   F. Posternak, M. Orusco, J. Csank-Brassert, J. Cox, T. Posternak, and P. Laugier, Regression of experimental tumours in mice by treatment with two cAMP analogues. *Dermatologica,* **153**, 96 (1976).

146.   J. J. Marchalonis and P. Smith, Effects of dibutrylcyclic AMP on the *in vitro* primary response of mouse spleen cells to sheep erythrocytes. *Aust. J. Exp. Biol. Med. Sci.,* **54**, 1 (1976).

Author Index

Numbers in parentheses indicate reference numbers. Pages in *italics* indicate where full references appear.

Subject Index